Prostate Diseases: Assessment and Therapeutics

Prostate Diseases: Assessment and Therapeutics

Editor: Blake Xavier

FOSTER
ACADEMICS
www.fosteracademics.com

www.fosteracademics.com

FOSTER ACADEMICS

Cataloging-in-Publication Data

Prostate diseases : assessment and therapeutics / edited by Blake Xavier.
p. cm.
Includes bibliographical references and index.
ISBN 978-1-64646-633-7
1. Prostate--Diseases. 2. Prostate--Diseases--Diagnosis. 3. Prostate--Diseases--Treatment. I. Xavier, Blake.
RC899 .P76 2023
616.65--dc23

Foster Academics,
118-35 Queens Blvd., Suite 400,
Forest Hills, NY 11375, USA

ISBN 978-1-64646-633-7 (Hardback)

Contents

Preface

The prostate gland refers to a type of male reproductive organ that creates fluids which nourish and shield sperm cells. Prostate cancer, prostatitis and benign prostatic hyperplasia (BPH) are the three most common types of prostate diseases. The symptoms of these diseases include blood in the sperm or urine, painful ejaculation, frequent urges to urinate, and dribbling of urine. A number of tests are used to diagnose prostate diseases including the PSA test, biopsies of the prostate, mid-stream urine (MSU) tests, etc. Depending on the type of prostatitis, antibacterial medications and supportive therapies can be used in the treatment. The treatment for BPH may include drugs to reduce the size of the prostate and relax the smooth muscle of the gland as well as surgery to create a permanently enlarged channel in the part of the urethra that passes through the prostate. This book is compiled in such a manner, that it will provide in-depth knowledge about the assessment and management of prostate diseases. Its extensive content provides the readers with a thorough understanding of these medical conditions.

This book unites the global concepts and researches in an organized manner for a comprehensive understanding of the subject. It is a ripe text for all researchers, students, scientists or anyone else who is interested in acquiring a better knowledge of this dynamic field.

I extend my sincere thanks to the contributors for such eloquent research chapters. Finally, I thank my family for being a source of support and help.

Editor

1

Unbiased data mining identifies cell cycle transcripts that predict non-indolent Gleason score 7 prostate cancer

Wendy L. Johnston[1*], Charles N. Catton[1,2] and Carol J. Swallow[3,4,5,6]

Abstract

Background: Patients with newly diagnosed non-metastatic prostate adenocarcinoma are typically classified as at low, intermediate, or high risk of disease progression using blood prostate-specific antigen concentration, tumour T category, and tumour pathological Gleason score. Classification is used to both predict clinical outcome and to inform initial management. However, significant heterogeneity is observed in outcome, particularly within the intermediate risk group, and there is an urgent need for additional markers to more accurately hone risk prediction. Recently developed web-based visualization and analysis tools have facilitated rapid interrogation of large transcriptome datasets, and querying broadly across multiple large datasets should identify predictors that are widely applicable.

Methods: We used camcAPP, cBioPortal, CRN, and NIH NCI GDC Data Portal to data mine publicly available large prostate cancer datasets. A test set of biomarkers was developed by identifying transcripts that had: 1) altered abundance in prostate cancer, 2) altered expression in patients with Gleason score 7 tumours and biochemical recurrence, 3) correlation of expression with time until biochemical recurrence across three datasets (Cambridge, Stockholm, MSKCC). Transcripts that met these criteria were then examined in a validation dataset (TCGA-PRAD) using univariate and multivariable models to predict biochemical recurrence in patients with Gleason score 7 tumours.

Results: Twenty transcripts met the test criteria, and 12 were validated in TCGA-PRAD Gleason score 7 patients. Ten of these transcripts remained prognostic in Gleason score 3 + 4 = 7, a sub-group of Gleason score 7 patients typically considered at a lower risk for poor outcome and often not targeted for aggressive management. All transcripts positively associated with recurrence encode or regulate mitosis and cell cycle-related proteins. The top performer was BUB1, one of four key MIR145-3P microRNA targets upregulated in hormone-sensitive as well as castration-resistant PCa. SRD5A2 converts testosterone to its more active form and was negatively associated with biochemical recurrence.

Conclusions: Unbiased mining of large patient datasets identified 12 transcripts that independently predicted disease recurrence risk in Gleason score 7 prostate cancer. The mitosis and cell cycle proteins identified are also implicated in progression to castration-resistant prostate cancer, revealing a pivotal role for loss of cell cycle control in the latter.

Keywords: Prostate cancer prognosticators, Gleason 3 + 4 = 7 prostate cancer, Biochemical recurrence, Castration-resistant prostate cancer, Biomarker, HES6, E2F2, Cell cycle, BUB1, SRD5A2

* Correspondence: wendyjohnstonchitin@gmail.com
[1]Radiation Medicine Program, Princess Margaret Cancer Centre, University Health Network, Toronto, ON, Canada
Full list of author information is available at the end of the article

Background

In developed countries, prostate cancer (PCa) is the most commonly diagnosed non-skin cancer in men and a leading cause of cancer death [1, 2]. Data compiled in 2010 for Canadian men, for example, showed a 14.1% lifetime risk for developing PCa, and a 3.5% probability of dying from PCa [3]. As such, PCa is second only to lung and bronchus for cancer-related mortality in men.

In PCa patients who have had their prostate removed, biochemical recurrence (BCR) of blood prostate-specific antigen (PSA) occurs in ~ 20–40% of cases within 10–15 years [4–6]. BCR is commonly used as a surrogate for metastatic PCa, since it is a necessary antecedent [7]. However, BCR can occur without radiological evidence of metastasis, and the reported PCa-specific mortality in patients with BCR is only 19–45% by 10–15 years [4, 6, 8]. Prostate tissue is androgen-sensitive, and treatments for metastatic PCa typically include androgen-deprivation. While initially successful, within 2 years ~ 70% of metastatic PCa becomes resistant to androgen deprivation (castration-resistant PCa [CRPC]), leading, almost invariably, to PCa-specific mortality (reviewed in [9]). Given the heterogeneous outcome in patients diagnosed with localized PCa, risk stratification of newly diagnosed patients with non-metastatic disease at presentation is critical to inform clinical management, and treatment options include observation and one or more of radical prostatectomy, radiotherapy, and androgen deprivation therapy [10, 11].

Twenty years ago, D'Amico and colleagues [12] proposed a classification scheme assessing risk for BCR following radical prostatectomy based on PSA, Gleason score and tumour category. Low risk was defined as PSA < 10 ng/ml, Gleason score < 6, and tumour T1-T2a; intermediate risk as PSA 10–20 ng/ml, and/or Gleason score 7, and/or T2b; and high risk as PSA > 20 ng/ml and/or Gleason score 8–10 and/or > T2c. Tumour sub-staging has since been abolished by the AJCC Eighth Edition and by the International Society for Urologic Pathology (https://www.ncbi.nlm.nih.gov/pubmed/27251951). However, tumours can still be stratified within groups; for example, patients with Gleason score 7 tumours are frequently sub-classified into 3 + 4 = 7 (3, primary, 4; secondary, patterns), or 4 + 3 = 7, since 3 + 4 = 7 has a 3-fold lower risk of lethal outcome than 4 + 3 = 7 [13]. Despite these refinements, significant heterogeneity is apparent in the observed incidence of BCR and the more clinically relevant PCa-specific mortality. Heterogeneity is particularly evident for intermediate risk patients, who comprise the largest group [14, 15]. Enhanced discrimination amongst these patients would facilitate more tailored management. As such, new biomarkers are required to accurately identify patients who are at a higher risk for aggressive disease and therefore merit more aggressive treatment, while at the same time allowing for patients with more indolent disease to be observed. Of particular interest are biomolecule markers isolated from tumours, blood, or urine, including proteins, coding and non-coding RNA, and genetic and epigenetic modifications. Unbiased co-discovery of molecules that act in shared cellular pathways might also suggest particularly vulnerable cell signaling pathways to target for therapeutic intervention.

Next generation sequencing with public sharing of data has yielded an enormous amount of genomic and transcriptomic information that is now available to PCa researchers worldwide [16, 17]. An unprecedented and still emerging picture of genome alterations, epigenetic landscape, and gene and protein expression in tumours and normal tissue has enabled the development of a number of PCa prognostic systems (reviewed in [18–20]). Interestingly, there is not much overlap between most previously identified biomarkers [20]. This may reflect, in part, different strategies for biomarker discovery. For example, some studies have queried restricted groups of genes (e.g., a subset of cell cycle genes [21], annotated PCa-associated genes [22], miRNA-regulated transcripts [23]), or different cell types (e.g. stromal cells [24]).

In this study, we exploit recently developed web-based tools and publicly available PCa transcriptome data to perform an unbiased query of multiple datasets, focusing on Gleason score 7 PCa. We identify 12 transcripts that predicted BCR (1 downregulated, 11 upregulated in tumours). Ten of these transcripts remained prognostic for poor outcome in patients with Gleason score 3 + 4 = 7 PCa. Importantly, this suggests a possible strategy to identify higher risk patients within a group that is, overall, considered at a low to intermediate risk for poor outcome. Multivariable logistic regression analysis within the 3 + 4 = 7 group showed combining either UBE2C or CCNB1, which are elevated in PCa, with SRD5A2, which is decreased in PCa, increased the prognostic power over and above any of the 3 transcripts alone. Ten of the 11 Gleason 7 (and all of the Gleason 3 + 4 = 7 sub-group) upregulated biomarkers are mitosis and cell cycle related genes that are also part of an E2F1 transcription-factor regulated cell cycle network that predicts lethal metastatic CRPC [25]. Therefore, in addition to predicting BCR, they are prognostic for PCa-specific mortality. Future studies comparing the performance of these transcripts with other biomarkers in new datasets will help determine their robustness in predicting, and potentially treating, non-indolent PCa.

Methods

A set of test transcripts was identified in an unbiased, stepwise fashion using 3 free, publicly available web-based data visualization and analysis tools that enable rapid genome-wide screening (Fig. 1a). In step 1, Cancer

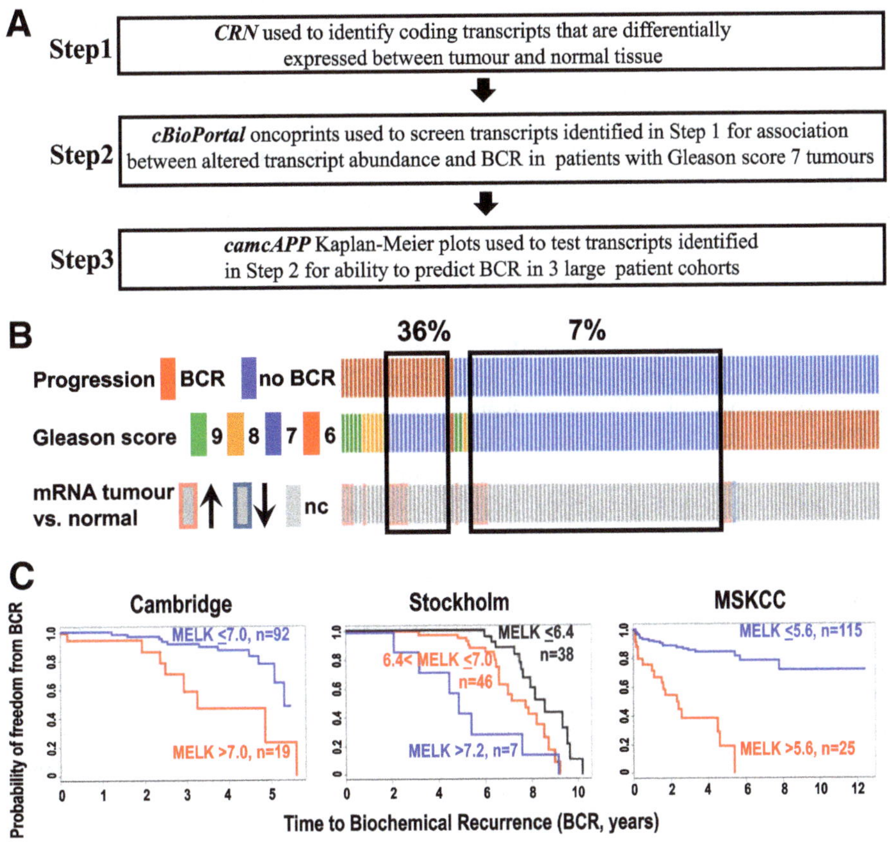

Fig. 1 Rapid generation of a transcript test set using 3 web-based tools: CRN, cBioPortal, and camcAPP. **a**) Outline of steps used to generate the transcript test set. **b**) cBioPortal oncoprint (step 2) example (MELK) indicates 36% of patients with Gleason score 7 tumours who experienced biochemical recurrence (BCR) had increased MELK transcript. In contrast, only 7% of those who remained BCR-free had increased transcript. Patients (individual bars) are aligned within the three rows**.** nc- no difference in tumour transcript abundance compared with normal tissue. **c**) camcAPP Kaplan-Meier plots (step 3) example (MELK) shows higher MELK expression is associated with shorter time to BCR in all three datasets. Grouping of samples determined by recursive partitioning (Hothorn et al., 2006). **b**, **c**) MSKCC data from Taylor et al., 2010. **c**) Cambridge and Stockholm data from Ross-Adams et al., 2015

RNA-Seq Nexus (CRN) TCGA-PRAD data (http://syslab4.nchu.edu.tw/) [26] was used to identify genes that had at least one isoform with altered transcript abundance in tumours, compared to normal controls ($p < 1.0\text{E-}04$). DAVID 6.8 Gene Name Batch Viewer (https://david.ncifcrf.gov/list.jsp) [27, 28] was used to remove duplicates. In step 2, genes identified in step 1 were queried for patient BCR status, tumour transcript abundance (z-score threshold of 2.0), and tumour Gleason score using cBioPortal, (http://www.cbioportal.org/) [29, 30] MSKCC 2010 data [31]. MSKCC data was used since it is the only cBioPortal prostate cancer dataset in which tumour transcript abundance is compared to normal tissue (other datasets compare patient tumour sample transcript abundance to all tumours that are diploid). In this cohort, 131 patients had primary tumour transcript data available, with 27 of these patients experiencing BCR. Of the 27, 14 had Gleason score 7 tumours and 4 had PSA 10–20 ng/ml. Taking into account the limited number of patients who experienced BCR, we chose to screen transcript abundance in patients with Gleason score 7 tumours. Batches of oncoprints for 50 genes were examined manually to identify transcripts that were increased or decreased in Gleason score 7 patients with BCR, compared to Gleason score 7 patients who remained free of BCR (Fig. 1b shows MELK as an example). In step 3, transcripts identified in Step 2 were then examined using camcAPP (http://bioinformatics.cruk.cam.ac.uk/apps/camcAPP/) [32]. Kaplan-Meier plots examining the relationship between transcript abundance and time to BCR were generated for each transcript using Cambridge, Stockholm, [33] and MSKCC [31] data (Fig. 1c shows MELK as an example). Genes for which the time to BCR could be separated by recursive partitioning [34] into distinct transcript abundance groups for all three datasets were designated the test set.

Expression (transcript per million; TPM) of test genes was examined in TCGA-PRAD normal tissues ($n = 52$), and tumours for which transcript abundance, BCR status, and reviewed Gleason score were available (n = 285). Details of sample acquisition and processing following radical prostatectomy at authorized tissue source sites are provided by TCGA-PRAD [35]. Reviewed Gleason score (assigned by TCGA genitourinary pathologists on prostatectomy specimens) was used to avoid possible collection site variability in scoring. Samples with zero or near zero (TPM < 1.6E-07) transcript abundance were removed from the analysis; these included 1 normal for DLGAP5 and CDK1, 3 normals for E2F2 and MELK, and 5 normals and 6 tumours for CDKN3. Univariate logistic regression (SAS 9.4) was performed to determine odds ratios (ORs), and ROC-AUC was calculated for each of the test transcripts, as well as for Gleason score and pre-operative PSA using easyROC http://www.biosoft.hacettepe.edu.tr/easyROC/ [36]. Multivariable logistic regression was performed on transcripts with increased abundance and ORs having p values < 0.05, and SRD5A2, which had decreased abundance, in Gleason score 7 (n = 158), Gleason score 4 + 3 = 7 (n = 70) and Gleason score 3 + 4 = 7 (n = 88) tumours. The multivariable model was restricted to include only 2 independent variables due to the limited number (n=13) of BCR events in patients with Gleason score 7 tumours. Pre-operative PSA concentration was only available for a subset of patients (88/156) that included only 4 patients with BCR, so was not included in the multivariable analysis. Future studies that include more samples with longer term follow-up (and hence, more BCR) will be helpful to test the independent contributions of PSA in patients with Gleason score 7 tumours.

Transcripts identified in the current study were examined for overlap with previously reported prognostic transcript signatures [21–23, 25, 33, 37–56]. Gene names were standardized using GeneCards http://www.genecards.org/ v4.5.0 Build 38, except for TSBP, for which 2 aliases were listed in GeneCards (CTR9, c6orf10), and Gene Ontology (GO terms) were determined using DAVID 6.8 https://david.ncifcrf.gov/home.jsp [27, 28]. Proportional Venn diagrams were generated using euler*APE* http://www.euler-diagrams.org/eulerAPE [57].

Results

A comparison of prostate cancer primary tumours (n = 497) vs. normal prostatic tissue samples (n = 52) revealed altered transcript abundance of at least one isoform of 8187 genes (Additional file 1: Table S1). Manual examination of these 8187 genes in MSKCC Gleason score 7 patients using cBioPortal oncoprints identified 1816 genes with differences in expression between patients without BCR (n = 60) and those with BCR (n = 14) (Additional file 1: Table S2). For each of the 1816 genes identified by the above algorithm, the Cambridge (n = 111), Stockholm (n = 92), and MSKCC (n = 140) datasets were interrogated for any correlation between transcript abundance and BCR-free survival across all Gleason scores. The level of expression of twenty-two individual genes predicted BCR-free survival in all three of the patient cohorts (Table 1). Two of these genes were eliminated from the test set due to discordance in the expression differential between data sets. In particular, for ANKMY1, higher BCR-free survival was observed in association with lower expression in the Cambridge and MSKCC datasets, but with higher expression in the Stockholm dataset. In the case of ALDH1A2, there were discordant results between the MSKCC cohort of Gleason score 7 patients queried using cBioPortal, and the group of patients in the Cambridge, Stockholm, and MSKCC datasets examined using camcAPP. The final test set of 20 transcripts included 13 with higher expression in tumour vs. normal tissue that were positively associated with BCR, and 7 with decreased expression in tumours that were negatively associated with BCR (Table 1).

When examined across Gleason scores 6 through 10, 14 of 20 test set genes yielded an OR, and 17 an ROC-AUC, that was prognostic (p < .05) for BCR in the TCGA-PRAD validation dataset (n = 285) (Additional file 1: Table S3). For half of the genes, the AUC was greater than for Gleason score or pre-operative PSA, examined in the same group of patients (Additional file 2). Within the group of Gleason score 7 patients in the TCGA-PRAD dataset (n = 158), 12 transcripts remained prognostic (Table 2, Fig. 2), with 1 negatively associated with BCR (SRD5A2) and 11 positively associated with BCR (BUB1, TPX2, NCAPG, UBE2C, MELK, CCNA2, CCNB1,CDK1, E2F2, DLGAP5, TMEM206,). Ten of the 11 transcripts positively associated with BCR encode proteins that are functionally annotated as related to mitotic and cell cycle (GO:0000082, GO:0051726), cell division (GO:0051301), or cell proliferation (GO:0008283). The proteins they encode also participate in an E2F1-dependent cell cycle network associated with CRPC, and 4 of the 11 (BUB1, NCAPG, CDK1, MELK) are implicated in miRNA (MIR145-3P)-dependent CRPC (Fig. 3). The 11th transcript encodes a membrane protein (TMEM206) that has recently been identified as important to control cell proliferation in colorectal cancer cells [58].

Ten of 12 transcripts that were prognostic in Gleason score 7 tumours remained prognostic in patients with Gleason 3 + 4 = 7 tumours (Table 3), and multivariable logistic regression analysis showed that combining CCNB1 or UBE2C with SRD5A2 slightly improved the predictive power of the model (Additional file 1: Table S4). In low risk (Gleason score 6) tumours, 9 transcripts remained prognostic, although the limited number of cases of BCR (n=3) in this group may limit its predictive power (Additional file 1: Table S5). Interestingly, in Gleason 4 + 3 = 7, only TMEM206 was prognostic (Additional

Table 1 Test set of 20 transcripts that predicted time until BCR

			Cambridge ($n = 111$)		Stockholm ($n = 92$)		MSKCC ($n = 140$)	
Transcript*	Chromosomal location	Fold change[c]	*p* value	RP cutoff [d]	*p* value	RP cutoff [d]	*p* value	RP cutoff [d]
TPX2	20q11.21	3.0	4.80E-05	< 6.96	5.40E-02	< 6.45	5.10E-07	< 6.38
BUB1	2q13	2.8	1.10E-02	< 6.26	9.10E-03	< 6.36	9.40E-07	< 6.27
CCNA2	4q27	2.5	1.00E-02	< 6.99	8.70E-03	< 7.16	6.70E-06	< 6.91
E2F2	1p36.12	1.9	2.90E-03	< 7.04	4.10E-02	< 6.62	1.40E-02	< 9.99
UBE2C	20q13.12	3.4	1.80E-03	< 7.52	5.80E-03	< 8.15	2.00E-06	< 6.62
NCAPG	4p15.31	2.7	2.70E-02	< 6.63	4.60E-03	< 6.77	5.50E-07	< 6.02
CDK1	10q21.2	2.1	3.70E-03	< 7.13	2.20E-03	< 7.13	1.40E-04	< 4.95
CDKN3	14q22.2	2.4	1.50E-02	< 6.83	4.50E-03	< 7.01	1.60E-07	< 5.12
DLGAP5	14q22.3	3.4	4.90E-03	< 6.61	1.90E-02	< 6.63	2.90E-06	< 5.45
MELK	9p13.2	3.3	2.40E-02	< 6.97	6.60E-04	< 6.45	3.50E-06	< 5.6
CCNB1	5q13.2	1.8	1.60E-02	< 7.05	3.00E-03	< 6.83	4.30E-04	< 6.98
TMEM206	1q32.3	1.3	2.90E-02	< 7.87	1.30E-02	< 7.22	2.50E-03	< 7.66
SHMT2	12q13.3	1.7	3.20E-02	< 10.4	3.50E-02	< 10.1	1.10E-03	< 8.57
ANKMY1[a]	2q37.3	1.03	4.90E-02	< 7.77	2.20E-03	> 7.29	2.70E-03	< 8.11
SRD5A2	2p23.1	− 3.7	9.10E-03	> 7.11	1.70E-03	> 6.53	1.60E-07	> 7.05
CSRP1	1q32.1	−2.9	1.60E-02	> 12	2.30E-02	> 10.9	2.00E-05	> 9.55
NFIB	9p23-p22.3	− 1.1	7.30E-03	> 11.5	1.90E-02	> 11.15	1.80E-04	> 9.23
PGM5	9q21.11	−3.6	5.70E-03	> 8.59	9.30E-03	> 10.8	4.10E-07	> 7.97
CNN1	19p13.2	−3.1	1.40E-02	> 8.99	3.00E-02	> 8.72	2.40E-07	> 8.72
DES	2q35	−3.1	2.40E-02	> 9.53	4.70E-02	> 8.32	2.70E-05	> 8.99
MPDZ	9p23	−1.4	1.10E-02	> 8.22	1.10E-02	> 7.44	3.40E-03	> 8.43
ALDH1A2[b]	15q21.3	− 3.2	3.30E-02	> 8.47	2.50E-02	> 7.55	6.40E-07	> 7.19

*The 20 transcripts shown in bold text were altered in tumours compared to normal tissue, and predicted time until BCR in Cambridge (Ross-Adams et al., 2015), Stockholm (Ross-Adams et al., 2015), and MSKCC (Taylor et al., 2010) datasets

[a]*ANKMY1* was excluded since results were discordant between the datasets

[b]*ALDH1A2* was excluded since results were discordant between cBioPortal and camcAPP portals

[c] total of all isoforms in tumour compared with normal (TCGA-PRAD)

[d] expression level cutoff for longer time to BCR, determined by recursive partitioning (RP) (Hothorn et al., 2006)

file 1: Table S6). The reason for the discrepancy between results for Gleason 3 + 4 = 7 and 4 + 3 = 7 is unclear. One possibility is that, with the exception of MELK, transcript abundance of positive prognosticators was higher in Gleason 3 + 4 = 7 than in Gleason 4 + 3 = 7 in patients with BCR (Additional file 1: Table S7). Future studies examining transcript abundance within regions of different pattern within the tumour may be helpful to explain these findings.

Discussion

PCa is a common disease with a heterogeneous clinical outcome that is difficult to predict using available risk stratification tools. Treatments such as prostatectomy, radiotherapy and androgen deprivation extend lifespan and improve the quality of life in patients with aggressive disease, but also cause unnecessary morbidity and loss of quality of life in those with indolent disease. Thus, a key goal in disease management is to develop biomarkers that accurately predict outcome. Variable outcome is especially evident in "intermediate risk" patients, making clinical decision-making particularly difficult within this group. To identify biomarkers that may be helpful for predicting outcome in this group, we took the approach of broadly querying publicly available transcriptome data using multiple distinct visualization and analysis data portals. We identify 12 genes, the expression of which predicted poor outcome (BCR) in patients with Gleason score 7 tumours. Eleven of the twelve genes have been identified as prognostic for PCa outcome in at least one other study (Additional file 1: Table S8), portending robustness. Importantly, 10/12 of the genes remained prognostic in Gleason score 3 + 4 = 7 tumours. Since Gleason 3 + 4 = 7 tumours are often projected to have a more favourable prognosis [59], the identification of transcripts that may stratify this group into higher and lower risk of poor outcome may be particularly helpful for clinical decision-making.

The top performer we identified in Gleason score 7 tumours, including Gleason 3 + 4 = 7, was BUB1. BUB1

Table 2 Univariate logistic regression and ROC-AUC analyses for predicting BCR in patients with Gleason score 7 tumours

Variable	Odds Ratio (OR)	95% CI OR	*P* value OR	ROC-AUC	SE AUC	*P* value AUC	Youden cut-off	Sensitivity	Specificity	PPV	NPV
(up in tumour)											
BUB1	1.31	0.908–1.889	1.48E-01	0.720	0.055	5.35E-05	1.22	0.92	0.58	0.16	0.99
TPX2	1.18	0.994–1.406	5.79E-02	0.732	0.066	4.53E-04	3.54	0.85	0.64	0.18	0.98
NCAPG	1.51	0.913–2.510	1.08E-01	0.711	0.065	1.08E-03	0.94	0.92	0.48	0.14	0.99
UBE2C	1.07	0.998–1.142	5.60E-02	0.713	0.067	1.42E-03	7.79	0.69	0.69	0.17	0.96
MELK	1.21	0.908–1.612	1.93E-01	0.687	0.065	3.97E-03	1.82	0.69	0.69	0.17	0.96
CCNA2	1.27	0.967–1.680	8.57E-02	0.694	0.069	5.04E-03	2.58	0.69	0.70	0.17	0.96
CCNB1	1.13	0.954–1.345	1.56E-01	0.685	0.066	5.20E-03	4.60	0.92	0.48	0.14	0.99
CDK1	1.07	0.969–1.181	1.81E-01	0.691	0.070	6.27E-03	4.97	0.77	0.62	0.15	0.97
E2F2	2.84	0.715–11.309	1.38E-01	0.682	0.068	7.55E-03	0.37	0.77	0.63	0.16	0.97
DLGAP5	1.24	0.766–2.014	3.80E-01	0.657	0.070	2.54E-02	0.65	0.85	0.46	0.12	0.97
TMEM206	1.15	0.999–1.321	5.10E-02	0.672	0.086	4.51E-02	9.11	0.85	0.52	0.14	0.97
CDKN3	1.14	0.936–1.387	1.93E-01	0.643	0.079	6.93E-02	2.04	0.92	0.39	0.12	0.98
SHMT2	1.01	0.990–1.038	2.52E-01	0.605	0.069	1.25E-01	56.64	0.69	0.57	0.13	0.95
(down in tumour)											
SRD5A2	0.90	0.786–1.021	9.85E-02	0.674	0.079	2.70E-02	7.98	0.92	0.44	0.13	0.99
CSRP1	0.998	0.996–1.001	1.30E-01	0.628	0.080	1.11E-01	417.97	0.54	0.72	0.15	0.95
PGM5	0.99	0.974–1.006	2.04E-01	0.592	0.085	2.84E-01	22.95	0.39	0.81	0.15	0.94
NFIB	0.98	0.941–1.029	4.68E-01	0.584	0.092	3.60E-01	27.09	0.69	0.56	0.12	0.95

Data are from TCGA-PRAD (TCGA, 2015). $n = 158$. CI-confidence interval, SE-standard error. Youden cut-off is the optimal point to separate biochemical recurrence (BCR) from non-BCR. PPV-positive predictive value, NPV-negative predictive value

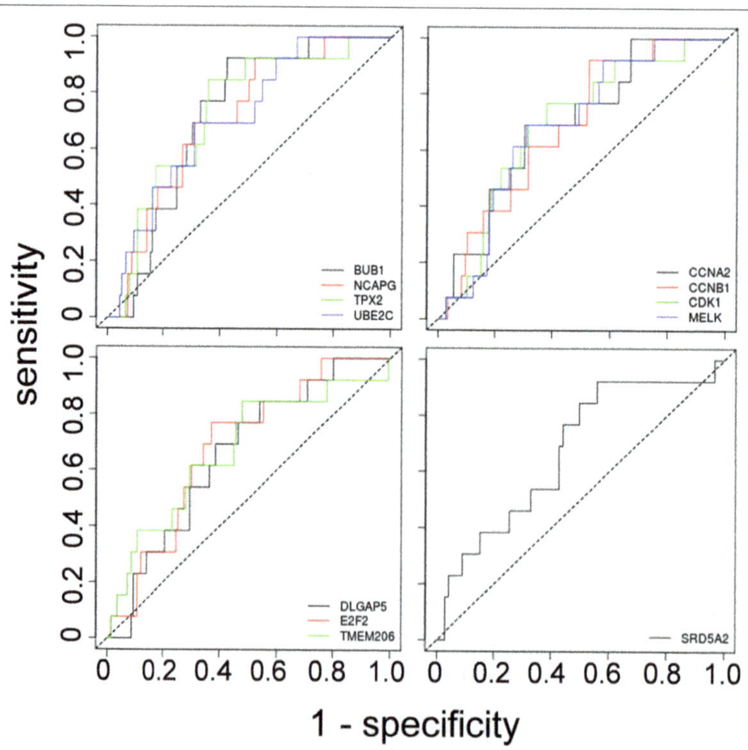

Fig. 2 Receiver Operating Characteristic (ROC) curves for transcripts predicting biochemical recurrence (BCR) in patients with Gleason score 7 tumours. ($n = 158$). BCR predicted by increased (BUB1, NCAPG, TPX2, UBE2C, CCNA2, CCNB1, CDK1, MELK, DLGAP5, E2F2, TMEM206), or decreased (SRD5A2) abundance of transcripts. See Table 2 for details. AUC-Area under the curve. Data from TCGA-PRAD (TCGA, 2015)

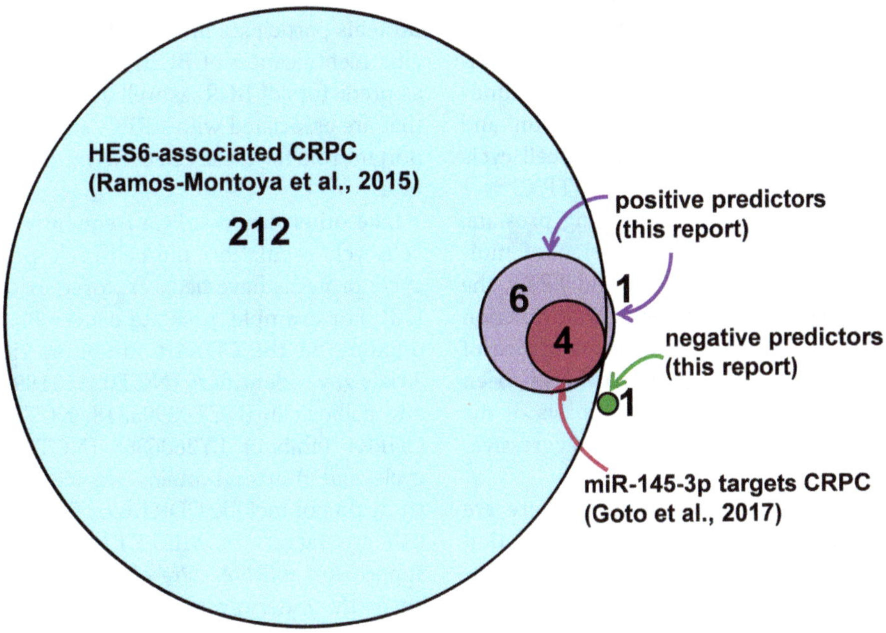

Fig. 3 The positive predictors of BCR in Gleason score 7 tumours also predict castration-resistant prostate cancer (CRPC). Ten of 11 positive predictors identified in this study encode cell cycle and mitosis proteins that are part of a HES6-associated E2F1-dependent signature of castration-resistant prostate cancer (CRPC). Four of the 10 are targeted by the miRNA miR-145-3p in CRPC. Total of numbers within or adjacent to each circle are the number of prognostic transcripts in each dataset

Table 3 Univariate logistic regression and ROC-AUC analyses for predicting BCR in patients with Gleason score 3 + 4 = 7 tumours

Variable	Odds Ratio (OR)	95% CI OR	*P* value OR	ROC-AUC	SE AUC	*P* value AUC	Youden cut-off	Sensitivity	Specificity	PPV	NPV
(up in tumour)											
BUB1	1.93	1.029–3.604	4.03E-02	0.865	0.045	4.75E-16	1.54	1.000	0.78	0.22	1.00
TPX2	1.40	1.055–1.852	1.98E-02	0.872	0.060	5.07E-10	4.09	1.000	0.74	0.19	1.00
NCAPG	2.72	1.071–6.915	3.55E-02	0.855	0.067	1.23E-07	1.33	0.800	0.83	0.22	0.99
UBE2C	1.20	1.051–1.369	7.00E-03	0.889	0.050	7.21E-15	7.79	1.000	0.80	0.23	1.00
MELK	1.72	0.939–3.152	7.89E-02	0.819	0.082	1.03E-04	2.17	0.800	0.86	0.25	0.99
CCNA2	1.83	1.113–3.000	1.71E-02	0.810	0.106	3.39E-03	2.63	0.800	0.80	0.19	0.99
CCNB1	1.63	1.109–2.383	1.27E-02	0.824	0.083	1.00E-04	4.69	1.000	0.57	0.12	1.00
CDK1	1.28	1.070–1.532	6.80E-03	0.863	0.090	5.50E-05	7.32	0.800	0.90	0.33	0.99
E2F2	5.98	0.824–43.408	7.70E-02	0.720	0.119	6.39E-02	0.37	0.800	0.70	0.14	0.98
DLGAP5	1.95	0.954–3.984	6.73E-02	0.855	0.066	6.61E-08	0.86	1.000	0.64	0.14	1.00
TMEM206	0.98	0.766–1.243	8.40E-01	0.545	0.154	7.72E-01	9.11	0.800	0.52	0.09	0.98
CDKN3	1.50	1.071–2.108	1.85E-02	0.708	0.187	2.65E-01	6.47	0.600	0.95	0.43	0.98
SHMT2	1.03	0.983–1.075	2.21E-01	0.740	0.093	9.94E-03	60.61	0.800	0.71	0.14	0.98
(down in tumour)											
SRD5A2	0.58	0.367–0.921	2.09E-02	0.884	0.079	1.03E-06	3.75	0.800	0.88	0.29	0.99
CSRP1	1.00	0.992–1.001	9.71E-02	0.752	0.132	5.66E-02	417.97	0.800	0.80	0.19	0.99
PGM5	0.97	0.930–1.007	1.04E-01	0.745	0.136	7.28E-02	18.57	0.600	0.90	0.27	0.97
NFIB	0.98	0.903–1.054	5.26E-01	0.578	0.129	5.45E-01	24.07	0.600	0.72	0.12	0.97

Data are from TCGA-PRAD (TCGA, 2015). $n = 88$. CI-confidence interval, SE-standard error. Youden cut-off is the optimal point to separate biochemical recurrence (BCR) from non-BCR. PPV-positive predictive value, NPV-negative predictive value encodes a mitotic checkpoint Ser/Thr kinase that has recently been implicated as a key regulator of prostate cancer progression [60]. TPX2 was also a top prognosticator and is a microtubule-associated protein that stimulates Ran-GTP-dependent microtubule nucleation and regulates Aurora A kinase during mitosis and cell cycle progression [61, 62]. Elevated expression of TPX2 is a common finding in human cancers, including prostate, and overexpression in vitro increases invasion of multiple cancer cell lines [63–65]. Like BUB1 and TPX2, the other transcripts positively associated with BCR function in the cell cycle and/or mitosis. Elevated abundance of cell cycle and mitosis transcripts has previously been shown to predict PCa outcome, and is the basis of the Prolaris commercial test for predicting PCa aggressiveness [21].

The cell cycle and mitosis genes identified here are associated with HES6-dependent E2F1 transcription factor-mediated CRPC [25]. HES6 is a transcription cofactor that physically interacts with E2F1 as well as the androgen receptor [25]. During the G1/S transition, cyclin-dependent kinases and cyclins phosphorylate the tumour suppressor retinoblastoma, resulting in a weakening of its interaction with E2F proteins [66]. E2F2 (as well as E2F1 and E2F3a) are then free to activate genes that promote S phase entry and cell cycle progression. In CRPC, HES6 is able to maintain androgen receptor activity in the absence of testosterone. In the current study E2F2, but not E2F1, was found to be prognostic for BCR, indicating E2F2 may be a more sensitive or earlier indicator of poor clinical outcome than the related family member, E2F1.

E2F2 transcription factor has been shown previously to be negatively regulated by the Let-7 family miRNA, MIRLET7A, leading to suppression of growth of PCa cells [67]. miRNAs are small RNA molecules that are bound by Argonaute proteins to form an RNA-induced silencing complex that targets specific mRNA(s), typically leading to translational repression [68]. The abundance of many miRNA is altered in PCa, and is prognostic for clinical outcome [69]. Some miRNA, such as MIRLET7A, act as tumour suppressors by targeting genes (e.g. E2F2), that enhance tumour growth. In contrast, others act as oncogenes by targeting tumour suppressors or cell death and differentiation pathway mRNAs [70]. MIR145-3P, a tumour suppressive miRNA, is decreased modestly in hormone-sensitive PCa, and decreased severely in CRPC, and low levels are associated with a shorter time to BCR [71]. Examining MIR145-3P in detail, Goto et al. identified four key MIR145-3P targets (BUB1, NCAPG, CDK1, MELK) [23]. All four are upregulated in hormone-sensitive PCa, and elevated even more in CRPC, and all are part of the group of cell cycle and mitosis genes identified in the current study, both in Gleason score 7, and in the Gleason score 3 + 4 = 7 subgroup. Given that thousands of proteins participate in the cell division cycle [72], the specific identification of BUB1, NCAPG, CDK1, and MELK as predictors of BCR, as well as key targets of MIR145-3P that are associated with CRPC, suggests a particularly important role for these cell cycle/mitosis genes in aggressive PCa.

Like other cancers, PCa frequently exhibits defects in cell cycle regulation and cell cycle progression and cell cycle proteins have been explored as therapeutic targets [73]. For example, prostate cancer Phase IB/II trials are ongoing for the CDK4/6 inhibitors ribociclib (ClinicalTrials.gov identifier: NCT02555189, NCT02494921) and palbociclib (NCT02905318, NCT02059213), and the CHEK1 inhibitor LY2606368 (NCT02203513). The cell cycle and mitosis proteins we identified in the present study do not include CDK4/6 or CHEK1. However, almost half are targets of MIRLET7A or MIR145-3P tumour suppressor miRNA. Pre-clinical and clinical trials are currently underway to determine the feasibility of using synthetic miRNA mimics (to compensate for decreased abundance of endogenous tumour suppressive miRNA) or antimiRNA (to block endogenous oncogenic miRNA) as therapeutic agents [70]. Diseases currently being targeted in clinical trials include hepatitis (NCT02508090, NCT02452814), lymphoma (NCT0250552) and mesothelioma (NCT02369198). The experimental evidence supports an important role in PCa progression of miRNA regulation of E2F2, BUB1, NCAPG, CDK1, and MELK. As such, in future studies it would be interesting to determine if the cell cycle and mitosis transcripts identified in the current study might prove to be effective targets for miRNA-based therapeutics in PCa patients.

SRD5A2 was decreased in tumours and negatively associated with BCR. SRD5A2 encodes a steroid 5-α-reductase 2 that converts testosterone to the more potent androgen receptor agonist, dihydrotestosterone. Multivariable logistic regression analysis showed that including CCNB1 or UBE2C and SRD5A2 as variables improved the predictive power in Gleason 3 + 4 = 7. CCNB1 encodes a cyclin B1 required during mitosis, and UBE2C encodes an E2 ubiquitin-conjugating enzyme important in cyclin destruction. These findings suggest it may be beneficial to pair predictors from distinct cellular pathways (cell cycle/mitosis plus androgen synthesis) to improve prognostication in Gleason score 3 + 4 = 7 PCa. SRD5A2 was previously identified in a candidate screen of 732 PCa-related genes [22] and forms part of the commercial Oncotype DX Genomic Prostate Score assay that predicts tumour aggressiveness in low and intermediate risk PCa. SRD5A2 was also identified by Rubicz et al. [50] in an unbiased screen for transcripts that improved prediction of PCa recurrence following radical prostatectomy when combined with Gleason score. Taken together, these findings suggest SRD5A2 may be a robust prognosticator of disease outcome in PCa. However, lower SRD5A2 transcript abundance has previously been reported to be associated with poor [50] or favourable [22] outcome. Moreover, altered SRD5A2 activity resulting from genetic polymorphisms or treatment with drugs such as finasteride has inconsistent effects on PCa outcome [74–76]. Accordingly, additional studies are warranted to clarify the role of SRD5A2 abundance in PCa outcome.

The average patient follow-up time in the TCGA validation dataset was short (< 2 years) [35], consistent with the transcripts identified in the current study as prognostic for early, aggressive disease progression. The small number of patients with BCR in this short follow-up time (13/158 Gleason score 7 cases), together with incomplete data for pre-operative PSA, precluded our testing for concurrent, independent roles for transcript abundance and PSA in the multivariable logistic regression analysis. In the future, prospective studies that include a larger number of patients with complete clinical information and long-term follow-up (15 years+) would be helpful to determine if the improvement in risk stratification we identified here is durable and reproducible.

Conclusions

In this study we identify SRD5A2, and 11 mitosis and cell cycle transcripts that predict PCa disease progression in patients with Gleason score 7 disease. The prognostic power of 10 of these transcripts extended to patients with Gleason 3 + 4 = 7 disease indicating they are excellent candidates for stratifying risk in this group of patients with disease that is often deemed likely to have a favourable outcome. Future studies, especially those including long-term clinical follow-up, will be helpful to confirm the robustness of their predictive power, as well as the therapeutic potential for pharmacologic or genetic intervention.

Additional files

Additional file 1: An excel file containing 8 spreadsheets: **Table S1.** (transcripts identified in Step 1 using CRN), **Table S2.** (transcripts identified in Step 2 using cBioPortal), **Table S3.** (univariate logistic regression and ROC-AUC analyses in patients with Gleason score 6–10 tumours), **Table S4.** (multivariable logistic regression analysis for predicting BCR in patients with Gleason score 3 + 4 = 7 using pairs of one upregulated and one downregulated transcript), **Table S5.** (univariate logistic regression and ROC-AUC analyses in patients with Gleason score 6 tumours), **Table S6.** (univariate logistic regression and ROC-AUC analyses in patients with Gleason score 4 + 3 = 7 tumours), **Table S7.** (mean transcript abundance in patients with BCR and without BCR, broken down by Gleason score), and **Table S8.** (description of the 12 transcripts that predicted BCR in the validation dataset. Includes citations for other studies that found these transcripts to be prognostic for PCa outcome). (XLSX 189 kb)

Additional file 2: Figure S1. showing ROC-AUC for test transcripts in patients with Gleason score 6–10 tumours. (JPG 1535 kb)

Abbreviations

BCR: Biochemical recurrence; CRPC: Castration-resistant prostate cancer; miRNA: microRNA; OR: Odds ratio; PCa: Prostate cancer; PSA: Prostate-specific antigen; ROC-AUC: Receiver operating characteristic area under the curve; TPM: Transcripts per million

Acknowledgements

The authors thank Dr. Haiyan Jiang, Senior Biostatistician, University Health Network, Toronto, Canada, for statistical help in generating univariate and multivariable models.

Author details

[1]Radiation Medicine Program, Princess Margaret Cancer Centre, University Health Network, Toronto, ON, Canada. [2]Department of Radiation Oncology, University of Toronto, Toronto, ON, Canada. [3]Lunenfeld-Tanenbaum Research Institute, Mount Sinai Hospital, Toronto, ON, Canada. [4]Department of Surgery, University of Toronto, Toronto, ON, Canada. [5]Institute of Medical Science, University of Toronto, Toronto, ON, Canada. [6]Laboratory Medicine and Pathobiology, University of Toronto, Toronto, ON, Canada.

References

1. Torre LA, Bray F, Siegel RL, Ferlay J, Lortet-Tieulent J, Jemal A. Global cancer statistics, 2012. CA Cancer J Clin. 2015;65(2):87–108.
2. Attard G, Parker C, Eeles RA, Schroder F, Tomlins SA, Tannock I, et al. Prostate cancer. Lancet. 2016;387(10013):70–82.
3. Canadian Cancer Statistics Advisory Committee. Canadian Cancer Statistics 2017. Toronto, ON: 2017 2017. Report No.
4. Brockman JA, Alanee S, Vickers AJ, Scardino PT, Wood DP, Kibel AS, et al. Nomogram predicting prostate Cancer-specific mortality for men with biochemical recurrence after radical prostatectomy. Eur Urol. 2015;67(6): 1160–7.
5. Stephenson AJ, Kattan MW, Eastham JA, Dotan ZA, Bianco FJ Jr, Lilja H, et al. Defining biochemical recurrence of prostate cancer after radical prostatectomy: a proposal for a standardized definition. J Clin Oncol. 2006; 24(24):3973–8.
6. Freedland SJ, Humphreys EB, Mangold LA, Eisenberger M, Dorey FJ, Walsh PC, et al. Risk of prostate cancer-specific mortality following biochemical recurrence after radical prostatectomy. JAMA. 2005;294(4):433–9.
7. Anscher MS. PSA kinetics and risk of death from prostate cancer: in search of the holy grail of surrogate end points. JAMA. 2005;294(4):493–4.
8. Bianco FJ Jr, Scardino PT, Eastham JA. Radical prostatectomy: long-term cancer control and recovery of sexual and urinary function ("trifecta"). Urology. 2005;66(5 Suppl):83–94.
9. Stuchbery R, McCoy PJ, Hovens CM, Corcoran NM. Androgen synthesis in prostate cancer: do all roads lead to Rome? Nature Reviews Urology. 2017; 14(1):49–58.
10. Mottet N, Bellmunt J, Bolla M, Briers E, Cumberbatch MG, De Santis M, et al. EAU-ESTRO-SIOG guidelines on prostate Cancer. Part 1: screening, diagnosis, and local treatment with curative intent. Eur Urol. 2017;71(4): 618–29.
11. Mohler JL, Armstrong AJ, Bahnson RR, D'Amico AV, Davis BJ, Eastham JA, et al. Prostate Cancer, version 1.2016. J Natl Compr Canc Netw. 2016;14(1):19–30.
12. D'Amico AV, Whittington R, Malkowicz SB, Schultz D, Blank K, Broderick GA, et al. Biochemical outcome after radical prostatectomy, external beam radiation therapy, or interstitial radiation therapy for clinically localized prostate cancer. JAMA. 1998;280(11):969–74.
13. Stark JR, Perner S, Stampfer MJ, Sinnott JA, Finn S, Eisenstein AS, et al. Gleason score and lethal prostate cancer: does 3 + 4 = 4 + 3? J Clin Oncol. 2009;27(21):3459–64.
14. Zumsteg ZS, Spratt DE, Pei I, Zhang Z, Yamada Y, Kollmeier M, et al. A new risk classification system for therapeutic decision making with intermediate-risk prostate cancer patients undergoing dose-escalated external-beam radiation therapy. Eur Urol. 2013;64(6):895–902.
15. Gnanapragasam VJ, Lophatananon A, Wright KA, Muir KR, Gavin A, Greenberg DC. Improving clinical risk stratification at diagnosis in primary prostate Cancer: a prognostic modelling study. PLoS Med. 2016;13(8): e1002063.
16. Jensen MA, Ferretti V, Grossman RL, Staudt LM. The NCI genomic data commons as an engine for precision medicine. Blood. 2017;130(4):453–9.

17. Metzker ML. Sequencing technologies - the next generation. Nat Rev Genet. 2010;11(1):31–46.
18. Gaudreau PO, Stagg J, Soulieres D, Saad F. The present and future of biomarkers in prostate Cancer: proteomics, genomics, and immunology advancements. Biomark Cancer. 2016;8(Suppl 2):15–33.
19. Lamy PJ, Allory Y, Gauchez AS, Asselain B, Beuzeboc P, de Cremoux P, et al. Prognostic biomarkers used for localised prostate Cancer management: a systematic review. Eur Urol Focus. 2017.
20. Sharma P, Zargar-Shoshtari K, Pow-Sang JM. Biomarkers for prostate cancer: present challenges and future opportunities. Future Science OA. 2016;2(1):FSO72.
21. Cuzick J, Swanson GP, Fisher G, Brothman AR, Berney DM, Reid JE, et al. Prognostic value of an RNA expression signature derived from cell cycle proliferation genes in patients with prostate cancer: a retrospective study. Lancet Oncol. 2011;12(3):245–55.
22. Klein EA, Cooperberg MR, Magi-Galluzzi C, Simko JP, Falzarano SM, Maddala T, et al. A 17-gene assay to predict prostate cancer aggressiveness in the context of Gleason grade heterogeneity, tumor multifocality, and biopsy undersampling. Eur Urol. 2014;66(3):550–60.
23. Goto Y, Kurozumi A, Arai T, Nohata N, Kojima S, Okato A, et al. Impact of novel miR-145-3p regulatory networks on survival in patients with castration-resistant prostate cancer. Br J Cancer. 2017;117(3):409–20.
24. Jia Z, Rahmatpanah FB, Chen X, Lernhardt W, Wang Y, Xia XQ, et al. Expression changes in the stroma of prostate cancer predict subsequent relapse. PLoS One. 2012;7(8):e41371.
25. Ramos-Montoya A, Lamb AD, Russell R, Carroll T, Jurmeister S, Galeano-Dalmau N, et al. HES6 drives a critical AR transcriptional programme to induce castration-resistant prostate cancer through activation of an E2F1-mediated cell cycle network. EMBO Mol Med. 2014;6(5):651–61.
26. Li JR, Sun CH, Li W, Chao RF, Huang CC, Zhou XJ, et al. Cancer RNA-Seq Nexus: a database of phenotype-specific transcriptome profiling in cancer cells. Nucleic Acids Res. 2016;44(D1):D944–51.
27. Huang da W, Sherman BT, Lempicki RA. Systematic and integrative analysis of large gene lists using DAVID bioinformatics resources. Nat Protoc 2009; 4(1):44–57.
28. Huang da W, Sherman BT, Lempicki RA. Bioinformatics enrichment tools: paths toward the comprehensive functional analysis of large gene lists. Nucleic Acids Res 2009;37(1):1–13.
29. Gao J, Aksoy BA, Dogrusoz U, Dresdner G, Gross B, Sumer SO, et al. Integrative analysis of complex cancer genomics and clinical profiles using the cBioPortal. Sci Signal. 2013;6(269):pl1.
30. Cerami E, Gao J, Dogrusoz U, Gross BE, Sumer SO, Aksoy BA, et al. The cBio cancer genomics portal: an open platform for exploring multidimensional cancer genomics data. Cancer Discov. 2012;2(5):401–4.
31. Taylor BS, Schultz N, Hieronymus H, Gopalan A, Xiao Y, Carver BS, et al. Integrative genomic profiling of human prostate cancer. Cancer Cell. 2010; 18(1):11–22.
32. Dunning MJ, Vowler SL, Lalonde E, Ross-Adams H, Boutros P, Mills IG, et al. Mining human prostate Cancer datasets: the "camcAPP" shiny app. EBioMedicine. 2017;17:5–6.
33. Ross-Adams H, Lamb AD, Dunning MJ, Halim S, Lindberg J, Massie CM, et al. Integration of copy number and transcriptomics provides risk stratification in prostate cancer: a discovery and validation cohort study. EBioMedicine. 2015;2(9):1133–44.
34. Hothorn T, Hornik K, Zeileis A. Unbiased recursive partitioning: a conditional inference framework. J Comput Graph Stat. 2006;15(3):651–74.
35. Cancer Genome Atlas Research Network. The molecular taxonomy of primary prostate Cancer. Cell. 2015;163(4):1011–25.
36. Goksuluk D, Korkmaz S, Zarasiz G, Karaagaoglu AE. easyROC: an interactive web-tool for ROC curve analysis using R language environment. The R journal. 2016;8(2):213–30.
37. Agell L, Hernandez S, Nonell L, Lorenzo M, Puigdecanet E, de Muga S, et al. A 12-gene expression signature is associated with aggressive histological in prostate cancer: SEC14L1 and TCEB1 genes are potential markers of progression. Am J Pathol. 2012;181(5):1585–94.
38. Bibikova M, Chudin E, Arsanjani A, Zhou L, Garcia EW, Modder J, et al. Expression signatures that correlated with Gleason score and relapse in prostate cancer. Genomics. 2007;89(6):666–72.
39. Bismar TA, Demichelis F, Riva A, Kim R, Varambally S, He L, et al. Defining aggressive prostate cancer using a 12-gene model. Neoplasia. 2006;8(1):59–68.
40. Chen X, Xu S, McClelland M, Rahmatpanah F, Sawyers A, Jia Z, et al. An accurate prostate cancer prognosticator using a seven-gene signature plus Gleason score and taking cell type heterogeneity into account. PLoS One. 2012;7(9):e45178.
41. Erho N, Crisan A, Vergara IA, Mitra AP, Ghadessi M, Buerki C, et al. Discovery and validation of a prostate cancer genomic classifier that predicts early metastasis following radical prostatectomy. PLoS One. 2013;8(6):e66855.
42. Glinsky GV, Berezovska O, Glinskii AB. Microarray analysis identifies a death-from-cancer signature predicting therapy failure in patients with multiple types of cancer. J Clin Invest. 2005;115(6):1503–21.
43. Irshad S, Bansal M, Castillo-Martin M, Zheng T, Aytes A, Wenske S, et al. A molecular signature predictive of indolent prostate cancer. Sci Transl Med. 2013;5(202):202ra122.
44. Long Q, Johnson BA, Osunkoya AO, Lai YH, Zhou W, Abramovitz M, et al. Protein-coding and microRNA biomarkers of recurrence of prostate cancer following radical prostatectomy. Am J Pathol. 2011;179(1):46–54.
45. Long Q, Xu J, Osunkoya AO, Sannigrahi S, Johnson BA, Zhou W, et al. Global transcriptome analysis of formalin-fixed prostate cancer specimens identifies biomarkers of disease recurrence. Cancer Res. 2014;74(12):3228–37.
46. Luca BA, Brewer DS, Edwards DR, Edwards S, Whitaker HC, Merson S, et al. DESNT: A Poor Prognosis Category of Human Prostate Cancer. European urology focus. 2017.
47. Rajan P, Stockley J, Sudbery IM, Fleming JT, Hedley A, Kalna G, et al. Identification of a candidate prognostic gene signature by transcriptome analysis of matched pre- and post-treatment prostatic biopsies from patients with advanced prostate cancer. BMC Cancer. 2014;14:977.
48. Ramaswamy S, Ross KN, Lander ES, Golub TR. A molecular signature of metastasis in primary solid tumors. Nat Genet. 2003;33(1):49–54.
49. Romanuik TL, Ueda T, Le N, Haile S, Yong TM, Thomson T, et al. Novel biomarkers for prostate cancer including noncoding transcripts. Am J Pathol. 2009;175(6):2264–76.
50. Rubicz R, Zhao S, Wright JL, Coleman I, Grasso C, Geybels MS, et al. Gene expression panel predicts metastatic-lethal prostate cancer outcomes in men diagnosed with clinically localized prostate cancer. Mol Oncol. 2017; 11(2):140–50.
51. Sharma NL, Massie CE, Ramos-Montoya A, Zecchini V, Scott HE, Lamb AD, et al. The androgen receptor induces a distinct transcriptional program in castration-resistant prostate cancer in man. Cancer Cell. 2013;23(1):35–47.
52. Varambally S, Yu J, Laxman B, Rhodes DR, Mehra R, Tomlins SA, et al. Integrative genomic and proteomic analysis of prostate cancer reveals signatures of metastatic progression. Cancer Cell. 2005;8(5):393–406.
53. Wu CL, Schroeder BE, Ma XJ, Cutie CJ, Wu S, Salunga R, et al. Development and validation of a 32-gene prognostic index for prostate cancer progression. Proc Natl Acad Sci U S A. 2013;110(15):6121–6.
54. Yu J, Yu J, Rhodes DR, Tomlins SA, Cao X, Chen G, et al. A polycomb repression signature in metastatic prostate cancer predicts cancer outcome. Cancer Res. 2007;67(22):10657–63.
55. Jhun MA, Geybels MS, Wright JL, Kolb S, April C, Bibikova M, et al. Gene expression signature of Gleason score is associated with prostate cancer outcomes in a radical prostatectomy cohort. Oncotarget. 2017;8(26):43035–47.
56. Sunkel B, Wu D, Chen Z, Wang CM, Liu X, Ye Z, et al. Integrative analysis identifies targetable CREB1/FoxA1 transcriptional co-regulation as a predictor of prostate cancer recurrence. Nucleic Acids Res. 2016;44(9):4105–22.
57. Micallef L, Rodgers P. eulerAPE: drawing area-proportional 3-Venn diagrams using ellipses. PloS One. 2014;9(7):e101717.
58. Zhao J, Zhu D, Zhang X, Zhang Y, Zhou J, Dong M. TMEM206 promotes the malignancy of colorectal cancer cells by interacting with AKT and extracellular signal-regulated kinase signaling pathways. J Cell Physiol. 2018. https://doi.org/10.1002/jcp.27751.
59. Morlacco A, Cheville JC, Rangel LJ, Gearman DJ, Karnes RJ. Adverse Disease Features in Gleason Score 3 + 4 "Favorable Intermediate-Risk" Prostate Cancer: Implications for Active Surveillance. Eur Urol. 72(3):442–7.
60. Jurmeister S, Ramos-Montoya A, Sandi C, Pertega-Gomes N, Wadhwa K, Lamb AD, et al. Identification of potential therapeutic targets in prostate cancer through a cross-species approach. EMBO Mol Med. 2018;10:e8274. https://doi.org/10.15252/emmm.201708274.
61. Neumayer G, Belzil C, Gruss OJ, Nguyen MD. TPX2: of spindle assembly, DNA damage response, and cancer. Cell Mol Life Sci. 2014;71(16):3027–47.
62. Zhang R, Roostalu J, Surrey T, Nogales E. Structural insight into TPX2-stimulated microtubule assembly. Elife. 2017;6:e30959. https://doi.org/10.7554/eLife.30959.

63. Gu JJ, Zhang JH, Chen HJ, Wang SS. TPX2 promotes glioma cell proliferation and invasion via activation of the AKT signaling pathway. Oncol Lett. 2016; 12(6):5015–22.
64. Hsu CW, Chen YC, Su HH, Huang GJ, Shu CW, Wu TT, et al. Targeting TPX2 suppresses the tumorigenesis of hepatocellular carcinoma cells resulting in arrested mitotic phase progression and increased genomic instability. J Cancer. 2017;8(8):1378–94.
65. Pan HW, Su HH, Hsu CW, Huang GJ, Wu TT. Targeted TPX2 increases chromosome missegregation and suppresses tumor cell growth in human prostate cancer. OncoTargets and therapy. 2017;10:3531–43.
66. Ruijtenberg S, van den Heuvel S. Coordinating cell proliferation and differentiation: antagonism between cell cycle regulators and cell type-specific gene expression. Cell Cycle. 2016;15(2):196–212.
67. Dong Q, Meng P, Wang T, Qin W, Qin W, Wang F, et al. MicroRNA let-7a inhibits proliferation of human prostate cancer cells in vitro and in vivo by targeting E2F2 and CCND2. PLoS One. 2010;5(4):e10147.
68. Wilczynska A, Bushell M. The complexity of miRNA-mediated repression. Cell Death Differ. 2015;22(1):22–33.
69. Kanwal R, Plaga AR, Liu X, Shukla GC, Gupta S. MicroRNAs in prostate cancer: functional role as biomarkers. Cancer Lett. 2017;407:9–20.
70. Rupaimoole R, Slack FJ. MicroRNA therapeutics: towards a new era for the management of cancer and other diseases. Nat Rev Drug Discov. 2017;16(3): 203–22.
71. Coarfa C, Fiskus W, Eedunuri VK, Rajapakshe K, Foley C, Chew SA, et al. Comprehensive proteomic profiling identifies the androgen receptor axis and other signaling pathways as targets of microRNAs suppressed in metastatic prostate cancer. Oncogene. 2016;35(18):2345–56.
72. Santos A, Wernersson R, Jensen LJ. Cyclebase 3.0: a multi-organism database on cell-cycle regulation and phenotypes. Nucleic Acids Res. 2015; 43(Database issue):D1140–4.
73. Otto T, Sicinski P. Cell cycle proteins as promising targets in cancer therapy. Nat Rev Cancer. 2017;17(2):93–115.
74. Cussenot O, Azzouzi AR, Nicolaiew N, Mangin P, Cormier L, Fournier G, et al. Low-activity V89L variant in SRD5A2 is associated with aggressive prostate cancer risk: an explanation for the adverse effects observed in chemoprevention trials using 5-alpha-reductase inhibitors. Eur Urol. 2007;52(4):1082–7.
75. Maier C. Editorial comment on: low-activity V89L variant in SRD5A2 is associated with aggressive prostate cancer risk: an explanation for the adverse effects observed in chemoprevention trials using 5-alpha-reductase inhibitors. Eur Urol. 2007;52(4):1088–9.
76. Prayer-Galetti T. Editorial comment on: low-activity V89L variant in SRD5A2 is associated with aggressive prostate cancer risk: an explanation for the adverse effects observed in chemoprevention trials using 5-alpha-reductase inhibitors. Eur Urol. 2007;52(4):1087–8.

2

Safety and effectiveness of high-power thulium laser enucleation of the prostate in patients with glands larger than 80 mL

Ching-Hsin Chang[1,2†], Tzu-Ping Lin[3†] and Jung-Yao Huang[4*]

Abstract

Background: The efficacy of thulium laser prostate enucleation (ThuLEP) for large prostates is unclear. This study aimed to explore the expanded utility of 150–200-W ThuLEP by studying patients with a large prostate (> 80 mL).

Methods: We retrospectively reviewed records of 125 patients with large prostate glands (> 80 mL) who underwent ThuLEP performed by a single surgeon from June 2012 to June 2016. The ThuLEP data from our previous pilot study were used as the control. Operative variables, patient profiles, preoperative and postoperative urine flow rates, prostate volume, and the international prostate symptom score (IPSS) were recorded and analyzed using Student's *t*-test, the *z*-test, and logistic regression analysis.

Results: Of 366 patients who underwent ThuLEP, 125 (34.15%) were enrolled. The ages and estimated prostate volumes were compared with those of the control. Overall, 39.2% underwent Foley placement and 4% received an anticoagulant agent preoperatively. Maximum urinary flow rates before and 3 and 12 months postoperatively were 9.93, 23.20, and 19.00 mL/s, respectively, which were generally equal to those of the control groups ($P = 0.68$, 0.18, 0.98, respectively). Preoperative and postoperative IPSSs were 27.09 and 7.35, respectively. The postoperative prostate-specific antigen was reduced by 85.59% in comparison to the preoperative level. The estimated prostate size was reduced by 74.17% postoperatively. The modified Clavien-Dindo classification system was used to identify the overall rate of complications, which was approximately 22.4%. The mortality rate was 0.8%.

Conclusions: High-power ThuLEP is safe and effective for patients with large prostate glands (> 80 mL). Prostate enucleation using a high-power thulium laser is feasible for patients who exhibit contraindications for surgery.

Keywords: Thulium laser, Enucleation, Large, Prostate, Bladder outlet obstruction, Open prostatectomy

Background

Open prostatectomy (OP) offers the highest probability of symptomatic improvement and the lowest failure rate of all treatment modalities for bladder outlet obstruction (BOO) due to benign prostatic hyperplasia (BPH) [1]. Despite considerable blood loss and prolonged recovery, OP has been the traditional treatment option for extremely large prostates [2, 3]. The previous American Urological Association (AUA) and European Urological Association (EAU) guidelines (in 2001 and 2003) suggest that OP should be the treatment of choice for patients with prostate volumes of 80–100 mL [4, 5].

Holmium laser enucleation of the prostate (HoLEP) has been adopted by many urologists worldwide because of the increased commercial availability (beginning in 1994) of high-powered holmium:yttrium-aluminum-garnet lasers. Since then, numerous single-center and multicenter large-scale series and randomized clinical trials have demonstrated its effectiveness and safety when used to treat BOO [6, 7]. HoLEP has been proven to be an endourological alternative to OP for large prostates [8]. Furthermore, beginning in 2013, HoLEP became the new "gold standard" because it was associated with a low operative blood loss, recatheterization rate, and reintervention rate, shorter hospital stay, and other benefits [9]. The section "Laser

* Correspondence: jyhuang431114@gmail.com
†Ching-Hsin Chang and Tzu-Ping Lin contributed equally to this work.
4Shutien Uro Clinic, Taipei, Taiwan
Full list of author information is available at the end of the article

treatments of the prostate" of the last EAU Male LUTS Guidelines (the 2018 edition) was adapted [10]. OP or endoscopic enucleation of the prostate such as holmium laser or bipolar enucleation of the prostate are the first choice of surgical treatment in men with a substantially enlarged prostate and moderate-to-severe LUTS. This treatment was strongly recommended for men with prostate size > 80 mL.

With the evolution of technology, thulium laser prostate enucleation (ThuLEP) has become a novel treatment option for BOO [11]. In 2005, the thulium laser entered clinical practice with a power of approximately 50–120 W, thereby offering advanced vaporization and hemostatic features [12, 13]. Thulium appears to provide improved vaporization ability, thereby ensuring smooth tissue incisions compared to those of the holmium laser. Holmiun laser can only be used in pulsed form; the thulium laser is continuous but pulsatile. This nature is enabling the surgeon to accurately remove the adenoma at the level of the surgical capsule because it is easier to distinguish the adenoma in this plane. Theoretically, regardless of the size of the prostate, ThuLEP can effectively clear the transition zone [11, 14].

The power of an advanced thulium device is 150–200 W. In our pilot study published in 2015, a high-power thulium laser was used to perform ThuLEP in patients from the general or unselected public. One year of follow-up showed that ThuLEP and traditional transurethral resection of the prostate (TURP) effectively alleviated subjective and objective voiding symptoms with a low rate of complications [15]. Limited evidence described favorable outcomes with ThuLEP that were comparable with those with OP, TURP, and HoLEP for prostates < 80 mL [16, 17]. The studies by Pearce at el and Gross et al. evaluated patients with prostates > 80 mL [18, 19]. The former study included only 25 patients (> 75 mL) [18], and these patients became one of the subgroups (24%, 266 in 1080 patients) in the latter study but were briefly discussed [19].

Limited number of randomized controlled trials with long-term follow-up support the efficacy of ThuLEP, there is a need for ongoing investigation of the technique [10]. Furthermore the efficacy of ThuLEP for large prostates is unclear.

To confirm ThuLEP as an endourological alternative to OP and HoLEP for numerous specific conditions, the application of ThuLEP for treating large prostates should be evaluated. Therefore, in this study, we assessed the outcomes (i.e., safety, feasibility) of ThuLEP for patients with a large prostate (> 80 mL).

Methods

We retrospectively reviewed data from 125 patients who underwent ThuLEP performed by a single surgeon (JYH) between June 2012 and June 2016. Approval was received from the institutional review board (VGHIRB 2016-03-007 AC), along with a waiver for informed consent.

All patients, regardless of the presence of malignancy, had a prostate gland that was larger than 80 mL in volume, as measured using transabdominal ultrasonography and the prolate ellipsoid volume formula. No exclusion criteria were applied during chart review. The Cyber 150 device (Quanta System, Solbiate Olona, Varese, Italy) was used with 150–200 W of energy in continuous mode (Fig. 1). The Piranha Morcellator device (Richard Wolf, Knittlingen, Germany) was used after the enucleation step. Postoperative Foley catheter irrigation was performed, and then the catheter was removed the day after surgery. Patients who underwent ThuLEP during our pilot study were considered as a control group [15]. Data regarding surgical variables, patient status, preoperative and postoperative urinary flow rates, prostate volume, and the international prostate symptom score (IPSS) were extracted from each patient's medical records. Follow-up consisted of written questionnaires that were sent in June 2017 and telephone interviews.

The database from published articles were introduced as the the OP, HoLEP, and ThuLEP control group [15, 20, 21]. Data were analyzed using Student's t-test, the z-test, and logistic regression analysis with MedCalc software (Medcalc, Mariakerke, Belgium). For all statistical comparisons, significance was assumed when $P < 0.05$.

Results

Of 366 patients (with all size of prostate glands) who underwent ThuLEP during a 4-year period, 125 (34.15%, with glands > 80 mL) were enrolled. Fifteen patients exhibited malignant pathological findings (Table 1). Compared to the ThuLEP group in the pilot study, patients in this study were younger (mean ± standard deviation, 71.85 ± 8.89 years; $P = 0.02$) and had a higher estimated prostate volume (106.80 ± 45.77 mL, range 80–332; $P < 0.001$) [15]. Additionally, patients in our study were generally older and had a larger prostate than did the general public. Of these patients, 39.2% underwent Foley placement, and 4% were treated with an anticoagulant agent preoperatively.

The preoperative IPSS was 27.09 ± 5.91, and the postoperative IPSS was 7.35 ± 5.89 in this study group. The control groups included the ThuLEP, HoLEP, and OP groups (Fig. 2) [15, 20]. These data indicated a higher preoperative IPSS and larger prostates in the study group, which were relieved after surgery, than in the control groups ($P < 0.001$, 0.51) (Table 2).

The maximum urinary flow rates before and at 3 and 12 months postoperatively were 9.93 ± 5.02, 23.20 ± 6.87, and 19.00 ± 18.30 mL/s, respectively, which were generally equal to those found during the pilot study ($P = 0.68$, 0.18, and 0.98, respectively) (Fig. 3a, b). The postoperative prostate-specific antigen (PSA) was reduced by 85.59 ± 14.92% compared to the preoperative level. The estimated

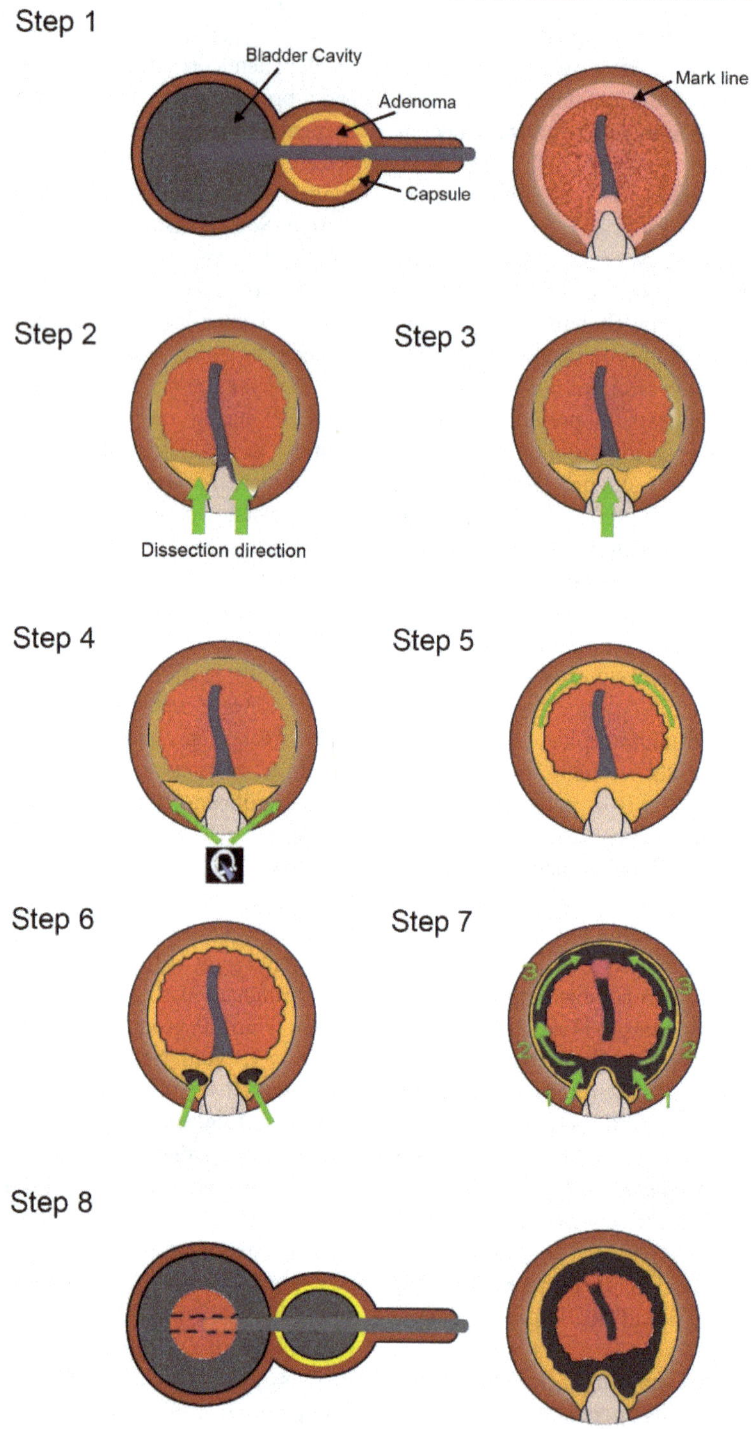

Fig. 1 Illustration of the thulium laser prostate enucleation (ThuLEP) surgical technique. Step 1: Creation of the working space: coagulate the mucosa along the proximal side of the sphincter, sparing the verumontanum, and create the marked line. Step 2: Cut and extend from the marked line to the capsule in the 5 o'clock and 7 o'clock directions. The marked line that is proximal to the verumontanum is spared (in the 6 o'clock direction). Step 3: Extend from the cutting edge in the 5 o'clock and 7 o'clock directions to the 6 o'clock direction. Step 4: Place the guiding tube on the scope sheath and keep dissecting from the 6 o'clock direction to the opposite side (in the 5 to 4 and 3 o'clock directions and in the 7 to 8 and 9 o'clock directions, respectively). Step 5: The tissue in the 12 o'clock direction is relatively thin. Be careful to not cut too deep or shallow while cutting in this direction. Step 6: Cut along the prostate capsule and make a window to the urinary bladder space in the 5 and 7 o'clock directions. Step 7: Extend the cutting edge from the 5 and 7 o'clock directions to the 6 o'clock direction. Extend the edge along the lateral wall in the 12 o'clock direction. Step 8: Push the adenoma tissue into the bladder space, check the bleeder, and then perform the morcellation procedure

Table 1 Baseline characteristics and comparisons with the control groups

	Our study			Pilot study: ThuLEP [15]		Pilot study: TURP [15]	
	Total	Malignancy	Benign		*P*-value**		*P*-value**
Patients	125	15	110	29		30	
Age, years	71.85 ± 8.89	78.81 ± 7.17	71.07 ± 8.68	76.1 ± 9.4	0.02	72.6 ± 7.4	0.62
PSA level, ng/mL	18.40 ± 37.35	37.03 ± 60.34	16.14 ± 33.26	5.0 ± 5.4	0.49	8.3 ± 7.9	0.47
Anticoagulant agent use	5 (4%)	0	5 (4.45%)	15 (51.7%)		6 (20.0%)	
Estimated prostate volume, mL	106.80 ± 45.77	106.80 ± 70.76	106.40 ± 41.25	57.2 ± 25.1	< 0.01	64.7 ± 32.5	< 0.01
Preoperative Foley placement	49 (39.2%)	5 (100%)	44 (40%)	3 (10.34%)		7 (23.33%)	
Transfusion rate	4 (3.2%)	1 (6.67%)	3 (2.72%)	4 (13.79%)		8 (26.67%)	
Reduction ratio of the PSA level 3 months postoperatively (%)	85.59 ± 14.92			39.21 ± 44.95	< 0.0001	70.22 ± 28.86	0.0047
Reduction ratio of the estimated prostate size postoperatively (%)	74.17 ± 11.27			47.24 ± 16.20	< 0.0001	49.01 ± 17.79	< 0.0001

PSA, prostate-specific antigen, ThuLEP, thulium laser enucleation of the prostate, TURP, transurethral resection of the prostate
**Compared with the total group using Student's t-test

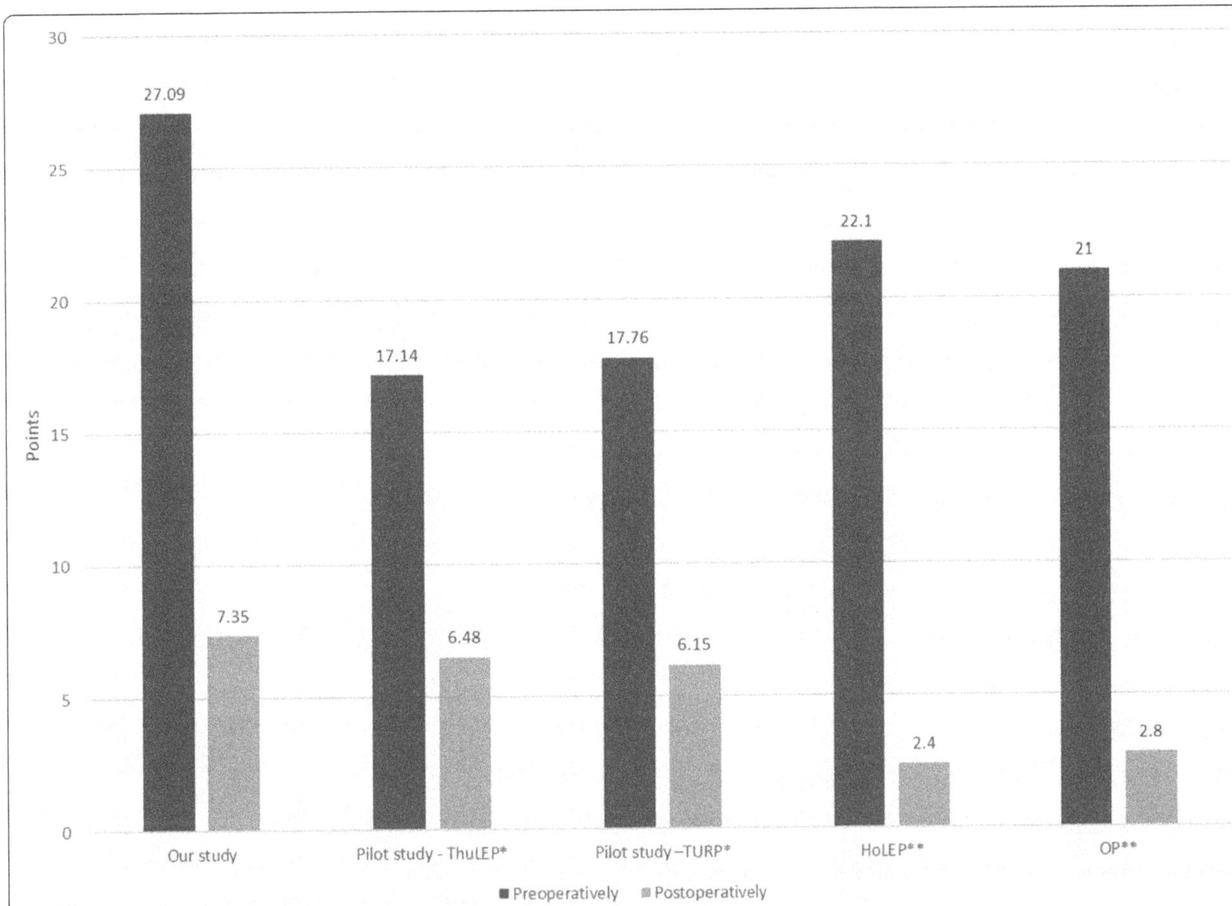

Fig. 2 Preoperative and postoperative IPSSs are decreased dramatically in all studies. The IPSSs were measured preoperatively and postoperatively. IPSS, international prostate symptom score; ThuLEP, thulium laser prostate enucleation; HoLEP, holmium laser enucleation of the prostate

Table 2 Perioperative profiles and comparisons

		Our study: Total (n = 125)	Pilot study: ThuVEP [15] (n = 29)		Pilot study: TURP [15] (n = 30)	
				P-value*		P-value*
IPSS, points	Preoperatively	27.09 ± 5.91	17.14 ± 5.08	< 0.01	17.76 ± 4.27	< 0.01
IPSS, points	Postoperatively	7.35 ± 5.89	6.48 ± 3.73	0.51	6.15 ± 4.43	0.49
PVR volume, mL	Preoperatively	329.76 ± 350.52	138.64 ± 127.74	0.01	90.91 ± 66.53	< 0.01
Maximum UFR, mL/s		9.93 ± 5.02	10.5 ± 4.86	0.68	10.84 ± 4.74	0.46
Mean UFR, mL/s		5.40 ± 2.18	5.02 ± 2.62	0.55	4.58 ± 2.15	0.13
PVR volume, mL	1 week postoperatively	60.67 ± 74.08				
Maximum UFR, mL/s		19.39 ± 12.01				
Mean UFR, mL/s		11.24 ± 6.38				
PVR volume, mL	1 month postoperatively	53.97 ± 36.05				
Maximum UFR, mL/s		17.92 ± 9.3				
Mean UFR, mL/s		11.09 ± 5.78				
PVR volume, mL	3 months postoperatively	38.67 ± 18.52	68.24 ± 37.54	< 0.01	69.50 ± 47.85	< 0.01
Maximum UFR, mL/s		23.20 ± 6.87	16.26 ± 7.72	0.18	22.77 ± 10.46	0.01
Mean UFR, mL/s		10.20 ± 3.77	7.50 ± 3.07	0.76	12.15 ± 6.20	0.04
PVR volume, mL	6 months postoperatively	48.22 ± 45.85				
Maximum UFR, mL/s		9.38 ± 13.98	16.53 ± 6.99	0.02	22.67 ± 10.40	0.06
Mean UFR, mL/s		18.28 ± 8.96	8.69 ± 3.62	0.60	11.51 ± 5.74	0.58
PVR volume, mL	12 months postoperatively	41.33 ± 42.02				
Maximum UFR, mL/s		19.00 ± 18.30	18.40 ± 7.13	0.98	23.34 ± 13.73	0.53
Mean UFR, mL/s		7.50 ± 4.71	9.68 ± 4.45	0.72	12.99 ± 8.38	0.34

The estimated prostate volume was calculated as the volume of the entire gland using the prolate elliptical formula (height × width × length × π/6). Overall, 10.4% of patients returned as outpatients and had uroflow data at more than 1 year postoperatively. IPSS, international prostate symptom score; PVR, postvoid residual volume; URF, urinary flow rate; ThuLEP, thulium laser enucleation of the prostate; TURP, transurethral resection of prostate
*Compared with the total group using Student's t-test

prostate size was reduced by 74.17 ± 11.27% postoperatively. These reduction rates were compatible with the characteristics of enucleation treatment.

The modified Clavien-Dindo classification system was used to identify complications following the pilot study [15, 22]. The overall complication rate was approximately 22.4%, whereas the mortality rate was 0.8% (Table 3). There were few differences between the OP, HoLEP, and ThuLEP control groups [20, 21], with only one case of mortality due to postoperative

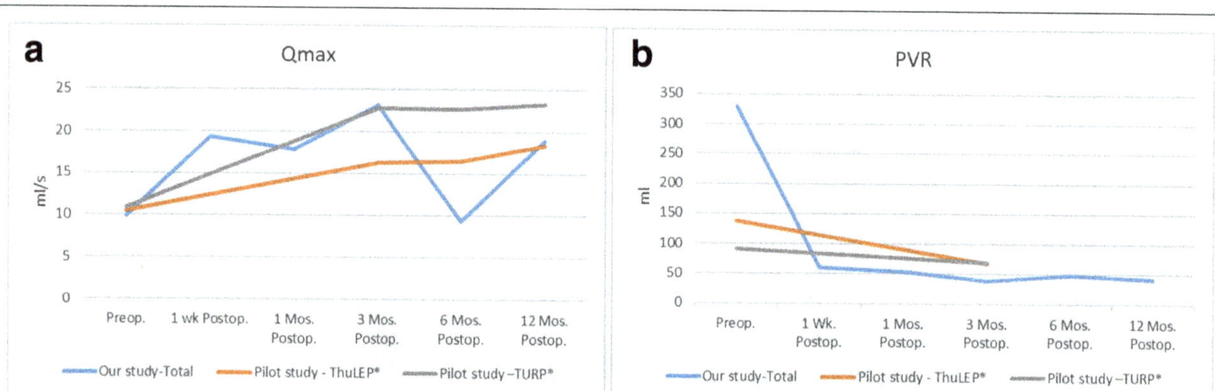

Fig. 3 Perioperative Qmax (**a**) and PVR urine volume (**b**). The average of (**a**) the Qmax (mL/s) and (**b**) PVR urine volume (mL) from this study and our pilot study at different time points (preoperatively and postoperatively at 1 week, 1 month, 3 months, 6 months, and 12 months). Qmax, maximum flow rate; PVR, postvoiding residual; Wk., week; Mos., months; Preop., preoperatively; Postop., postoperatively; ThuLEP, thulium laser prostate enucleation; HoLEP, holmium laser enucleation of the prostate

Table 3 Modified Clavien-Dindo classification system for reporting complications of prostate procedures

Grade	Modified Clavien-Dindo system for TURP	Our study		HoLEP [21]	OP [21]	ThuVEP [20]
		(*n*)	Incidence (%)			
1	Hematuria clot retention requiring bladder irrigation/clot evacuation/catheter traction	2	1.6	5	5	16.65
	Catheter block because of retained TUR chip	0	0	5	5	
	Failed trial without catheter with acute urinary retention requiring bedside recatheterization (CIC)	12	9.6			
2	Hemorrhage/hematuria requiring transfusion	4	3.2	0	13.3	4.34
	Urinary incontinence requiring a antimuscarinic agent	3	2.4			
3	Bladder neck contracture or urethral stricture, required surgical intervention	6	4.8	1.7	3.3	8.25
4	Acute myocardial infarction requiring admission to the ICU	0	0	0	1.7	0.79
	TUR syndrome requiring admission to ICU	0	0			
5	Death	1	0.8			0
Total		28	22.4	15	26.7	30.03

OP, open prostatectomy, CIC, clean intermittent catheterization, ICU, intensive care unit, HoLEP, holmium laser enucleation of the prostate, ThuLEP, thulium laser enucleation of the prostate, TURP, transurethral resection of prostate, TUR, transurethral resection

stroke 1 day later. The telephone follow-up time was 26.62 ± 13.76 months, and the completion rate of the postoperative IPSS questionnaire was 54.4%.

Discussion

Urologists evaluate prospective BOO methods to ensure that they can be *extended* and *focused*. Such steps have been applied to all techniques that are commonly used today, such as OP, monopolar and bipolar TURP, photoselective vaporization techniques, and different laser therapies.

Extension of a technique involves its application across races and geographic regions. To achieve this, the learning curve for the technique should not be steep. The focus refers to its use in different groups, such as the elderly, patients with large glands, patients with heart disease, or those who use anticoagulants. After these two types of tests, the novel tool can be qualified and used in clinical practice.

Our pilot study demonstrated the ability of ThuLEP to be extended, and this study presented its ability to be focused [23]. To our knowledge, this is the first study to highlight 2 topics: the high-power thulium laser device and large prostates (> 80 mL). We used 80 mL as the cut-off value because that is the standard size of a large prostate according to the guidelines [4, 5]. This standard was applied to many endoscopic surgical procedures and different kinds of lasers (such as HoLEP) [9, 24]. Several previous studies discussed ThuLEP for patients with large prostates [25, 26]. However, their cut-off values varied (60 mL, 70 mL, and 100 mL) [27]. Our study was useful and crucial for determining the surgical management of patients with prostate volumes > 80 mL causing BOO secondary to BPH.

When analyzing this study's results, we attempted to ensure consistent demographic characteristics; therefore, we used control patient data from our pilot study. Following the case series analysis protocol, we compared several OP, HoLEP, and ThuLEP studies (Table 4) [20, 21]. Generally, our patients were younger, had bigger prostates, and exhibited more extensive urine retention. The reduction ratio of the estimated prostate size (%) in our study was 74.17 ± 11.27, which is comparable to the ratio reported by previous studies (82% for OP; 85% for HoLEP; and 61% for ThuVEP). The postvoiding residual (PVR) urine volume slope in our study was − 0.9265 (Fig. 4). However, in studies using OP, HoLEP, and ThuVEP, PVR urine volume slopes were − 13.411, − 9.64738, and − 41.1333, respectively (data not shown). These differences in PVR urine volumes and the incidence of complications may be due to differences in the collection method used. However, these incidence data were difficult to compare statistically because the patient population, surgeon, and technique were variable.

Our measured complication rate may be related to the large number of failed trials, as indicated by the increased number of patients who experienced urine retention postoperatively. These subgroups of complications were not considered in other studies (Table 3). Similarly, Gross et al. reported the complications of 266 patients with a large prostate [19]. The rates of acute urinary retention, re-operation, transfusion, and mortality were 7.5, 5.3, 2.6, and 0%, respectively. These rates seem to be slightly lower than those in our study (9.6, 4.8, 3.2, and 0.9%, respectively). The association between using of high-power Laser and the complications, especially the bladder neck stenosis, was not clear and required further evaluation. However, most importantly, only 1 case of mortality occurred

Table 4 Comparisons of perioperative profiles

		Our study: Total	HoLEP [21]		OP [21]		ThuVEP [20]	
				P-value*		*P*-value*		*P*-value*
Patients, N		125	60		60		1382	
Preoperative IPSS, points		27.09 ± 5.91	22.1 ± 3.3	< 0.0001	21.0 ± 3.6	< 0.0001	18.6 ± 7.6	< 0.0001
Postoperative IPSS, points		7.35 ± 5.89	2.4 ± 1.9	< 0.0001	2.8 ± 3.9	< 0.0001		
PVR volume, mL	Preoperatively	329.76 ± 350.52	280 ± 273	0.2915	292 ± 191	0.3438	156.3 ± 195.4	< 0.0001
Maximum UFR, mL/s		9.93 ± 5.02	3.8 ± 3.6	< 0.0001	3.6 ± 3.8	< 0.0001	10.7 ± 6.5	0.11
Mean UFR, mL/s		5.40 ± 2.18						
PVR volume, mL	1 week postoperatively	60.67 ± 74.08	10.2 ± 22.4	< 0.0001				
Maximum UFR, mL/s		19.39 ± 12.01	24.7 ± 3.3	< 0.0001				
Mean UFR, mL/s		11.24 ± 6.38						
PVR volume, mL	1 month postoperatively	53.97 ± 36.05	6.3 ± 18.7	< 0.0001	3.8 ± 8.7	< 0.0001		
Maximum UFR, mL/s		17.92 ± 9.3	26.9 ± 7.9	< 0.0001	26.6 ± 6.1	< 0.0001		
Mean UFR, mL/s		11.09 ± 5.78						
PVR volume, mL	3 months postoperatively	38.67 ± 18.52	7.2 ± 18.8	< 0.0001	3.0 ± 7.7	< 0.0001	32.9 ± 67.2	0.0186
Maximum UFR, mL/s		23.20 ± 6.87	27.6 ± 7.0	< 0.0001	27.3 ± 6.2	< 0.0001	19.2 ± 10.6	< 0.0001
Mean UFR, mL/s		10.20 ± 3.77						
PVR volume, mL	6 months postoperatively	48.22 ± 45.85	4.4 ± 11	< 0.0001	2.1 ± 6.0	< 0.0001		
Maximum UFR, mL/s		9.38 ± 13.98	29.9 ± 8.8	< 0.0001	27.0 ± 0.5	< 0.0001		
Mean UFR, mL/s		18.28 ± 8.96						
PVR volume, mL	12 months postoperatively	41.33 ± 42.02	5.8 ± 16.7	< 0.0001	6.4 ± 12.3	< 0.0001		
Maximum UFR, mL/s		19.00 ± 18.30	27.4 ± 9.7	< 0.0001	28.3 ± 7.5	< 0.0001		
Mean UFR, mL/s		7.50 ± 4.71						
Reduction ratio of the estimated prostate size postoperative (%)		74.17 ± 11.27	82		85		61	

IPSS, international prostate symptom score, Qmax, maximum urinary flow rate, OP, open prostatectomy, PVR, postvoid residual volume, UFR, urinary flow rate.
*Comparison with our study using a two-tailed z-test

in our study, which showed an uncertain relationship with the operation.

Randomized clinical trials are most suitable for testing the efficacy and safety of various methods. However, there have been only a few such studies. Although our study demonstrated the experience of real-world patients, the traceability of our patients was limited and impacted data collection. We sent questionnaires and conducted telephone interviews to avoid any error due to selection bias. The methods used to collect patient data in previous multicenter and national studies were unavailable, likely because they are time-consuming and resource-intensive [20].

There were a few limitations to our study. We encountered patients who elected to undergo the surgical procedure described in this study after seeking a second opinion at our clinic. For example, some patients had undergone Foley catheterization performed by their general physician or another urologist. The mean PSA level from the benign subgroup was 16.14 ± 33.26 ng/mL, which is very high compared to that reported in the literature before enucleation [16, 17]. However, the PSA density was equal to that in the pilot study. Thus, this result might reflect the presence of a larger prostate size or urinary retention with catheterization preoperatively.

Moreover, some patients were unable to undergo extensive follow-up at our clinic and returned to their general physicians. The high variation in follow-up (mean ± standard deviation, 26.62 ± 13.76 months) reflects this trend. Certain patients who were unhappy with the outcomes often visited the clinic more frequently and for a longer period. This may have affected our measurements of surgical outcomes (Fig. 3a, b). By excluding data of those who answered our questionnaires by mail or telephone, only 13 patients (10.4%) returned as outpatients and had uroflow data at more than 1 year postoperatively. Although our

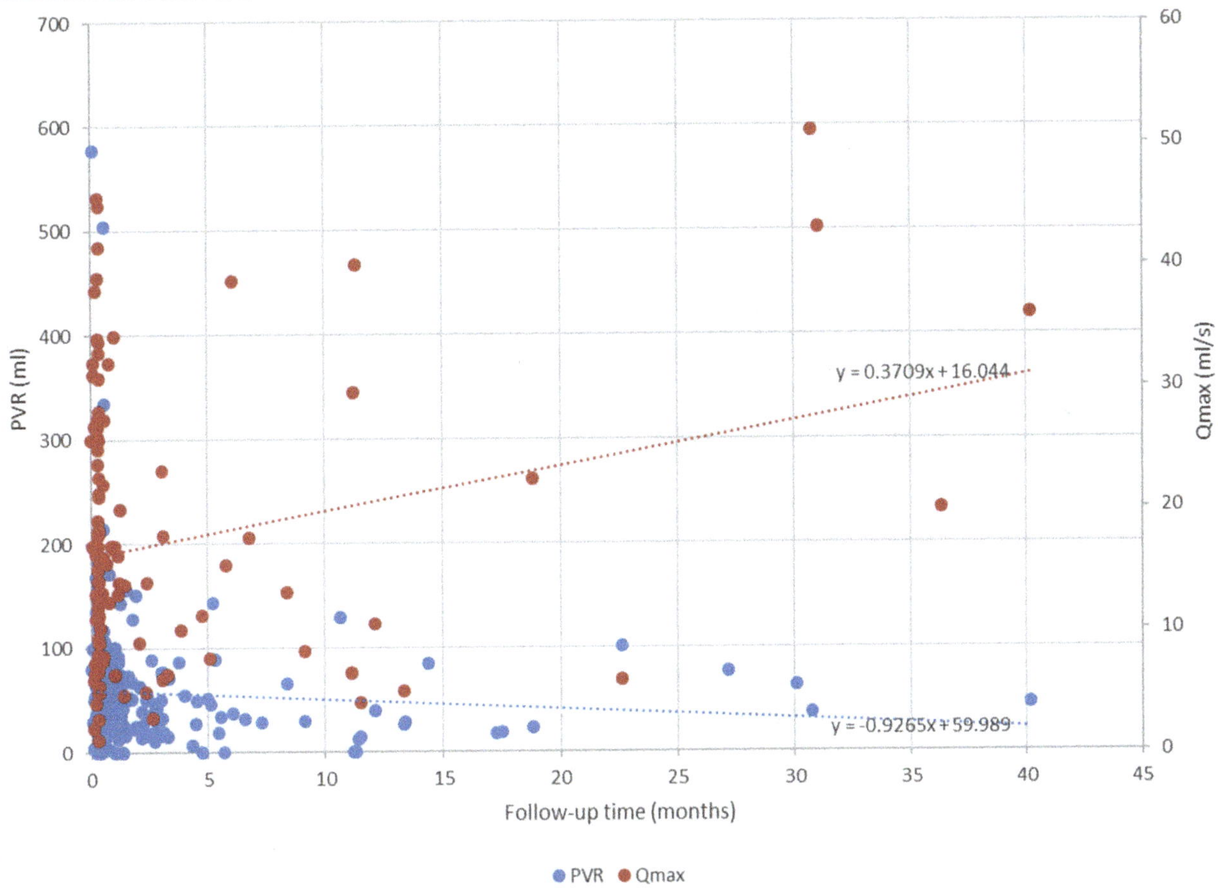

Fig. 4 Perioperative PVR and Qmax. The PVR urine volume (mL, blue dots) and Qmax of uroflowmetry (mL/min, red dots) are shown based on the chart review. A regression line is drawn. PVR, postvoiding residual; Qmax, maximum urinary flow rate

short-term postoperative outcomes appeared promising, further investigations of long-term efficacy are needed.

Conclusions

The latest guideline and consensus demonstated OP or holmium laser or bipolar enucleation of the prostate are the first choice of surgical treatment in men with moderate-to-severe LUTS, and prostate size > 80 mL. Although OP and HoLEP have been described for large prostates, our study confirmed that ThuLEP is a suitable endourological alternative. High-power ThuLEP (i.e., approximately 150–200 W) is safe and effective for patients with large prostates (> 80 mL).

Therefore, promising outcomes associated with ThuLEP suggested that enucleation using a high-power laser is feasible for patients with large prostate > 80 mL.

Abbreviations

AUA: American Urological Association; BOO: Bladder outlet obstruction; BPH: Benign prostatic hyperplasia; EAU: European Urological Association; HoLEP: Holmium laser enucleation of the prostate; IPSS: International prostate symptom score; OP: Open prostatectomy; PSA: Prostate-specific antigen; PVR: Postvoiding residual; ThuLEP: Thulium laser prostate enucleation.; TURP: Transurethral resection of the prostate

Acknowledgements

None.

Authors' contributions

TPL contributed to the project development and manuscript editing. CHC contributed to the data management and manuscript writing. JYH contributed to the project development and data collection. All authors read and approved the final manuscript.

Author details

[1]Taipei Medical University Hospital, Taipei, Taiwan. [2]Institute of Microbiology and Immunology, National Yang-Ming University, Taipei, Taiwan. [3]Taipei Veterans General Hospital, Taipei, Taiwan. [4]Shutien Uro Clinic, Taipei, Taiwan.

References

1. Kuntz RM. Current role of lasers in the treatment of benign prostatic hyperplasia (BPH). Eur Urol. 2006;49(6):961–9.
2. Wilson LC, Gilling PJ, Williams A, Kennett KM, Frampton CM, Westenberg AM, Fraundorfer MR. A randomised trial comparing holmium laser enucleation versus transurethral resection in the treatment of prostates larger than 40 grams: results at 2 years. Eur Urol. 2006;50(3):569–73.
3. Naspro R, Suardi N, Salonia A, Scattoni V, Guazzoni G, Colombo R, Cestari A, Briganti A, Mazzoccoli B, Rigatti P, et al. Holmium laser enucleation of the prostate versus open prostatectomy for prostates >70 g: 24-month follow-up. Eur Urol. 2006;50(3):563–8.

4. de la Rosette JJ, Alivizatos G, Madersbacher S, Perachino M, Thomas D, Desgrandchamps F, de Wildt M. European Association of U: EAU Guidelines on benign prostatic hyperplasia (BPH). Eur Urol. 2001;40(3):256–63 discussion 264.
5. Committee AUAPG. AUA guideline on management of benign prostatic hyperplasia (2003). Chapter 1: diagnosis and treatment recommendations. J Urol. 2003;170(2 Pt 1):530–47.
6. Gilling PJ, Aho TF, Frampton CM, King CJ, Fraundorfer MR. Holmium laser enucleation of the prostate: results at 6 years. Eur Urol. 2008;53(4):744–9.
7. Elzayat EA, Elhilali MM. Holmium laser enucleation of the prostate (HoLEP): the endourologic alternative to open prostatectomy. Eur Urol. 2006;49(1):87–91.
8. Kuntz RM, Lehrich K, Ahyai SA. Holmium laser enucleation of the prostate versus open prostatectomy for prostates greater than 100 grams: 5-year follow-up results of a randomised clinical trial. Eur Urol. 2008;53(1):160–6.
9. van Rij S, Gilling PJ. In 2013, holmium laser enucleation of the prostate (HoLEP) may be the new 'gold standard'. Curr Urol Rep. 2012;13(6):427–32.
10. EAU Guidelines. In., edn. the EAU Annual Congress Copenhagen 2018. ISBN: EAU Guidelines Office; 2018.
11. Herrmann TR, Bach T, Imkamp F, Georgiou A, Burchardt M, Oelke M, Gross AJ. Thulium laser enucleation of the prostate (ThuLEP): transurethral anatomical prostatectomy with laser support. Introduction of a novel technique for the treatment of benign prostatic obstruction. World J Urol. 2010;28(1):45–51.
12. Fried NM, Murray KE. High-power thulium fiber laser ablation of urinary tissues at 1.94 microm. J Endourol. 2005;19(1):25–31.
13. Chung JS, Kang PM, Seo WI, Oh CK, Kim SC, Park SH, Choi JH, Yoon JH, Kang DI, Chung JI. Thulium laser (RevoLix) vaporesection versus vapoenucleation with morcellator (piranha) for the treatment of benign prostatic obstruction: a propensity-matched multicenter analysis. Int J Urol. 2014;21(11):1156–61.
14. Zarrabi A, Gross AJ. The evolution of lasers in urology. Ther Adv Urol. 2011; 3(2):81–9.
15. Chang CH, Lin TP, Chang YH, Huang WJ, Lin AT, Chen KK. Vapoenucleation of the prostate using a high-power thulium laser: a one-year follow-up study. BMC Urol. 2015;15:40.
16. Zhang F, Shao Q, Herrmann TR, Tian Y, Zhang Y. Thulium laser versus holmium laser transurethral enucleation of the prostate: 18-month follow-up data of a single center. Urology. 2012;79(4):869–74.
17. Swiniarski PP, Stepien S, Dudzic W, Kesy S, Blewniewski M, Rozanski W. Thulium laser enucleation of the prostate (TmLEP) vs. transurethral resection of the prostate (TURP): evaluation of early results. Cent European J Urol. 2012;65(3):130–4.
18. Pearce SM, Pariser JJ, Malik RD, Famakinwa OJ, Chung DE. Outcomes following thulium vapoenucleation of large prostates. Int Braz J Urol. 2016; 42(4):757–65.
19. Gross AJ, Netsch C, Knipper S, Holzel J, Bach T. Complications and early postoperative outcome in 1080 patients after thulium vapoenucleation of the prostate: results at a single institution. Eur Urol. 2013;63(5):859–67.
20. Bach T, Wolbling F, Gross AJ, Netsch C, Tauber S, Pottek T, Wulfing C, Brunken C. Prospective assessment of perioperative course in 2648 patients after surgical treatment of benign prostatic obstruction. World J Urol. 2017; 35(2):285–92.
21. Kuntz RM, Lehrich K. Transurethral holmium laser enucleation versus transvesical open enucleation for prostate adenoma greater than 100 gm.:: a randomized prospective trial of 120 patients. J Urol. 2002;168(4 Pt 1):1465–9.
22. Mitropoulos D, Artibani W, Graefen M, Remzi M, Roupret M, Truss M. European Association of Urology Guidelines P: reporting and grading of complications after urologic surgical procedures: an ad hoc EAU guidelines panel assessment and recommendations. Eur Urol. 2012;61(2):341–9.
23. Netsch C, Tiburtius C, Bach T, Knipper S, Gross AJ. Association of prostate size and perioperative morbidity in thulium:YAG vapoenucleation of the prostate. Urol Int. 2014;93(1):22–8.
24. Naspro R, Gomez Sancha F, Manica M, Meneghini A, Ahyai S, Aho T, Fiori C, Vavassori I, LF DAP, Pansadoro V, et al. From "gold standard" resection to reproducible "future standard" endoscopic enucleation of the prostate: what we know about anatomical enucleation. Minerva Urol Nefrol. 2017;69(5):446–58.
25. Rausch S, Heider T, Bedke J, Kruck S, Schwentner C, Fischer K, Stenzl A, Kalble T. Analysis of early morbidity and functional outcome of thulium: yttrium-aluminum-garnet laser enucleation for benign prostate enlargement: patient age and prostate size determine adverse surgical outcome. Urology. 2015;85(1):182–8.
26. Iacono F. Efficacy and safety profile of a novel technique, ThuLEP (thulium laser enucleation of the prostate) for the treatment of benign prostate hypertrophy. Our experience on 148 patients. BMC Surg. 2012;12(Suppl 1):S21.
27. Gross AJ, Orywal AK, Becker B, Netsch C. Five-year outcomes of thulium vapoenucleation of the prostate for symptomatic benign prostatic obstruction. World J Urol. 2017;35(10):1585–93.

3

The importance of sexuality, changes in erectile functioning and its association with self-esteem in men with localized prostate cancer

Caren Hilger[1*], Martin Schostak[2], Stephan Neubauer[3], Ahmed Magheli[4], Thomas Fydrich[5], Silke Burkert[1,6] and Friederike Kendel[1]

Abstract

Background: Treatment for localized prostate cancer (PCa) can cause long-term changes in erectile functioning. However, data on the importance of sexuality and possible consequences of altered erectile functioning on self-esteem in men with localized PCa are lacking.

Methods: Self-report questionnaires were completed by 292 men with PCa, initially managed with active surveillance (AS) or radical prostatectomy (RP). Independent t-tests were conducted to evaluate group differences. A sequential multiple regression model was fitted to analyze the associations between the importance of sexuality, changes in erectile functioning and impairment of self-esteem. Interaction effects were tested using simple slope analyses.

Results: Participants were 70 ± 7.2 years old and 66.5% rated sex as being "rather/very important". The two groups differed markedly in changes in erectile functioning, importance of sexuality and impairment of self-esteem ($p < .001$), with higher values in RP patients. Regression analysis showed that after adjustment for control variables and importance of sexuality, changes in erectile functioning were still associated with impairment of self-esteem ($B = .668$, $SE = .069$, $p < .001$). The interaction of changes in erectile functioning and importance of sexuality reached significance ($B = .318$, $SE = .062$, $p < .001$).

Conclusions: RP patients report more changes in erectile functioning than AS patients. Moreover, in men with localized PCa, erectile functioning and self-esteem are closely related. Sexuality seems to be important for the majority of these men. Physicians should address the possibility of erectile dysfunction and its potential effects on psychological well-being before the treatment decision.

Keywords: Active surveillance, Erectile functioning, Importance of sexuality, Localized prostate cancer, Radical prostatectomy, Self-esteem

* Correspondence: caren.hilger@charite.de
[1]Institute of Medical Psychology, Charité Universitätsmedizin Berlin, D-10117 Berlin, Germany
Full list of author information is available at the end of the article

Background

Men who are diagnosed with localized prostate cancer (PCa) have to choose among treatment options that differ considerably in their invasiveness, [1] ranging from active surveillance (AS) to radical prostatectomy (RP). In AS, treatment is delayed until a predefined histological or biochemical disease progression occurs, or until the patient choses a different treatment strategy due to other reasons, for example, cancer-related anxiety. [2] One of the most important reasons that men opt for AS is the possible impairment of sexual function as a side effect of invasive treatment. [3] Negative effects of RP on sexual function compared to AS have been summarized in systematic reviews [4, 5] and were confirmed by the latest results from the randomized controlled trial ProtecT that compared RP to AS directly. [6] Recent research has also highlighted a close association of PCa treatment and psychosexual outcomes, such as sexual bother [7] and an impaired sense of masculinity. [8] However, most studies dealing with sexuality in PCa patients still focus on the physiological aspects of sexuality despite the fact that an impairment of erectile function has far-reaching consequences on men's quality of life. [9, 10] For most men, sexuality is a vital aspect of their male identity and an impairment of erectile functioning may also affect their self-esteem (i.e. men's appraisal of their individual abilities combined with a sense of self-worth [11]). [12–14]

Prostate cancer is typically a disease of older men. [16] Therefore, one may assume that an impairment of erectile functioning is negligible in most PCa patients. Eventually, at the time of diagnosis, men are an average of about 70 years old. [17] However, to draw the conclusion that sexuality plays a subordinate role in the process of decision-making could mean to adapt the stereotype of sex unjustifiably being "unseemly, even unnatural in the old." [15] Indeed, sexual activity decreases with increasing age. Nevertheless, most older men still seem to experience sexual desire [15, 18] and also report being sexually active. [9, 19]

Although the relationship between erectile dysfunction and self-esteem has been subject to previous studies [13, 20], no study, to the best of our knowledge, has examined this association in men with localized PCa undergoing different treatment options. Additionally, data on the importance of sexuality in this population are lacking. The diagnosis of PCa might represent a critical life-event for some men. One could therefore assume that the diagnosis entails a change in men's priorities: PCa and its treatment may become the main focus whereas other aspects of quality of life, such as sexuality, may become of diminishing relevance. In fact, studies with colorectal cancer patients showed that the importance of sexuality decreased due to the cancer experience [21]. It remains unclear, however, whether this also applies to men with localized PCa. Our study therefore seeks to find out how important sexuality actually is for men with localized PCa. In addition, PCa treatment and RP in particular can result in an abrupt change of erectile functioning (in contrast to a normative, more gradual worsening of erectile functioning with increasing age). This does not allow for anticipating non-normative changes in erectile functioning for men with localized PCa after invasive treatment, which could also have an impact on self-esteem.

This study seeks to close a twofold gap: On the one hand, we wanted to assess the consequences of erectile dysfunction on PCa patients' self-esteem and, on the other hand, we wanted to shed light on the importance of sexuality in this population of older men with PCa. More specifically, we aimed at (1) comparing perceived changes in erectile functioning, self-esteem, and the importance of sexuality in men having opted for either RP or AS, and (2) assessing how changes in erectile functioning for the worse affect PCa patients' self-esteem, considering the importance of sexuality.

Methods

Study design, procedure and participants

The study was nested within the prospective, multicenter, observational HAROW study, which included patients newly diagnosed with localized PCa between July 2008 and July 2013. [22] The present study was conducted in 2014: 378 men who had chosen RP as their primary treatment were matched based on the time since treatment decision to 378 men who had opted for AS. Men who opted for radiation therapy were excluded from this study as it aimed at comparing the two extremes of possible treatment strategies (AS = minimally invasive vs. RP = maximally invasive). All men contacted had agreed to take part in future studies. Men in the high risk category, as defined by D'Amico and colleagues, [23] were excluded from the study to improve the balance of the two treatment groups (see Kendel and colleagues for more details [24]). Those participants who gave written consent to the follow-up were mailed a self-report questionnaire. The average time from treatment decision to follow-up was 42 ± 16.6 months (range: 1–6 years).

The final sample comprised 292 men (150 RP patients, 142 AS patients). All participants had given informed consent prior to the study. IRB approval was obtained from the Charité – Universitätsmedizin Berlin (EA 1/242/13).

Materials and main outcome measures

Baseline clinical parameters were abstracted from case report forms. Changes in erectile functioning (*"Did your erectile function change due to your prostate cancer or its treatment?"*) and impairment of self-esteem due to decreased erectile functioning (*"If your erectile function has decreased, did this impair your self-esteem?"*) were measured using items adapted from Johannson and colleagues.

[25] The item measuring subjective importance of sexuality (*"How important is sexuality for you?"*) was adapted from van den Bergh and colleagues. [26] A five-point Likert scale was used for the item on impairment of self-esteem (range 0–4 with 0 indicating no changes in erectile functioning and therefore no impairment of self-esteem, 1 indicating changes in erectile functioning but no impairment of self-esteem due to these changes and 2–4 indicating changes in erectile functioning with lower to high impairment of self-esteem). For all other items, a four-point Likert scale (range 1–4) was used, with higher levels indicating higher expressions of the specific characteristic.

Previous studies have demonstrated that erectile dysfunction is not necessarily associated with decreased sexual satisfaction. [9] Therefore, satisfaction with sexual life was assessed as a control variable. The item (*"Overall, how satisfied are you with your current sex-life?"*) was adapted from van den Bergh and colleagues. [26] A five-point Likert scale was used for the item on satisfaction with sexual life (range 1–5, higher levels indicating higher expressions of satisfac tion).

Statistical analysis

The RP and AS patients were compared regarding relevant sociodemographic variables and cancer characteristics. Chi^2-tests were run for categorical variables and independent t-tests were conducted for continuous variables to compare (a) changes in erectile functioning, (b) impairment of self-esteem (c) the importance of sexuality and (d) satisfaction with sexual life between the two groups. Cohen's d as a measure of effect size was calculated for group comparisons. Bivariate correlations between variables were calculated. A sequential multiple regression analysis was conducted to evaluate the relationship between sociodemographic characteristics, clinical variables, the importance of sexuality and changes in erectile functioning with the criterion self-esteem. Covariates were entered first, followed by the importance of sexuality, changes in erectile functioning and finally the interaction term. Within all regression models, collinearity diagnostics indicated no multicollinearity among the independent variables. For moderation analyses, [27] predictor variables and the constituents of the respective interaction terms were centered around their grand means. In moderation models, covariates were entered first, followed by the importance of sexuality as moderator and changes in erectile functioning as predictor, and finally by the interaction term. To display and test the interaction effects, simple slopes were tested. [28] Low and high values of the continuous moderators were generated by adding or subtracting one standard deviation from the centered mean of the respective moderator. Moderation analyses were conducted using the PROCESS macro for SPSS (model 1). [29] An alpha level of $p < 0.05$ was considered significant for all analyses.

Results

Of the 292 men with PCa included in this study, 150 (51.4%) had chosen RP as the initial treatment and 142 (48.6%) were still under AS. Table 1 presents the sociodemographic data, clinical characteristics and descriptive statistics based on the two different treatment groups. Table 2 displays correlations between the variables under study. Fewer men after RP (69%) were classified as low-risk compared with men under AS (88%). The two groups differed in age, marital status, occupation, and initial cancer risk classification (Table 1). The RP patients reported significantly more changes in erectile functioning (t (246.8) = – 10.11, $p < .001$; $d = 1.2$), and greater impairment of self-esteem (t (269) = – 4.19, $p < .001$, $d = .51$) than men under AS. On average, men under AS considered sexuality as being less important

Table 1 Sample characteristics and sexuality

	Total ($n = 292$)	RP ($n = 150$)	AS ($n = 142$)	P
Age, yrs., *M (SD)*	70 (7.2)	67.9 (6.8)	72.2 (7.1)	< .001
Living with partner, *n* (%)	268 (92.4)	140 (94)	128 (90.8)	.031
Higher education, *n* (%)	116 (40)	61 (40.9)	54 (38.3)	.737
Still working vs. retired, *n* (%)	40 (13.8)	28 (18.8)	12 (8.5)	.04
Time since treatment decision (months), *M (SD)*	42 (16.6)	41.7 (16.3)	42.3 (17.1)	.774
Risk classification[1]				< .001
Gleason-Score (low), *n* (%)	221 (76.7)	85 (57.8)	136 (96.5)	< .001
PSA, *M (SD)*	6.2 (3.2)	6.9 (2.8)	5.5 (3.3)	< .001
Number of comorbidities, *M (SD)*	1.8 (1.5)	1.8 (1.5)	1.8 (1.5)	.713
Importance of sexuality, *M (SD)*	2.8 (0.8)	2.9 (0.8)	2.6 (0.85)	< .001
Changes in erectile functioning, *M (SD)*	3 (0.99)	3.5 (0.7)	2.5 (0.99)	< .001
Impairment of self-esteem, *M (SD)*	1.8 (1.15)	2.1 (1.1)	1.5 (1.1)	< .001
Satisfaction with sexual life, *M (SD)*	2.8 (1)	2.7 (1.1)	3 (0.9)	.002

AS, active surveillance, RP, radical prostatectomy; [1] Risk classification based on D'Amico and colleagues [23]

Table 2 Correlations between study variables

Variables	2	3	4	5	6	7	8	9	10	11	12	13
1. Impairment of self-esteem	.55**	.26**	.20**	−.08	−.07	.01	.11	.04	−.04	.08	.09	−.56**
2. Changes in erectile functioning	–											
3. Importance of sexuality	.23**	–										
4. Importance* changes EF	−.12	−.14*	–									
5. Age	−.16**	−.34**	.19**	–								
6. Living with partner	.04	.13*	−.05	−.03	–							
7. Higher education	.58	.03	−.04	−.03	.10	–						
8. Still working	.09	.23**	<−.01	−.59**	.08	.06	–					
9. Time since treatment decision	−.01	−.01	.03	.21**	−.08	.06	−.13*	–				
10. Gleason-Score (low)	−.27**	−.13*	.04	.09	.01	−.01	−.03	.02	–			
11. PSA	.17**	<.01	−.04	.06	−.07	−.02	−.10	−.03	−.13*	–		
12. Number of comorbidities	.11	−.07	.01	.07	−.04	−.05	<.01	.05	−.04	−.11	–	
13. Satisfaction with sexual life	−.42**	−.09	−.20**	−.01	−.01	.01	−.01	.04	.04	−.16**	−.06	–

*$p < .05$; **$p < .01$

compared to the RP patients (t (278.4) = – 3.54, $p < .001$; d = .42). Across both groups, 66.5% of men rated sexuality as "rather or very important" (59% of the AS patients, 73.5% of the RP patients). The AS patients reported being more satisfied with their sexual life compared to RP patients (t (277.4) = 3.17, $p = .002$, $d = .38$). The correlation between satisfaction with sexual life and changes in erectile functioning was $r = -.42$ ($p < .001$, Table 2).

Table 3 Multiple regression of impairment of self-esteem on the importance of sexuality and changes in erectile functioning: final model ($n = 277$)

Variables	*B*	*S.E.*	*β*	ΔR^2 (ad. R^2)
Sociodemographic characteristics				
Age	.002	.011	.009	
Living with a partner	−.511	.216	−.117	
Higher education	−.05	.115	−.021	
Still working vs. retired	.137	.204	.042	.033
Group: RP vs. AS	.016	.143	.007	.06
Tumor risk category				
Gleason-Score (4–6)	.305	.141	.116	
PSA	.004	.019	.012	.002
Time since treatment decision (months)	.004	.004	.056	.004
Number of comorbidities	.039	.039	.051	.01
Importance of sexuality	.252	.074	.184	.048**
Changes in erectile functioning	.668	.069	.567	.207***
Importance of sexuality*changes in erectile functioning	.318	.062	.257	.062***
			$R^2 = .426$ Adjusted $R^2 = .398$ $F = 14.93$***	

B, unstandardized regression coefficient, *S.E.*, standard error; *β*, standardized regression coefficient, *AS*, active surveillance, *RP*, radical prostatectomy; **$p < .01$; ***$p < .001$

Multiple regression analysis

Sequential multiple regression was used to determine whether the importance of sexuality and changes in erectile functioning predicted impairment of self-esteem (Table 3). ΔR^2 refers to the amount of variance in the criterion (*impairment of self-esteem*), which is explained by the respective variables entered into the regression model at each step. Sociodemographic variables were entered in the first step and did not explain the variance of impairment of self-esteem significantly ($p = .08$). R^2 was significantly different from zero in the second step including *treatment group* ($\Delta R^2 = .06$, $p < .001$), but not in the third to fifth step including *PSA* and *Gleason-Score* ($\Delta R^2 = .002$, $p = .725$), *time since treatment decision* ($\Delta R^2 = .004$, $p = .271$) and *number of comorbidities* ($\Delta R^2 = .01$, $p = .1$). Again, R^2 was significantly different from zero when including *importance of sexuality* ($\Delta R^2 = .048$, $p < .001$) and *changes in erectile functioning* ($\Delta R^2 = .207$, $p < .001$). After the inclusion of *changes in erectile functioning*, the control variable *treatment group* was no longer significant. The interaction term of *importance of sexuality*changes in erectile functioning* also contributed significantly to an explanation of the variance ($\Delta R^2 = .062$, $p < .001$).

The final model explained 42.6% of variance ($R^2 = .426$; adjusted $R^2 = .398$), meaning that more than a third of the variability in impairment of self-esteem is predicted by our model. The pattern of results suggests that changes in erectile functioning predicted more than a fifth (20.7%) of the variability in impairment of self-esteem, whereas the contribution of the importance of sexuality was small (4.8%).

Moderation analysis

Moderation analysis revealed that the importance of sexuality moderated effects of changes in erectile

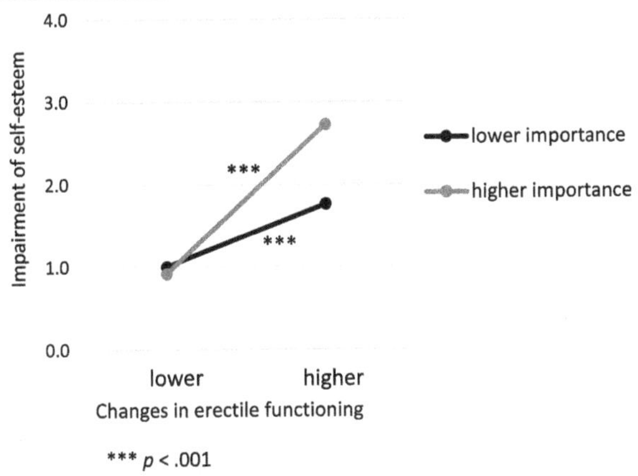

Fig. 1 The association of changes in erectile functioning and impairment of self-esteem is stronger for men who report a higher importance of sexuality

functioning on impairment of self-esteem (Table 3). Simple slope analyses showed that for both individuals with higher ($B = .93$, $t = 10.43$, $p < .001$) and lower importance of sexuality ($B = .40$, $t = 4.78$, $p < .001$) changes in sexual functioning more strongly affect their self-esteem, however this effect was weakened with lower importance of sexuality (Fig. 1). We additionally tested the conditional effect of changes in erectile functioning on impairment of self-esteem if participants reported that sexuality was "not at all" important to them. Then the effect was not significant ($B = .11$, $t = .85$, $p = .4$), i.e. if sexuality is of no importance changes in erectile functioning and self-esteem are not associated.

Discussion

Our study aimed at evaluating the importance of sexuality and the relationship of erectile functioning and self-esteem among older men with localized PCa under different treatment strategies. We have identified three key findings: Firstly, age and, even more so, an invasive treatment for PCa are predictive of changes in erectile functioning. Secondly, even after adjustment for socio-demographic and clinical variables, changes in erectile functioning prove to be a strong predictor of self-esteem. Thirdly, the existing relationship between erectile functioning and self-esteem seems to be stronger in those men, for whom sexuality is more important.

Our finding that RP is associated with poorer erectile functioning is supported by findings of RCTs that provide evidence for the invasive procedure being a causal factor. [6, 30] In addition, the results of our study show that men after AS consider sexuality as being less important compared to men after RP. This finding may appear counterintuitive at first sight as one could assume that AS is predominantly chosen by those men who value sexuality as more important. However, due to the cross-sectional design of our study we cannot identify the time at which sexuality became more important for RP patients. We suggest that the higher importance of sexuality for men after RP manifested after surgery: erectile dysfunction is a common side-effect of RP and men and their partners have to cope with this problem in the long-term. In this process, sexuality may become a present, yet sensitive topic in men's everyday-life, which vice versa might change men's attitude towards sexuality.

Erectile functioning is a strong predictor for self-esteem

Erectile functioning explains more than a fifth of the variance in self-esteem across both groups, after adjusting for sociodemographic variables, group assignment and the importance of sexuality. We challenged the common stereotype portraying older people as "asexual" by integrating the importance of sexuality in our study. [18] It is often assumed that older people may no longer consider sexuality an important aspect of their life and would, therefore, see a worsening of their sexual functioning as irrelevant. Our results contradict this stereotype: two thirds of the men, who were on average 70 years of age, rated sexuality as being "rather or very important". However, even after adjusting for the importance of sexuality, there was a stable association between worsened sexual functioning and impaired self-esteem. This means that even men who consider sexuality as less important could experience an impairment of their self-esteem due to changes in erectile functioning. This finding corresponds with the results from a qualitative study by Gannon and colleagues, who supposed that the ability to perform penetrative sex may be essential for male identity, independent of a man's actual sexual activity. [31] Only in the small group of men (7% of our sample), who reported that sexuality was of *no* importance to them, there was no association between erectile functioning and self-esteem.

Changes in erectile functioning may have different consequences for men with localized PCa

Our results show a strong association of erectile functioning and self-esteem for men with localized PCa. Moreover, altered erectile functioning and satisfaction with sexual life are negatively correlated in our sample. In a study with men from the general population Braun and colleagues demonstrated that only 14% of men aged 60 to 69 years report having ED and being dissatisfied with their sex life. [9] In our study, however, almost 40% of men who report at least some changes in erectile functioning state that they are "dissatisfied or very dissatisfied" with their sex life. Thus, the consequences of erectile dysfunction might be different for men with localized PCa compared to men without PCa. After the diagnosis, men might address actual or anticipated erectile dysfunction as a possible consequence of invasive PCa treatment. The intensive preoccupation with implications of erectile dysfunction may thus strengthen the association of erectile functioning and self-esteem, whereas for men without PCa a decrease in erectile functioning may be a simple expression of a normal aging process.

Strengths and limitations

The strengths of this study are a high external validity by using a non-interventional, multicenter design, the length of the follow-up and the sample size which represents one of the largest samples for the comparison of RP and AS. Additionally, our study focuses on the psychosocial aspects of sexuality. While most studies addressing sexuality in men with localized PCa focus more on physiological aspects, we aimed to investigate the psychological aspects of an altered sexuality. We selected our items measuring men's sexual life accordingly. However, the study is subject to some limitations. (1) The cross-sectional and observational design does not allow for causal interpretations. For example, it remains speculative whether a change in erectile functioning for the worse leads to an impairment of self-esteem, or whether there are additional confounding variables. To deal with possible selection biases due to the non-randomization, we controlled for several sociodemographic and clinical variables, which did not explain a significant amount of variance. As opposed to a randomized study, strengths of our observational design are a high external validity and an exceptional participant rate. (2) Our data are based on the participants' self-reports of erectile functioning and we did not validate the latter by objective measures (e.g. medical records). However, the focus of the study was on men's subjective experience, which, particularly regarding sexuality, seems more important than objective parameters. [32] (3) Information on the psychometric properties of measurement of sexuality used in our study is still lacking. (4) Impairment of self-esteem was assessed in the context of erectile functioning. As 90% of our sample report having experienced at least some degree of changes in erectile functioning it seems reasonable to measure self-esteem in this way. However, the amount of variance in self-esteem explained by erectile functioning in our findings may be artificially inflated as a consequence. Thus, independent measures of (impaired) self-esteem should also be taken into account in future research. (5) We did not assess whether men with impaired sexual functioning made use of erection restoration treatments, which could have had an impact on our results. Therefore, this aspect should be included and analysed in future studies. Moreover, we are well aware that a differentiation between homosexual and heterosexual men's sexuality is desirable. The importance of sexuality and erectile functioning particularly when predicting self-esteem could differ among these subgroups. Therefore, our findings may not gene ralize regarding homosexual men. Finally, our sample comprises a cohort that was operated in the years 2008 to 2013. Since then, great progress has been made in the field of nerve-sparing PCa surgery. Hence, compared to the present situation, the differences between AS and RP patients in this study may be more pronounced, and emphasis should be given to the relationship between erectile functioning, the importance of sexuality and self-esteem rather than to the absolute differences.

Implications

Our results have some implications for future research. Firstly, questionnaires on male sexuality in PCa patients to date, focus primarily on the function rather than psychological aspects of sexuality. An effort should be made to develop questionnaires that comply with a broader definition of sexuality as a holistic construct [15] and meet the particularities of older men or PCa patients. Widely accepted and validated questionnaires would also facilitate a comparison of results. Secondly, longitudinal studies in this field are desirable to gain a deeper insight into the interplay of age, sexuality, self-esteem and other psychosocial variables in men with PCa over time. As erectile functioning is only one facet of the sexual response cycle that can be affected by invasive PCa treatment more items assessing sexual functioning should be included. Similarly, self-esteem is only one example for the connection between sexual functioning and psychological well-being. Future research should take this into account.

Other implications refer to clinical practice. Previous studies have shown that psychosocial interventions providing information or emotional support can improve psychological outcomes in men with localized PCa. [33] However, men with localized PCa stated not being in need of psychosocial interventions in a qualitative study. [34] Thus, despite of being potentially beneficial for men with localized PCa the preliminary setting of psychosocial interventions may not meet men's needs. We therefore suggest low-threshold services to counsel men on PCa treatment, possible physiological side-effects and associated psychological consequences. This could be put into practice using online tools or by extending the role of the urologist: For men with localized PCa, the urologist is usually the first and probably the most important specialist contact person. With urologists not only giving medical but also psychological advice PCa patients would receive comprehensive consulting without having to make additional efforts. A specific clinical implication of our study concerning medical practice is to structure the doctor-patient conversation about sexuality. Many men still have difficulties discussing this topic with their physician. However, they feel their physician should address it on his or her own volition. The discussion about adverse effects of an invasive treatment should comprise the psychological impact of an impairment of erectile functioning to reach a fully informed decision. Furthermore, the physician is crucial for rebutting stereotypes for men who experience an impairment of erectile functioning due to invasive treatment or age. The physician may discuss with the patient that the stereotype of older people being asexual, focusing mainly on the degree of erectile functioning, is based on a "too narrow definition of sexuality." [18] Professionals could encourage their patients to maintain their sexual life and, when being sexually active, to use "what they have." [15] Low-threshold services (e.g. online consulting tools) and interventions aiming to improve the communication of sensitive (psychological) topics should be conceptualized and tested in future research.

Conclusions

The effect of erectile dysfunction on men's self-esteem is a neglected topic in PCa research that deserves attention in both clinical practice and research. Changes in erectile functioning may become particularly important if they occur due to a PCa treatment. Our results emphasize the importance of sexuality for men with PCa. Therefore, medical advice on PCa treatment should encompass the strong association of erectile dysfunction and self-esteem in men with PCa. This topic should be addressed as a possible consequence of invasive treatment.

Abbreviations

AS: Active surveillance; E.g: Exempli gratia; I.e: Id est.; PCa: Prostate cancer; RP: Radical prostatectomy

Acknowledgements

We thank the study participants who provided their time and showed great interest in this study. We would particularly like to thank Hans-Jörg Fiebrandt and the German Association of Prostate Cancer Self-Help for their encouragement. We would like to thank the Stiftung Männergesundheit Foundation for their cooperation.

Authors' contributions

FK and CH conceptualized the study and developed the research questions. FK and CH were also responsible for the acquisition of data. FK, SH, and CH analyzed and interpreted the data; AM, MS, SN, and TF also contributed to the interpretation of data. FK and CH drafted the article which was then revised by SH, SN, MS, AM, and TH. All authors read and approved the final manuscript.

Author details

[1]Institute of Medical Psychology, Charité Universitätsmedizin Berlin, D-10117 Berlin, Germany. [2]Department of Urology and Pediatric Urology, Otto von Guericke University Magdeburg, Magdeburg, Germany. [3]Department of Urology, Klinik am Ring Cologne, Cologne, Germany. [4]Department of Urology, Vivantes Klinikum am Urban Berlin, Berlin, Germany. [5]Institute of Psychology, Humboldt-Universität zu Berlin, Berlin, Germany. [6]Department of Psychology, University of Applied Sciences Europe, Berlin, Germany.

References

1. Agency for Healthcare Research and Quality (US). Therapies for clinically localized prostate cancer. Update of a 2008 systematic review: Rockville (MD) 2014.
2. Latini DM, Hart SL, Knight SJ, Cowan JE, Ross PL, Duchane J, Carroll PR. The relationship between anxiety and time to treatment for patients with prostate cancer on surveillance. J Urol. 2007;178:826–32.
3. Bellardita L, Valdagni R, van den Bergh R, Randsdorp H, Repetto C, Venderbos LDF, Lane JA, Korfage IJ. How does active surveillance for prostate cancer affect quality of life? A systematic review. Eur Urol. 2015;67:637–45.
4. Wilt TJ, MacDonald R, Rutks I, Shamliyan TA, Taylor BC, Kane RL. Systematic review: comparative effectiveness and harms of treatments for clinically localized prostate cancer. Ann Intern Med. 2008;148:435–48.
5. Chou R, Croswell JM, Dana T, Bougatsos C, Blazina I, Fu R, Gleitsmann K, Koenig HC, Lam C, Maltz A, Rugge JB, Lin K. Screening for prostate cancer: a review of the evidence for the U.S. preventive services task force. Ann Intern Med. 2011;155:762–71.
6. Donovan JL, Hamdy FC, Lane JA, Mason M, Metcalfe C, Walsh E, Blazeby JM, Peters TJ, Holding P, Bonnington S, Lennon T, Bradshaw L, Cooper D, Herbert P, Howson J, Jones A, Lyons N, Salter E, Thompson P, Tidball S, Blaikie J, Gray C, Bollina P, Catto J, Doble A, Doherty A, Gillatt D, Kockelbergh R, Kynaston H, Paul A, Powell P, Prescott S, Rosario DJ, Rowe E, Davis M, Turner EL, Martin RM, Neal DE. Patient-reported outcomes after monitoring, surgery, or radiotherapy for prostate cancer. N Engl J Med. 2016;375:1425–37.
7. Zaider T, Manne S, Nelson C, Mulhall J, Kissane D. Loss of masculine identity, marital affection, and sexual bother in men with localized prostate cancer. J Sex Med. 2012;9:2724–32.
8. Chambers SK, Chung E, Wittert G, Hyde MK. Erectile dysfunction, masculinity, and psychosocial outcomes: a review of the experiences of men after prostate cancer treatment. Transl Androl Urol. 2017;6:60–8.
9. Braun M, Wassmer G, Klotz T, Reifenrath B, Mathers M, Engelmann U. Epidemiology of erectile dysfunction: results of the 'Cologne male Survey'. Int J Impot Res. 2000;12:305–11.
10. Wittmann D, Carolan M, Given B, Skolarus TA, Crossley H, An L, Palapattu G, Clark P, Montie JE. What couples say about their recovery of sexual intimacy after prostatectomy: toward the development of a conceptual model of couples' sexual recovery after surgery for prostate cancer. J Sex Med. 2015; 12:494–504.
11. Mruk CJ. Defining self-esteem as a relationship between competence and worthiness: how a two-factor approach integrates the cognitive and affective dimensions of self-esteem. Pol Psychol Bull. 2013;44:157–64.
12. McMahon CG. Erectile dysfunction. Int Med J. 2014;44:18–26.
13. Mulhall J, Althof SE, Brock GB, Goldstein I, Junemann K-P, Kirby M. Erectile dysfunction: monitoring response to treatment in clinical practice - recommendations of an international study panel. J Sex Med. 2007;4:448–64.
14. Kogel AM, Dinkel A, Marten-Mittag B, Baron J, Albers P, Arsov C, Hadaschik B, Hohenfellner M, Imkamp F, Kuczyk M, Gschwend JE, Herkommer K. Selbstbild und erektile Dysfunktion 45-jahriger Manner. Ergebnisse eines Begleitprojekts der PROBASE-Studie. Urologe A. 2016;55:1321–8.
15. DeLamater JD, Sill M. Sexual desire in later life. J Sex Res. 2005;42:138–49.
16. Siegel RL, Miller KD, Jemal A. Cancer statistics, 2015. CA Cancer J Clin. 2015; 65:5–29.
17. Robert-Koch-Institut. Bericht zum Krebsgeschehen in Deutschland 2016 2016. http://www.krebsdaten.de/Krebs/DE/Content/Publikationen/Krebsgeschehen/Krebsgeschehen_download.pdf?__blob=publicationFile . (January 2019).
18. Kenny RT. A review of the literature on sexual development of older adults in relation to the asexual stereotype of older adults. CJFY. 2013;5:91–106.
19. Corona G, Rastrelli G, Maseroli E, Forti G, Maggi M. Sexual function of the ageing male. Best Pract Res Clin Endocrinol Metab. 2013;27:581–601.
20. Lowy M, Collins S, Bloch M, Gillman M, Lording D, Sutherland P, Wang H, Stecher V. Quality of erection questionnaire correlates: change in erection quality with erectile function, hardness, and psychosocial measures in men treated with sildenafil for erectile dysfunction. J Sex Med. 2007;4:83–92.
21. Reese JB, Haythornthwaite JA. Importance of sexuality in colorectal cancer: predictors, changes, and response to an intimacy enhancement intervention. Support Care Cancer. 2016;24:4309–17.
22. Herden J, Eminaga O, Wille S, Weissbach L. Treatment of incidental prostate cancer by active surveillance: results of the HAROW study. Urol Int. 2015;95:209–15.
23. D'Amico AV, Whittington R, Malkowicz SB, Cote K, Loffredo M, Schultz D, Chen M-H, Tomaszewski JE, Renshaw AA, Wein A, Richie JP. Biochemical outcome after radical prostatectomy or external beam radiation therapy for patients with clinically localized prostate carcinoma in the prostate specific antigen era. Cancer. 2002;95:281–6.
24. Kendel F, Helbig L, Neumann K, Herden J, Stephan C, Schrader M, Gaissmaier W. Patients' perceptions of mortality risk for localized prostate cancer vary markedly depending on their treatment strategy. Int J Cancer. 2016;139:749–53.

25. Johansson E, Steineck G, Holmberg L, Johansson J-E, Nyberg T, Ruutu M, Bill-Axelson A. Long-term quality-of-life outcomes after radical prostatectomy or watchful waiting. The Scandinavian prostate Cancer Group-4 randomised trial. Lancet Oncol. 2011;12:891–9.
26. van den Bergh R, Korfage IJ, Roobol MJ, Bangma CH, de KHJ, Steyerberg EW, Essink-Bot M-L. Sexual function with localized prostate cancer: active surveillance vs radical therapy. BJU Int. 2012;110:1032–9.
27. Aiken LS, West SG. Multiple regression. Testing and interpreting interactions, vol. XI. 4th ed. Newbury Park Calif: Sage Publ; 1996. p. 212 S.
28. Preacher KJ, Curran PJ, Bauer DJ. Computational tools for probing interaction effects in multiple linear regression, multilevel modeling, and latent curve analysis. J Educ Behav Stat. 2006:437–48.
29. Hayes AF. PROCESS: a versatile computational tool for observed variable mediation, moderation, and conditional process modeling [white paper]. 2012. http://www.afhayes.com/public/process2012.pdf
30. Steineck G, Helgesen F, Adolfsson J, Dickman PW, Johansson J-E, Norlen BJ, Holmberg L. Quality of life after radical prostatectomy or watchful waiting. N Engl J Med. 2002;347:790–6.
31. Gannon K, Guerro-Blanco M, Patel A, Abel P. Re-constructing masculinity following radical prostatectomy for prostate cancer. Aging Male. 2010;13:258–64.
32. Owczarek K. The concept of quality of life. Acta Neuropsychol. 2010;8:207–13.
33. Weber BA, Sherwill-Navarro P. Psychosocial consequences of prostate cancer: 30 years of research. Geriatr Nurs. 2005;26:166–75.
34. Oliffe JL, Davison BJ, Pickles T, Mróz L. The self-management of uncertainty among men undertaking active surveillance for low-risk prostate cancer. Qual Health Res. 2009;19:432–43.

4

Transurethral resection of the prostate versus prostatic artery embolization in the treatment of benign prostatic hyperplasia

Yu-Li Jiang[1,2*] and Lu-Jie Qian[1,2]

Abstract

Background: To compare the clinical efficiency and safety of transurethral resection of the prostate (TURP) and prostatic artery embolization (PAE) for the treatment of Benign prostatic hyperplasia (BPH).

Methods: We searched PUBMED, EMBASE and the Cochrane Central Register for studies from May 1998 to May 2018 for studies comparing the efficiency and safety of TURP with PAE. Four studies met the inclusion criteria for our meta-analysis. After data extraction and quality assessment, we used RevMan 5.2 to pool the data.

Results: A total of four studies involving 506 patients were included in our meta-analysis. The pooled data showed that the Qmax was higher in TURP group than PAE with a significant difference (WMD:4.66, 95%CI 2.54 to 6.79, $P <$ 0.05). The postoperative QOL was lower in the TURP than PAE group (WMD: -0.53, 95%CI -0.88 to − 0.18, $P < 0.05$). The postoperative prostate volume was significantly smaller in the TURP than PAE group (WMD: -8.26, 95%CI -12.64 to − 3.88, $P < 0.05$). The operative time was significantly shorter in the TURP than PAE group (WMD: -10.55, 95%CI -16.92 to − 4.18, $P < 0.05$). No significant difference was found in the postoperative IPSS and complications between TURP and PAE ($P > 0.05$, WMD:1.56, 95%CI -0.67 to 3.78, $p = 0{,}05$, OR:1.54, 95%CI 1.00 to2.38, respectively).

Conclusions: TURP could achieve improved Qmax and QoL compared to PAE. Therefore, for patients with BPH and lower urinary tract symptoms (LUTS), TURP was superior to PAE.

Keywords: Benign prostatic hyperplasia, Transurethral resection of the prostate, Prostatic artery embolization, Meta-analysis

Background

Benign prostatic hyperplasia (BPH) is common among elderly males, affecting 50% at the age of 60 years [1, 2]. The main manifestations of BPH are intermittently decreased urinary stream, nocturia and urgency, which are also called lower urinary tract symptoms (LUTS), and BPH accounts for 60% of LUTS in 50–60-year-old men [1]. Treatment options for BPH often include medical waiting, minimally invasive approaches, alpha-1-Blocker, or surgical therapies. Medical treatment, which has been considered first-line treatment, can include the use of 5-reductase inhibitors; these inhibitors have been demonstrated to reduce prostate volumes by more than 30 ml [3]. Surgical treatments (transurethral resection of the prostate or open surgery) are used for treatment in the event of failed medical management [4]. Transurethral resection of the prostate (TURP) is considered the gold standard of treatment for men with prostate volumes of 30–80 ml, and it is also appropriate for those with prostate volumes > 80 ml [1, 5]. However, the complications of TURP include sexual dysfunction, retrograde ejaculation, postoperative hemorrhage, continent urinary retention, TURP syndrome and urinary stricture [6, 7]. Prostatic artery embolization (PAE) has been suggested as a minimally invasive interventional radiological procedure [8]. In PAE, injection of microspheres or

* Correspondence: renren108@126.com
[1]Department of Urology, The Affiliated Hospital of Hang Zhou Normal University, Hangzhou 310015, China
[2]School of Medicine, Hang Zhou Normal University, Hangzhou 310016, China

small particles or directly into the prostatic arteries bilaterally or unilaterally could result in ischemia or an enlarged prostate [9]. Michlle et al. first reported that embolization of hypogastric arteries (PAE) could be used to control severe prostate hemorrhage caused by BPH [10].

Several studies had compared the clinical outcomes and safety of TURP with PAE [11–14]. Schreuder et al. reported a systematic review of the use of TURP and PAE for treating BPH [15]. Ray et al. recently reported an observational study comparing the efficiency and safety of TURP and PAE for treating BPH [13]. Feng et al. reported a meta-analysis of 20 studies about PAE for treating BPH [16]. However, no meta-analysis was previously performed to compare the clinical efficiency and safety of TURP and PAE.

At present, no standards or guidelines exist for evaluating the clinical efficacy of TURP and PAE for treating BPH. Therefore, we thought it necessary to perform a meta-analysis to evaluate the optimal treatment by comparing the clinical outcomes and safety between TURP and PAE. The purpose of this study is to compare the efficiency and perioperative safety with the quantitative data for the clinical efficacy and safety of PAE or TURP in treating BPH.

Methods

Search strategy

This meta-analysis was performed according to the Preferred Reporting Items for systemic Reviews and meta-analysis (PRISMA) statement. We searched PUBMED, EMBASE and the Cochrane Central Register for relevant studies published in English from May 1998 to May 2018. We used the following search terms: "BPH", "benign prostate hyperplasia", "prostatic arterial embolization". We also used the combined Boolean operators "AND" or "OR" in the Title/Abstract.

Inclusion and exclusion criteria

The two investigators reviewed the articles. The inclusion criteria were as follows: (1) comparative analysis of TURP and PAE for treating BPH; (2) BPH patients treated with TURP and PAE; (3) follow-up duration longer than 12 months; and (4) articles with the IPSS, Qmax, Qol, postoperative prostate, volume, and operative time. The exclusion criteria were as follows: (1) case reports, reviews, editorial comments, meeting abstracts and articles without applicable data; (2) studies with insufficient data, such as missing the SD (standard deviation) and number and (3) studies that were not comparative in nature. The process of identifying relevant studies is summarized in Fig. 1.

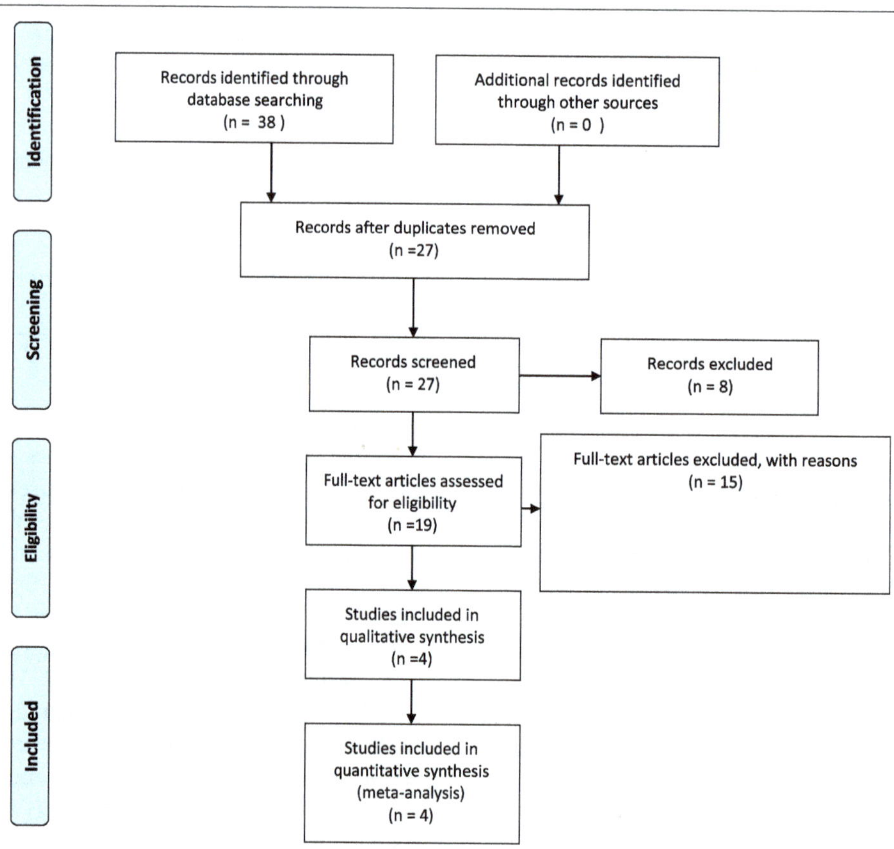

Fig. 1 Flow diagram of the process for the selection of relevant studies

Table 1 Basic characteristics of the included studies

Study	Year	Design	IPSS		prostate volume(ml)		Study group	
			TURP	PAE	TURP	PAE	TURP(n)	PAE(n)
Gao	2014	RCT	23.1	22.8	63.5	64.7	57	57
Qiu	2017	P, S	23.9	24.5	68.7	64.6	40	17
Ray	2018	R, M	21.63	21.3	101.2	65.6	216	89
Carnevale	2016	RCT	27.6	25.3	56.6	63.0	15	15

P Prospectively study, *RCT* Randomised controlled trial, *S* Sigle center, *R* Retrospectively study, *M* Mutli-centers

Data extraction

Two authors reviewed the relevant studies. The two authors extracted data, such as the IPSS, Qmax, and QOL score. The following data were recorded: (1) baseline comparative data; (2) clinical outcomes; and (3) postoperative complications. Two reviewers (YLJ and LJQ) assessed the quality of the included studies.

Statistical analysis

We used Review Manager Version 5.2 software with the Mantel-Haenszel method (The Cochrane Collaboration, Oxford, UK) and Stata 12.0 to perform the analysis of the included data. We used Cochran's Q to evaluate the heterogeneity; Q < 50% or $P > 0.01$ was indicative of little heterogeneity. However, Q > 50% or $P < 0.01$ was indicative of heterogeneity. For quantitative data, we used the weight mean difference (WMD) and 95% confidence interval (CI) or standard mean difference (SMD) and 95%CI to calculate continuous data. We used the odds ratio (OR) and 95%CI to evaluate binary data. The statistical significance level was 0.05.

Results

Four studies were included in our study [11–14]. The process of obtaining these studies is summarized in Fig. 1. From the selected databases, 38 studies were obtained. After screening the titles and abstracts, 11 studies were excluded. After detailed processing, 23 studies were excluded. Finally, 4 studies were included in our meta-analysis. Table 1 summarizes basic characteristics of the included studies.

Quality assessment of the included studies

We used the New-Ottawa Scale (NOS) to evaluate the included studies. The NOS scores were evaluated using a 9-point system. An NOS score of 7 or above is considered as higher quality, and an NOS score of 3 or below was believed to have a lower quality. For RCT, we assessed the risk of bias according to the Cochrane Collabortation handbook, version 5.0. Table 2 shows quality assessment of the included studies.

IPSS

The pooled data of preoperative IPSS indicated no statistical differences between the TURP group and PAE group ($n = 506$, WMD: 0.69, 95%CI: -0.33 to 1.71, $I^2 = 0$; $p = 0.18$, fixed-effects model, Fig. 2). Data related to the postoperative IPSS were available in two studies No significant difference between the TURP and PAE groups was noted ($n = 87$, WMD: 1.56, 95%CI: -0.67 to 3.78, $I^2 = 88\%$; $p = 0.17$, fixed-effects model, Fig. 3).

Qmax

The pooled data of preoperative Qmax indicated no statistical differences between the TURP group and PAE group ($n = 506$, WMD: 0.21, 95%CI: -0.47 to 0.89, $I^2 = 68\%$; $p = 0.54$, fixed-effects model, Fig. 4). The postoperative Qmax was higher in the TURP group than in the

Table 2 Quality assessment of the included studies

Study	Design	Selection				Comparability	Outcome			Total
		Representativeness of exposed cohort	Selective of nonexposed Cohort	Ascertainment of exposure	Outcome not present at start		Assessment of outcome	Adequate follow-up length	Adequacy of follow-up	
Qiu	P, S	*	*	*	*	*	*	*	*	8
Ray	R, M	*	*	*	*	*	*	*	*	8
		Randomization	Allocation concealment		Blinding			Quality level		
Carnevale	RCT	Adequate	Unclear		Unclear			Unclear		
Gao	RCT	Adequate	Unclear		Unclear			Unclear		

P Prospectively study, *RCT* Randomised controlled trial, *R* Respectively study, *M* mutli-centers
The symbol "*" represents score

Study or Subgroup	TURP Mean	TURP SD	TURP Total	PAE Mean	PAE SD	PAE Total	Weight	Mean Difference IV, Fixed, 95% CI
Carnevale2016	27.6	3.2	15	25.3	3.6	15	17.4%	2.30 [-0.14, 4.74]
Gao2014	23.1	5.8	57	22.8	5.9	57	22.5%	0.30 [-1.85, 2.45]
Qiu2017	24.5	4.5	40	23.9	4.9	17	14.1%	0.60 [-2.11, 3.31]
Ray2018	21.6	5.8	89	21.3	6.7	216	46.0%	0.30 [-1.20, 1.80]
Total (95% CI)			**201**			**305**	**100.0%**	**0.69 [-0.33, 1.71]**

Heterogeneity: Chi² = 2.07, df = 3 (P = 0.56); I² = 0%
Test for overall effect: Z = 1.33 (P = 0.18)

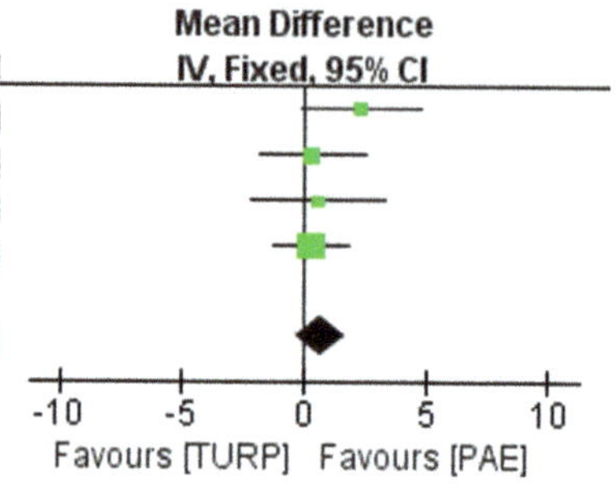

Fig. 2 Forest plot for the preoperative IPSS between the TURP and PAE for BPH

PAE group ($n = 87$, 55 patients were in the TURP group, 32 patients were in the PAE group, WMD: 4.66, 95%CI: 2.54 to 6.79, $I^2 = 96\%$, $P < 0.05$, fixed-effects model, Fig. 5).

Qol

Two studies reported the Qol. The Qol was lower in the TURP group than in the PAE group (n = 87; 55 patients were in the TURP group and 32 patients were in the PAE group, WMD; − 0.53, 95%CI; − 0.88 to − 0.18, I^2 = 67%; $p < 0.05$, fixed-effects model, Fig. 6).

Prostate volume

The pooled data of preoperative prostate volume indicated statistical differences between the TURP group and PAE group ($n = 506$, WMD: -4.19, 95%CI: -8.06 to − 0.32, $I^2 = 94\%$; $p = 0.03$, fixed-effects model, Fig. 7). Data related to the postoperative prostate volume were available in two studies. The postoperative prostate volume was smaller in the TURP group than in the PAE group ($n = 87$; 55 patients were in the TURP group and 32 patients were in the PAE group, WMD; − 8.26, 95%CI; − 12.64 to − 3.88, $I^2 = 76\%$; $p < 0.05$, fixed-effects model, Fig. 8).

Operative time

Two studies reported the operative time. The operative time was shorter in the TURP group than in the PAE group ($n = 137$; 68 patients were in the TURP group and 69 patients were in the PAE group, WMD; − 10.55, 95%CI; − 16.92 to − 4.18, $I^2 = 97\%$; $p = 0.001$, fixed-effects model, Fig. 9).

Complications

Two studies reported complications. No statistically significant difference between the TURP and PAE groups was noted ($n = 412$, 142 patients were in the TURP group, 270 patients were in PAE group, OR; 1.54, 95%CI; 1.00 to 2.38, $I^2 = 95\%$; $p = 0.05$, fixed-effects model, Fig. 10).

Discussion

In the present study, we included four clinical studies with at least a 12-month follow-up. The present systematic review and meta-analysis was performed to compare the efficiency of TURP and PAE for the treatment of BPH. In addition, our study was the first meta-analysis to compare the efficiency and safety of TURP and PAE for the treatment of BPH.

Our meta-analysis demonstrated that patients with BPH had comparable basic characteristics. The present study compared the short-term follow-up outcomes among patients undergoing TURP versus PAE. These patients shared comparable common baseline characteristics. In our study, the IPSS and complications were not significantly different for patients undergoing TURP versus PAE. The Qol, Qmax, operative time, and postoperative volume were better in TURP than in PAE.

Study or Subgroup	TURP Mean	TURP SD	TURP Total	PAE Mean	PAE SD	PAE Total	Weight	Mean Difference IV, Fixed, 95% CI
Carnevale2016	6.1	8.6	15	12.8	8	15	14.0%	-6.70 [-12.64, -0.76]
Qiu2017	13.1	3.5	40	10.2	4.5	17	86.0%	2.90 [0.50, 5.30]
Total (95% CI)			**55**			**32**	**100.0%**	**1.56 [-0.67, 3.78]**

Heterogeneity: Chi² = 8.62, df = 1 (P = 0.003); I² = 88%
Test for overall effect: Z = 1.37 (P = 0.17)

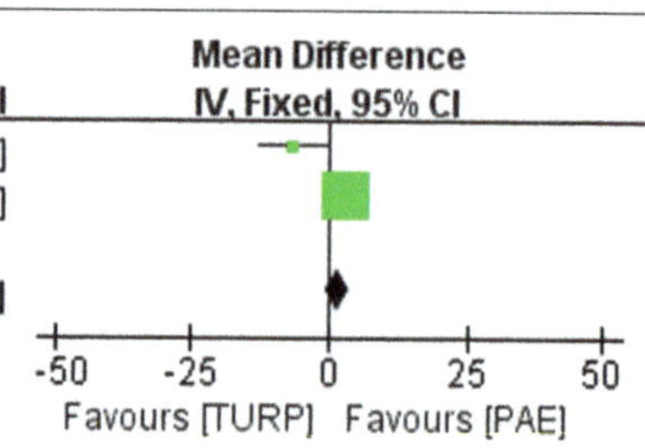

Fig. 3 Forest plot for the postoperative IPSS between the TURP and PAE for BPH

Study or Subgroup	TURP Mean	TURP SD	TURP Total	PAE Mean	PAE SD	PAE Total	Weight	Mean Difference IV, Fixed, 95% CI
Carnevale2016	9.7	3.8	15	7	3.6	15	6.6%	2.70 [0.05, 5.35]
Gao2014	7.3	2.3	57	7.8	2.5	57	59.8%	-0.50 [-1.38, 0.38]
Qiu2017	9.4	3.1	40	9.5	3.7	17	11.6%	-0.10 [-2.10, 1.90]
Ray2018	10.36	6.3	89	8.8	4.718	216	22.0%	1.56 [0.11, 3.01]
Total (95% CI)			**201**			**305**	**100.0%**	**0.21 [-0.47, 0.89]**

Heterogeneity: Chi² = 9.30, df = 3 (P = 0.03); I² = 68%
Test for overall effect: Z = 0.61 (P = 0.54)

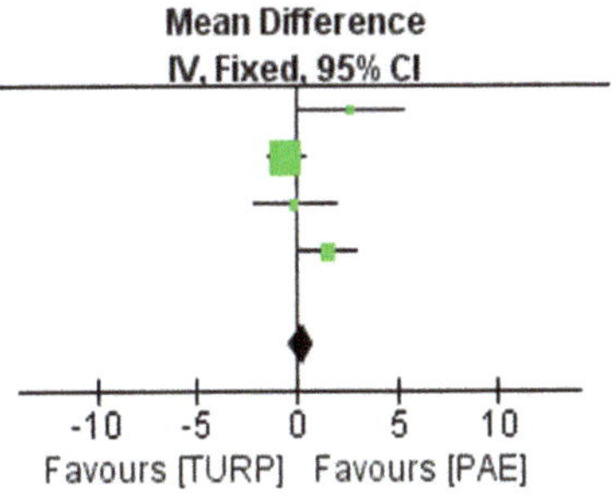

Fig. 4 Forest plot for the preoperative Qmax between the TURP and PAE for BPH

Study or Subgroup	TURP Mean	TURP SD	TURP Total	PAE Mean	PAE SD	PAE Total	Weight	Mean Difference IV, Fixed, 95% CI
Carnevale2016	27.1	8.7	15	10.1	6.5	15	14.9%	17.00 [11.50, 22.50]
Qiu2017	24.3	3.7	40	21.8	4.2	17	85.1%	2.50 [0.20, 4.80]
Total (95% CI)			**55**			**32**	**100.0%**	**4.66 [2.54, 6.79]**

Heterogeneity: Chi² = 22.75, df = 1 (P < 0.00001); I² = 96%
Test for overall effect: Z = 4.31 (P < 0.0001)

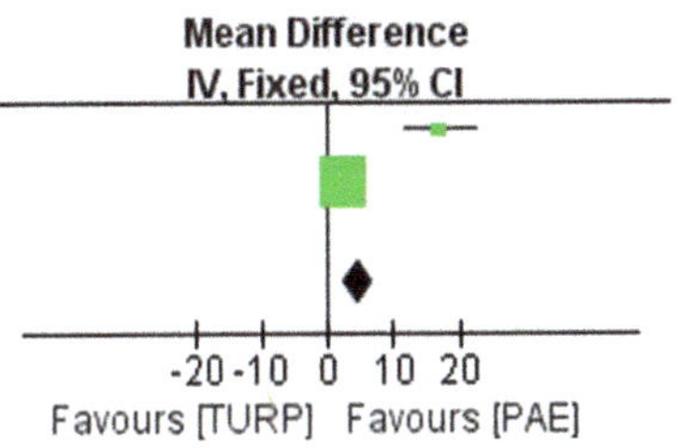

Fig. 5 Forest plot for for the postoperative Qmax between the TURP and PAE for BPH

Study or Subgroup	TURP Mean	TURP SD	TURP Total	PAE Mean	PAE SD	PAE Total	Weight	Mean Difference IV, Fixed, 95% CI
Carnevale2016	0.9	1.4	15	2.2	1.2	15	14.3%	-1.30 [-2.23, -0.37]
Qiu2017	1.7	0.6	40	2.1	0.7	17	85.7%	-0.40 [-0.78, -0.02]
Total (95% CI)			**55**			**32**	**100.0%**	**-0.53 [-0.88, -0.18]**

Heterogeneity: Chi² = 3.06, df = 1 (P = 0.08); I² = 67%
Test for overall effect: Z = 2.94 (P = 0.003)

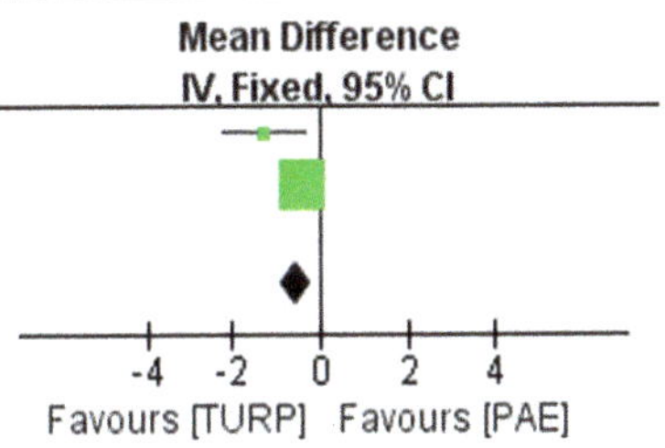

Fig. 6 Forest plot for Qol between the TURP and PAE for BPH

Study or Subgroup	TURP Mean	TURP SD	TURP Total	PAE Mean	PAE SD	PAE Total	Weight	Mean Difference IV, Fixed, 95% CI
Carnevale2016	56.6	21.5	15	63	17.8	15	7.5%	-6.40 [-20.53, 7.73]
Gao2014	63.5	18.6	57	64.7	19.7	57	30.3%	-1.20 [-8.23, 5.83]
Qiu2017	68.7	9.2	40	64.6	10.2	17	47.3%	4.10 [-1.52, 9.72]
Ray2018	65.6	31.5	89	101.2	57.1	216	14.9%	-35.60 [-45.64, -25.56]
Total (95% CI)			**201**			**305**	**100.0%**	**-4.19 [-8.06, -0.32]**

Heterogeneity: Chi² = 46.73, df = 3 (P < 0.00001); I² = 94%
Test for overall effect: Z = 2.12 (P = 0.03)

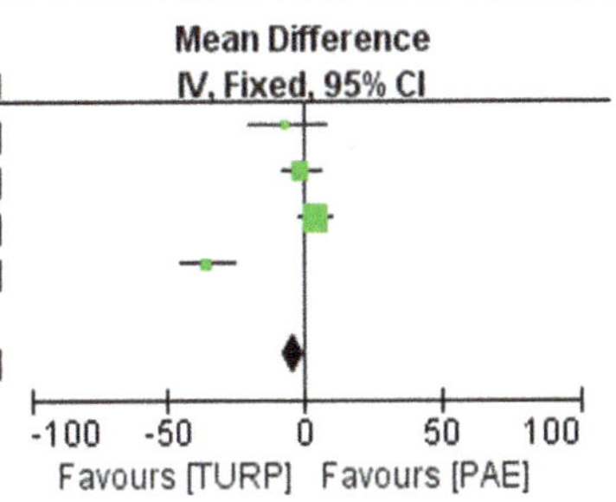

Fig. 7 Forest plot for the preoperative prostate volume between the TURP and PAE for BPH

Study or Subgroup	TURP Mean	TURP SD	TURP Total	PAE Mean	PAE SD	PAE Total	Weight	Mean Difference IV, Fixed, 95% CI
Carnevale2016	32.9	4.6	15	42	7.5	15	96.8%	-9.10 [-13.55, -4.65]
Qiu2017	32	11.4	40	15	50.9	17	3.2%	17.00 [-7.45, 41.45]
Total (95% CI)			**55**			**32**	**100.0%**	**-8.26 [-12.64, -3.88]**

Heterogeneity: Chi² = 4.24, df = 1 (P = 0.04); I² = 76%
Test for overall effect: Z = 3.70 (P = 0.0002)

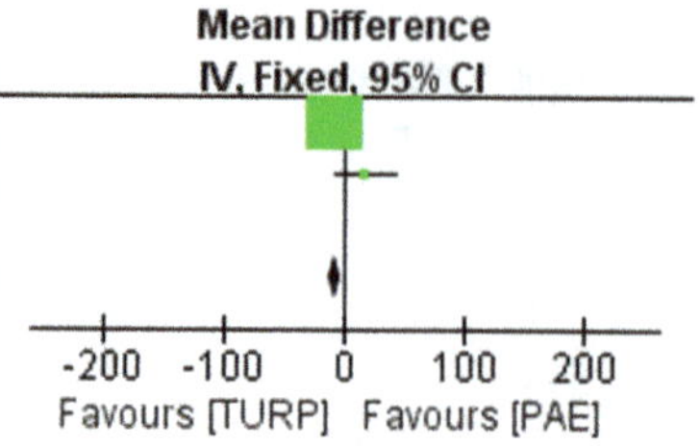

Fig. 8 Forest plot for for the postoperative prostate volume between the TURP and PAE for BPH

Feng et al. performed a meta-analysis that reported only one method for the efficiency and safety of PAE [16]. Their meta-analysis indicated that the IPSS and Qol score showed great improvement after PAE ($P <$ 0.05). However, this study did not compare the TURP and PAE groups. Schreuder et al. published a review about the management of BPH [15].

In present study, no statistically significant difference in the preoperative Qmax between the 2 groups ($p >$ 0.05, Fig. 4). The Qmax could be as a parameter to compare the clinical efficacy between the TURP group and PAE group. We found that the postoperative Qmax was higher in the TURP group than in the PAE group (P < 0.05, Fig. 5). This may be from the TURP achieving a radical resection of an enlarged volume. It may take longer after PAE to achieve the histopathologic changes associated with destruction of the prostate vasculature [17]. However, the PAE could not make a big change for non-radical removal of the prostate volume. Similarly, Carnevale et al. reported that the Qmax of patients in the TURP group was higher than in the PAE group. In our study, the Qmax of patients had a better change after PAE, which was related to apoptosis in the prostate tissue. Bagla et al. reported a single-arm trial involving 18 patients who received PAE, demonstrating that the Qmax was decreased in the sixth-month follow up compared with the first and third months [18]. This may also be attributed to the recurrence of new enlarged prostate tissue.

The pooled studies showed statistically significant difference in the preoperative prostate volume between the 2 groups ($p > 0.05$, Fig. 7). This may due to the selction bias among the four studies. Our study demonstrated that the residual prostate volume was smaller in the TURP group than in the PAE group. The direct resection of pathologically protruding prostate tissue could instantaneously achieve satisfactory urodynamics outcomes. The PAE group could have a later decrease in the prostate volume. Other studies reported a similar outcome [14, 19]. Pisco et al. reported that the postoperative prostate volume was associated with clinical efficiency [20]. Amouyal et al. reported that improvement of urodynamics was not associated with the clinical outcome [21]. Tinto et al. reported a single-arm PAE trial wherein the PVR significantly improved after PAE. They reported on 103 patients undergoing PAE for BPH [22]. They demonstrated that the PVR was much changed after PAE.

The pooled studies showed no statistically significant difference in the preoperative IPSS between TURP group and PAE group ($p > 0.05$, Fig. 2). Our study reported that the two groups could achieve a similar IPSS score for BPH treatment ($p > 0.05$, Fig. 3). Qiu et al. reported that the TURP group had a lower IPSS score than the PAE group ($P = 0.021$) [12]. Similarly, Carnevale et al. reported that the score was lower for patients in the PAE group than in the TURP group. Additionally, the posttreatment IPSS was lower for patients in the TURP group than for patients in the PAE group ($p = 0.012$ and $p = 0.0007$, respectively) [14]. Pisco et al. reported improvement of 20 ml/s in the Qmax and 12 points in the IPSS score together [20].

With respect to the Qol, the TURP group had a lower score than the PAE group, demonstrating that the TURP

Study or Subgroup	TURP Mean	TURP SD	TURP Total	PAE Mean	PAE SD	PAE Total	Weight	Mean Difference IV, Fixed, 95% CI
Carnevale2016	61.7	17	15	144.8	50.1	15	5.7%	-83.10 [-109.87, -56.33]
Gao2014	83.5	17.5	53	89.7	17.1	54	94.3%	-6.20 [-12.76, 0.36]
Total (95% CI)			**68**			**69**	**100.0%**	**-10.55 [-16.92, -4.18]**

Heterogeneity: Chi² = 29.90, df = 1 (P < 0.00001); I² = 97%
Test for overall effect: Z = 3.25 (P = 0.001)

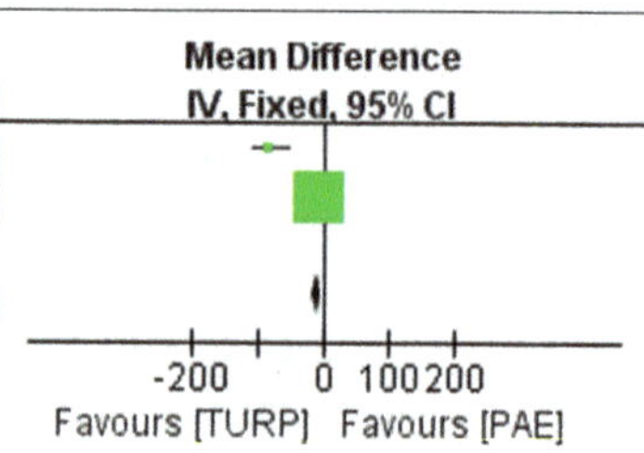

Fig. 9 Forest plot for operative time between theTURP and PAE for BPH

Study or Subgroup	TURP Events	TURP Total	PAE Events	PAE Total	Weight	Odds Ratio M-H, Fixed, 95% CI
Gao2014	17	53	30	54	59.7%	0.38 [0.17, 0.83]
Ray 2018	72	89	122	216	40.3%	3.26 [1.80, 5.90]
Total (95% CI)		**142**		**270**	**100.0%**	**1.54 [1.00, 2.38]**
Total events	89		152			

Heterogeneity: $Chi^2 = 18.38$, df = 1 ($P < 0.0001$); $I^2 = 95\%$
Test for overall effect: $Z = 1.95$ ($P = 0.05$)

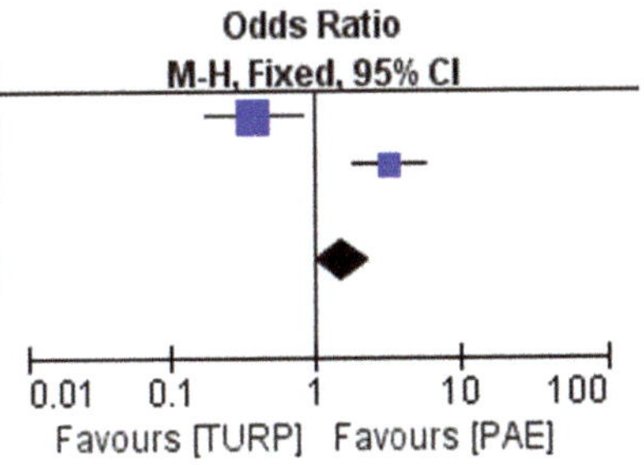

Fig. 10 Forest plot for complications between the TURP and PAE for BPH

group could achieve a higher life quality. Ray et al. reported that the Qol score changed from baseline of 14.4 to 12 for the last follow-up, which was 2.00 in PAE, and the score changed from 4.9 in the beginning to 1.5 in the last follow-up [13]. Tinto et al. reported that the Qol score improved slightly from 4.11 to 2.01 at 12 months. This observation changed little in the next 12 months.

Our study showed no statistically significant difference in complications between the TURP and PAE groups (Fig. 10). However, Gao et al. demonstrated that the complication rate was higher after PAE [11]. In addition to blood transfusion, acute urinary retention was higher in the PAE group. Grosso et al. reported that studies on PAE described few complications, while bleeding, sexual dysfunction, and incontinence were more common with TURP [23].

The operation time was shorter in the TURP group than in the PAE group. This may be from unfamiliarity with the complicated anatomy. Wang et al. reported that the artery of prostate was a variant [24]. Additionally, TURP, unlike PAE, was a routine surgical method to treat with BPH for most centers.

Our study also had several limitations. First, not all included studies were RCTs, which may decrease the quality of evidence. Additionally, the sample size of patients was low. Second, publication and selection bias should also be considered when interpreting the results. Third, the included studies had a shorter follow-up period. This may contribute to worse outcomes for the PAE group. PAE may require a long follow-up time. Additionally, the studies that included PAE may have different embolization standards. This design may contribute to bias. Moreover, the four studies involved unilateral embolization, bilateral artery embolization or combined unilateral and bilateral embolization, which also increases the heterogeneity. We could not eliminate all sources of heterogeneity.

Conclusions

In our meta-analysis, the efficiency of TURP for treating BPH was better than that of PAE. Our meta-analysis shows that PAE is an efficient and safe procedure that achieves better improvement in urodynamics and Qol. Our meta-analysis indicates that TURP is superior to PAE in clinical efficiency improvement. More multi-center high quality RCTs with large sample size are needed to verify the clinical efficiency of TURP and PAE for the treatment of BPH.

Abbreviations

BPH: Benign prostatic hyperplasial; CI: Confidence interval; IIEF: International index of erectile function; IPSS: International prostate symptom score; LUTS: Lower urinary tract symptoms; OR: Odds ratio; PAE: Prostatic arterial embolization; PVR: Postvoid residual volume; Qmax: Maximum urinary flow rate/peak urinary flow rate; QoL: Quality of life; TURP: Transurethral resection of the prostate; WMD: Weight mean difference

Acknowledgements

Not applicable.

Authors' contributions

YLJ and LJQ designed the study. YLJ wrote the manuscript. YLJ and LJQ analyzed the data. LJQ and YLJ searched the articles. Both authors read and approved the final manuscript.

References

1. Oelke M, Bachmann A, Descazeaud A, Emberton M, Gravas S, Michel MC, et al. EAU guidelines on the treatment and follow-up of non-neurogenic male lower urinary tract symptoms including benign prostatic obstruction. Eur Urol. 2013;64:118–40.
2. Garraway WM, Collins GN, Lee RJ. High prevalence of benign prostatic hypertrophy in the community. Lancet. 1991;338:469–71.
3. Sarma AV, Wei JT. Clinical practice. Benign prostatic hyperplasia and lower urinary tract symptoms. N Engl J Med. 2012;367:248–57.
4. Bachmann A, Muir GH, Wyler SF, Rieken M. Surgical benign prostatic hyperplasia trials: the future is now! Eur Urol. 2013;63:677–9 discussion 9-80.
5. Joshi HN, De Jong IJ, Karmacharya RM, Shrestha B, Shrestha R. Outcomes of transurethral resection of the prostate in benign prostatic hyperplasia comparing prostate size of more than 80 grams to prostate size less than 80 grams. Kathmandu Univ Med J (KUMJ). 2014;12:163–7.
6. Pavone C, Abbadessa D, Scaduto G, Caruana G, Scalici Gesolfo C, Fontana D, et al. Sexual dysfunctions after transurethral resection of the prostate (TURP): evidence from a retrospective study on 264 patients. Arch Ital Urol Androl. 2015;87:8–13.
7. Pasha MT, Khan MA, Jamal Y, Wahab F, Naeemullah. Postoperative Complications With Glycine And Sterile Distilled Water After Transurethral Resection Of Prostate. J Ayub Med Coll Abbottabad. 2015;27:135–9.
8. Abt D, Hechelhammer L, Mullhaupt G, Markart S, Gusewell S, Kessler TM, et al. Comparison of prostatic artery embolisation (PAE) versus transurethral resection of the prostate (TURP) for benign prostatic hyperplasia: randomised, open label, non-inferiority trial. BMJ. 2018;361:k2338.

9. Lin YT, Amouyal G, Correas JM, Pereira H, Pellerin O, Del Giudice C, et al. Can prostatic arterial embolisation (PAE) reduce the volume of the peripheral zone? MRI evaluation of zonal anatomy and infarction after PAE. Eur Radiol. 2016;26:3466–73.
10. Mitchell ME, Waltman AC, Athanasoulis CA, Kerr WS Jr, Dretler SP. Control of massive prostatic bleeding with angiographic techniques. J Urol. 1976;115: 692–5.
11. Gao YA, Huang Y, Zhang R, Yang YD, Zhang Q, Hou M, et al. Benign prostatic hyperplasia: prostatic arterial embolization versus transurethral resection of the prostate--a prospective, randomized, and controlled clinical trial. Radiology. 2014;270:920–8.
12. Qiu Z, Zhang C, Wang X, Cheng K, Liang X, Wang D, et al. Clinical evaluation of embolization of the superior vesical prostatic artery for treatment of benign prostatic hyperplasia: a single-center retrospective study. Wideochir Inne Tech Maloinwazyjne. 2017;12:409–16.
13. Ray AF, Powell J, Speakman MJ, Longford NT, DasGupta R, Bryant T, et al. Efficacy and safety of prostate artery embolization for benign prostatic hyperplasia: an observational study and propensity-matched comparison with transurethral resection of the prostate (the UK-ROPE study). BJU Int. 2018;122:270-82.
14. Carnevale FC, Iscaife A, Yoshinaga EM, Moreira AM, Antunes AA, Srougi M. Transurethral resection of the prostate (TURP) versus original and PErFecTED prostate artery embolization (PAE) due to benign prostatic hyperplasia (BPH): preliminary results of a single center, prospective, urodynamic-controlled analysis. Cardiovasc Intervent Radiol. 2016;39:44–52.
15. Schreuder SM, Scholtens AE, Reekers JA, Bipat S. The role of prostatic arterial embolization in patients with benign prostatic hyperplasia: a systematic review. Cardiovasc Intervent Radiol. 2014;37:1198–219.
16. Feng S, Tian Y, Liu W, Li Z, Deng T, Li H, et al. Prostatic arterial embolization treating moderate-to-severe lower urinary tract symptoms related to benign prostate hyperplasia: a meta-analysis. Cardiovasc Intervent Radiol. 2017;40:22–32.
17. Camara-Lopes G, Mattedi R, Antunes AA, Carnevale FC, Cerri GG, Srougi M, et al. The histology of prostate tissue following prostatic artery embolization for the treatment of benign prostatic hyperplasia. Int Braz J Urol. 2013;39:222–7.
18. Bagla S, Martin CP, van Breda A, Sheridan MJ, Sterling KM, Papadouris D, et al. Early results from a United States trial of prostatic artery embolization in the treatment of benign prostatic hyperplasia. J Vasc Interv Radiol. 2014;25:47–52.
19. Sun F, Sanchez FM, Crisostomo V, Diaz-Guemes I, Lopez-Sanchez C, Uson J, et al. Transarterial prostatic embolization: initial experience in a canine model. AJR Am J Roentgenol. 2011;197:495–501.
20. Pisco JM, Rio Tinto H, Campos Pinheiro L, Bilhim T, Duarte M, Fernandes L, et al. Embolisation of prostatic arteries as treatment of moderate to severe lower urinary symptoms (LUTS) secondary to benign hyperplasia: results of short- and mid-term follow-up. Eur Radiol. 2013;23:2561–72.
21. Amouyal G, Thiounn N, Pellerin O, Yen-Ting L, Del Giudice C, Dean C, et al. Clinical results after prostatic artery embolization using the PErFecTED technique: a single-center study. Cardiovasc Intervent Radiol. 2016;39:367–75.
22. Bilhim T, Pisco J, Rio Tinto H, Fernandes L, Campos Pinheiro L, Duarte M, et al. Unilateral versus bilateral prostatic arterial embolization for lower urinary tract symptoms in patients with prostate enlargement. Cardiovasc Intervent Radiol. 2013;36:403–11.
23. Grosso M, Balderi A, Arno M, Sortino D, Antonietti A, Pedrazzini F, et al. Prostatic artery embolization in benign prostatic hyperplasia: preliminary results in 13 patients. Radiol Med. 2015;120:361–8.
24. Wang MQ, Guo LP, Zhang GD, Yuan K, Li K, Duan F, et al. Prostatic arterial embolization for the treatment of lower urinary tract symptoms due to large (>80 mL) benign prostatic hyperplasia: results of midterm follow-up from Chinese population. BMC Urol. 2015;15:33.

5

Prostate-specific antigen (PSA) and distress - a cross-sectional nationwide survey in men with prostate cancer

Ulrika Rönningås[1,2,3*], Per Fransson[4,5], Maja Holm[3] and Agneta Wennman-Larsen[1,3]

Abstract

Background: The prostate-specific antigen (PSA) -value is often used during the prostate cancer trajectory as a marker of progression or response to treatment. Concerns about PSA-values are often expressed by patients in clinical situations. Today there is a lack of larger studies that have investigated the association between PSA-value and distress. The aim was to investigate the association between PSA-values and distress adjusted for sociodemographic factors, hormonal therapy and quality of life (QoL), among men with prostate cancer.

Methods: In this cross-sectional survey of 3165 men with prostate cancer, members of the Swedish Prostate Cancer Federation, answered questions about sociodemographic factors, PSA, distress, QoL and treatments. Descriptive statistics, and bivariate and multivariable analyses were performed. The result was presented based on four PSA-value groups: 0–19, 20–99, 100–999, and ≥ 1000 ng/ml.

Results: Of the men, 53% experienced distress. An association between distress and PSA-values was found where higher PSA-values were associated with higher OR:s for experiencing distress in the different PSA-groups: 0–19 ng/ml (ref 1), 20–99 ng/ml (OR 1.25, 95% CI 1.01–1.55), 100–999 ng/ml (OR 1.47, 95% CI 1.12–1.94), ≥1000 ng/ml (OR 1.77, 95% CI 1.11–2.85). These associations were adjusted for sociodemographic factors and hormonal therapy. In the multivariable analyses, beside PSA-values, higher levels of distress were associated with being without partner or hormonal therapy. When adding QoL in the multivariable analysis, the association between PSA and distress did not remain significant.

Conclusion: These results indicate that the PSA-values are associated with distress, especially for those with higher values. However, to be able to support these men, continued research is needed to gain more knowledge about the mechanisms behind the association between emotional distress and PSA-values.

Keywords: Prostate cancer, Prostatic neoplasm, PSA, Prostate-specific antigen, Distress, Quality of life

Background

Among Swedish men, prostate cancer is the most common type of cancer comprising 33% of all cancer cases [1]. The prostate-specific antigen (PSA)-test is not specific to prostate cancer, but the value may increase when cancer is present and the PSA-test is used for detection of cancer. The value is used in diagnostics to evaluate the severity of the tumor, but is also used throughout the disease trajectory during monitoring and treatment [2].

The PSA-values are often divided into different PSA-groups and the groupings are decisive in risk analysis at detection, recurrence and progression of the prostate cancer. Despite the relevance of measuring PSA in all stages of the disease few studies have been conducted regarding the importance and impact that the PSA-values have for the men with prostate cancer. The existing studies are small and mainly qualitative and most report these findings as incidental. Interviews with men with prostate cancer receiving curative treatment showed that PSA-tests and values dominated the narratives of many

* Correspondence: ulrika.ronningas@ki.se
[1]Division of Insurance Medicine, Department of Clinical Neuroscience, Karolinska Institutet, 171 77 Stockholm, Sweden
[2]Department of Oncology, Sundsvall County Hospital, 851 86 Sundsvall, Sweden
Full list of author information is available at the end of the article

participants'. The men tended to focus on the numeric value of the PSA and they often compared PSA-values with each other [3]. Roth and Passik [4] introduces the concept of a specific anxiety related to PSA, *PSA-anxiety*, among men with prostate cancer when studying overall anxiety in this group. Another study [5] showed that survivors of prostate cancer with high scores on fear of recurrence also had higher levels of PSA-anxiety and lower health-related quality of life (QoL).

In one interview study, men with localized prostate cancer described the PSA-tests as a lifeline and that they had a feeling of being healthy when the PSA-value was low and stable [6]. Shen et al. [7] interviewed men with biochemical recurrence in relation to their experience and affective responses regarding increasing PSA-values and treatment options. Most men experienced more worry and fear of death when they learned about the rising PSA-values than they did when their cancer was initially diagnosed. They were also more worried before a physician's appointment if they knew PSA-values were to be discussed. Many of them kept track of the PSA-values, checked the doubling time and had determined their own PSA-limits when they thought a new treatment was to begin.

In a small questionnaire study [8] on how patients with prostate cancer knew if their disease was progressing, 77% of the 52 men reported PSA-levels as one of the indicators. The study showed that many men with prostate cancer defined changes in disease through their PSA-value instead of their physical and functional status. For some men a decrease in the PSA-value was a more important goal than a reduction of disease symptoms [8]. In an interview study of men with castration-resistant prostate cancer the researchers found that the men graded PSA-anxiety and fatigue as being most important when grading complications and QoL issues [9]. Nanton, Dochertry, Meystre and Dale [10] suggest that there is an uncertainty about what happens during the prostate cancer journey regarding the disease and treatment, which may generate anxiety and distress. Worry and anxiety as signs of distress may be related to fear of the future [10]. Along the cancer continuum, distress is frequent, and several factors, have been shown to be involved in terms of distress in cancer, such as psychological, social and spiritual factors [11]. Symptoms of distress, e.g., worry and fear about the future, thoughts of illness and death, and also concerns about physical symptoms, can be disabling and lead to depression, anxiety and panic disorders [11]. Other factors that have been shown to be associated with distress in men with prostate cancer are ongoing hormone treatment [12], and younger age, where younger cancer survivors tend to have higher fear of recurrence than older cancer survivors [13]. Another study suggests a more complex situation, where overall distress and anxiety decreases with age at the same time as depressive symptoms increase [14].

In conclusion, there are few studies about PSA-values from the men's perspective and most of them are either small quantitative studies or interview studies. In addition, the PSA-value and its impact on the men have mostly been reported as incidental findings. As mentioned, some studies have shown that men with prostate cancer may experience PSA-anxiety in relation to PSA-tests, when having increasing PSA-values and before attending appointments with their physician [3, 5, 7–9]. However, to our knowledge, there is a lack of larger studies that have investigated the association between PSA-values and distress, and what importance the different levels of PSA have, regarding the men's distress, especially when the PSA-values are high or extremely high.

Therefore, the aim of this study was to investigate the association between PSA-value and distress among men with prostate cancer, adjusted for sociodemographic factors, hormonal therapy (surgical or medical) and overall QoL.

Methods

Data were obtained from an overall cross-sectional study where a questionnaire was sent to members of the Swedish Prostate Cancer Federation (SPCF) in collaboration with one of the authors (PF) in 2012 on the initiative of the SPCF [15]. The questionnaire was distributed to all 6389 members. Members in the federation consist of men with prostate cancer and their family members/relatives, professionals as well as individuals who join the federation in support of it. Out of the 6389 distributed questionnaires, 3512 (55%) were returned. Of the returned questionnaires 3165 (90%) were received from members who reported that they had been diagnosed with prostate cancer. Hence, answers from these 3165 men were used in the analysis reported here.

Data collection

Some questions for this study was taken from a validated questionnaire developed by Fransson, Tavelin and Widmark [16] whereas others, were developed for the project in close cooperation with the SPCF [15]. The questions used in the present study are concerning age, marital status, level of education, time since diagnosis, type of treatments, the latest PSA-value, distress and overall QoL. Distress was measured by the question "Do you have any problems with worry/anxiety/feelings of depression?" with the response options "Never", "Sometimes", "Often" and "Always". QoL was measured by the question "How would you estimate your QoL today?"

with the answers on a numeric rating-scale from 0, "Very bad" to 10, "Excellent".

For the multivariable analysis, distress was dichotomized into: those who never experienced distress and those who experienced distress sometimes/often/always. QoL was dichotomized by the median (7) into: 0–6 and 7–10. Age was dichotomized by the median (73) into: 41–73 years and 74–95 years. Marital status was dichotomized into: married/cohabiting/in a relationship and divorced/widowed/single. Education level was categorized in three groups: elementary school, high school, and university. Years since prostate cancer diagnosis were dichotomized by the median (6) into: 0–6, and 7–43 years. Hormonal therapy was dichotomized into: "no hormonal therapy (no surgical or ongoing medical)" and "hormonal therapy (surgical or ongoing medical)". PSA-values were categorized into four groups according to a grouping suggested by Koo et al. [17]: 0–19 ng/ml; 20–99 ng/ml; 100–999 ng/ml; and ≥ 1000 ng/ml, –where the values ≥1000 ng/ml are considered to be extremely high.

Data analysis

Data analysis was conducted using IBM SPSS 23 (Statistical Package for the Social Science). Data were analysed using descriptive statistics regarding age, marital status, education, years since diagnosis, hormonal therapy and latest known PSA-value. Listwise deletion was applied to manage missing values. A logistic regression analysis with 95% CI was used to explore the association between distress and latest known PSA-value adjusted for sociodemographic factors, hormonal therapy and overall QoL. The logistic regression analysis was performed in three models; first as a bivariate analysis (Model 1). In Model 2, all significant variables ($p < 0.05$) from Model 1 were included simultaneously except for QoL. This strategy was chosen because distress is assumed to be part of the concept of overall QoL to avoid over-adjustment in the first step. In Model 3, QoL was included for the purpose of adjusting for wellbeing other than distress, including physical aspects of wellbeing. Model 3 should be interpreted carefully because there is a theoretical overlap between the concepts of distress and QoL, where distress may be a part of the overall concept of QoL [18].

Table 1 Sociodemographic and medical characteristics of 3 165 men with prostate cancer: frequencies, percentages, mean, standard deviation (SD), median, range

Age (years)	Mean (*SD*)	72.8 (*7.2*)	
	Median (*Interquartile*)	73 (*10*)	
	Missing	*n* = 24	0.8%
	Range	41–95	
Years since diagnosis (years)	Mean (*SD*)	6.9 (*4.4*)	
	Median (*Interquartile*)	6 (*5*)	
	Missing	*n* = 114	3.6%
	Range	0–43	
Quality of Life[a]	Mean	6.9	
	Median	7	
	Quality of Life 0–6	*n* = 1112	35.7%
	Quality of Life 7–10	*n* = 2006	64.3%
	Missing	*n* = 47	1.5%
		n	%[b]
Marital status	Married/cohabiting	2525	8.0
	Divorced	78	2.6
	Widowed	182	6.1
	Single	101	3.4
	In a relationship	84	2.8
	Missing	195	6.2
Education	Elementary school	1213	40.0
	High school	886	29.2
	University	937	30.9
	Missing	129	4.1
PSA – latest value (ng/ml)	0–19	2336	73.8
	20–99	473	14.9
	100–999	267	8.4
	1000–	89	2.8
	Missing	0	0.0
Hormonal therapy	No	2556	81.8
	Yes	609	19.2
	Missing	0	0.0
Distress	Never	1455	46.6
	Sometimes	1468	47.0
	Often	166	5.3
	Always	31	1.0
	Missing	45	1.4

[a]Higher values indicate better QoL
[b]Totals i some cases do not amount to 100% due to the use of rounding

Results

Sample characteristics

Of the 3165 men, the median age was 73 years (min–max, 41–95), and 80% (2609/3165) of the participants were in a relationship. Regarding the participants' levels of education, 38% (1213/3165) had completed elementary school, 28% (886/3165) had completed high school and 30% (937/3165) had a university education (Table 1).

The time since diagnosis of prostate cancer varied between 0 and 43 years, with a mean value of almost 7 years and a median of 6 years. All the men had reported their latest PSA-value. The largest group (74%) had relatively low PSA-values (0–19 ng/ml), while 3% had extremely high PSA-values (≥1000 ng/ml). About 46% (1455/3165) stated that they "never" experienced distress, while about 53% (1665/3165) experienced distress "sometimes", "often" or "always". Most men (64%, 2006/3165), reported good QoL (Table 1).

Associations between PSA-level and distress

In the bivariate analysis (Model 1), higher PSA-values were significantly associated with more distress compared to lower levels of PSA (0–19 ng/ml) (Table 2). Not being in a relationship, having ongoing hormonal therapy or low overall QoL were also associated with higher levels of distress, while those with a university-level education had less distress compared to those with elementary school (Table 2). No association was found between distress and the number of years since the prostate cancer diagnosis, or age (Table 2).

In the first step in the multivariable analysis (Model 2) when adjusted for education, marital status and hormonal therapy but not QoL, the odds ratio (OR) for having distress significantly increased with higher PSA-values (PSA-group 20–99 ng/ml, OR 1.25 (95% CI 1.01–1.55), PSA-group 100–999 ng/ml, OR 1.47 (95% CI 1.12–1.94), PSA group ≥1000 ng/ml, OR 1.77 (95% CI 1.11–2.85)). The significant association between marital status, hormonal therapy and distress also remained (Table 2). In Model 3, in which QoL was included, there was an association between QoL and distress, OR 4.33 (95% CI 3.62–5.17) while the association between distress and PSA-values and the association between distress and marital status, ongoing hormonal therapy and PSA-values was not significant (Table 2).

Table 2 Crude and adjusted odds ratios (OR) with 95% confidence interval (95%CI), for associations between distress and PSA, sociodemographic factors, hormonal therapy (surgical or medical) and overall QoL ($n = 3165$)

Variable	Model 1[a]			Model 2[b]			Model 3[c]		
	OR	(95% CI)	*p*	OR	(95% CI)	*p*	OR	(95% CI)	*p*
Age $n = 3141$									
41–73	1			-			-		
74–95	0.90	(0.78–1.04)	0.14						
Years since diagnosis $n = 3051$									
0–6	1			-			-		
7–43	1.10	(0.96–1.27)	0.18						
Quality of life $n = 3118$									
7–10	1			-			1		
0–6	4.49	(3.81–5.29)	**0.00**				4.33	(3.62–5.17)	**0.00**
Marital status $n = 2970$									
Married/cohabiting/in a relationship	1			1			1		
Single/widowed/divorced	1.50	(1.19–1.88)	**0.00**	1.40	(1.10–1.77)	**0.01**	1.16	(0.90–1.49)	0.25
Education $n = 3036$									
Elementary school	1			1			1		
High school	1.04	(0.87–1.24)	0.83	1.06	(0.89–1.28)	0.50	1.21	(1.00–1.47)	**0.05**
University	0.83	(0.70–0.99)	**0.02**	0.85	(0.71–1.01)	0.07	1.00	(0.83–1.21)	0.98
PSA (ng/ml) $n = 3165$									
0–19	1			1			1		
20–99	1.36	(1.11–1.66)	**0.00**	1.25	(1.01–1.55)	**0.04**	1.21	(0.96–1.51)	0.10
100–999	1.54	(1.19–2.01)	**0.00**	1.47	(1.12–1.94)	**0.01**	1.25	(0.93–1.68)	0.14
1000–	2.19	(1.38–3.47)	**0.00**	1.77	(1.11–2.85)	**0.02**	1.17	(0.70–1.94)	0.55
Hormonal therapy $n = 3165$									
No	1			1			1		
Yes	1.42	(1.18–1.71)	**0.00**	1.35	(1.11–1.65)	**0.00**	1.12	(0.91–1.39)	0.28

$p \leq 0.05$, significant values in bold

[a]Model 1: Bivariate association between all variables and distress

[b]Model 2: Association between PSA-value and distress adjusted for all significant independent variables in Model 1 excluding QoL

[c]Model 3: Association between PSA-values and distress adjusted for all significant independent variables in Model 1 also including QoL

Discussion

The results show that higher PSA-values were associated with higher likelihood for experiencing distress. Not living in a relationship and hormonal therapy were factors also associated with reported distress as well as overall QoL.

About half of the men in this study experienced distress at least sometimes and there was an association between distress and PSA-values in the groups, PSA 20–99 ng/ml, PSA 100–999 ng/ml and PSA ≥ 1000 ng/ml. The association between PSA-value and distress was positive, i.e. higher PSA-values were associated with higher OR:s for experiencing distress. Lofters et al.'s [8] results showed that PSA-values were strongly correlated with anxiety. Medium to severe anxiety before receiving the results of a PSA-test was also reported by a third of the men with metastatic prostate cancer in their study [8]. An association between rising PSA-values and increasing anxiety among men 6–18 months after prostatectomy has also been shown [19]. PSA-values seem to affect men diagnosed with prostate cancer in a similar way in which the cancer antigen (CA) 125-values affect women diagnosed with gynecological cancer. Parker et al. [20] described that women often knew their CA 125-value, many wrote the value down and tracked the values over time and they also reported that the values affected their mood. Parker et al.'s study also showed that the more metastases the women had the more they were preoccupied with the CA 125-values [20]. In this study, we did not have data on metastases and can therefore only speculate on whether men with metastases, who probably have higher PSA-values, are more preoccupied with their PSA than men without metastases. However, in the group of men with extremely high PSA-values (≥1000), we do know that they have a metastatic prostate cancer, even if not detected, and the disease may affect the men, with more physical symptoms as well. Distress induced by higher PSA-values may be related to fear of recurrence and progression, and the laboratory referral for PSA-test may eventually work as a trigger for fear of recurrence or progression of the disease. Results from a study by Simard, Simard and Ivers (2013) showed that around 10% of patients diagnosed with cancer reported high scores for fear of recurrence and, and also reacted more to "triggers" for fear of recurrence as well as had more psychological distress [21]. "Triggers" in this case are things leading to intrusive thoughts and fear of recurrence, for example, reading a newspaper and seeing an advertisement about cancer treatment or during a physical examination [13, 21]. When patients with metastatic disease were asked about their opinion about discontinuing PSA-tests, more than 50% responded that it would feel as though the physician had given up on them; only one patient thought it would be a relief [8]. In the questionnaire for the present study, all men reported their last PSA-value, even those who reported a longer period since their diagnosis. Together with hormonal therapy, it was the only variable with no missing data, which may indicate the importance of PSA-values and the impact that the hormonal therapy had on these men.

In both the bivariate and in the adjusted analyses, it was shown that other factors besides PSA-values were also associated with distress, e.g., men who lived without a partner had a higher likelihood of being distressed. One explanation may be that; even if men who live in a relationship and who have high PSA-values may be distressed, they may also receive more support from their partner, which could in turn reduce the level of distress. In a previous interview study of men with prostate cancer who were living without a partner, a higher need for information and support regarding treatment alternatives was also found when compared to men who were living in a relationship [22]. However, the level of partner support may also affect the experienced distress, where men reporting low partner support have been shown to experience the same level of distress as those who do not have a close relationship [23]. Men not living in a relationship experienced more social isolation and many of them did not seek support actively. Nonetheless, the authors described that during interviews descriptions of anxiety and fear of dying appeared even though the men did not always recognise the emotional distress affecting them [24].

Hormonal therapy was also a factor associated with distress in this study. This result is in line with those of Sharpley, Bitsika, Wooten and Christie [25], which show that men receiving hormonal therapy had higher scores regarding anxiety and depression, compared to men who had completed the hormonal therapy or who had never had hormonal therapy [25]. It would have been interesting to know which type of hormonal therapy was given to the men in the present study and at what stage of the disease. Distress may be experienced differently if the hormonal therapy is adjuvant or if it has a palliative intent. Unfortunately, we did not have access to data on type of hormonal therapy for the men in the present study, thus this could be a question for future studies.

When adding QoL into the models the association between distress and PSA-levels were no longer significant. This may be due to a possible dependency between QoL and distress, where QoL is an overall concept that also covers aspects of distress. Overall QoL had a stronger association with distress than PSA-values, which may be interpreted as the notion that there are more aspects of health that may affect the level of distress in this group of patients. Dale et al. [18] describe that it is possible that an increasing PSA-value may increase the worry and anxiety-level, which in turn may affect health-related QoL [18]. When comparing early-stage prostate cancer and advanced-stage prostate cancer with bone metastases, those in the late-stage group had more anxiety [26]. The PSA-value is also often important in treatment evaluation and may also in that sense be related to overall QoL. Distress could also be another aspect affecting QoL. As mentioned earlier, distress may be a part of the overall concept of QoL because there is a theoretical overlap between the concepts of distress and QoL [18] and therefore the results of this analysis should be interpreted cautiously.

A bit surprisingly, the present study did not show an association between distress and age, whereas earlier studies have shown that in newly diagnosed men with localized prostate cancer, younger age was associated with greater distress [27] and younger cancer survivors also had a higher fear of cancer recurrence [13], which may also be associated with distress. Previous results based on the same sample as in the present study have also shown that younger men had more thoughts of suicide than older men with prostate cancer [15]. The rather high age (mean 72.8) with few young men (SD 7) in the present sample could however explain the lack of association between age and distress.

A clinical implication of the results in the present study is that there may be a need to pay more attention to men living without a partner and/or who receive hormonal therapy (surgical or ongoing medical) when awaiting PSA results. This may be an important aspect to consider for the treating physician, and for the patient access to a specialist nurse may also be helpful in order to receive relevant information and support [28].

Strengths and limitations

One strength of this study is the large nationwide sample, providing a large spread in age, 41–95 years, and in years since diagnosis, 0–43 years. Hence, the data include various generations and were drawn both from newly diagnosed men and those diagnosed many years ago. Although, men who are members of the SPCF may be a selected group, earlier research [29] has shown that data from members of prostate cancer associations are likely to correspond with data from other studies within the wider prostate cancer population regarding symptoms, QoL and disease status [29]. Earlier research has also shown that men do not become members of patient associations due to distress or, as for women, due to psychosocial needs related to having cancer. For men with prostate cancer, the motives were rather that they wanted the information and activities the associations could provide [30]. Data from prostate cancer patients' associations have also been used in previous studies of this population in the Nordic Countries [29, 31, 32]. A limitation in this study is however that we do not know how many of the non-responders were men with prostate cancer and how many that were supportive members of the federation and therefore we cannot estimate the actual response rate. There is a possibility that more supportive members were non-responders due to the cancer-related questions.

A limitation of this study is also that the questions in the questionnaire were not specifically developed for the aim of the present study. One example is that distress was measured by the question "Do you have any problems with worry/anxiety/feelings of depression?" which covers three aspects of distress. This may be problematic if only one of the aspects were experienced. A strength may, on the other hand, be that the question covers many aspects of overall distress, thus it does not exclude men who experienced any of the aspects.

It would also have been interesting to control for data on other factors that may cause distress, such as physical symptoms and/or comorbidity. It would have been interesting to compare other aspects of wellbeing than QoL, i.e. performance status or physical functioning.

It would also have been advantageous to verify data on disease status and PSA-values from medical records which was not possible due to the nationwide sample with anonymous answers. There may be a possibility that the distress would have been even more prominent when measured closer to the PSA-testing. Another strength would also have been to have data on stage or status of the disease. In this case, a low PSA-level may both indicate that the disease is cured, in a stable, controlled phase, e.g., after initial treatment, or in a state where successful life-prolonging treatment is given. Thus, by treatment and treatment outcome, patients may move between the different PSA-groups. However, we do know that those with the highest PSA-values do have a more severe disease.

Conclusion

An association between PSA-values and distress was found, where higher PSA-values were associated with higher likelihood of distress. Other factors, such as hormonal therapy and not living in a relationship, were also found to be associated with distress, as was overall QoL. However, to be able to support these men to reduce distress related to PSA-values, which is also a marker of progression, more detailed knowledge is needed on the complex mechanisms behind the experienced distress, and also on the role of PSA-values for understanding the disease from the men's perspective.

Abbreviations

PSA: Prostate Specific Antigen; QoL: Quality of Life; SPCF: Swedish Prostate Cancer Federation

Acknowledgements
The authors also wish to acknowledge the contribution to this article by the late Olav Lindqvist, Ph.D.

Authors' contributions
UR and AWL drafted the study and conducted the analyses. UR wrote the manuscript. PF collected data, drafted the study and reviewed the manuscript. MH and AWL reviewed the manuscript. All authors approved the final version of the manuscript.

Author details
[1]Division of Insurance Medicine, Department of Clinical Neuroscience, Karolinska Institutet, 171 77 Stockholm, Sweden. [2]Department of Oncology, Sundsvall County Hospital, 851 86 Sundsvall, Sweden. [3]Department of Nursing Science, Sophiahemmet University, 114 86 Stockholm, Sweden. [4]Department of Nursing, Umeå University, 901 87 Umeå, Sweden. [5]Cancercentrum, Norrlands University Hospital, 901 85 Umeå, Sweden.

References
1. Cancer incidence in Sweden 2014 [In Swedish]. [https://www.socialstyrelsen.se/globalassets/sharepoint-dokument/artikelkatalog/statistik/2015-12-26.pdf].
2. Lynch T, Burgess M. Prostate-specific antigen test: an informed choice. Prim Health Care. 2011;21(3):16–21.
3. Appleton L, Wyatt D, Perkins E, Parker C, Crane J, Jones A, Moorhead L, Brown V, Wall C, Pagett M. The impact of prostate cancer on men's everyday life. Eur J Cancer Care. 2015;24(1):71–84.
4. Roth A, Passik S. Anxiety in men with prostate cancer may interfere with effective managment of the disease. Prim Care Cancer. 1996;16:30.
5. van de Wal M, van Oort I, Schouten J, Thewes B, Gielissen M, Prins J. Fear of cancer recurrence in prostate cancer survivors. Acta Oncol. 2016;55(7):821–7.
6. Hedestig O, Sandman P-O, Widmark A, Rasmussen BH. Meanings of prostate-specific antigen testing as narrated by men with localized prostate cancer after primary treatment. Scand J Urol Nephrol. 2008;42(2):101–9.
7. Shen MJ, Nelson CJ, Peters E, Slovin SF, Hall SJ, Hall M, Herrera PC, Leventhal EA, Leventhal H, Diefenbach MA. Decision-making processes among prostate Cancer survivors with rising PSA levels: results from a qualitative analysis. Med Decis Making. 2015;35(4):477–86.
8. Lofters A, Juffs HG, Pond GR, Tannock IF. "PSA-itis": knowledge of serum prostate specific antigen and other causes of anxiety in men with metastatic prostate Cancer. J Urol. 2002;168(6):2516–20.
9. Eton DT, Shevrin DH, Beaumont J, Victorson D, Cella D. Constructing a conceptual framework of patient-reported outcomes for metastatic hormone-refractory prostate cancer. Value Health. 2010;13(5):613–23.
10. Nanton V, Docherty A, Meystre C, Dale J. Finding a pathway: information and uncertainty along the prostate cancer patient journey. Br J Health Psychol. 2009;14(3):437–58.
11. Holland JC, Andersen B, Breitbart WS, Compas B, Dudley MM, Fleishman S, Fulcher CD, Greenberg DB, Greiner CB, Handzo GF, et al. Distress management. J Natl Compr Cancer Netw. 2010;8(4):448–85.
12. Sharpley CF, Christie DR, Bitsika V. Do hormone treatments for prostate cancer cause anxiety and depression? Int J Clin Oncol. 2014;19(3):523–30.
13. Simard S, Thewes B, Humphris G, Dixon M, Hayden C, Mireskandari S, Ozakinci G. Fear of cancer recurrence in adult cancer survivors: a systematic review of quantitative studies. J Cancer Surviv. 2013;7(3):300–22.
14. Nelson CJ, Weinberger MI, Balk E, Holland J, Breitbart W, Roth AJ. The chronology of distress, anxiety, and depression in older prostate cancer patients. Oncologist. 2009;14(9):891–9.
15. Lehuluante A, Fransson P. Are there specific health-related factors that can accentuate the risk of suicide among men with prostate cancer? Support Care Cancer. 2014;22(6):1673–8.
16. Fransson P, Tavelin B, Widmark A. Reliability and responsiveness of a prostate cancer questionnaire for radiotherapy-induced side effects. Support Care Cancer. 2001;9(3):187–98.
17. Koo KC, Park SU, Kim KH, Rha KH, Hong SJ, Yang SC, Chung BH. Predictors of survival in prostate cancer patients with bone metastasis and extremely high prostate-specific antigen levels. Prostate Int. 2015;3(1):10–5.
18. Dale W, Bilir P, Han M, Meltzer D. The role of anxiety in prostate carcinoma: a structured review of the literature. Cancer. 2005;104(3):467–78.
19. Tavlarides AM, Ames SC, Diehl NN, Joseph RW, Castle EP, Thiel DD, Broderick GA, Parker AS. Evaluation of the association of prostate cancer-specific anxiety with sexual function, depression and cancer aggressiveness in men 1 year following surgical treatment for localized prostate cancer. Psychooncology. 2013;22(6):1328–35.
20. Parker PA, Kudelka A, Basen-Engquist K, Kavanagh J, de Moor J, Cohen L. The associations between knowledge, CA125 preoccupation, and distress in women with epithelial ovarian cancer. Gynecol Oncol. 2006;100(3):495–500.
21. Simard S, Savard J, Ivers H. Fear of cancer recurrence: specific profiles and nature of intrusive thoughts. J Cancer Surviv. 2010;4(4):361–71.
22. Kazer MW, Harden J, Burke M, Sanda MG, Hardy J, Bailey DE. The experiences of unpartnered men with prostate cancer: a qualitative analysis. J Cancer Surviv. 2011;5(2):132–41.
23. Kamen C, Mustian KM, Heckler C, Janelsins MC, Peppone LJ, Mohile S, McMahon JM, Lord R, Flynn PJ, Weiss M, et al. The association between partner support and psychological distress among prostate cancer survivors in a nationwide study. J Cancer Surviv. 2015;9(3):492–9.
24. Ettridge KA, Bowden JA, Chambers SK, Smith DP, Murphy M, Evans SM, Roder D, Miller CL. "Prostate cancer is far more hidden...": Perceptions of stigma, social isolation and help-seeking among men with prostate cancer. Eur JCancer Care. 2018;27(2):e12790.
25. Sharpley CF, Bitsika V, Wootten AC, Christie DR. Differences in major depressive disorder and generalised anxiety disorder symptomatology between prostate cancer patients receiving hormone therapy and those who are not. Psychooncology. 2014;23(12):1350–5.
26. Johanes C, Monoarfa RA, Ismail RI, Umbas R. Anxiety level of early- and late-stage prostate cancer patients. Prostate Int. 2013;1(4):177–82.
27. Orom H, Nelson CJ, Underwood W 3rd, Homish DL, Kapoor DA. Factors associated with emotional distress in newly diagnosed prostate cancer patients. Psychooncology. 2015;24(11):1416–22.
28. King AJL, Evans M, Moore THM, Paterson C, Sharp D, Persad R, Huntley AL. Prostate cancer and supportive care: a systematic reviewand qualitative synthesis of men's experiences and unmet needs. Eur J Cancer Care. 2015; 24:618–34.
29. Fransson P. Quality of life for members of Swedish prostate Cancer patient associations. Cancer Nurs. 2008;31(1):23–31.
30. Carlsson C, Baigi A, Killander D, Larsson US. Motives for becoming and remaining member of patient associations: a study of 1,810 Swedish individuals with cancer associations. Support Care Cancer. 2005;13(12): 1035–43.
31. Fossa SD, Bengtsson T, Borre M, Ahlgren G, Rannikko A, Dahl AA. Reduction of quality of life in prostate cancer patients: experience among 6200 men in the Nordic countries. Scand J Urol. 2016;50(5):330–7.
32. Fossa SD, Dahl AA. Global quality of life after curative treatment for prostate Cancer: what matters? A study among members of the Norwegian prostate Cancer patient association. Clin Genitourin Cancer. 2015;13(6):518–24.

6

Sustained density of neuroendocrine cells with aging precedes development of prostatic hyperplasia in spontaneously hypertensive rats

Yuki Kyoda*, Koji Ichihara, Kohei Hashimoto, Ko Kobayashi, Fumimasa Fukuta and Naoya Masumori

Abstract

Background: Neuroendocrine (NE) cells may have an impact on the development and initial growth of benign prostatic hyperplasia (BPH) according to previous human studies.

Methods: To explore the relationship of NE cells and BPH development, we compared the density of NE cells and also prostatic weight in spontaneously hypertensive rats (SHR), which develop by aging, and Wistar-Kyoto rats (WKY) as control. The total weights of the epithelium and stroma in the ventral lobes of 8-, 12, 16-, 28- and 56-week-old SHR and WKY were calculated using Image J software. NE cells in the ventral prostatic ducts (VPd) were quantified using immunohistochemical staining for serotonin.

Results: Although there was no significant difference in the estimated total weight of the epithelium and stroma in the ventral lobes adjusted by body weight (ES weight) between the two groups at 8, 12 and 16 weeks of age, ES weight was significantly greater in the SHR group than in the WKT group at 28 and 56 weeks. The density of NE cells in the VPd decreased with aging in the WKY group, whereas it was sustained until 16 weeks and then decreased with aging in the SHR group. The difference in the density between the two groups was most marked at 16 weeks of age.

Conclusion: In the natural history of BPH, NE cells may play an important role in the initial development of BPH because sustained density of NE cells in the VPd precedes the development of prostatic hyperplasia.

Keywords: Neuroendocrine cell, Prostatic hyperplasia, Spontaneously hypertensive rat

Background

Benign prostatic hyperplasia (BPH) is a common disease that causes lower urinary tract symptoms in elderly men. However, we do not precisely know its etiology, although chronic inflammation, the change of hormonal status and aging have an influence on it [1–3].

Neuroendocrine (NE) cells are one of epithelial cells of the prostate. Their function is to maintain homeostasis in the prostate by producing a variety of neurosecretory products having growth-promoting activities, including serotonin (5-HT), calcitonin, parathyroid hormone-related peptides and so on [4, 5]. In addition, NE cells are involved in carcinogenesis and progression of prostate cancer as well as development of castration resistance prostate cancer 6–8]. On the other hand, few studies have examined the relationship between NE cells and human BPH [9–11]. Cockett et al. reported that there were many NE cells in and around small adenomatous nodules, which are the main pathological finding of BPH, whereas there are few NE cells in large adenomatous nodules [9]. Furthermore, we retrospectively quantified the density of NE cells in the transition zone (TZ) of the human prostate, where adenomatous nodules mainly appear [10]. Since the density of NE cells in the TZ containing small adenomas with normal epithelium and stroma around them in the TZ was higher than in the TZ containing large adenoma or no adenoma, we hypothesized that NE cells might have an influence on the initial growth of BPH.

* Correspondence: kyohday@sapmed.ac.jp
Department of Urology, Sapporo Medical University School of Medicine, S. 1, W. 16, Chuo-ku, Sapporo 060-8543, Japan

The epithelium of the rat prostate is different from that of the human prostate because the rat epithelium lacks NE cells [12]. NE cells in the Sprague-Dawley rats are distributed only in the urethra and the periurethral ducts, which link the urethra and the prostatic lobes, but not in the prostatic lobes. The density of NE cells in the periurethral ducts of the Wistar rat peaks in puberty and then decreases as the rats become older [13]. It is known that Sprague-Dawley and Wistar rats have no findings of prostatic hyperplasia with aging. On the other hand, no studies have reported on NE cells in the periurethral ducts of the spontaneously hypertensive rat (SHR), which is a model of BPH. SHR have been widely studied as an experimental model of hypertension and revealed their features of benign adenomatous hyperplasia in the ventral prostate of old SHR [14]. Previous studies demonstrated hyperplastic changes in the ventral prostate from young to older SHR, and close associations between the degree of its hyperplasia and aging in SHR [14–16]. The development of prostatic hyperplasia may result from both epithelial and stromal growth in SHR with age and may be predominantly expressed as a glandular type in SHR [16]. Thus, we compared the density of NE cells of the Wistar Kyoto rat (WKY), normotensive counterparts of SHR, to that of the SHR to investigate the relationship between NE cells and prostatic hyperplasia. Moreover, since few studies have reported when the hyperplasia begins in the prostate of SHR, we histologically evaluated the time of the initial development of prostatic hyperplasia by using image analysis software.

Methods

All surgical procedures and experimental protocols complied with institutional guidelines and were reviewed and approved by the Animal Care and Use Committee of Sapporo Medical University (#15–026).

Animals and experimental procedure

In this study, 8-, 12-, 16-, 28- and 56-week-old male SHR and WKY rats purchased from CHARLES RIVER LABORATORIES JAPAN, INC. (Yokohama, Japan) were used. They were bred in specific pathogen free room. The number of rats analyzed for each age group was five for both the SHR and WKY groups. Their body weights were measured and they were euthanized under isoflurane (2–4%) anesthesia by cervical dislocation. Thereafter, an abdominal incision was made to identify the abdominal cavity and they underwent cystoprostatectomy with simultaneous partial urethrectomy by cutting of the urethra axially at the level of pubic height. Each specimen was microscopically divided into 7 parts: 2 ventral lobes, 2 dorsolateral lobes, 2 coagulating glands, an ampullary gland, 2 seminal vesicles, the bladder and part of the urethra in saline. The weight of bilateral ventral lobes was measured using an electronic analytical scale.

Histopathological examination

The divided specimens were fixed in 15% neutral-buffered formalin (Wako Pure Chemical Industries, Ltd., Osaka, Japan) for 48–96 h. The specimens were then embedded in paraffin, cut into 5-μm sections and stained with hematoxylin and eosin (Fig. 1) [10].

Immunohistochemical staining was carried out using polyclonal antibodies for serotonin. It was done on 4-μm-thick paraffin sections cut from the formalin-fixed tissues. Heat-induced epitope retrieval was performed in Tris-EDTA buffer (10 mM Tris Base, 1 mM EDTA solution, 0.05% Tween 20, pH 9.0). The sections were then incubated in 3% H2O2 for 10 min to eliminate endogenous peroxidase activity. The primary rabbit anti-serotonin polyclonal antibody (1,20,000 Immunostar, Stillwater, MN) and a horseradish peroxidase-conjugated anti-rabbit secondary antibody were used at room temperature for 60 min and 30 min, respectively [10]. Color development

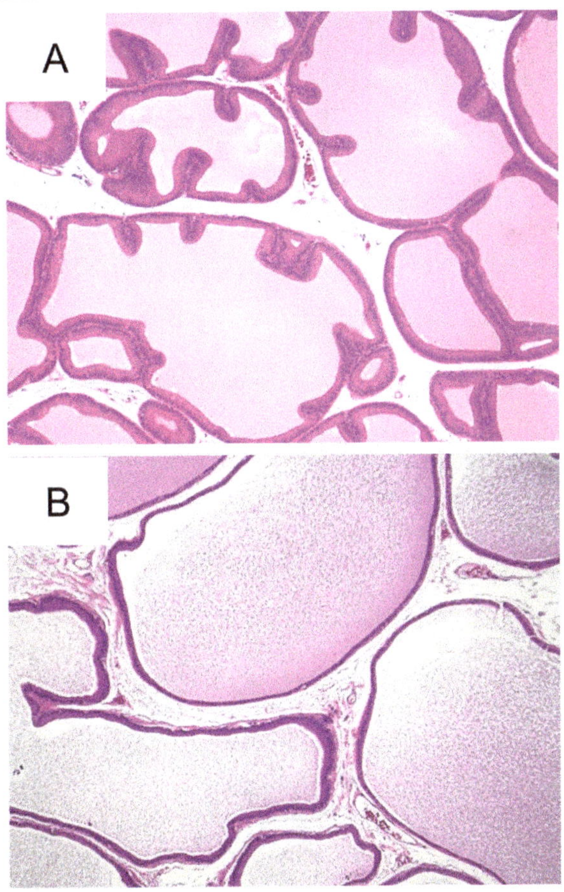

Fig. 1 Observation of epithelia and stromal cells in ventral prostate using hematoxylin and eosin staining. **a**: 56-week-old SHR, Spontaneously hypertensive rat; **b**: 56-week-old WKY, Wistar Kyoto rat. (× 200)

was accomplished with 3,3′-diaminobenzidine. The nuclei were then counterstained with hematoxylin. Only manifest cytoplasmic staining was defined as a positive reaction. Negative controls were incubated with normal rabbit serum instead of the primary antibody [10].

Histological analysis of hyperplasia of the prostate

Rats have much more lumen and matrix in the prostate than humans. Thus, the whole weight of the rat ventral lobes does not reflect hyperplasia histologically. Five randomly selected areas from one of bilateral ventral lobes captured by microscopy under 200-fold magnification. The percent areas of epithelium and stroma, the lumen, and matrix were calculated using Image J software (Rasband, W.S., ImageJ, U. S. NIH, Bethesda, Maryland) (Fig. 2). We estimated the total weight of the epithelium and stroma in the ventral lobe adjusted by body weight (ES weight) as follow; (percent area of epithelium and stroma x weight of bilateral ventral lobes)/body weight of rat (mg/g).

Analysis of density of NE cells

We evaluated the density of NE cells in the epithelia of the ventral prostatic ducts (VPd) in a cross section of the urethra. This section, which was 1.5 mm from the bladder contained a urethra, 10 to 16 ventral prostatic ducts (VPd), 32 to 40 dorsolateral prostatic ducts (DLPd), 2 coagulating gland ducts (CGd), 2 seminal vesicle ducts (SVd) and 2 deferent ducts (DD) (Fig. 3). NE cells were distributed in the epithelia of the periurethral ducts and urethra. The density of NE cells in the VPd was calculated as the ratio of serotonin-positive NE cells among the total number of epithelial cells, which was manually counted in high power fields of a microscope (BZ-9000, KEYENCE, Tokyo, Japan).

Statistical analysis

Statistical comparisons were made using the unpaired t-test and Mann-Whitney U-test. $P < 0.05$ was considered to be statistically significant. These analyses were performed using SPSS®, v. 23.0 (SPSS Inc., Chicago, IL).

Results

The weights of the ventral lobes in SHR were significantly lower than in WKY except in rats 28 weeks old, although their body weights were nearly the same (Table 1).

Evaluation of estimated total weight of epithelium and stroma in ventral lobe of the prostate

Image J quantified the areas of the epithelium and stroma, lumen, and matrix in the prostatic ventral lobes of SHR and WKY (Table 2). The percent area of epithelium and stroma in SHR was significantly larger than that of WKY for each age week analyzed. In WKY, the percent area of epithelium and stroma were less than that of the lumen and matrix for all ages.

The ES weights are shown in Fig. 4. Although there were no differences in the ES weights between SHR and WKY at 8, 12 and 16 weeks of age, significant differences were observed at 28 and 56 weeks of age ($p = 0.034$ and $p = 0.014$).

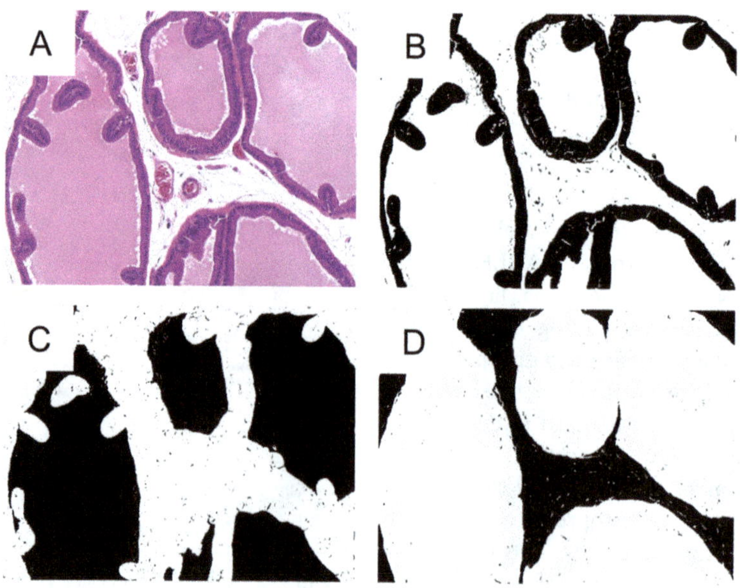

Fig. 2 Histological evaluation of the ventral lobe of the rat prostate. Percent areas of epithelium and stroma, lumen, and matrix in 5 randomly selected areas from one of bilateral ventral lobes were calculated using Image J software. **a**: Hematoxylin and eosin stain; **b**: Black area, epithelium and stroma; **c**: Black area, lumen; **d**: Black area, matrix. (× 200)

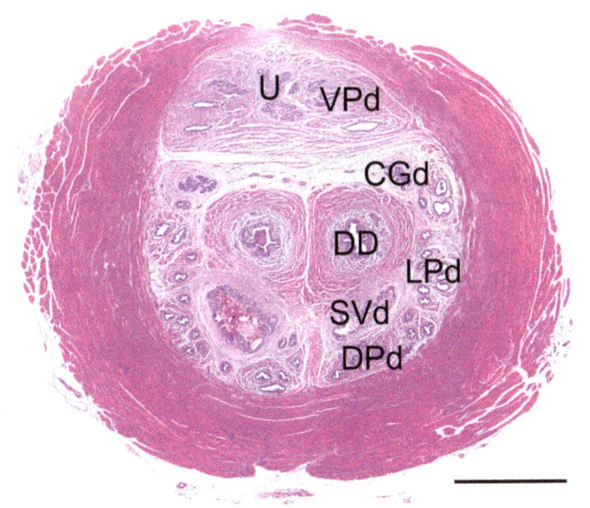

Fig. 3 Cross section of proximal urethra consisting of the periurethral ducts around the urethra. CGd, coagulating gland duct; DD, deferent duct; DPd, dorsal prostatic duct; LPd, lateral prostatic duct; SVd, seminal vesicle duct; U, urethra; VPd, ventral prostatic duct. Scale bar: 1 mm

Density of NE cells in the ventral prostatic ducts

Figure 5 shows immunohistochemical staining of serotonin in the VPd. The density of NE cells in the VPd decreased with aging in the WKY group, whereas it was sustained until 16 weeks of age and then decreased with aging in the SHR group (Fig. 6). The difference in the density between the two groups was greatest at 16 weeks of age.

Discussion

Our previous study using human prostates demonstrated that NE cells were plentiful in the TZ having a small

Table 1 Body weights and weights of ventral lobes in rat

Weight	SHR[a] (*n* = 5)	WKY[b] (*n* = 5)	*P* value
Mean body weight (g) ± S.E.			
8 weeks old	228 ± 9.7	216 ± 5.1	0.521
12 weeks old	314 ± 11.7	298 ± 12.8	0.823
16 weeks old	338 ± 6.6	338 ± 5.8	> 0.999
28 weeks old	378 ± 13.5	396 ± 7.5	0.344
56 weeks old	444 ± 13.3	456 ± 6.9	0.340
Bilateral ventral lobes (mg) ± S.E.			
8 weeks old	203 ± 18.8	303 ± 15.6	0.021
12 weeks old	384 ± 15.5	560 ± 40.0	0.016
16 weeks old	425 ± 10.4	580 ± 38.4	0.008
28 weeks old	595 ± 44.7	772 ± 40.7	0.056
56 weeks old	585 ± 51.7	832 ± 62.2	0.032

[a]Spontaneously hypertensive rat
[b]Wistar Kyoto rat

Table 2 Percent areas of epithelium and stroma, lumen, and matrix of ventral lobes in rat

Percent area (mean ± S.E.)	SHR[a] (*n* = 5)	WKY[b] (*n* = 5)	*P* value
Epithelium and stroma			
8 weeks old	42.7 ± 3.1	28.8 ± 1.9	0.016
12 weeks old	39.5 ± 2.1	24.0 ± 2.1	0.008
16 weeks old	36.3 ± 1.1	24.7 ± 2.6	0.008
28 weeks old	33.2 ± 4.6	21.8 ± 3.4	0.008
56 weeks old	41.8 ± 5.6	22.4 ± 2.5	0.016
Lumen			
8 weeks old	32.3 ± 3.4	41.6 ± 1.6	0.056
12 weeks old	39.1 ± 2.1	48.6 ± 2.3	0.016
16 weeks old	37.1 ± 0.8	48.4 ± 4.6	0.151
28 weeks old	43.0 ± 4.3	51.3 ± 3.8	0.032
56 weeks old	39.1 ± 4.2	44.2 ± 4.1	0.421
Matrix			
8 weeks old	25.0 ± 3.2	29.6 ± 2.0	0.222
12 weeks old	21.3 ± 2.2	27.4 ± 1.8	0.056
16 weeks old	26.6 ± 1.0	26.9 ± 4.1	0.690
28 weeks old	23.8 ± 2.0	26.9 ± 1.7	0.548
56 weeks old	19.1 ± 2.9	33.4 ± 2.9	0.016

[a]Spontaneously hypertensive rat
[b]Wistar Kyoto rat

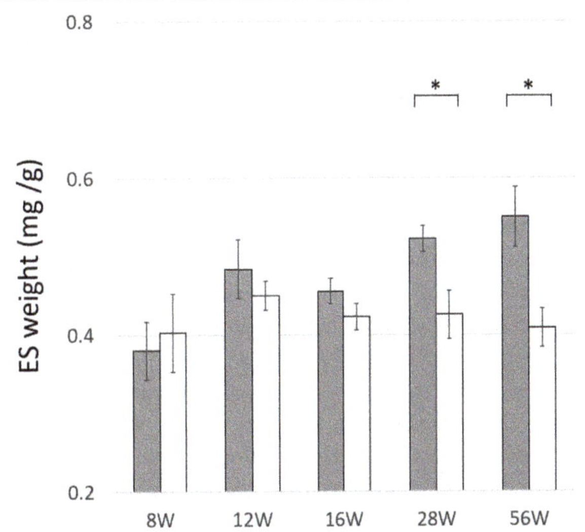

Fig. 4 Estimated total weight of epithelium and stroma in the ventral lobe per body in rats. Grey columns, SHR; white columns, WKY. The estimated total weights of the epithelium and stroma in the ventral lobe per body weight (mean ± S.E.) in SHR vs. WKY were 0.38 ± 0.04 vs. 0.40 ± 0.05 in 8-week old rats ($p = 0.624$), 0.48 ± 0.04 vs. 0.45 ± 0.02 in 12-week old rats ($p = 0.303$), 0.46 ± 0.02 vs. 0.42 ± 0.02 in 16-week old rats ($p = 0.090$), 0.52 ± 0.02 vs. 0.43 ± 0.03 in 28-week old rats ($p = 0.03$) and 0.55 ± 0.04 vs. 0.41 ± 0.02 in 56-week-old rats ($p = 0.014$). Significant differences in weight were observed between SHR and WKY at 28 and 56 weeks of age

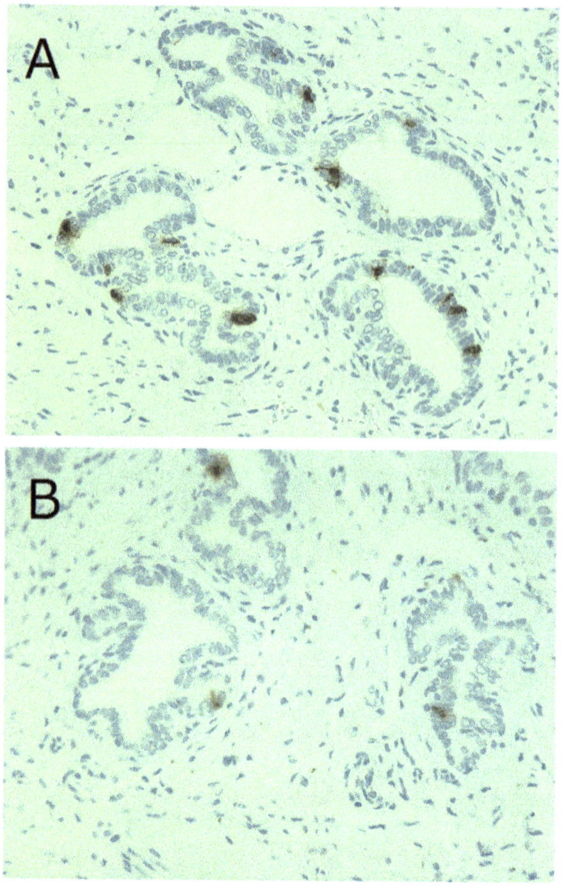

Fig. 5 Immunohistochemical staining of serotonin in the ventral prostatic ducts. Ventral prostatic ducts of (**a**): 16-week-old SHR and (**b**): 16-week-old WKY. (× 400)

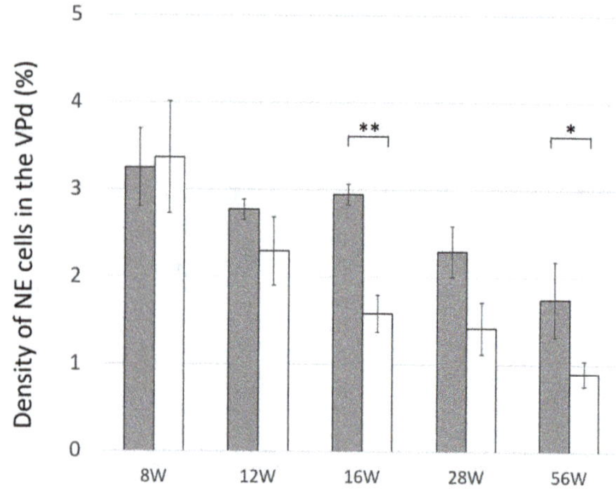

Fig. 6 Density of NE cells in the epithelium of ventral prostatic ducts. Grey columns, SHR; white columns, WKY. The density of serotonin-positive NE cells to all epithelial cells (mean ± SE) (%) in SHR vs. WKY were 3.25 ± 0.44 vs. 3.37 ± 0.64 in 8-week old rats (p = 0.882), 2.77 ± 0.12 vs. 2.30 ± 0.39 in 12-week old rats (p = 0.117), 2.95 ± 0.12 vs. 1.58 ± 0.21 in 16-week old rats ($p < 0.001$), 2.29 ± 0.29 vs. 1.42 ± 0.30 in 28-week old rats (p = 0.069) and 1.75 ± 0.43 vs. 0.90 ± 0.14 in 56-week old rats (p = 0.043). The density of NE cells in the VPd decreased with aging in the WKY group, whereas it was sustained by 16 weeks old, then decreased with aging in the SHR group. There was the most remarkable difference in the density between the two groups at 16 weeks old ($p < 0.001$)

adenomatous nodule compared to the TZ having no adenomatous nodule or a large adenomatous nodule [10]. Thus, we hypothesized that NE cells had an impact on the initial growth of BPH in a paracrine fashion. In the present study using animal models, we found that the density of NE cells in the VPd was much larger in 16-week-old SHR than in WKY rats. After the age of 16 weeks, the difference in the ES weight in the ventral lobes of SHR and WKY became remarkable. Thus, sustained density of NE cells in the VPd preceded development of prostatic hyperplasia. The main factors initiating BPH are not known, although many factors such as chronic inflammation, for instance, which influences the growth of adenoma in the progressive period, have been reported [1]. NE cells may influence the initial growth of prostatic hyperplasia as one of the initiators, although they have negligible or negative impact on it in the progressive period. Carvalho-Dias et al. reported that 5-HT, one of the products by NE cells is decreased in BPH through modulation of androgen receptor [17].

Based on the ES weights in the ventral lobes, the present study showed a progressive degree of prostatic hyperplasia in SHR. The rat prostate contains more fluid in the lumen than the human one, so it is incorrect to consider that the whole weight of the ventral lobes reflects the degree of prostatic hyperplasia because it is easily influenced by fluid weight rather than actual histological weight. In fact, the mean weight of the bilateral ventral lobes in SHR had a tendency to be lower than that of the WKY rat even when the SHR histologically had hyperplasia in the ventral lobes. On the other hand, the ES weight estimated by adjustment of the percent area of the epithelium and stroma, as well as the body weight of the rat, was greater in SHR than in WKY at 28 weeks and older. Although a few reports have examined prostatic hyperplasia in SHR, no report has clarified the beginning of the histological progression of the hyperplasia because they did not examine the histology before 15 weeks of age [16, 18]. We considered that the difference of the ES weight in the ventral lobes between SHR and WKY rats represented the histological progression of hyperplasia in the prostate with aging.

Rats have no NE cells in the ventral lobe, which corresponds to the TZ of the human prostate [12]. NE cells that are present in the periurethral duct work in a paracrine fashion and may have an effect on the epithelial and stromal cells of the ventral lobe via the duct. In the VPd, there are many open-type NE cells that release serotonin into the lumen [12]. Closed-type NE cells, on the other hand, release it into the inter- and subepithelial spaces. The presence of NE cells is restricted to the terminal (periurethral) portion of the tributary ducts of the lateral and ventral lobes, which are located in the initial segment of the pelvic urethra [8]. Therefore, we evaluated the periurethral duct in the portion where VPds join the urethra. Furthermore, it would be appropriate to evaluate the NE cells in the VPd, because NE cells are more frequent in the periurethral ducts than in the peripheral parts of the gland in the human prostate [9].

There are several limitations in the present study. Firstly, we adopted the SHR as a BPH model. Though this is a common model it has a serious drawback in that the SHR predominantly has epithelium in the prostate compared to stroma in the human prostate and the prostate slightly enlarges. However, we have no alternative ideal animal model of BPH. Second, we only used serotonin as an immunohistochemical marker to evaluate NE cells. It is impossible to detect all NE cells in the prostate even though multiple NE markers are used because, of the more than 200 secretory products, there is no universal one that every NE cell secretes [5]. In the present study, we selected serotonin as a representative NE marker according to previous reports using rats [12]. Finally, a critical limitation of the present study is that we do not know how prostatic NE cells work for the development of prostatic hyperplasia, because we could not demonstrate direct evidence to support the NE cells in the VPd promoted the growth of the ventral lobes which are located above the VPd. However, we believe the present study, which demonstrates that sustained density of NE cells in the VPd precedes the development of prostatic hyperplasia in rats, provides a clue suggesting that NE cells have an impact on the initial growth of BPH as we hypothesized in our previous human study [10].

Conclusions

NE cells may have an impact on the initial growth of BPH. However, further studies are needed to clarify their function in BPH.

Abbreviations

BPH: Benign prostatic hyperplasia; CGd: Coagulating gland ducts; DD: Deferent ducts; DLPd: Dorsolateral prostatic ducts; ES weight: Estimated total weight of the epithelium and stroma in the ventral lobes adjusted by body weight; NE: Neuroendocrine; SHR: Spontaneously hypertensive rats; SVd: Seminal vesicle ducts; TZ: Transition zone; VPd: Ventral prostatic ducts; WKY: Wistar-Kyoto rats

Acknowledgements

The authors thank to Mr. Kim Barrymore for advice on English usage of this article. All authors have permission to use their full names.

Authors' contributions

YK was a major contributor in writing the manuscript. FF and NM made the contribution to the design of the work. YK, KI, KK and KH contributed to the analysis and the interpretation of data. YK have drafted the work and NM substantively revised it. All authors read and approved the final manuscript.

References

1. Robert G, Descazeaud A, Nicolaïew N, Terry S, Sirab N, Vacherot F, et al. Inflammation in benign prostatic hyperplasia: a 282 patients' immunohistochemical analysis. Prostate. 2009;69:1774–80.
2. Mishra VC, Allen DJ, Nicolaou C, Sharif H, Hudd C, Karim OM, et al. Does intraprostatic inflammation have a role in the pathogenesis and progression of benign prostatic hyperplasia? BJU Int. 2007;100:327–31.
3. Roberts RO, Jacobson DJ, Rhodes T, Klee GG, Leiber MM, Jacobsen SJ. Serum sex hormones and measures of benign prostatic hyperplasia. Prostate. 2004;61:124–31.
4. Bonkhoff H. Neuroendocrine cells in benign and malignant prostate tissue: morphogenesis, proliferation, and androgen receptor status. Prostate Suppl. 1998;8:18–22.
5. Xue Y, Smedts F, Verhofstad A, Debruyne F, de la Rosette J, Schalken J. Cell kinetics of prostate exocrine and neuroendocrine epithelium and their differential interrelationship: new perspectives. Prostate Suppl. 1998;8:62–73.
6. Masumori N, Thomas TZ, Chaurand P, Case T, Paul M, Kasper S, et al. A probasin-large T antigen transgenic mouse line develops prostate adenocarcinoma and neuroendocrine carcinoma with metastatic potential. Cancer Res. 2001;61:2239–49.
7. Jin RJ, Wang Y, Masumori N, Ishii K, Tsukamoto T, Shappell SB, et al. NE-10 neuroendocrine cancer promotes the LNCaP xenograft growth in castrated mice. Cancer Res. 2004;64:5489–95.
8. Uchida K, Masumori N, Takahashi A, Itoh N, Kato K, Matusik RJ, et al. Murine androgen-independent neuroendocrine carcinoma promotes metastasis of human prostate cancer cell line LNCaP. Prostate. 2006;66:536–45.
9. Cockett AT, di Sant'Agnese PA, Gopinath P, Schoen SR, Abrahamsson PA. Relationship of neuroendocrine cells of prostate and serotonin to benign prostatic hyperplasia. Urology. 1993;42:512–9.
10. Kyoda Y, Ichihara K, Hashimoto K, Kobayashi K, Fukuta F, Masumori N. Distribution of neuroendocrine cells in the transition zone of the prostate. Adv Urol. 2017;2017:8541697.
11. Nascimento-Viana JB, Carvalho AR, Nasciutti LE, Alcántara-Hernández R, Chagas-Silva F, Souza PA, et al. New multi-target antagonists of α1A-, α1D-adrenoceptors and 5-HT1A receptors reduce human hyperplastic prostate cell growth and the increase of Intraurethral pressure. J Pharmacol Exp Ther. 2016;356:212–22.
12. Aumuller G, Doll A, Wennemuth G, Dizeyi N, Abrahamsson PA, Wilhelm B. Regional distribution of neuroendocrine cells in the urogenital duct system of the male rat. Prostate. 2012;72:326–37.
13. Rodríguez R, Pozuelo JM, Martín R, Henriques-Gil N, Haro M, Arriazu R, et al. Presence of neuroendocrine cells during postnatal development in rat prostate: immunohistochemical, molecular, and quantitative study. Prostate. 2003;57:176–85.
14. Golomb E, Rosenzweig N, Eilam R, Abramovici A. Spontaneous hyperplasia of the ventral lobe of the prostate in aging genetically hypertensive rats. J Androl. 2000;21:58–64.
15. Lujan M, Ferruelo A, Paez A, Moreno A, Berenguer A. Prostate apoptosis after doxazosin treatment in the spontaneous hypertensive rat model. BJU Int. 2004;93:410–4.
16. Yamashita M, Zhang X, Shiraishi T, Uetsuki H, Kakehi Y. Determination of percent area density of epithelial and stromal components in development of prostatic hyperplasia in spontaneously hypertensive rats. Urology. 2003;61:484–9.
17. Carvalho-Dias E, Miranda A, Martinho O, Mota P, Costa Â, Nogueira-Silva C, et al. Serotonin regulates prostate growth through androgen receptor modulation. Sci Rep. 2017;7:15428.
18. Zhang X, Na Y, Guo Y. Biologic feature of prostatic hyperplasia developed in spontaneously hypertensive rats. Urology. 2004;63:983–8.

7

Epidemic investigation of benign prostatic obstruction with coexistin overactive bladder in Shanghai Pudong New Area and its impact on the health-related quality of life

Qing-Tong Yi*, Min Gong*, Chu-Hong Chen, Wei Hu and Ru-Jian Zhu

Abstract

Background: We aimed to investigate the prevalence, relative risk factors, and the impact on the health-related quality of life (HRQoL) of benign prostatic obstruction (BPO) with coexisting overactive bladder (OAB) in men aged over 50 and living in Shanghai Pudong New Area.

Methods: Using a multi-stage sampling and descriptive epidemiological method, 1632 men were selected from among the general population. Participants completed an evaluation of lower urinary tracts symptoms (LUTS), including international prostate symptom score (IPSS) and quality of life (QoL) questionnaires. Erectile function was assessed using the International Index of Erectile Function-5 (IIEF-5) questionnaire. In addition, the Overactive Bladder Symptom Score (OABSS) and King's health questionnaire (KHQ) were used to assess the impact of BPO with coexisting OAB on the HRQoL. Maximum flow rate (Q_{max}), postvoid residual urine volume (PVR) and prostate-specific antigen (PSA) were also recorded.

Results: A total of 1476 men with complete data were analyzed. The overall prevalence of BPO with coexisting OAB was 39.6%. Age and prostate volume were associated risk factors for BPO with coexisting OAB. In addition, BPO with coexisting OAB negatively impacted the HRQoL, with increased IPSS, QoL, OABSS, and KHQ scores and decreased IIEF-5 scores compared to that in patients with BPO without OAB.

Conclusions: Q_{max}, PVR and serum PSA did not predict whether the patients had a combined BPO + OAB or not. The prostate volume and age were associated risk factors for BPO with coexisting OAB. BPO is a progressive disease and may be one of the risk factors for OAB.

Keywords: Benign prostatic obstruction, Epidemic investigation, Health-related quality of life, Overactive bladder

Background

Benign prostatic obstruction (BPO) is one of the most common urinary disorders leading to lower urinary tracts symptoms (LUTS) in middle-aged and elderly men. LUTS can be divided into storage, voiding and post-micturition symptoms. Overactive bladder (OAB) features urinary urgency, usually with frequency and nocturia, and with or without urge urinary incontinence [1, 2]. Currently, the relationship between BPO and OAB remains unclear, and large epidemic investigations of BPO with coexisting OAB are lacking worldwide. Therefore, we performed a sample survey of men aged ≥50 years in Shanghai Pudong New Area, to investigate the prevalence of BPO with coexisting OAB. In addition, we investigated the associated risk factors and the impact of BPO with coexisting OAB on the health-related quality of life (HRQoL).

BPO commonly coexists with OAB and consequently decreases the QoL in men. The following factors should be considered in the study of patients with lower urinary tract function: observations of patients (symptoms), quantification of symptoms, physician's observations (anatomy, function and compliance), QoL measures, and socioeconomic evaluations [3].

* Correspondence: yiqt926@sina.com; mg813@hotmail.com
Department of Urology, Shanghai Pudong Hospital, Fudan University Pudong Medical Center, Shanghai, China

Patient-reported outcomes (PROs) refer to any report from the patient regarding their health and treatment status. It includes reports of patient symptoms, physical, psychological and social functional status, healthy behavior, different tendencies expressed by patients for different treatments, a desire to participate (or not participate) in a treatment, patient satisfaction with treatment, doctor-patient communication and cooperative treatment [4]. PROs can accurately reflect the subjective feelings of patients with OAB, and can be used to assess the impact of OAB on the QoL of patients and treatment response [5]. BPO and OAB questionnaires, including international prostate symptom score (IPSS), QoL, Overactive Bladder Symptom Score (OABSS) and OAB scale are commonly used in clinical practice. The IPSS and OABSS mainly reflect changes in the symptoms of LUTS, while the QoL reflects the degree of suffering. The OABSS scoring table includes four OAB-related symptom issues (urinary urgency, frequency, nocturia and urge urinary incontinence) and the total score is sum these individual item scores [6]. Furthermore, the OABSS score is highly correlated with the IPSS score.

The HRQoL is an assessment of how an individual's well-being may be affected over time by a disease, disability or disorder. The current concept of the HRQoL acknowledges that individuals place their actual situation in relation to their personal expectations. King's health questionnaire (KHQ), a kind of PROs, has high validity and reliability and is now widely accepted as a useful instrument for evaluating the HRQoL of OAB patients [7]. KHQ consists of two subscales: HRQoL and lower urinary symptoms severity. HRQoL consists of nine domains: general health, incontinence impact and seven limitations including role, physical, social, personal, emotion, sleep/energy, and severity measures. Lower urinary symptoms severity scale contains ten questions and the higher the score, the more severe the symptoms [8]. In the present study, the WHO-QOL cross-cultural quality of life questionnaire translation method was used to translate the original KHQ into Chinese [9, 10].

Participants were asked to complete questionnaires which mentioned above regarding personal information, urination, sexual function, and the QoL.

Methods

Subjects and sampling methods

This survey was a cross-sectional study conducted from October 2012 to September 2016. Using standard formula, we calculated the sample size based on a two-sided t-test with a significance level of 5%. According to the total prevalence rate of benign prostatic hyperplasia (BPH) in males over 50 years old in Pudong New Area (62.9%) [11], we calculated the sample size to be 1434. Permanent residents aged 50 years or more from 10 subdistricts/towns in Pudong New Area who met BPO diagnostic criteria were included. A multi-stage stratified random sampling was used to select the geographic regions; three-stage sampling including district-subdistrict, town-committee or village was used. Ten subdistricts or towns in Pudong New Area were randomly selected; four neighborhood or village committees were then randomly selected from each selected subdistrict or town. Patients diagnosed with BPO were chosen according to the residents' health records at the community health centers. The neighborhood/village committee, as a unit, informed the selected patients of the study. Selected patients with voluntary participation were finally enrolled.

The inclusion criteria were as follows meanwhile: the presence of voiding or/and post-micturition symptoms, prostate volume ≥ 25 mL on transrectal ultrasonography, maximum urinary flow rate (Qmax) ≤15 mL/s. A series of tests were conducted in the community health centers, including a medical history inquiry, physical examination, urinalysis, prostate-specific antigen (PSA) assessment, imaging of the urinary system, and uroflowmetry, to exclude other disorders that could cause LUTS (e.g., neurogenic bladder dysfunction, detrusor overactivity, detrusor sphincter dyssynergia, foreign body in the bladder or urethra, bladder neoplasms, prostatic neoplasms, vesical calculus, bladder neck contracture, small capacity bladder, urethral stricture, chronic pelvic pain syndrome, urinary tract infection, etc.). Exclusion criteria included patients of BPO with no symptoms, a post-void residual urine volume of more than 50 mL, severe mental disorder (except anxiety or depression), previous prostate or bladder surgery, and the use of medications affecting urination.

Inquiry content and data collection

In addition to the clinical examination, participants completed a field questionnaire survey, which collected data regarding personal information, urination, sexual function, and the QoL. LUTS severity was evaluated using IPSS and QoL questionnaires. IIEF-5 was used to assess penile erectile function. For patients with BPO and coexisting OAB, the OABSS and KHQ were used to assess the impact of OAB on the QoL. Questionnaires were checked to ensure completeness and were supplemented with the examination results.

Diagnostic criteria of BPO with coexisting OAB

Patients with BPO who had OAB symptoms were defined as BPO with coexisting OAB. The OAB diagnostic criteria were as follows: total OABSS ≥3 and urgent micturition ≥2, with duration of more than 3 months. Based on the IPSS and OABSS, the patients were divided into a mild (IPSS score 0~7 or OABSS score 3~5), moderate (IPSS score 8~19 or OABSS score 6~11), and severe groups (IPSS score 20~35 or OABSS score 12~15) [6, 12].

Quality control

All investigators were professionally trained. The questionnaires were reviewed twice and 1% of patients were selected for a revisit. The database was built using excel software with double entry and was subjected to verification and logic error checking. When any problems were detected, the original records were checked and the corresponding contents were revised as appropriate.

Statistics

Statistical analyses were performed using SPSS 18.0 software (SPSS Inc. Chicago). Categorical variables are described as numbers and percentages. Group comparisons were performed using the chi-squared test for classification data and the t-test and analysis of variance for continuous data. For quantitative variables with non-normal distribution, group comparisons were performed using Mann–Whitney U test. Binomial logistic regression analyses were performed to determine the risk factors of BPO with coexisting OAB. *P* value < 0.05 was considered statistically significant.

Ethical approval was given by the medical ethics committee of Shanghai Pudong Hospital and informed consent was obtained from the participants in all cases.

Results

General characteristics of the study population and prevalence of BPO with coexisting OAB

A total of 1632 participants were recruited from 10 subdistricts or towns in Shanghai Pudong New Area during October 2012 to September 2016. A complete dataset was achieved in 1476 participants; 156 participants were dropped due to incomplete information. A total of 697 participants lived in cities, while 779 lived in the suburbs. General characteristics of the study population were shown in Tables 1 and 2. The prostate volume, the IPSS and QOL scores were significantly higher, and the IIEF-5 score was significantly lower, in patients with BPO and coexisting OAB compared to those in patients without coexisting OAB($P < 0.05$) (Table 1).

The overall prevalence of BPO with coexisting OAB was 39.6% (584/1476) in men over 50 years old in Shanghai Pudong New Area. The prevalence of BPO with coexisting OAB increased with age, with a significantly higher prevalence in the 70–79, 80–89, and ≥ 90 years age groups compared to that in the 50–59 years age group ($P < 0.05$). In addition, a higher prevalence of BPO with coexisting OAB was observed in participants with anxiety-depression compared to that in normal participants ($P < 0.05$). Moreover, an increasing trend in the prevalence of BPO with coexisting OAB was observed in participants with higher BMI or diabetes, though both of which have no significant different (Table 2).

Comparison among different age groups in BPO with coexisting OAB

IPSS, QoL, OABSS, and KQH scores significantly increased while the IIEF-5 score significantly decreased with increasing age ($P < 0.05$). However, there were no significant differences among different age groups in aspects of prostate volume, serum PSA, testosterone, Qmax, PVR and BMI ($P > 0.05$). The QoL items most affected included the general health status, severity of urinary problems, and sleep/energy. In all, the quality of life of patients with BPO with coexisting OAB decreased with increasing age (Table 3).

Impact of LUTS severity on HRQoL in patients with BPO and coexisting OAB

With increased LUTS severity, IPSS, QoL, OABSS, and KHQ scores increased, while IIEF-5 scores decreased ($P < 0.05$). Thus, the QoL in patients with BPO and coexisting OAB declined with LUTS severity. The QoL items most affected included the general health

Table 1 General characteristics of the study population

Variable	BPO without OAB (*n* = 892)	BPO with coexisting OAB (*n* = 584)	*P* value
Prostate volume (mL)	55.6 ± 20.7	62.7 ± 26.5	0.005
Serum PSA (ng/mL)	3.6 ± 0.8	3.7 ± 0.7	0.624
Testosterone (nmol/L)	14.2 ± 4.6	13.9 ± 4.3	0.196
Qmax (mL/s)	10.2 ± 3.9	10.1 ± 3.8	0.162
PVR (mL)	19.8 ± 17.3	20.5 ± 18.7	0.820
BMI (kg/m2)	24.3 ± 3.7	24.6 ± 4.1	0.461
IPSS (score)	19.2 ± 6.8	23.5 ± 7.3	0.000
QoL (score)	3.9 ± 0.9	4.6 ± 1.2	0.000
IIEF-5 (score)	9.9 ± 2.3	9.0 ± 1.7	0.036

BPO Benign prostatic obstruction, *OAB* Overactive bladder syndrome, *PSA* Prostate-specific antigen, *Qmax* Maximum flow rate, *PVR* Postvoid residual urine volume, *IPSS* International prostate symptom score, *QoL* Quality of life, *IIEF-5* International index of erectile function-5, *OABSS* Overactive bladder symptom score

Table 2 Prevalence of BPO with coexisting OAB

Group	Sample size (n)	BPO with coexisting OAB (n)	Prevalence (%)	OR	*P* Value
Age (years)					
50~	288	81	28.1	1	
60~	363	124	34.2	1.33	0.142
70~	545	243	44.6	2.10	0.002
80~	247	119	48.2	2.37	0.002
90~	33	17	51.5	2.72	0.014
BMI (kg/m^2)					
< 24	381	167	43.8	1	
24~	337	154	45.7	1.07	0.808
≥ 27	317	152	47.9	1.18	0.552
Diabetes					
No	1255	488	38.9	1	
Yes	221	96	43.4	1.21	0.209
Emotional State					
Normal	1361	521	38.3	1	
Anxiety/ depression	115	63	54.8	1.95	0.036
Total	1476	584			

BMI Body mass index, *BPO* Benign prostatic obstruction, *OAB* Overactive bladder, *OR* Odds ratio

perception, severity of the micturition problem, and sleep/energy status (Table 4).

Risk factors of BPO with coexisting OAB

Univariate logistic regression analyses revealed that the prevalence of BPO with coexisting OAB increased with the age, prostate volume, PVR and serum PSA ($P < 0.05$). The prevalence of BPO with coexisting OAB was higher in participants with diabetes mellitus. The prevalence of BPO with coexisting OAB was 1.09 times higher in obese participants (47.9%; BMI ≥27 kg/m^2) compared to that in normal participants (43.8%; BMI < 24 kg/m^2) (Table 5).

A multivariate logistic regression analysis revealed that BPO with existing OAB was associated with the age and prostate volume ($P < 0.05$). With increasing age or prostate volume, LUTS, IPSS, QoL, and OABSS scores increased, while IIEF-5 scores decreased (Table 6).

Discussion

LUTS have traditionally been related to bladder outlet obstruction (BOO), which is often caused by benign prostatic enlargement (BPE) resulting from the histologic condition of BPH. BPO and OAB are common clinical and public health concerns, causing male urinary dysfunction and affecting the QoL, whether occurring alone or in combination [2, 13, 14]. OAB occurs in 11.8% of adults over 18 years old, and LUTS morbidity and severity increase along with age [15]. The symptoms of OAB are the most bothersome symptoms in patients with LUTS induced by BPH and the effect of LUTS during the urine storage period is greater than that during the urination period [16]. In addition, BPH-related LUTS are one of the main reasons for a decline in patient QoL, and are associated with increased prostate volume which leads to BOO [13, 14]. It has been reported that 30 to 60% of cases with BOO caused by BPO will appear as OAB symptoms, and 30 to 40% of cases of BOO combined with OAB still show up as OAB symptoms after the release of BOO [17]. Moreover, OAB morbidity is positively correlated with the degree of BOO [18]. Thus, BPH, OAB, and LUTS are closely related to each other, and all are positively correlated with age.

At present, large-sample epidemiological studies of the prevalence of BPO with coexisting OAB and related factors are lacking. In our study, an epidemiological survey of the BPO population aged ≥50 years in Pudong New Area was conducted using a multistage, stratified, random sampling method to better understand the prevalence of BPO with coexisting OAB, the related risk factors and its impact on the QoL. The results demonstrated that the overall prevalence of BPO with coexisting OAB was 39.6% (584/1476), close to previous reports [18]. Interestingly, we found a higher prevalence of BPO with coexisting OAB in participants with anxiety-depression. This suggested that we should pay attention to the mental health of patients and necessary psychological interventions could be performed to treat patients with anxiety and depression to improve overall efficacy. Furthermore, those who had diabetes or obesity had an increasing trend in the prevalence of BPO with

Table 3 Comparisons among different age groups in BPO with coexisting OAB ($\overline{x} \pm s$)

Age Group	50~years (*n* = 81)	60~years (*n* = 124)	70~years (*n* = 243)	80~year (*n* = 119)	90~years (*n* = 17)
Prostate volume (mL)	57.7 ± 24.1	56.9 ± 16.3	62.8 ± 26.5	69.6 ± 34.1	77.1 ± 20.4
P Value		0.214	0.235	0.358	0.347
Serum PSA (ng/mL)	3.2 ± 0.7	3.4 ± 0.6	3.7 ± 0.9	3.9 ± 1.2	4.2 ± 1.1
P Value		0.541	0.512	0.336	0.357
Testosterone (nmol/L)	17.2 ± 6.4	16.0 ± 5.7	12.7 ± 5.2	9.2 ± 3.9	7.1 ± 3.2
P Value		0.544	0.112	0.054	0.05
Qmax (mL/s)	11.5 ± 4.2	10.1 ± 3.4	10.1 ± 3.8	9.5 ± 4.1	8.8 ± 3.4
P Value		0.337	0.463	0.425	0.372
PVR (mL)	10.0 ± 4.2	12.6 ± 5.3	18.4 ± 6.7	26.8 ± 8.2	29.3 ± 8.8
P Value		0.130	0.688	0.393	0.246
BMI (kg/m2)	24.3 ± 3.6	25.2 ± 4.0	24.7 ± 4.2	23.9 ± 3.9	25.5 ± 2.3
P Value		0.051	0.221	0.768	0.095
IPSS	9.1 ± 3.3	14.3 ± 2.7	18.6 ± 3.9	24.7 ± 5.4	27.8 ± 6.6
P Value		0.031	0.028	0.000	0.001
QoL	4.2 ± 0.7	4.4 ± 0.7	4.7 ± 0.9	5.0 ± 1.2	5.4 ± 1.5
P Value		0.042	0.040	0.038	0.001
IIEF-5	10.5 ± 1.4	9.2 ± 0.9	7.7 ± 0.7	6.1 ± 0.8	5.6 ± 1.0
P Value		0.040	0.003	0.000	0.000
OABSS	7.2 ± 3.1	8.4 ± 3.6	9.1 ± 3.4	10.7 ± 4.0	11.6 ± 3.7
P Value		0.046	0.009	0.000	0.000
KHQ	23.4 ± 6.5	23.2 ± 7.3	28.6 ± 9.1	30.0 ± 9.5	28.7 ± 10.6
P Value		0.988	0.042	0.028	0.005
General health status	25.6 ± 8.9	25.3 ± 8.4	28.4 ± 9.7	28.6 ± 7.7	27.0 ± 10.6
P Value		0.596	0.048	0.000	0.000
Severity of urinary problems	29.4 ± 9.1	29.4 ± 10.2	29.5 ± 9.1	31.3 ± 9.7	26.5 ± 8.9
P Value		0.735	0.500	0.548	0.681
Role limitations	18.6 ± 8.8	18.3 ± 6.2	18.2 ± 5.9	19.8 ± 7.7	19.1 ± 7.5
P Value		0.996	0.451	0.007	0.633
Physical limitations	3.6 ± 2.0	3.2 ± 2.1	2.9 ± 1.5	3.2 ± 2.6	3.3 ± 1.8
P Value		0.793	0.659	0.594	0.771
Social limitations	16.9 ± 7.1	18.3 ± 7.9	19.7 ± 9.5	18.8 ± 9.1	18.9 ± 7.7
P Value		0.009	0.048	0.006	0.011
Personal relationships	2.2 ± 0.9	2.3 ± 0.9	2.2 ± 0.9	2.3 ± 1.0	2.2 ± 1.0
P Value		0.218	0.500	0.17	0.500
Emotions	8.3 ± 5.1	7.5 ± 3.7	6.9 ± 3.7	9.3 ± 5.3	7.0 ± 2.9
P Value		0.633	0.742	0.564	0.530
Sleep/Energy	29.8 ± 11.5	29.0 ± 9.3	37.5 ± 11.3	34.0 ± 9.8	33.5 ± 7.5
P Value		0.707	0.000	0.000	0.001
Coping urination problems	14.8 ± 4.8	15.5 ± 6.7	18.4 ± 8.0	15.9 ± 5.1	18.4 ± 6.1
P Value		0.467	0.001	0.058	0.000

BPO Benign prostatic obstruction, *OAB* Overactive bladder syndrome, *PSA* Prostate-specific antigen, Q_{max} Maximum flow rate, *PVR* Postvoid residual urine volume, *IPSS* International prostate symptom score, *QoL* Quality of life, *IIEF-5* International index of erectile function-5, *OABSS* Overactive bladder symptom score, *KHQ* King's health questionnaire. *P* Value vs 50~ years

Table 4 The impact of LUTS severity on the HRQoL in patients with BPO and coexisting OAB ($\bar{x} \pm s$)

Impact on HRQoL (score)	Mild LUTS (*n* = 227)	Moderate LUTS (*n* = 254)	Severe LUTS (*n* = 103)
IPSS	5.4 ± 2.2	14.7 ± 3.5	26.3 ± 6.7
P Value		0.000	0.000
QoL	3.3 ± 0.5	4.6 ± 0.7	5.4 ± 1.1
P Value		0.000	0.000
IIEF-5	10.5 ± 1.4	7.7 ± .07	5.6 ± 1.0
P Value		0.017	0.009
OABSS	3.6 ± 1.3	9.5 ± 3.2	12.8 ± 3.9
P Value		0.036	0.012
KHQ	21.7 ± 6.3	26.8 ± 8.5	30.9 ± 11.4
P Value		0.001	0.000
General health status	20.4 ± 7.2	25.9 ± 9.5	28.3 ± 10.9
P Value		0.002	0.021
Severity of urinary problems	22.5 ± 11.6	27.6 ± 8.5	30.5 ± 9.2
P Value		0.001	0.001
Role limitations	13.8 ± 7.9	16.2 ± 8.3	19.9 ± 7.8
P Value		0.000	0.000
Physical limitations	2.6 ± 1.9	2.9 ± 1.5	3.3 ± 1.8
P Value		0.654	0.728
Social limitations	15.2 ± 7.1	17.8 ± 9.2	19.2 ± 7.9
P Value		0.000	0.000
Personal relationships	1.7 ± 0.7	2.3 ± 0.9	2.1 ± 0.9
P Value		0.059	0.633
Emotions	7.3 ± 4.6	7.7 ± 3.9	8.9 ± 3.2
P Value		0.742	0.684
Sleep/Energy	20.8 ± 7.5	28.3 ± 8.7	33.9 ± 11.6
P Value		0.008	0.001
Coping urination problems	12.7 ± 4.4	16.4 ± 8.0	18.8 ± 6.7
P Value		0.024	0.018

BPO Benign prostatic obstruction, *OAB* Overactive bladder syndrome, *IPSS* International prostate symptom score, *QoL* Quality of life, *IIEF-5* International index of erectile function-5, *OABSS* Overactive bladder symptom score, *KHQ* King's health questionnaire. *P* Value vs mild LUTS

Table 5 Univariate regression analysis of risk factors for BPO with coexisting OAB

Variable	B	SE	P	OR	EXP(B)95%CI
Age	0.002	0.006	0.000	1.032	[1.016,1.4321]
Prostate volume	0.215	0.053	0.000	1.013	[1.008,1.375]
Q_{max}	0.028	0.129	0.670	0.990	[0.755,1.252]
PVR	0.005	0.005	0.000	1.010	[1.006,1.016]
Serum PSA	0.017	0.104	0.000	1.040	[1.007,1.426]
Testosterone	0.500	0.447	0.650	0.973	[0.253,1.458]
Diabetes	0.025	0.138	0.200	1.213	[0.794,1.357]
BMI Level	0.098	0.109	0.280	1.084	[0.891,1.373]

Q_{max} Maximum urine flow rate, *PVR* Postvoid residual urine volume, *PSA* Prostate specific antigen, *BMI* Body mass index, *BPO* Benign prostatic obstruction, *OAB* Overactive bladder syndrome, *OR* Odds ratio

Table 6 Multivariate logistic regression analysis of risk factors for BPO with coexisting OAB

Variable	B	SE	P	OR	EXP(B)95%CI
Age	0.047	0.010	0.000	1.049	[1.012,1.524]
Prostate volume	0.010	0.004	0.011	1.010	[1.003,1.013]
Q_{max}	0.019	0.024	0.433	1.019	[0.779,1.318]
BMI	0.023	0.026	0.372	1.023	[0.746,1.425]
Anxiety	0.205	0.370	0.579	1.227	[0.980,1.336]
Diabetes	0.275	0.970	0.354	1.316	[0.825,1.344]

Q_{max} Maximum urine flow rate, *BMI* Body mass index, *BPO* Benign prostatic obstruction, *OAB* Overactive bladder syndrome. Variable levels: Diabetes: Yes = 1, No = 0; BMI: BMI < 24 kg/m^2 = 1, 24 ≤ BMI < 27 kg/m^2 = 2, ≥27 kg/m^2 = 3. *SE* Standard error, *OR* Odds ratio coexisting OAB, indicating that reducing weight and controlling blood sugar may help prevent and reduce the occurrence of BPO with coexisting OAB.

Previously reported risk factors for the clinical progression of BPH include age, serum PSA, prostate volume, Q_{max}, PVR, IPSS, chronic inflammation of the prostate, metabolic syndrome, intravesical prostatic protrusion, prostate transition zone volume, and transition zone index [19–25]. The etiology of OAB and its correlation with BPO remains unclear. There are many factors affecting the occurrence and development of BPH, OAB and LUTS. The present results showed that IPSS, QoL scores, prostate volume, PVR and LUTS increased with increasing age in patients with BPO, while the Q_{max} and IIEF-5 score decreased. In addition, BMI and IPSS and QoL scores were higher while IIEF-5 scores were lower, in patients with BPO and coexisting OAB compared to that in patients with BPO only. In contrast, there was no significant difference in prostate volume, Q_{max}, PVR, serum PSA, and testosterone levels between the two groups. These findings indicated that Q_{max}, PVR and serum PSA did not predict whether the patients had a combined BPO + OAB or not. In addition, the prostate volume and age were associated risk factors for BPO with coexisting OAB. Thus, we believe that BPO is a progressive disease and may be one of the risk factors for OAB.

The present results showed that the QoL items affected by BPO with coexisting OAB most were those regarding the general health status, the severity of the urinary problems, and sleep/energy. With an increase in LUTS severity, the IPSS, QoL, OABSS and KHQ scores increased, while the Q_{max} and IIEF-5 scores decreased. Age and prostate volume are not only risk factors for BPO with coexisting OAB, but are also for sexual dysfunction. Moreover, LUTS affects sexual function, including sexual desire, erectile function, ejaculation status and sexual satisfaction, with a positive correlation between the severity of LUTS and sexual dysfunction [26]. Thus, BPO, OAB, and LUTS are independent risk factors for sexual dysfunction. Among LUTS, those with the most impact on the sexual function of patients with BPO, were nocturnal polyuria, dysuria and frequent micturition.

The treatment goal of BPO with coexisting OAB is to improve the clinical symptoms and QoL. All men with LUTS should be formally assessed prior to any allocation of treatment in order to establish symptom severity classification. Treatment can be tailored according to the severity of disease and individualized for cost-effective management [27].

There were several limitations in the study. There is evidence to suggest that prostate volume less than 25 ml can still have significant obstruction and intravesical prostatic protrusion is a better and more reliable predictor of BPO [28, 29]. However, we did not record this data. The samples included cannot cover all patients (sampling bias) and a systematic error due to distortions or incompleteness in memory may exist (memory bias).

Conclusions

In summary, Q_{max}, PVR and serum PSA did not predict whether the patients had a combined BPO + OAB or not. The prostate volume and age were associated risk factors for BPO with coexisting OAB. BPO is a progressive disease and may be one of the risk factors for OAB. All men with LUTS should be formally assessed and treatment can be tailored according to the symptom severity classification.

Abbreviations

BOO: Bladder outlet obstruction; BPE: Benign prostatic enlargement; BPH: Benign prostatic hyperplasia; BPO: Benign prostatic obstruction; HRQoL: Health-related quality of life; IIEF-5: International Index of Erectile Function-5; IPSS: International prostate symptom score; KHQ: King's health questionnaire; LUTS: Lower urinary tracts symptoms; OAB: Overactive bladder; OABSS: Overactive Bladder Symptom Score; PROs: Patient-reported outcomes; PSA: Prostate-specific antigen; PVR: Postvoid residual urine volume; Q_{max}: Maximum flow rate

Acknowledgements

None.

Authors' contributions

Q-TY: Study design, project development and manuscript drafting. MG: Study design, project development and data collection. C-HC: Project development and data collection. WH: Project development and data collection. R-JZ: Project development and data collection. All authors have read and approved the manuscript.

References

1. Wein AJ, Rovner ES. Definition and epidemiology of overactive bladder. Urology. 2002;60(1):7.
2. Abrams P, Cardozo L, Fall M, Griffiths D, Rosier P, Ulmsten U, Kerrebroeck PV, Victor A, Wein A. The standardization of terminology of lower urinary tract function: report from the standardisation subcommittee of the International Continence Society. Neurourol Urodyn. 2002;21(2):167–78.
3. Mattiasson A, Djurhuus JC, Fonda D, Lose G, Nordling J, Stöhrer M. Standardization of outcome studies in patients with lower urinary tract dysfunction: a report on general principles from the standardisation committee of the international continence society. Neurourol Urodyn. 1998; 17(3):249–53.
4. Bradley C, Psychol C. Patient-reported outcome measures: use in medical product development to support labeling claims FDA draft guidance or industry 2006. Health Qual Life Outcomes. 2006;4(1):79.
5. Doward LC, Mckenna SP. Defining patient-reported outcomes. Value Health. 2004;7(S1):S4.
6. Homma Y, Yoshida M, Seki N, Yokoyama O, Kakizaki H, Gotoh M, Yamanishi T, Yamaguchi O, Takeda M, Nishizawa O. Symptom assessment tool for overactive bladder syndrome--overactive bladder symptom score. Urology. 2006;68(2):318–23.
7. Duckett JR, Hall S. A new questionnaire to assess the quality of life of urinary incontinent women. Br J Obstet Gynaecol. 1997;104(12):1374–9.
8. Reese PR, Pleil AM, Okano GJ, Kelleher CJ. Multinational study of reliability and validity of the King's health questionnaire in patients with overactive bladder. Qual Life Res. 2003;12(4):427–42.
9. Guillemin F, Bombardier C, Beaton D. Cross-cultural adaptation of health-related quality of life measures: literature review and proposed guidelines. J Clin Epidemiol. 1993;46(12):1417–32.

10. Chou CL, Chuang YC, Wang CC, Kuo HC. Validity of the traditional Chinese version of the King's health questionnaire for Taiwanese patients with an overactive bladder. Urol Sci. 2010;21(4):180–4.
11. Quan S, Ning J, Guozeng W, Yulong Z, Jing Z, Li J, Yan G, Menqing X, Ma J. Epidemiological survey of BPH in men over 50 years old in Pu Dong new area. Chin J Androl. 2006;20(7):36–8.
12. Barry MJ, Jr FF, O'Leary MP, Bruskewitz RC, Holtgrewe HL, Mebust WK, Cockett AT. The American urological association symptom index for benign prostatic hyperplasia. The measurement committee of the American Urological Association. J Urol. 1992;148(5):1549–57.
13. Moorthy P, Lapitan MCQuek PL, Lim PH. Prevalence of overactive bladder in Asian men: an epidemiological survey. BJU Int. 2004;93(4):528–31.
14. Höfner K. Symptomatic and quality of life response to tolterodine in subgroups of men with overactive bladder symptoms and presumed non-obstructive benign prostatic hyperplasia. World J Urol. 2010;28(3):353.
15. Irwin DE, Milsom I, Hunskaar S, Reilly K, Kopp Z, Herschorn S, Coyne K, Kelleher C, Hampel C, Artibani W. Population-based survey of urinary incontinence, overactive bladder, and other lower urinary tract symptoms in five countries: results of the EPIC study. Eur Urol. 2006;50(6):1306.
16. Peters TJ, Donovan JL, Kay HE, Abrams P, Rosette JJMCH, Porru D, Thuroff JW. The international continence society "benign prostatic hyperplasia" study: the bothersomeness of urinary symptoms. J Urol. 1997;157(3):885–9.
17. Lee JY, Kim HW, Lee SJ, Koh JS, Suh HJ, Chancellor MB. Comparison of doxazosin with or without tolterodine in men with symptomatic bladder outlet obstruction and an overactive bladder. BJU Int. 2015;49(1):194–5.
18. Knutson T, Edlund C, Fall M, Dahlstrand C. BPH with coexisting overactive bladder dysfunction--an everyday urological dilemma. Neurourol Urodyn. 2001;20(3):237.
19. Mcconnell JD, Roehrborn CG, Bautista OM, Jr AG, Dixon CM, Kusek JW, Lepor H, Mcvary KT, Jr NL, Clarke HS. The long-term effect of doxazosin, finasteride, and combination therapy on the clinical progression of benign prostatic hyperplasia. N Engl J Med. 2003;349(25):2387–98.
20. Jiménez-Cruz F. Identifying patients with lower urinary tract symptoms/ benign prostatic hyperplasia (LUTS/BPH) at risk for progression. Eur Urol Suppl. 2003;2(7):6–12.
21. Lowe FC, Batista J, Berges R, Chartier-Kastler E, Conti G, Desgrandchamps F, Dreikorn K, O'Leary M, Perez M, Speakman M. Risk factors for disease progression in patients with lower urinary tract symptoms|[sol]|benign prostatic hyperplasia (LUTS|[sol]|BPH): a systematic analysis of expert opinion. Eur Urol Suppl. 2005;8(3):206.
22. Roehrborn CG, Mcconnell JD, Saltzman B, Bergner D, Gray T, Narayan P, Cook TJ, Johnson-Levonas AO, Quezada WA, Waldstreicher J. Storage (irritative) and voiding (obstructive) symptoms as predictors of benign prostatic hyperplasia progression and related outcomes. Eur Urol. 2002; 42(1):1–6.
23. Roehrborn C. 10 the impact of acute or chronic inflammation in baseline biopsy on the risk of progression in the MTOPS study. Eur Urol Suppl. 2005;4(3):5–5.
24. Kwon H, Kang HC, Lee JH. Relationship between predictors of the risk of clinical progression of benign prostatic hyperplasia and metabolic syndrome in men with moderate to severe lower urinary tract symptoms. Urology. 2013;81(6):1325–9.
25. Zhang K, Xu Z, Jing Z, Wang H, Zhang D, Shi B. Clinical significance of Intravesical prostatic protrusion in patients with benign prostatic enlargement. Urology. 2007;70(6):1096–9.
26. Li MK, Garcia LA, Rosen R. Lower urinary tract symptoms and male sexual dysfunction in Asia: a survey of ageing men from five Asian countries. BJU Int. 2005;96(9):1339.
27. Keong Tatt F. Decision making in the management of benign prostatic enlargement and the role of transabdominal ultrasound. Int J Urol. 2010; 17(12):974–9.
28. Akihide H, Shoji S, Ken F, Akira Y, Tatsuya A, Yoshihisa F. Comparison of parameters to determine the cause of urinary disturbance in men with prostate volume less than 20 milliliters. Int J Urol. 2010;9(10):554–9.
29. Chia SJ, Heng CTChan SP, Foo KT. Correlation of intravesical prostatic protrusion with bladder outlet obstruction. BJU Int. 2015;91(4):371–4.

8

The association of pathogenic factors of metabolic syndrome on serum prostate-specific antigen levels

Bo-Wen Xia†, Si-Cong Zhao†, Zong-Ping Chen, Chao Chen, Tian-Shu Liu, Fan Yang and Yong Yan*

Abstract

Background: Metabolic syndrome (MetS) and serum prostate-specific antigen (PSA) levels are correlated. To investigate the underlying effect of MetS on PSA levels, the relationship between the major pathogenic factors of MetS and serum PSA levels was studied.

Methods: A total of 506 ostensibly healthy men who underwent routine health check-ups were recruited to this study. We evaluated the effect of the major pathogenic factors of MetS, which included insulin resistance, a subclinical inflammatory state and sexual hormone changes, on serum PSA levels by using linear regression analysis and multivariate analysis after adjusting for age, BMI and prostate volume.

Results: When simultaneously adjusting for age, BMI, prostate volume and high-density lipoprotein cholesterol, serum insulin levels and SHBG levels were inversely correlated with serum PSA levels ($P = 0.049$ and $P = 0.004$, respectively), and testosterone levels were positively correlated with serum PSA levels ($P = 0.039$). In multivariate regression models, serum insulin levels and serum SHBG levels were significantly associated with serum PSA levels (both $P < 0.001$).

Conclusions: Among the major pathogenic factors of metabolic syndrome, insulin resistance and sexual hormone changes may be the most significant contributors to the decline in serum PSA levels.

Keywords: Metabolic syndrome, Prostate-specific antigen, Insulin resistance, Sex hormone binding globulin, Screening

Background

Prostate cancer (PCa) is the second most common cancer in the world, with nearly 1.3 million new cases and neerly 0.4 million PCa-associated deaths worldwide in 2018, and becoming the 5th leading cause of cancer-associated death in men [1]. Serum prostate-specific antigen (PSA) testing has been take for worldwide as a screening and diagnostic tool for PCa management [2]; however, the sensitivity and specificity of serum PSA levels are limited, as many factors, for instance age, obesity, prostate volume (PV), and benign prostate diseases, may significantly affect PSA levels [3].

Metabolic syndrome (MetS) is considered as a complicated clinical disease characterized by a combination of multiple metabolic disorders, which include obesity, hypertension, dyslipidemia, hyperglycemia and insulin resistance [4]. MetS is prevalent worldwide and has become a major social and public health issue in the last 2 decades. Previous studies demonstrated that MetS may be involved in the onset and progression of certain types of cancer including carcinoma of the liver, colon, breast, bladder, prostate, etc. [5]. Additionally, studies that aimed to improve PCa management have also demonstrated the specific relationship between MetS and PSA levels [6–8]. Our previous study made investigate the association between MetS and serum PSA levels. We first found that the diagnosis of MetS decreased serum PSA levels by 11.3% compared to the absence of MetS after adjustment with a larger PV in MetS patients, at the

* Correspondence: yyshijitan@126.com
†Bo-Wen Xia and Si-Cong Zhao contributed equally to this work.
Department of Urology, Beijing Shijitan Hospital, Capital Medical University, 10th Tieyi Road, Haidian District, Beijing 100038, China

same time, there is a linear relationship between the decrease of PSA and the number of components of metabolic syndrome [9].

However, the detailed effect of MetS on PSA levels is still unclear. In the recent period of time, increasing evidence has suggested insulin resistance (IR), a subclinical inflammatory state and sex hormone changes may be the major pathogenic factors involved in MetS [4]. Historically, IR was considered the key feature of MetS, and the effect of IR significantly increased the prevalence of MetS [10].

Second, previous studies clearly demonstrated that there was a causal relationship between changes in serum sex hormone levels and MetS, as MetS was accompanied by sex hormone imbalances [11–13]. Finally, MetS was also considered a low-grade systematic inflammatory state that may enable the body to release more subclinical inflammatory factors, such as IL-6, CRP and TNF-α [14–17]. Interestingly, although a systematic study has not been carried out so far, individual studies have shown that the abovementioned major pathogenic factors involved in MetS may play a role in serum PSA levels [18–20].

As the underlying mechanism connecting MetS to PSA levels is complicated and undefined, there is a compelling need for further understanding these topics. Therefore, the aim of the present study was to clarify the underlying mechanism connecting MetS to serum PSA levels by using multivariate regression models.

Methods

From October 2014 to August 2015, by routine physical examination programs, 506 men over 45 years old were recruited consecutively to the study. By completing a standardized, structured questionnaire, subjects who were diagnosed with urethritis and prostatitis, urethral stricture, and neurogenic bladder, and who had a history of urological surgery or trauma and malignant diseases of the urinary system were excluded from this study. Additionally, subjects were also excluded if they had received anticholinergics, 5α-reductase inhibitors or hormone replacement therapy. These study protocols were approved by the the ethics committee of Beijing shijitan hospital affiliated to capital medical university and China railway corporation, and all subjects received informed consent and agreed in writing prior to registration.

All subjects completed the International Prostate Symptom Sore (I-PSS) questionnaire after Chinese translation, and the medical history of subjects was collected using a standardized, structured questionnaire. Anthropometric measurements, including blood pressure (mmHg), body weight (kg), height (cm) and waist circumference (cm), were measured by trained nurses using a standardized protocol. Body mass index (BMI) was calculated by using the formula (Square of weight/height). The PV (cm3) was measured by suprapubic ultrasonography (3.5 MHz, Hitachi EUB-400, Tokyo, Japan) using the formula for the volume of an ellipse (height×width×length×π/6).

Before undergoing direct recording electronic, a 10-mL, 12-h fasting blood specimen was drawn for biochemical analyses after the participants had been relaxed sitting for 15 min. The biochemical index analysis included PSA, fasting blood glucose (FBG), triglycerides, low-density lipoprotein cholesterol (LDL-C), high-density lipoprotein cholesterol (HDL-C) and total cholesterol. Insulin, 5α-dihydrotestosterone (DHT), sex hormone-binding globulin (SHBG), estradiol, testosterone, leptin, resistin, adiponectin, Il-6, CRP and TNF-α were measured using enzyme-linked immunosorbent assay methods. The IR index was derived using the HOMA arithmetic: FBG (mg/dL) × Insulin (μU/mL)/405 [21].

We defined MetS using the criteria established by the 2009 joint statement from the International Diabetes Federation Task Force on Epidemiology and Prevention; National Heart, Lung and Blood Institute; American Heart Association; World Heart Federation; International Atherosclerosis Society; and International Association for the Study of Obesity [4]. According to that report, MetS was diagnosed based on the simultaneous occurrence of at least three of the following five risk factors: waist circumference ≥ 90 cm; triglyceride levels≥150 mg/dL or drug treatment for elevated triglyceride levels; HDL cholesterol≤40 mg/dL or drug treatment for low HDL cholesterol; elevated blood pressure (systolic blood pressure ≥ 130 mmHg, diastolic blood pressure ≥ 85 mmHg or antihypertensive drug treatment with a history of hypertension); and FBG levels≥100 mg/dL or drug treatment for elevated FBG levels.

Continuous variables are shown as the mean ± SD, and categorical variables are shown as numbers and percentages. We divided subjects into two groups based on the presence of MetS. The clinical characteristics were compared using an independent t test for continuous variables and a chi-square test for categorical variables. Multivariate linear regression models were used to evaluate the effect of MetS-related factors on serum PSA levels. Furthermore, we divided subjects into four groups based on the quartile serum levels of insulin and SHBG to investigate whether there was a linear difference in the mean PSA level among the groups by using ANOVA. Data were analyzed using SPSS software version 13.0 for Windows (SPSS Inc., Chicago, IL, USA), and two-tailed P values < 0.05 were considered significant.

Results

The baseline characteristics of the subjects are presented in Table 1. The mean age was 69.3 ± 8.3 years. The overall prevalence of MetS in the entire cohort was 37.5% (190/506). Age, BMI, waist circumference, blood pressure (which included the systolic pressure and diastolic pressure), FBG, triglycerides, PV, IPSS score, HOMA index and leptin levels were significantly higher in subjects with MetS than in subjects without MetS (all $P < 0.01$). HDL-C, TNF-α and testosterone levels were significantly lower in subjects with MetS than in subjects without MetS (all $P < 0.05$).

In Table 2, results shows that among the MetS components only HDL-C was positively and significantly correlated with serum PSA levels after adjusting for age, BMI and PV ($P = 0.046$).

Table 1 Baseline characteristics

Characteristics	Overall(506)	Mets(190)	non-Mets(316)	*P*-value
Age	69.27 ± 8.31	70.63 ± 7.93	68.46 ± 8.44	**0.004†**
BMI, kg/m^2	24.70 ± 3.10	25.26 ± 2.93	24.36 ± 3.16	**0.002†**
Waist circumference, cm	86.91 ± 8.69	89.00 ± 8.44	85.66 ± 8.61	**<0.001†**
SBP, mmHg	137.61 ± 15.52	146.74 ± 13.05	132.13 ± 14.27	**<0.001†**
DBP, mmHg	79.22 ± 10.56	81.77 ± 10.65	77.69 ± 10.22	**<0.001†**
Elevated blood pressure, *n* (%)	72.1	95.8	50.1	**<0.001‡**
FBG, mg/dL	102.14 ± 25.45	113.04 ± 31.37	95.59 ± 18.25	**<0.001†**
Triglycerides,mg/dL	160.38 ± 138.81	225.63 ± 191.67	121.15 ± 68.81	**<0.001†**
HDL-C, mg/dL	47.29 ± 11.45	40.20 ± 8.65	51.56 ± 10.80	**<0.001†**
LDL-C, mg/dL	111.86 ± 30.59	109.86 ± 29.27	113.07 ± 31.34	0.253†
PV, cm^3	24.57 ± 7.15	26.31 ± 7.83	23.53 ± 6.50	**<0.001†**
Q_{max}, mL/s	15.41 ± 6.09	11.96 ± 4.31	17.50 ± 6.07	**<0.001†**
PSA, ng/mL	1.35 ± 1.12	1.36 ± 1.10	1.35 ± 1.14	0.940†
IPSS	13.04 ± 7.62	14.26 ± 7.34	12.30 ± 7.71	**0.005†**
Insulin, pmol/L	51.68 ± 31.08	52..93 ± 29.74	50.93 ± 31.88	0.484†
HOMA IR	2.15 ± 1.35	2.42 ± 1.52	1.98 ± 1.21	**<0.001†**
Leptin, ng/mL	3.51 ± 2.83	4.21 ± 2.79	3.09 ± 2.77	**<0.001†**
Resistin, ng/mL	29.70 ± 18.29	29.05 ± 16.39	30.09 ± 19.35	0.518†
Adiponectin, μg/mL	2.99 ± 1.70	2.99 ± 1.65	2.99 ± 1.72	0.991†
CRP, mg/L	2.20 ± 4.31	2.24 ± 3.58	2.18 ± 4.70	0.871†
IL-6, pg/mL	1.87 ± 5.47	1.97 ± 7.44	1.81 ± 3.84	0.755†
TNF-α, pg/mL	43.52 ± 9.63	42.20 ± 9.41	44.31 ± 9.69	**0.017†**
DHT, pg/mL	380.87 ± 230.30	370.63 ± 208.30	387.05 ± 242.73	0.438†
SHBG, nmol/L	70.71 ± 35.21	67.39 ± 33.34	72.72 ± 36.20	0.100†
Estradiol, pg/mL	38.70 ± 17.10	40.29 ± 19.50	37.74 ± 15.43	0.117†
Testosterone, ng/mL	4.61 ± 1.75	4.31 ± 1.36	4.79 ± 1.92	**0.001†**
E2/T	9.67 ± 8.66	10.23 ± 5.89	9.33 ± 9.96	0.261†
Number of MetS components, *n*				
0	–		48 (9.5%)	–
1	–		126 (24.9%)	–
2	–		142 (28.1%)	–
3	–	116 (22.9%)		–
4	–	63 (12.5%)		–
5	–	11 (2.2%)		–

MetS Metabolic syndrome, *BMI* Body mass index, *SBP* Systolic blood pressure, *DBP* Diastolic blood pressure, *FBG* Fasting blood glucose, *HDL* High-density lipoprotein, *LDL* Low-density lipoprotein, *PV* Prostate volume, *CRP* C-reactive protein, *IL-6* Interleukin 6, *TNF-α* Tumor Necrosis Factor alpha, *DHT* 5α-Dihydrotestosterone, *SHBG* Sex hormone binding globulin; *P* were calculated by independent t-test† and chi-squared test‡; Bold indicates statistically significant values

Table 2 Relationship between MetS and PSA

Characteristics	B	*t*	95% CI	†*P*-value
Waist circumference, cm	− 0.043	− 0,444	− 0.232, 0.147	0.657
Triglycerides, mg/dL	− 0.026	− 0.567	− 0.114, 0.063	0.571
HDL-C, mg/dL	0.089	1.998	0.001, 0.177	**0.046**
SBP, mmHg	0.080	1.673	−0.014, 0.173	0.095
DBP, mmHg	0.001	0.002	−0.091, 0.091	0.998
FBG, mg/dL	0.015	0.339	−0.073, 0.103	0.735
MetS	0.052	0.547	−0.134, 0.238	0.584

CI Confidence interval, *SBP* Systolic blood pressure, *DBP* Diastolic blood pressure, *FBG* Fasting blood glucose, *HDL* High-density lipoprotein; †*P*-value were calculated according to Multivariate linear regression analyses; Bold indicates statistically significant values

As shown in Table 3, after adjustment with age, BMI, PV and HDL-C in separate multivariate linear regression models, the data showed that serum insulin levels, SHBG and serum testosterone levels were significantly and linearly correlated with PSA levels (all $P < 0.05$). Serum testosterone levels were positively associated with serum PSA levels, while serum insulin levels and SHBG were negatively associated with serum PSA levels. Interestingly, when serum insulin levels, SHBG and serum testosterone levels were simultaneously adjusted in addition to adjusting age, BMI, PV and HDL-C, serum insulin and SHBG levels still showed significant and negative relationships with serum PSA levels (both $P < 0.05$).

Finally, we divided subjects into four groups based on the quartile serum levels of insulin and SHBG to investigate whether there were differences in the trend of serum PSA levels among the groups (Fig. 1). After adjusting for age, BMI, PV and HDL-C, the mean PSA level significantly and gradually decreased as serum insulin and SHBG levels increased (both P for this trend < 0.05).

Discussion

The results of the study indicated that insulin resistance and SHBG levels play a important role in the lower serum PSA levels in MetS patients. Previously, researchers have noted that the presence of MetS is associated with the risk of PCa development, but there was controversy over the correlation between MetS and the risk of PCa [22, 23]. The heterogeneity of previous research conclusions among different studies may be caused by the differences in sample sizes, baseline characteristics, MetS diagnostic criteria and follow-up time. However, considering the influence of MetS on the serum PSA level, this may be one of the reasons for the deviations in the correlation between MetS and the risk of PCa.

A study noted that although screening serum PSA levels can improve the detection rate of PCa, it has a relatively small impact on PCa-specific mortality, and researchers have suggested that when screening serum PSA levels, it is necessary to fully consider the problems of missed diagnosis and overdiagnosis [3]. The causes of these problems may involve the excessive interference of serum PSA levels.

In a study by Choi et al. [7], the serum PSA levels in the MetS group were lower than those in the control group (1.15 ± 0.91 vs. 1.26 ± 0.76 ng/ml, $P = 0.006$), and after adjusting for PV and plasma volume, the results

Table 3 Analysis of MetS-related affect PSA

Characteristics	B	95% CI	†*P*-value	B	95% CI	‡*P*-value
Insulin	−0.241	− 0.492, 0.009	**0.049**	− 0.172	−0.272, -0.073	**<0.001**
HOMA index	0.076	−0.169, 0.321	0.542			
DHT	−0.089	−0.184, 0.006	0.068			
SHBG	−0.182	−0.305, -0.058	**0.004**	−0.163	− 0.284, -0.042	**<0.001**
Estradiol	0.062	−0.028, 0.153	0.177			
Testosterone	0.128	0.006, 0.251	**0.039**	0.083	−0.032, 0.198	0.158
Leptin	−0.033	0.159, 0.093	0.607			
Resistin	0.061	−0.030, 0.153	0.186			
Adiponectin	0.041	−0.058, 0.140	0.412			
CRP	0.032	−0.064, 0.129	0.510			
IL-6	−0.072	−0.175, 0.031	0.169			
TNF-α	−0.025	−0.122, 0.072	0.617			

Abbreviations as in Table 1 and Table 2

†*P*-values were separately calculated three different statistics model according to multivariate linear regression analyses after adjustment of age, BMI, prostate volume and HDL-C;The model 1 include Insulin and HOMA index;The model 2 include DHT, SHBG, Estradiol, Testosterone; The model 3 include Leptin, Resistin, Adiponectin, CRP, IL-6, TNF-α;

‡*P*-value were calculated statistics model include Insulin, SHBG, Testosterone according to multivariate linear regression analyses after adjustment of age, BMI, prostate volume and HDL-C;

Bold indicates statistically significant

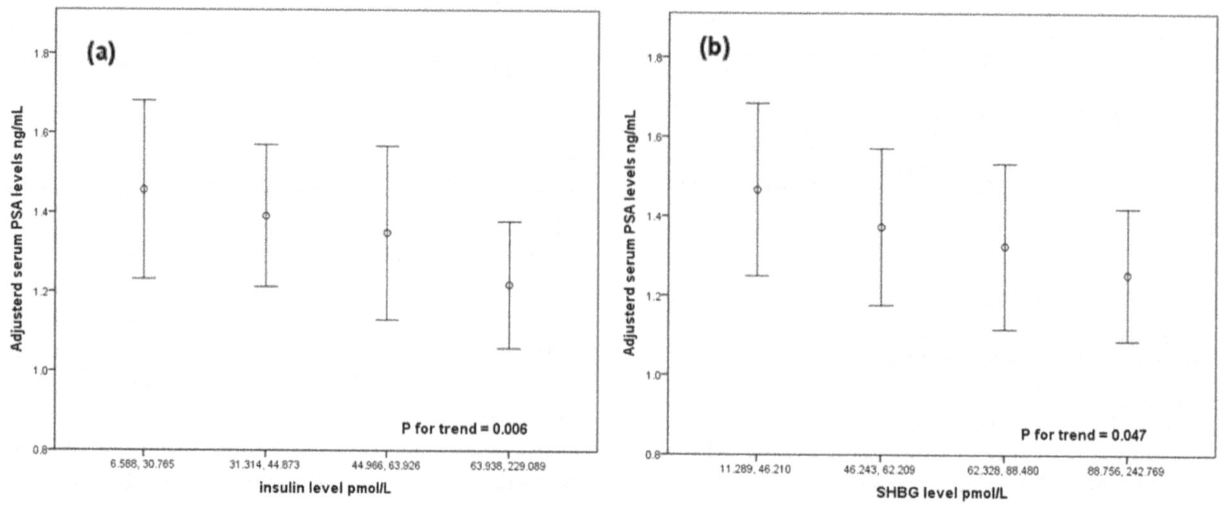

Fig. 1 Adjustment with age, BMI, PV and HDL-C, the mean PSA level decreased as (**a**) serum insulin and (**b**) SHBG levels increased

were also significantly correlated. Research has suggested that MetS is an independent risk factor for decreased serum PSA levels (serum PSA levels fell by 4.1%, $P =$ 0.046). A recent study from our research team demonstrated that serum PSA levels in the MetS group were lower than those in the non-MetS group (1.11 ± 0.79 vs. 1.21 ± 0.76 ng/ml, $P = 0.026$) and that MetS was an independent risk factor for a decrease in serum PSA levels, which can reduce the serum PSA level by 11.3%. We also reported that as the number of abnormal components in MetS increases, the serum PSA level presents a trend of progressive decline. This study was based on a sample of 45,540 healthy men aged 55 to 59 [9]. However, the serum PSA level was not associated with MetS in our study, which may have been due to the small sample size. However, based on our previous studies with large samples, it MetS is believed to be correlated with PSA declines.

A considerable number of studies have confirmed that MetS aggravates the degree of IR, and IR is not only the driving factor of MetS but is also one of the main pathogenic factors [10]. In a study of Parekh et al. on the relationship between physiological indicators and serum PSA concentration, their results showed that the serum PSA concentration was significantly and negatively correlated with IR ($p = 0.04$) after adjusting for age, BMI, and race [18]; Choi et al. [6] reached a similar conclusion in their study. However, previous studies failed to consider the large PV of MetS patients. Our results indicated a significant and negative association between insulin concentrations and PSA ($P = 0.049$) after adjustment with age, BMI, PV and HDL-C. Furthermore, the mean serum PSA levels showed a significantly declining trend with increasing insulin levels, as presented in Fig. 1a (P for trend =0.006). We believe that changes in the insulin level caused by IR are one of the pathogenic factors that play a crucial role in the influence of MetS on serum PSA levels.

Sofikerim et al. [24] analyzed 210 subject whose serum PSA level was less than 2.5 ng/ml and pointed out that there was no significant correlation between the serum PSA level with the serum testosterone and serum free testosterone concentration. A similar study demonstrated that there was no linear correlation between the serum testosterone concentration and the serum PSA level, and testosterone replacement therapy did not cause changes in the serum PSA level [25]. It is worth noting that Rastrelli et al. indicated a strong positive correlation between testosterone with PSA levels in subject with low testosterone; additionally, a similar idea was proposed in a previous study, in which researchers suggested that a natural decrease in serum androgen levels might alter PSA levels [26, 27]. Conversely, several studies have found a correlation between SHBG and the risk of MetS; as a carrier that combines and transports sexual steroids, changes in the SHBG level may better reflect changes in sexual hormone levels [11–13]. Considering the interaction between sex hormones, estradiol and DHT were also taken into account when we analyzed these data. Our results showed that the testosterone levels were positively associated with PSA levels after adjustment with age, BMI, PV and HDL-C, while SHBG was negatively correlated with serum PSA levels in the sex hormone factor group ($P = 0.039$, $P = 0.004$, respectively). The mean PSA levels tended to decrease as the concentration of SHBG increased (P for trend =0.047), as shown in Fig. 1b. We found that SHBG levels could be a better indicator than testosterone and estrogen, which should be considered further when examining the MetS-PSA relationship.

The pathology caused by MetS leads to chronic inflammation and changes in the serum levels of inflammatory factors and adipokines, including leptin, adiponectin, CRP, IL-6, TNF-α, etc. [14–17]. McDonald et al. found a correlation between serum CRP levels and elevated PSA levels (OR = 1.19; 95% CI, 1.06–1.33), suggesting that systemic inflammatory markers are associated with PSA elevation in the absence of prostate disease [19]. However, there was no significant association between serum leptin and adiponectin with PSA levels in previous studies [20, 28]. We found no association between subclinical inflammatory mediators and serum PSA levels, but the current results do not completely negate the influence of systemic inflammation on serum PSA levels, which may be caused by the interaction of inflammatory markers, such as leptin and adiponectin. Thus, we still need to conduct more detailed research and analysis to further clarify the correlation between serum PSA and inflammatory mediators.

Finally, indicators that had a significant correlation with the serum PSA level in previous studies were included in the multiple linear regression model after adjustment with for age, BMI, PV, HDL-C. There was a significant, negative correlated between insulin and SHBG with serum PSA levels (all $P < 0.001$). Previous research has indicated that SHBG are negatively correlated with glycosylated hemoglobin in people without diabetes, which indicates that there may be a relationship between SHBG and glucose homeostasis changes before diabetes [29]. Similar researches have found that there is a negative correlation between SHBG with insulin levels, insulin resistance, and diabetes risk, and researchers believe that low serum SHBG is an independent risk factor for type 2 diabetes [30]. Although the relationship between SHBG and insulin resistance needs to be further explored, it can be concluded that both insulin resistance and SHBG levels play a crucial role in the changes in serum PSA levels in MetS patients.

There are still some limitations in the present study because MetS leads to considerable, complicated pathophysiologic changes. However, according to existing research results, we narrowed the scope of this study. Due to the interaction between pathogenic factors, the current results may ignore the impact of a single pathogenic factor, so we still need to further explore the influence of single pathogenic factors on serum PSA levels. In addition, since prostate biopsy was not included in our health examination plan, we cannot explicitly exclude the existence of prostate cancer, but because the average PSA levels of our target population were low, even a small number of patients with early PCa would not affect the results of the current study.

Conclusions

The decrease in serum PSA levels in MetS patients is mainly related to insulin resistance and serum SHBG levels. Urologists need to pay attention to this effect to comprehensively evaluate patient serum PSA levels, and subsequent studies need to further refine the serum PSA correction formula for MetS patients based on research results and to explore the physiological mechanism of this process.

Abbreviations

BMI: Body mass index; CRP: C-reactive protein; DHT: 5α-Dihydrotestosterone; FBG: Fasting blood glucose; HDL-C: High-density lipoprotein cholesterol; LDL: Low-density lipoprotein cholesterol; MetS: Metabolic syndrome; Pca: Prostate cancer; PSA: Prostate-specific antigen; PV: Prostate volume; SHBG: Sex hormone binding globulin

Acknowledgements

Not Applicable.

Authors' contributions

XBW, ZSC, YY have made substantial contributions to the designed of the work and analyzed and interpreted of the data and drafted the manuscript and revised it. CZP, CC, YF and LTS have made contributions to collection of the data. All authors read and approved the final manuscript.

Authors' information

Bo-Wen Xia: Postgraduate of Capital Medical University.
Si-Cong Zhao, Zong-Ping Chen, Chao Chen, Tian-Shu Liu, Fan Yang: Doctor of Capital Medical University.
Yong Yan: Chief physician; Professor and doctoral supervisor of Capital Medical University; Doctor of Universitat Dusseldorf; Doctor of Peking University.

References

1. Bray F, Ferlay J, Soerjomataram I, et al. Global cancer statistics 2018: GLOBOCAN estimates of incidence and mortality worldwide for 36 cancers in 185 countries. CA Cancer J Clin. 2018;68(6):394–424.
2. Carter HB, Albertsen PC, Barry MJ, et al. Early detection of prostate cancer: AUA guideline. J Urol. 2013;190(2):419–26.
3. Ilic D, Djulbegovic M, Jung JH, et al. Prostate cancer screening with prostate-specific antigen (PSA) test: a systematic review and meta-analysis. BMJ. 2018;362:k3519.
4. Alberti KG, Eckel RH, Grundy SM, et al. Harmonizing the metabolic syndrome: a joint interim statement of the international diabetes federation task force on epidemiology and prevention; National Heart, Lung, and Blood Institute; American Heart Association; world heart federation; international atherosclerosis society; and International Association for the Study of obesity. Circulation. 2009;120(16):1640–5.
5. Esposito K, Chiodini P, Colao A, et al. Metabolic syndrome and risk of cancer: a systematic review and meta-analysis. Diabetes Care. 2012;35(11): 2402–11.
6. Choi HC, Park JH, Cho BL, et al. The illusion of prostate-specific antigen decline in patients with metabolic syndrome and insulin resistance. BJU Int. 2011;108(11):1756–61.
7. Choi WS, Heo NJ, Paick JS, et al. Prostate-specific antigen lowering effect of metabolic syndrome is influenced by prostate volume. Int J Urol. 2016;23(4): 299–304.
8. Kim YJ, Cho YJ, Oh JE, et al. The association between metabolic syndrome and prostate-specific antigen levels. Int J Urol. 2008;15(10):905–9.
9. Zhao S, Xia M, Tang J, et al. Actual lowering effect of metabolic syndrome on serum prostate-specific antigen levels is partly concealed by enlarged prostate: results from a large-scale population-based study. BJU Int. 2017; 120(4):482–9.

10. Weiss R, Dziura J, Burgert TS, et al. Obesity and the metabolic syndrome in children and adolescents. N Engl J Med. 2004;350(23):2362–74.
11. Bhasin S, Jasjua GK, Pencina M, et al. Sex hormone-binding globulin, but not testosterone, is associated prospectively and independently with incident metabolic syndrome in men: the Framingham heart study. Diabetes Care. 2011;34(11):2464–70.
12. Brand JS, van der Tweel I, Grobbee DE, et al. Testosterone, sex hormone-binding globulin and the metabolic syndrome: a systematic review and meta-analysis of observational studies. Int J Epidemiol. 2011;40(1):189–207.
13. Sa EQ, Sa FC, Oliveira KC, et al. Association between sex hormone-binding globulin (SHBG) and metabolic syndrome among men. Sao Paulo Med J. 2014;132(2):111–5.
14. Gacci M, Vignozzi L, Sebastianelli A, et al. Metabolic syndrome and lower urinary tract symptoms: the role of inflammation. Prostate Cancer Prostatic Dis. 2013;16(1):101–6.
15. Ackermann D, Jones J, Barona J, et al. Waist circumference is positively correlated with markers of inflammation and negatively with adiponectin in women with metabolic syndrome. Nutr Res. 2011;31(3):197–204.
16. Pravenec M, Kajiya T, Zidek V, et al. Effects of human C-reactive protein on pathogenesis of features of the metabolic syndrome. Hypertension (Dallas, Tex : 1979). 2011;57(4):731–7.
17. Esteghamati A, Noshad S, Khalilzadeh O, et al. Contribution of serum leptin to metabolic syndrome in obese and nonobese subjects. Arch Med Res. 2011;42(3):244–51.
18. Parekh N, Lin Y, Marcella S, et al. Associations of lifestyle and physiologic factors with prostate-specific antigen concentrations: evidence from the National Health and nutrition examination survey (2001-2004). Cancer Epidemiol Biomark Prev. 2008;17(9):2467–72.
19. McDonald AC, Vira MA, Vidal AC, et al. Association between systemic inflammatory markers and serum prostate-specific antigen in men without prostatic disease - the 2001-2008 National Health and nutrition examination survey. Prostate. 2014;74(5):561–7.
20. Burton A, Martin RM, Holly J, et al. Associations of adiponectin and leptin with stage and grade of PSA-detected prostate cancer: the ProtecT study. Cancer Causes Control. 2013;24(2):323–34.
21. Matthews DR, Hosker JP, Rudenski AS, et al. Homeostasis model assessment: insulin resistance and beta-cell function from fasting plasma glucose and insulin concentrations in man. Diabetologia. 1985;28(7):412–9.
22. Xiang YZ, Xiong H, Cui ZL, et al. The association between metabolic syndrome and the risk of prostate cancer, high-grade prostate cancer, advanced prostate cancer, prostate cancer-specific mortality and biochemical recurrence. J Exp Clin Cancer Res. 2013;32:9.
23. Gacci M, Russo GI, De Nunzio C, et al. Meta-analysis of metabolic syndrome and prostate cancer. Prostate Cancer Prostatic Dis. 2017;20(2):146–55.
24. Sofikerim M, Oruc O, Eskicorapci S, et al. Correlation of serum androgens and pituitary hormone levels with serum PSA less than 2.5 ng/ml. Sci World J. 2007;7:1128–33.
25. Reis LO, Denardi F, Faria EF, et al. Correlation between testosterone and PSA kinetics in metastatic prostate Cancer patients treated with diverse chemical castrations. Am J Mens Health. 2015;9(5):430–4.
26. Rastrelli G, et al. Serum PSA as a predictor of testosterone deficiency. J Sex Med. 2013;10(10):2518–28.
27. Morgentaler A, Bruning CR, DeWolf WC. Occult prostate cancer in men with low serum testosterone levels. JAMA. 1996;276(23):1904–6.
28. Fowke JH, Matthews CM, Buchowski MS, et al. Association between prostate-specific antigen and leptin, adiponectin, HbA1c or C-peptide among African-American and Caucasian men. Prostate Cancer Prostatic Dis. 2008;11(3):264–9.
29. Brand JS, Wareham NJ, Dowsett M, et al. Associations of endogenous testosterone and SHBG with glycated haemoglobin in middle-aged and older men. Clin Endocrinol. 2011;74(5):572–8.
30. Ding EL, Song Y, Malik VS, et al. Sex differences of endogenous sex hormones and risk of type 2 diabetes: a systematic review and meta-analysis. JAMA. 2006;295(11):1288–99.

9

Post-radical prostatectomy urinary incontinence: Is there any discrepancy between medical reports and patients' perceptions?

Rafael Castilho Borges[1*], Marcos Tobias-Machado[1], Estefânia Nicoleti Gabriotti[1], Francisco Winter dos Santos Figueiredo[2], Carlos Alberto Bezerra[1] and Sidney Glina[1]

Abstract

Background: Post-radical prostatectomy urinary incontinence (PPI) negatively affects the quality of life of patients. Accurate identification of the problem by physicians is essential for adequate postoperative management. In this study we sought to access whether there is, for urinary incontinence, any discrepancy between medical reports and the perception of patients.

Methods: We performed a retrospective analysis of medical records of 337 patients subjected to radical retropubic prostatectomy (RRP) between 2005 and 2010. Sociodemographic variables were collected, as well as continence status over the course of treatment. Next, we contacted patients by phone to determine continence status at present and at time of their last appointment, as well as to apply ICIQ – SF questionnaire. Poisson regression model with robust variance was used to estimate the factors associated with discrepancy, using the stepwise backward strategy. Software used was Stata® (StataCorp, LC) version 11.0.

Results: There is discrepancy between medical reports and patients' perceptions in 42.2% of cases. This discrepancy was found in 56% of elderly patients and 52% of men with low schooling, with statistical significance in these groups ($p = 0.069$ and 0.0001, respectively), whereas in multivariate regression analysis the discrepancy rate was significantly higher in black men (discrepancy rate of 52.6%) with low schooling ($p = 0.004$ and 0.043, respectively).

Conclusion: There is discrepancy between medical reports and the perception of black men with low schooling in respect to post-radical prostatectomy urinary incontinence and a need for more thorough investigation of this condition in patients that fit this risk profile.

Keywords: Urinary continence, Prostatic neoplasm, Prostatectomy, Quality-of-life, Patient-reported symptoms, Medical report

Background

Post-radical prostatectomy urinary incontinence (PPI) negatively affects quality of life of a great part of men subjected to surgical management of prostate cancer [1]. Six months after diagnosis, 66.4% of patients surgically treated in the cohort Prostate Cancer Outcomes Study (PCOS) considered the condition a problem; of these, 15.2% rated it as moderate to severe [2]. In a quality of life assessment of patients subjected to the same treatment, incontinence was significantly associated with increased confusion, depression and anger, and inversely related to physical and psychological well-being [3]. A total of 28 and 18% of patients in surgical arm of SPCG-4 study had moderate to severe discomfort secondary to daytime or nighttime urine loss, respectively [4].

The need for procedures to treat this complication is also somewhat frequent. Kim et al. noted that 6% of 16,348 men over 66 years, submitted to radical prostatectomy, required

* Correspondence: rafa_cborges@hotmail.com
[1]Department of Urology, Faculdade de Medicina do ABC, No.2000, Avenue Lauro Gomes, Santo André 09051-040, Brazil
Full list of author information is available at the end of the article

at least one procedure for incontinence within 6 months on average after surgery, and 15% of those had to undergo more than one type of procedure [5]. There is progressive improvement of the problem within 12 months, but 30 to 40% of patients have persistent incontinence [6, 7] and 8.4% go on to develop severe incontinence within 18 months after surgical procedure [2].

The increasing attention given to quality of life-related aspects of patients undergoing surgical treatment for prostate cancer mandates that data be collected as accurately as possible, with proper identification and management of postoperative complications. Development of an effective and consistent assessment of symptoms is critical, not only to understand the patients' experiences, but also to provide vital information for conduction of clinical care, and avoid or minimize any unfavorable impacts associated with treatment.

Although it is clear that appropriate postoperative care depends on the accurate identification of symptoms by physicians, evidence shows that physicians generally tend to underestimate patients' symptoms [8], including those with prostate cancer [9]: these inconsistencies may lead to ineffective treatment plans and disparity between patients' expectations and the real impact on their functional status.

Discrepancy between physicians' and patients' perceptions of post-radical prostatectomy urinary incontinence has been rarely investigated in literature, but is important in terms of its potential socioeconomic and clinical impacts: it may delay the early identification and management of this condition, prolong patient discomfort and lead to increased public healthcare spending.

In this sense, our study aims to determine whether there is any difference in prevalence of PPI based on medical evaluations and patients' perception', and which are the factors associated with this discrepancy.

Methods

We performed a retrospective analysis of the medical records of patients subjected to non-nerve-sparing radical retropubic prostatectomy between 2005 and 2010. Inclusion criteria included were standard RRP for clinical stage T1 or T2 prostate cancer performed more than 5 years before the beginning of the study, continent patients before surgery with a life expectancy of at least 10 years and a ECOG Scale of Performance Status 0 or 1. The variables age (adults, elderly), race (caucasian, mulatto, black), level of schooling (illiterate, low or high level of schooling, depending on completion of primary education), disease status according to D'Amico Risk Classification for Prostate Cancer, preoperative continence status, and physician-reported postoperative continence status were assessed, as well as information relative to the last appointment such as: date and if patients were discharged from outpatient follow-up or referred to a voiding dysfunction team.

Patients were excluded due to death, presence of added co-morbidities that may be the reason of incontinence (diabetes mellitus and neurologic diseases), preoperative history of overactive bladder and/or postsurgery symptoms of urge incontinence, adjuvant or salvage radiation therapy, development of stenosis of uretrovesical anastomosis requiring surgical procedures (endoscopic urethrotomy or endoscopic bladder neck resection) since this may compromise interpretation of post-surgical continence status. Next, we contacted subjects over phone to ask about their continence status at present and at the time of their last appointment/hospital discharge. Incontinent patients subjectively rated their condition (mild, moderate and severe), ICIQ – SF questionnaire was applied and patients were categorized according to the number of pads used daily: 0 pad; 1 security pad; 1 pad; 2 pads; 3 or more pads. The subjective severity rate of incontinence scale was based on the level of bothering caused by the condition.

We assessed: 1) incontinence rates as reported by physicians in patient records, reported by patients at the time of discharge and at present, as well as severity classification (using the questionnaire and pad usage); 2) discrepancy between medical records and patients' perceptions regarding post-surgical incontinence; 3) subgroups of patients in which this discrepancy is more frequent. Physician's reports to define presence or absence of urinary incontinence are based on pad usage by patients (sizes and numbers of pads were checked), and definition of continence was use of no pads.

To describe qualitative variables, we used absolute and relative frequencies, respectively. To assess the association between sociodemographic characteristics and discrepancy between physicians' and patients' views, we used the chi-square test. To estimate the magnitude of this association, multivariate Poisson regression model with robust variance was used. Level of significance was set at 5%. The software program used was Stata (StataCorp, LC) version 11.0.

Patients' informed consent was obtained over telephone; the patients received an information letter prior to the informed consent; verbal consent to participate in the study was recorded on the phone calls; patient's identity, answers and information on medical records were kept confidential. The study was performed according to the Declaration of Helsinki and approved by the Research Ethics Committee of *Faculdade de Medicina do ABC* (no. 3.031.751).

Results

During the period of the study, 337 radical prostatectomies were performed in our institution. Twenty-three patients were subjected to laparoscopic radical prostatectomy and were excluded of study; 54 were excluded due to death, presence of added co-morbidities that could have been the reason of incontinence (diabetes mellitus and neurologic diseases), adjuvant or salvage radiation therapy, or development of stenosis of uretrovesical anastomosis requiring surgical procedures; in 27 men successfully phone call was not possible; 5 patients refused to participate of study and 16 were excluded due to insufficient data. After exclusion we were left with 212 subjects. Of those, 115 (54.3%) were Caucasian, most were illiterate or had a low level of schooling (primary education) (62.7%), and 78,8% were elderly (cut-off: 65 years-old); median age was 65 years (interquartile range 60–69); mean time of physicians' report of continence status at the last appointment was 17 months; most patients ($n = 174$; 82%) were discharged after a follow-up of at least 1 year. These patients went on to be followed up in primary care services. Incontinent patients underwent pelvic floor muscle training and 28% of all men received it. Eight percent remained under follow-up with urologic oncology group for other reasons (Table 1). Table 2 shows the preoperative continence status: 98.6% of patients were continent.

According to medical charting, most patients (62.7%) were continent at their last appointment, whereas 70% of patients reported on phone interview that they still had urine loss symptoms at that moment. At time of phone call 46.2% of men ($n = 98$) referred the persistence of incontinence. Phone calls were made in 2017 and mean period from operation and last visit to phone call was 9 and 6.4 years, respectively. The largest portion of patients (43.9%) who still presented incontinence subjectively rate it as moderate, whereas through ICIQ-SF evaluation the complication is rated as severe or very severe in 80% of cases (score 7 and over). According to ICIQ-SF questionnaire applied at last physicians visit, 12.3, 52.8 and 34.9% of men were rated as having mild, moderate and severe incontinence, respectively (Table 2).

Twenty-five, 25.4, 37.2 and 12.4% of incontinent patients at phone call referred usage of one security pad, one pad, 2 pads and 3 or more pads, while according to medical reports the rates were 47, 33.3, 13.6, 6.1%, respectively.

Fifty-four percent of the 174 men who were discharged said they were incontinent at time of discharge. Sixty-five percent of patients who were incontinent at that time were considered as continent by physicians in the medical records.

Table 1 Demographic and clinical characteristics

Variables	N	%
Race		
Caucasian	115	54.3
Mulatto	69	32.5
Black	28	13.2
Level of schooling		
Low	133	62.7
High	79	37.3
Age range		
Adults	45	21.2
Elderly	167	78.8
D'Amico Risk Classification		
Low	29	13.7
Intermediate	25	11.8
High	157	74.1
Absence of neoplasm	1	0.5
Referral		
Discharge	174	82.1
Voiding dysfunction	21	9.9
Oncology	17	8

Table 2 Pre- and postoperative continence status

Variables	N	%
Pre-RRP incontinence		
Absent	209	98.6
Present	1	0.5
Use of urinary catheter	2	0.9
Post-RRP incontinence at last visit (physician's report)		
Absent	133	62.7
Present	58	27.4
Not informed	21	9.9
Post-RRP incontinence at last visit (patients' report)		
Absent	56	30.4
Present	128	69.6
Post-RRP incontinence at phone call		
Absent	114	53,8
Present	98	46,2
Subjective severity rate of incontinence		
Mild	35	35.7
Moderate	43	43.9
Severe	20	20.4
ICIQ – SF at last visit (psysician's report):		
Mild	26	12,3
Moderate	112	52,8
Severe	74	34,9
ICIQ – SF at phone call (patients' report):		
Mild	2	2
Moderate	17	17.4
Severe	79	80.6

RRP Retropubic radical prostatectomy

In general, there is divergence between medical reports and patients' perceptions in 42.2% of cases, and in all of them, the discrepancy was established due to physicians reporting as continent patients who said they were incontinent at time of the report. Aiming to determine the characteristics that put subjects at risk for this discrepancy, we evaluated whether variables race, age range and level of schooling were significantly associated with it (Table 3): univariate analysis reveals that only the age range (elderly patients) and level of schooling (low schooling) showed a statistically significant relationship ($p = 0.069$ and 0.0001, respectively).

Discrepancy was more frequent in black subjects, however with no statistical significance. In multivariate analysis, the percentage discrepancy relationship was greater in black subjects (IRR 17.8 95% CI 2.57 to 123.3; $p = 0.004$) with low schooling (IRR 1.54, 95%CI 1.01 to 2.35; $p = 0.043$) when compared to Caucasian subjects with high schooling (Table 4).

Discussion

We found a clear discrepancy between physicians' conclusions and patients' perceptions of PPI, which is surprising if we consider that such complication has significant negative impact on quality of life of patients, and most of these patients will live for a long time following initial diagnosis and treatment [1]. Despite the correct identification and management of this condition by physicians being vital and possible, multiple barriers affect medical management of PPI, starting with considerable divergences in literature regarding the incidence of incontinence and the most appropriate definition of the condition [10].

Table 3 Variables related to discrepancy (univariate analysis)

Variables	Discrepancy		*p*
	No	Yes	
Race			
Caucasian	57 (62.0)	35 (38.0)	0.419
Mulatto	30 (54.6)	25 (45.4)	
Black	9 (47.4)	10 (52.6)	
Age range			
Adult	15 (44.1)	19 (55.9)	0.069
Elderly	81 (61.3)	51 (38.6)	
Level of schooling			
Low	64 (48.1)	69 (51.9)	< 0.001
High	32 (97)	1.0 (3)	
D'Amico Risk classification			
Low	13 (50)	13 (50)	0.332
Intermediate	13 (72.2)	5 (27.8)	
High	69 (57)	52 (43)	

Table 4 Variables related to discrepancy (multivariate regression)

Variables	% Discrepancy (95%CI)	p^*
Low level of schooling	18.0 (3.0; 123.0)	0.004
Elderly	0.75 (0.55; 1.00)	0.073
Race		
Caucasian	Ref.	Ref.
Mulatto	1.0 (0.96; 2.0)	0.084
Black	2.0 (1.0; 2.0)	0.043

95%CI 95% confidence interval, *Ref* Reference category
*Poisson regression model with robust variance

The reported incidence of PPI falls between 6 and 69% [11–13]. This substantial variation is explained by the multiple methodologies used for assessment of incontinence, patient selection, diagnostic criteria and varying degrees of severity [14]. One of the major confounding factors is the very definition of incontinence. Definition of incontinence by the status of used pads is an important objective metric; however, there are different definitions based on this status, which include no pads, use of a safety pad or up to one pad per day.

Liss et al. showed that fully continent men (no pads used) have a lower symptom score and better quality of life, when compared to those who required use of a safety pad or one pad per day (score 5.8 ± 0.3 vs 7.6 ± 0.7 and 9.2 ± 0.6; respectively) [15]. In a prospective study from Oslo, with a cohort of 735 patients (including men with preoperative incontinence), PPI rate was 74% within 12 months, using "absence of pads" as the definition of continence. Severe incontinence was present in 3% of men, but when the stratification proposed by Ellison et al. was used, rates increased to 25% [16].

These studies do not support inclusion of a safety pad or one pad per day in definition of post-radical prostatectomy continence, and it must be strict: 0 pads. The high incontinence rate (60.7%) in our study population may be a reflection of the adoption of this definition which, although more rigorous, seems to be more truthful based on previous studies.

Initial management of PPI comprises detailed history taking, physical examination, objective evaluation of symptoms, and a voiding diary. According to European Association of Urology guideline [17], some tests such as urine chemistry and bladder ultrasound, including measurement of post-void residual volume, must be included. The guideline states that standardized questionnaires are valuable as additional tools, particularly in the clinical trial setting. There are multiple validated tools available: International Consultation on Incontinence-Short Form [18], Patient's Global Impression of Improvement Score [19] and the UCLA/RAND-Prostate Cancer Index Urinary Function Score [20].

As described by Avery et al. ICIQ-SF is a brief, but robust assessment of impact of urinary incontinence, which may be quickly completed with little data loss (1.6% on average), and most items show moderate to strong concordance with other questionnaires [18]. In our study, we subjectively determined PPI severity as reported by patients, and applied the ICIQ-SF questionnaire by phone to assess the current severity of the condition. Most patients (43.9%) rate their incontinence as moderate, however, 80.6% of subjects score as severe/very severe based on the questionnaire. Improvement rate of 23,4% has been shown in literature between 24 and 48 months after radical prostatectomy [21]. In our study, despite the overall improvement in incontinence rate over time according to patients' report (from 70 to 46,2% between last visit and phone call), the incontinence's profile declined since the proportion of patients with severe incontinence increased from 35 to 80,6%. We hypothesize that this may be related to the long follow-up of our study and the impact of increasing age in incontinence's severity. Evaluating the change patterns of urinary incontinence over a 5-year time span in 827 subjects, Iglesias et al reported a progression of slight and moderate incontinence to moderate and severe degrees, whereas severe UI remained unchanged in 40.1% [22].

Although validated questionnaires are considered important tools for measuring subjective phenomena (such as symptoms and quality of life in an objective way), we could find in this study a clearly discrepancy between men's impression of continence and questionnaire results as 20.6% of them rated the incontinence as severe versus 80.6% through ICIQ-SF evaluation.

There are reports in literature of discrepancy between patients' subjective impression of continence status and more objective criteria; investigating differences in objective and subjective grade of incontinence after radical prostatectomy Kontour and colleagues reported that 34.4% of 479 men who underwent radical prostatectomy felt incontinent by phone interview while only 14.9% of men were incontinent following the objective criteria (24 h pad test) [23].

Discrepancy between physicians' and patients' evaluation of clinical domains related with quality of life of urology or prostate cancer patients has been assessed in previous studies. In a study of 2252 patients in CaPSURE database, significant differences were noted between physicians' and patients' evaluations in different domains, including urinary function: 21% of patients had impaired urinary function/incontinence according to physicians, whereas 97.2% of patients reported the condition [9].

Physicians tend to underestimate the incidence of symptoms when compared to patients' reports. Jarernsiripornkul et al. found that only 22.6% of 716 symptoms were documented in medical records of 103 patients 1 year after receiving treatment [8]. Vistad et al., when investigating 147 cervical cancer survivors showed that physician-reported prevalence rates of grade 3–4 intestinal, bladder and vaginal morbidity were lower than those reported by patients [24]. Moreover, incontinent men tend not to discuss the condition with physicians: when evaluating 840 male veterans in primary care clinics, Smoger and colleagues reported that only 32% had discussed incontinence with their medical provider but 75% desired evaluation and treatment; conclusion was that although incontinence impacts quality of life and although men with incontinence desired treatment, they seldom discussed the problem with medical providers [25].

The results of these studies are in line with our results: 62,7% were continent as reported by physicians, while 70% of patients said they were incontinent at the time of the record.

In respect to racial differences in functional outcomes of patients diagnosed with prostate cancer or subjected to treatment for this condition, studies show a trend towards poorer results in black subjects. An analysis of 1178 patients enrolled in CaPSURE database shows that black men diagnosed with prostate cancer have statistically and clinically worse clinical features at presentation, and lower health-related quality of life, although no statistically significant differences were found in urinary function domain [26].

On the other hand, Johnson et al., when studying more than 2000 patients of Prostate Cancer Outcomes Study showed that black subjects have better bladder control 5 years after radical prostatectomy (urinary function score of 78.5 vs. 72.4) and lower probability of having problems with incontinence [27]. An analysis of 3708 men from CEASAR study showed a considerable decrease in post-radical prostatectomy urinary incontinence scores ("26-item Expanded Prostate Index Composite – EPIC") in the presence of active surveillance or radiation therapy and, although this association was seen for all racial groups, there was a greater decrease in black subjects when compared with Caucasians. Notwithstanding, there were no race-related differences in the chance of moderate/severe discomfort relative to global urinary function [28].

The fact that black men have worse urinary incontinence scores but the same level of discomfort as that of Caucasians may be in line with our study and explain the significant association we found between the black race and the discrepancy between medical records and patient-reported symptoms. Black men, by presenting the same level of discomfort despite the poorer incontinence score, may have even lower levels of discomfort when compared to Caucasians with milder grades of the condition, to the point of not reporting it to physicians.

In our study, we identified a significantly higher discrepancy rate in subjects with low schooling. Litwin et al. demonstrated, when investigating recovery of quality of life indices after radical prostatectomy, that education level was inversely associated with the probability of restoration of baseline urinary function. It was speculated that men with higher schooling might have been more straightforward in their answers to urinary function-related items of the questionnaire. This assumption could possibly explain our findings [29]. On the other hand, in our region, black and mixed-race individuals unfortunately have lower levels of schooling than Caucasians, which could also explain the higher incontinence rates.

This study, by revealing the underestimation of post-surgical urinary incontinence by physicians and identifying a patient profile for which this underestimation is more frequent, demonstrates the need for more careful postoperative management and assessment of urinary function, particularly for patients who fit this profile. Accurate identification of the symptom would allow for appropriate management and early initiation of treatment in patients with persistent incontinence, mitigating the impairment in quality of life caused by the condition.

Our study has limitations, starting with its retrospective nature, in addition to the small number of patients enrolled. A potential bias is the length time one, as there was a long time between last visit and phone call, in such a way that patients' impression of continence status could not be exact. Another important limitation is that the race classification used in this study is not appropriate to completely describe the ethnic/racial identity of each individual, since sociocultural differences are not accurately accounted for; individual, environmental and social characteristics may be even more important than race or ethnicity. Generalization of results is limited by the great variability of population and previously mentioned characteristics, particularly sociocultural differences and differences in the makeup of our population, when compared to others in the same country or around the world.

Conclusion

The factors associated with discrepancy between medical reports and perceptions of patients subjected to radical retropubic prostatectomy regarding urinary incontinence were race and level of schooling. Black men with low schooling are at higher risk for discrepancy and, therefore, postoperative assessment of urinary function must be more careful in these patients, since underestimation of the problem by physicians may negatively affect their quality of life.

Abbreviations

ICIQ-SF: International Consultation on Incontinence Questionnaire – Short Form; PPI: Post-radical prostatectomy urinary incontinence; RRP: Retropubic radical prostatectomy

Acknowledgements

Not applicable.

Author details

[1]Department of Urology, Faculdade de Medicina do ABC, No.2000, Avenue Lauro Gomes, Santo André 09051-040, Brazil. [2]Department of Epidemiology and Data Analysis, Faculdade de Medicina do ABC, No.2000, Avenue Lauro Gomes, Santo André 09051-040, Brazil.

References

1. Talcott JA, Rieker P, Propert KJ, Clark JA, Wishnow KI, Loughlin KR, Richie JP, et al. Patient-reported impotence and incontinence after nerve-sparing radical prostatectomy. J Natl Cancer Inst. 1997;89:1117–23.
2. Stanford J, Feng Z, Hamilton A. Urinary and sexual function after radical prostatectomy for clinically localized prostate cancer. JAMA. 2000;283(3): 354–60.
3. Braslis KG, Santa-Cruz C, Brickman AL, Solloway MS. Quality of life 12 months after radical prostatectomy. Br J Urol. 1995;75:48–53.
4. Johansson E, Steineck G, Holmberg L, Johansson JE, Nyberg T, Ruutu M, et al. Long-term quality-of-life outcomes after radical prostatectomy or watchful waiting: the Scandinavian prostate cancer group-4 randomised trial. Lancet Oncol. 2011;12:891–9.
5. Kim PH, Pinheiro LC, Atoria CL, Eastham JA, Sandhu JS, Elkin EB. Trends in the use of incontinence procedures after radical prostatectomy: a population based analysis. J Urol. 2013;189(2):602–8.
6. Herschorn S, Bruschini H, Comiter C, Grise P, Hanus T, Kirschner-Hermanns R, et al. Committee of the International Consultation on incontinence. Surgical treatment of stress incontinence in men. Neurourol Urodyn. 2010;29(1):179–90.
7. Herschorn S, Bosch JL, Bruschini H, Hanus T, Low A, Schick E. Surgical treatment of urinary incontinence in men. In: Abrams P, Cardozo L, Khoury S, Wein A, editors. Second International Consultation on Incontinence. Plymouth: Health publications ltd; 2002. p. 785–821.
8. Jarernsiripornkul N, Krska J, Capps PA, Richards RM, Lee A. Patient reporting of potential adverse drug reactions: a methodological study. Br J Clin Pharmacol. 2002;53:318–25.
9. Litwin MS, Lubeck DP, Henning JM, Carroll PR. Differences in urologist and patient assessments of health related quality of life in men with prostate cancer: results of the capsure database. J Urol. 1998;159:1988–92.
10. Sacco E, Prayer-Galetti T, Pinto F, Fracalanza S, Betto G. Urinary incontinence after radical prostatectomy: incidence by definition, risk factors and temporal trend in a large series with a long-term follow-up. BJU Int. 2006; 97(6):1234–41.
11. Poon M, Ruckle H, Bamshad BR, Tsai C, Webster R, et al. Radical retropubic prostatectomy: bladder neck preservation versus reconstruction. J Urol. 2000;163:194.
12. Bishoff JT, Motley G, Optenberg SA, Stein CR, Moon KA, et al. Incidence of fecal and urinary incontinence following radical perineal and retropubic prostatectomy in a national population. J Urol. 1998;160:454.
13. Kretschmer A, Hubner W, Sandhu JS, Bauer RM. Evaluation and management of postprostatectomy incontinence: a systematic review of current literature. Eur Urol Focus. 2016;2(3):245–59.
14. Wei JT, Dunn RL, Marcovich R, Montie JE, Sanda MG. Prospective assessment of patient reported urinary continence after radical prostatectomy. J Urol. 2000;164:744–8.
15. Liss MA, Osann K, Canvasser N, Chu W, Chang A, Gan J, et al. Continence definition after radical prostatectomy using urinary quality of life: evaluation of patient reported validated questionnaires. J Urol. 2010;183:1464–8.
16. Holm HV, Fosså SD, Hedlund H, Schultz A, Dahl AA. How should continence and incontinence after radical prostatectomy be evaluated? A prospective study of patient-ratings and changes over time. J Urol. 2014;192:1155–61.

17. Lucas MG, Bosch RJ, Burkhard FC, Cruz F, Madden TB, Nambiar AK, et al. EAU guidelines on assessment and nonsurgical management of urinary incontinence. Eur Urol. 2012;62:1130–42.
18. Avery K, Donovan J, Peters TJ, Shaw C, Gotoh M, Abrams P. ICIQ: a brief and robust measure for evaluating the symptoms and impact of urinary incontinence. Neurourol Urodyn. 2004;23:322–30.
19. Yalcin I, Bump RC. Validation of two global impression questionnaires for incontinence. Am J Obstet Gynecol. 2003;189:98–101.
20. Litwin MS, Hays RD, Fink A, Ganz PA, Leake B, Brook RH. The UCLA prostate Cancer index: development, reliability, and validity of a health-related quality of life measure. Med Care. 1998;36:1002–12.
21. Glickman L, Godoy G, Lepor H. Changes in continence and erectile function between 2 and 4 years after radical prostatectomy. J Urol. 2009;181(2):731–5.
22. Iglesias FJG, Ocerín JM C y, JPM M, Gama VE, Pérez LM, et al. Prevalence and psychosocial impact of urinary incontinence in older people of a Spanish rural population. J Gerontol A Biol Sci Med Sci. 2000;55(4):207–14.
23. Kontur SC, Schatzl G, Valimberti E, Marberger M. Differences in objective and subjective grade of incontinenc e after radical prostatectomy - a long term follow up study. Eur Urol Suppl. 2010;9(6):623.
24. Vistad I, Cvancarova M, Fossa SD, Kristensen GB. Postradiotherapy morbidity in long-term survivors after locally advanced cervical cancer: how well do physicians' assessments agree with those of their patients? Int J Radiat Oncol Biol Physics. 2008;71(5):1335–42.
25. Smoger SH, Felice TL, Kloecker GH. Urinary incontinence among male veterans receiving care in primary care clinics. Ann Intern Med. 2000;132(7): 547–51.
26. Lubeck DP, Kim H, Grossfeld G, Ray P, Penson DF, Flanders SC, et al. Health related quality of life differences between black and white men with prostate cancer: data from the cancer of the prostate strategic urologic research endeavor. J Urol. 2001;166:2281–5.
27. Johnson TK, Gilliland FD, Hoffman RM, Deapen D, Penson DF, Stanford JL, et al. Racial/ethnic differences in functional outcomes in the 5 years after diagnosis of localized prostate cancer. J Clin Oncol. 2004;22:4193–201.
28. Tyson MD, Alvarez J, Koyama T, Hoffman KE, Resnick MJ, Wuf X, et al. Racial variation in patient-reported outcomes following treatment for localized prostate cancer: results from the CEASAR study. Eur Urol. 2017;72(2):307–14.
29. Litwin MS, McGuigan KA, Shpall AI, Dhanani N. Recovery of health related quality of life in the year after radical prostatectomy: early experience. J Urol. 1999;161(2):515–9.

10

Is there any association between prostate-specific antigen screening frequency and uptake of active surveillance in men with low or very low risk prostate cancer?

Kerri Beckmann[1,2*], Netty Kinsella[1,3], Henrik Olsson[4], Anna Wallerstedt Lantz[4], Tobias Nordstrom[4], Markus Aly[4,5], Jan Adolfsson[4,6], Martin Eklund[4] and Mieke Van Hemelrijck[1,7]

Abstract

Background: Patient-related factors such as concern about cancer are believed to influence both men's decisions to undergo prostate specific antigen (PSA) testing and to have definitive treatment if diagnosed with low risk prostate cancer (PCa). The potential link between screening frequency and choice of active surveillance (AS) for low risk disease has not been studied previously. Our aim was to investigate whether there is any association between PCa screening frequency or previous negative prostate biopsy and uptake of AS among men with low risk PCa.

Methods: This register-based study included all men ≤75 years from Stockholm who were diagnosed with low risk PCa from 2008 to 2014 ($n = 4336$). Pre-diagnostic PSA testing and biopsy histories were obtained from the Stockholm PSA and Biopsy Register, a population-based register for the Stockholm country. The association between previous screening/biopsy history and AS uptake (based on primary treatment recorded in the National Prostate Cancer Register) was examined using multivariable logistic regression.

Results: Forty seven percent of men with low risk PCa underwent AS. Uptake was associated with older age, very low risk disease, more recent diagnosis and absence of family history. None of the screening/biopsy measures (testing frequency, mean interval, PSA velocity, highest pre-diagnostic PSA or prior negative biopsy) were associated with uptake of AS among men with low risk PCa. Generalisability to settings with different policies and practices may be limited.

Conclusion: We found no evidence that screening frequency and negative biopsy influence uptake of AS among Swedish men with low risk PCa. Further research is required to determine factors that still present barriers for men taking up AS.

Keywords: Active surveillance, PSA testing, Screening, Prostate biopsy, Prostate neoplasm

Background

The incidence of prostate cancer (PCa) has been increasing over the past two decades in a large number of countries, primarily due to the availability and uptake of prostate-specific antigen (PSA) testing as a means of early detection [1]. While prostate specific antigen PSA testing has considerable value in clinical follow-up after diagnosis, its utility with respect to detecting PCa is contentious' [2]. Most professional society guidelines do not recommend population-based PSA screening, due to increased risk of overdiagnosis and overtreatment, but do support shared decision making between physicians and men who are concerned about PCa risk [3].

Increased availability and use of PSA testing as a screening tool has led to an increase in the incidence of low and intermediate risk disease as well as stage

* Correspondence: Kerri.beckmann@kcl.ac.uk; kerri.beckmann@unisa.edu.au
1Translational Oncology & Urology Research, Comprehensive Cancer Centre, King's College London, 3rd Floor, Bermondsey Wing, Guy's Hospital, London SE1 9RT, UK
2University of South Australia, Centre for population Health Research Adelaide Australia, Adelaide, Australia
Full list of author information is available at the end of the article

migration in PCa across a number of countries [4], with a large proportion of PSA-detected cancers classified as low-grade/low-volume indolent disease, with little metastatic potential [5]. Many clinical practice guidelines now recommend active surveillance (AS) for low risk PCa, in an attempt to reduce the unnecessary morbidity of overtreatment [6]. Even so, variation in the uptake of AS occurs between and within countries [7, 8].

Recent reviews have identified several factors that appear to drive the uptake of AS [9–12]. These include patient related factors, family and social supports, clinician factors, health systems and health policy [9]. Concern about cancer progression and control of cancer are commonly mentioned as factors that impact choice to undertake AS [12, 13]. Similar factors have been reported to drive PSA screening, where men identify concerns about cancer, the need for peace of mind and control over one's health as reasons for undergoing PSA testing [14, 15]. Hence, the choice to undergo PSA testing, and to have definitive treatment if diagnosed with PCa, may be correlated through a common concern to optimize health outcomes. On the other hand, men with prior experience of prostate biopsy may be deterred from choosing AS due to negative adverse side effects following biopsy [16, 17], or because they have less confidence in the accuracy of biopsy procedures to detect cancer progression [18]. Several interview and internet content-based studies have suggested the psychological burden associated with ongoing monitoring during active surveillance, as well as the morbidity associated with repeat biopsy, may be linked to reduced uptake AS [19]. However, other studies have emphasized the process of repeated monitoring while on active surveillance as reassuring [20].

To our knowledge, the question of whether frequency of PSA testing or a negative prostate biopsy before diagnosis influence the uptake of AS has not previously been addressed. The primary aim of this study was to determine whether frequency of pre-diagnostic PSA testing was associated with uptake of AS among men diagnosed with low or very low risk PCa. Our secondary aims were to determine whether the experience of a negative prostate biopsy or changes in PSA levels prior to diagnosis influenced the likelihood of choosing AS. The quantitative findings of this work will add to the qualitative studies investigating patient and physician behaviour, so that combined they can help us develop better educational and supportive tools for patients and healthcare professionals.

Methods

To assess the relationship between PSA screening history and uptake of AS we utilized data from the Stockholm PSA and Biopsy Register, a population-based register which contains information on every PSA test and prostate biopsy for men residing in Stockholm County since 2003. PSA test results and biopsy reports were obtained from the three official laboratories within the Stockholm region (Karolinska University Laboratory, Aleris and Unilabs) providing near complete population coverage of all PSA and biopsy tests undertaken in the county since the start of the register [21]. All PSA and biopsy data were provided electronically, directly from laboratory records to the register. Data were also collected on demographic characteristics, all PCa diagnoses, history of PCa among first degree male relatives and hospitalisations (since 1998), through linkages with established national registries using the unique Swedish personal identification number. A previous quality study of the National Prostate Cancer Register (NPCR), which was the source of cancer related information, indicates coverage of 98% of PCa cases compared with the National Cancer Register, and on average 90% completeness of clinical variables collected [22].

In Sweden there is no formal PCa screening program. However, non-symptomatic men can request a "screening" test from their general physician. Hence data on PSA tests in this study include a mixture of tests relating to symptoms and testing based on requests from patients. However, they pertain only to PSA tests undertaken before diagnosis. In addition, treatment choices in Sweden are usually made through shared decision-making between patient and treating clinician.

Our study cohort consisted of all men residing in the Stockholm County between 2008 and 2014 who were diagnosed with low risk PCa, defined as PSA < 10 ng/ml, Gleason score < =6, and clinical stage T1–2. Men aged over 75 years at diagnosis were excluded. This cohort was chosen to represent men with 10 years life expectancy who would have been eligible for AS according to Swedish guidelines [23].

The main outcome of interest was uptake of AS. For our main analyses we derived the measure of AS uptake from the NPCR [24] based on primary treatment reported to the register 6 months post-diagnosis. When treatment data were missing ($n = 485$, 11%) men were considered not to have undergone AS. For sensitivity analyses, we reclassified AS based on linkage with the inpatient register to identify men who had undergone radical prostatectomy or radiotherapy as inpatients within 6 months of diagnosis. This resulted in reclassification of four men from the AS group to active treatment and 476 men with unknown treatment to the AS group. This reclassification assumes that men were on AS if treatment data were missing in NPCR and no active treatment was identified in the inpatient register.

Measures of pre-diagnosis PSA and biopsy history were derived from the Stockholm PSA and Biopsy Register. These included: total number of PSA tests; total

Table 1 Cohort characteristics

Characteristics N = 4336	Active surveillance		p-value
	no	yes	
Total - n (%)	2298 (53)	2038 (47)	
Age - mean (SD)	62.2 (6.6)	63.9 (5.7)	< 0.001
Cancer characteristics- median (IQR)			
PSA at diagnosis	5 (3.8–6.6)	4.6 (3.4–6.1)	< 0.001
Max cancer length	5 (2–11)	2 (1–4)	< 0.001
Positive cores	2 (1–4)	1 (1–2)	< 0.001
Prostate volume	35 (26–46)	40 (30–51)	< 0.001
Stage:			
T1c - n (%)	1800 (78)	1827 (90)	< 0.001
T2 - n (%)	498 (22)	211 (10)	
Risk Category (Swedish guidelines) - n (%):			
Very low risk	552 (24)	1114 (55)	< 0.001
Low risk	1746 (76)	924 (45)	
Reason for presentation - n (%)			
Health check	1412 (61)	1542 (76)	< 0.001
LUTS	397 (17)	297 (15)	
Other symptoms	257 (11)	153 (8)	
Unknown	218 (10)	41 (2)	
Comorbidity (CCI at diagnosis)			
0	2012 (88)	1764 (86)	0.531
1	179 (8)	178 (9)	
2	75 (3)	72 (4)	
3+	30 (1)	32 (2)	
Year of diagnosis - n (%)			
2008	337 (15)	127 (6)	< 0.001
2009	413 (18)	160 (8)	
2010	323 (14)	154 (8)	
2011	242 (11)	178 (9)	
2012	247 (11)	209 (10)	
2013	313 (14)	415 (20)	
2014	423 (18)	795 (39)	
Education level - n (%)			
< High school	323 (14)	320 (16)	0.073
High school	940 (41)	867 (43)	
Post high school< 3 yrs	330 (14)	296 (15)	
University	687 (30)	541 (27)	
missing	18 (1)	14 (1)	
Civil Status			
Not married/widowed	749 (33)	719 (35)	0.063
Married/partner	1549 (67)	1319 (65)	
History of PCa in family - n (%)			
No	1713 (75)	1621 (80)	< 0.001
Yes	583 (25)	415 (20)	

Table 1 Cohort characteristics *(Continued)*

Characteristics N = 4336	Active surveillance		p-value
	no	yes	
TREATMENTS - n (%)			
Active surveillance	0 (0)	2038 (100)	
Curative	1604 (69)	0 (0)	
Watchful waiting	209 (9)	0 (0)	
Treatment unknown	485 (21)	0 (0)	

number of PSA tests excluding any likely repeat tests for abnormal/inconclusive results (i.e. tests within 60 days of the previous PSA test); highest total PSA; PSA velocity (defined as change in total PSA/year from first test to PSA at diagnosis); and number of prior negative biopsies. Biopsies performed within 60 days of diagnosis were considered part of diagnostic workup and were excluded. For the main analysis, all measures were derived for the five-year period before PCa diagnosis to ensure equivalence with respect to period of observation.

Data on potential confounders included: age and year of diagnosis; Charlson comorbidity index (CCI) [25], civil status (married, not married); education level (<high school, high school, post-secondary and university); family history of PCa (any first-degree family member had PCa); symptoms at presentation (yes/no); and risk category (e.g. very low versus low risk). In accordance with Swedish guidelines, very low risk PCa was defined as those with T1c disease, ≤4 positive cores (of ≥8 cores) and PSA density (total PSA/prostate volume) < 0.15 μl/cm^3. Most men would have been assessed through 8–10 core TRUS biopsy prior to treatment decision. Use of MRI was not specified in the Swedish guidelines during the study period and thus has not been considered as a contributing factor in this study.

Multivariable logistic regression models were undertaken to determine the relationship between number of previous PSA tests and uptake of AS in the eligible cohort, with simultaneous adjustment for all confounders and prior number of negative biopsies. Separate models were also conducted for each of the specific PSA measures, and adjusted odds ratio and 95% confidence intervals are reported. Further subgroup analyses were undertaken according to risk category (very low, low risk) and period of diagnosis (2008–2010, 2011–2012, 2013–2014). Finally, we undertook the following sensitivity analyses to assess impact of potential errors in outcome and exposure measures: 1) analyses using all PSA and biopsy data from 2003 to include all available data, 2) analyses excluding men who did not have primary treatment recorded in NPCR, and 3) analysis with treatment reassigned according to linkage with the inpatient register.

Ethics approval was obtained from the Stockholm Regional Ethics Committee.

Results

Of the 4336 eligible participants, 2038 (47%) had AS recorded as the primary treatment for PCa. Table 1 shows the cohort characteristics according to whether participants underwent AS. Those who choose AS were slightly older, presented less frequently with symptoms, and had lower volume disease (e.g. fewer positive cores, lower maximum core length, and higher percent with very low risk disease). There was a strong trend toward more men taking up AS in the later years, especially 2013–2014.

PSA testing and prostate biopsy history are shown in Table 2 according to AS status. The two treatment groups were similar with respect to mean number of previous PSA tests, maximum total PSA, minimum free to total PSA ratio, and number of previous prostate biopsies. The mean PSA velocity was slightly lower for men who underwent AS.

Results of multivariable logistic regression analysis examining the effect of frequency of PSA tests and prior number of prostate biopsies on uptake of AS are shown in Table 3. Uptake of AS was more likely among older age groups (odds ratio [OR]: 1.69; 95% confidence interval [CI]: 1.37–2.20, 65-69 yrs. versus 55-59 yrs) and those with very low risk PCa (OR: 2.95; 95%CI: 2.49–3.40) and less likely among men with a family history of PCa (OR: 0.82; 95%CI: 0.69–0.97) and men who were married (OR: 0.80; 95%CI: 0.67–0.93). The odds of AS uptake also increased with more recent years of diagnosis. No association was observed with respect to either number of PSA tests or prostate biopsies during the 5 years before diagnosis.

Results for associations between specific PSA/biopsy measures and uptake of AS are shown in Table 4. There was no association between uptake of AS and pre-diagnostic total PSA concentration or PSA velocity prior to diagnosis. Odds were slightly elevated for any prior negative biopsy (OR: 1.11, 95%CI: 0.90–1.38), though the difference was not statistically significant. Results were similar when considering low and very low risk categories separately. Similarly, analyses for different diagnostic periods showed no association for PSA screening or biopsy history in any period. (Table 5).

Sensitivity analyses

Results were essentially unchanged from our main findings for all PSA test and biopsy measures in each of the sensitivity analyses undertaken. These included when AS status was reclassified based in hospital admission data, when cases with unknown treatment were excluded, and when PSA and biopsy history included all available data from 2003 rather than the 5-year period before diagnosis. (Additional file 1: Table S1).

Discussion

Our study is the first to explore whether frequency of PSA testing, PSA results or the experience of a negative prostate biopsy influence uptake of AS among men diagnosed with low risk PCa. We found no association between uptake of AS and frequency of PSA testing, PSA velocity or highest total PSA concentration prior to diagnosis. Uptake of AS was also not associated with a history of previous negative biopsy. Our findings applied equally to men with low or very low risk disease and across time periods. Equivalent results from our sensitivity analysis investigating the influence of missing data

Table 2 PSA testing and prostate biopsy history in the 5 years prior to diagnosis of prostate cancer

Measures	Active surveillance		*p*-value
	no	yes	
Prior PSA tests - *Mean (sd)*			
Total no. PSA tests	4.0 (2.6)	3.9 (2.7)	0.322
No. PSA tests excluding confirmatory tests	3.3 (2.3)	3.2 (2.2)	0.597
Screening interval (days)[a]	304 (281)	333 (313)	0.003
Mean pre-diagnostic total PSA level	4.6 (1.9)	4.3 (2.1)	0.001
Highest pre-diagnostic total PSA level	5.8 (3.1)	5.4 (3.6)	0.001
PSA velocity (ng/mL/year)[a]	0.46 (1.6)	0.42 (1.7)	0.001
No. biopsies prior to diagnosis *No. (%)*			
None	2001 (87)	1771 (87)	0.934
1	235 (10)	211 (10)	
2	48 (2)	46 (2)	
3+	14 (1)	10 (0.5)	

[a]among men with 2 or more tests during previous 5 years

Table 3 Factors associated with uptake of up active surveillance, among men with low and very low risk prostate cancer in Stockholm Sweden 2008–2014

Factors	crude			adjusted[a]		
	OR	95% CI	*p*-value	OR	95% CI	*p*-value
Age group						
< 55 yrs	0.64	0.49–0.84	< 0.001	0.61	0.46–0.81	< 0.001
55-59 yrs	1.00	ref	–	1.00	ref	–
60-64 yrs	1.14	0.90–1.29	0.170	1.19	0.96–1.49	0.117
65-69 yrs	1.80	1.50–2.15	< 0.001	1.69	1.37–2.10	< 0.001
70-74 yrs	1.37	0.74–0.98	0.005	1.70	1.30–2.21	< 0.001
Civil status						
Not married	1.00	ref	–	1.00	ref	
Married	0.89	0.78–1.01	0.063	0.80	0.67–0.93	0.004
Education level						
Less than high school	1.07	0.87–1.32	0.436	1.06	0.86–1.31	0.565
Completed High school	1.00	ref	–	1.00	ref	–
3 yrs. post high school	0.97	0.81–1.17	0.376	0.96	0.78–1.20	0.738
University	0.85	0.73–0.99	0.019	0.87	0.73–1.03	0.104
Family history of PCa						
No	1.00	ref	–	1.00	ref	–
Yes	0.75	0.65–0.87	< 0.001	0.82	0.69–0.97	0.023
CCI						
0	1.00	ref	–	1.00	ref	–
1	1.15	0.92–1.43	0.235	0.98	0.76–1.26	0.785
2+	1.17	0.88–1.55	0.567	1.05	0.76–1.47	0.785
Presented with symptoms/LUTS						
no	1.00	ref	–	1.00	ref	–
yes	0.63	0.54–0.72	< 0.001	0.88	0.74–1.03	0.113
Prostate volume	1.01	1.01–1.02	< 0.001	1.00	1.00–1.01	0.197
Risk category						
Low	1.00	ref	–	1.00	ref	
Very low	3.81	3.35–4.34	< 0.001	2.95	2.49–3.40	< 0.001
Diagnosis year (cont. 2008–2014)	1.34	1.30–1.38	< 0.001	1.35	1.30–1.40	< 0.001
No. PSA tests in past 5 yrs (cont.)	0.75	0.65–0.87	0.322	0.99	0.97–1.02	0.672
No. negative biopsies in past 5 yrs (cont.)	1.01	0.88–1.14	0.947	1.11	0.94–1.30	0.214

CCI Charlson comorbidity index, *CI* confidence interval, *LUTS* lower urinary tract symptoms, *OR* odds ratio, *PCa* prostate cancer, *PSA* prostate specific antigen, *ref.* reference
[a]simultaneously adjusted for all factors

indicate robust findings despite some missing treatment information.

Uptake of AS was higher among older men, those with very low risk disease and those more recently diagnosed, while it was lower among those with a family history of PCa. These findings are encouraging as they indicate increased uptake over time and among those most likely to be over-treated. Increasing trends toward AS among men with low risk PCa have been reported in a number of large cohorts, though considerable variations remains between countries, practices and physicians [7]. Current estimates of AS uptake range from 74% in Sweden in 2014 (Swedish National Prostate Cancer Register [8]), 40% in USA in 2010–13 (Cancer of the Prostate Strategic Urologic Research Endeavor [26]), 40% in Australia in 2012 (Victorian Prostate Cancer Registry [27]) to 21% in Canada in 2010 (Ontario Cancer Registry [28]). The rate of uptake in our study (47%) is within the range of contemporary cohorts worldwide. However, the relatively high rate of uptake in Sweden may limit the generalizability of our findings to other countries.

Table 4 Adjusted ORs for different measure of PSA testing/results associated with uptake of AS in men with low/very low risk PCa (History for the 5-year period before diagnosis)

PSA and Biopsy measures	OR	95% CI	*p*-value
Total number of PSA tests (continuous)	0.99	0.96–1.02	0.672
Total number of PSA tests excluding repeat tests (test within 60 days of previous test)	0.99	0.96–1.03	0.597
Highest pre-diagnostic total-PSA level (per ng/mL)	0.98	0.95–1.02	0.332
Mean PSA velocity (earliest to diagnostic PSA level)	0.98	0.96–1.01	0.133
Any previous negative prostate biopsy	1.11	0.90–1.38	0.329
Total number of previous biopsies (continuous)	1.04	0.88–1.21	0.669

CI confidence interval, *OR* odds ratio, *PSA* prostate specific antigen
ORs derived from separate multivariable logistic regression models adjusted for age, education level, civil status, CCI, family history, symptoms, diagnosis year and risk category (and number of previous PSA tests/biopsies)

Our finding of no association between AS uptake and frequency of PSA testing does not support the hypothesis that screening frequency and choice of treatment are linked through patient health-seeking behaviours, at least not for men residing in Stockholm. While anxiety and cancer worry have been suggested as potential factors influencing frequency of PSA testing, as well as choice of PCa treatment [12, 13], evidence for their effect on screening and treatment decisions is tenuous. Quantitative studies examining the relationship between anxiety and PSA screening have yielded mixed results, including positive [29] and negative [30] associations with higher anxiety, a U-shaped relationship [31] and no association [14]. Similarly, fear of disease progression and wanting control over cancer are commonly mentioned reasons for not choosing AS in several qualitative studies [13], but there is little quantitative evidence demonstrating the influence of such psychological factors on uptake of AS.

Several recent studies and reviews have highlighted the importance of more systemic factors on uptake of AS, such as physician's recommendation [11], and local or national policies and practices [8, 9, 11, 19]. For example, clinician bias for active treatment can reduce uptake of AS [9, 10, 12], while good patient-physician relationships, shared decision-making, a multidisciplinary approach and specific policies supporting AS facilitate greater uptake of AS [9, 10]. In the current study, AS uptake increased sharply in the later years. The strong endorsement of AS for low risk PCa in the 2013 update of Swedish guidelines is likely to explain this trend, lending support for the argument that clinician recommendation and the health policy environment have a major influence on uptake of AS [8]. Lack of data on treating clinician precluded direct assessment of clinician variability in the current study.

In addition, we found no evidence to support the hypothesis that having had a prior negative biopsy influences the decision to undergo AS. Nor did we find any evidence that higher serum PSA levels or higher PSA velocity prior to diagnosis, which may increase patients' concerns about the potential for disease progression, influenced the uptake of AS in men diagnosed with low risk disease. We had expected that having had a previous biopsy would be negatively associated with uptake of AS due to some men having experienced pain, discomfort or side effects, such as hematuria, infection and sepsis, which can affect up to 1 in 3 men undergoing biopsy [16, 17]. Equally, uptake of AS might be reduced due to a lack of confidence in biopsy procedures if it was

Table 5 Adjusted ORs for uptake of AS in relation to previous number of PSA tests and any prior negative biopsy, stratified by 1) risk and 2) period of diagnosis (History for the 5-year period before diagnosis)

Stratified by:	Number of PSA tests			Number of biopsies		
	OR	95% CI	*p*-value	OR	95% CI	*p*-value
Risk category						
Very low risk (*n* = 1568)	0.99	0.96–1.04	0.681	1.06	0.78–1.38	0.702
Low risk (*n* = 2292)	0.99	0.96–1.03	0.984	1.14	0.94–1.38	0.187
Year of diagnosis						
2008–2010 (n = 1,339)	0.98	0.94–1.03	0.485	1.21	0.95–1.56	0.121
2011–2012 (*n* = 818)	1.02	0.98–1.07	0.366	0.93	0.71–1.21	0.594
2013–2014 (*n* = 1703)	0.99	0.93–1.05	0.791	1.00	0.73–1.37	0.995

CI confidence interval, *OR* odds ratio, *PSA* prostate specific antigen
ORs derived from separate multivariable logistic regression models adjusted for age, education level, civil status, CCI, family history, symptoms, diagnosis year and risk category (simultaneous adjustment for no. PSA tests and biopsy)

perceived that cancer had been missed at an earlier biopsy [18]. Our findings do not indicate a negative association between prior history of biopsy and AS uptake.

Diagnostic and surveillance pathways for men with PCa cancer are rapidly evolving, particularly with respect to the use of MRI to detect significant cancer and to monitor disease progression [32]. Further research is required to determine whether this provides men with increased reassurance and confidence to commence AS.

The strengths of the study are its large size and the population-based nature of the data with accurate linkage resulting in complete coverage of all PSA testing and biopsy procedures undertaken in the Stockholm County since 2003. While some inaccuracy in exposure measures is possible given a small proportion of men may have undergone testing in another County during the study period, the effects are likely to be negligible. Primary treatment data were extracted from national registries for Stockholm residents so that treatment outside the County but within Sweden would be captured. Hence, our findings of no association are unlikely to be due to lack of power or misclassification of exposure, which would bias toward null findings. Furthermore, a substantial proportion of men in the study population had no treatment record at 6 months. However, sensitivity analyses using all available data and various adjusted measures of AS yielded consistent results. Since our study did not include assessment of any psychological measures (e.g. anxiety or cancer concern) we cannot draw direct conclusions that such factors are not influential in decision making around screening or treatment. The lack of data on treating clinician is a further limitation, given the potential influence physicians have on patients' treatment decisions. Finally, generalisability of these findings outside of Sweden may be limited, given the rates of AS uptake are relatively high in Sweden and that PSA testing and AS are likely to be driven by health care system-specific factors as well as the local policy environment (i.e. clinical guidelines) [9].

Conclusion

We found no evidence that pre-diagnostic PSA screening frequency or negative biopsies influence uptake of AS among Swedish men with low risk PCa. Given uptake of AS is not yet 100%, further research is required to determine what factors still present barriers for men taking up AS.

Additional file

Additional file 1: Table S1. Sensitivity analyses. Adjusted ORs for different measures of PSA/biopsy history associated with uptake of AS in men with low/very low risk PCa. (DOCX 15 kb)

Acknowledgements

This project would not have been possible without the efforts of Magnus Törnblom, Stefan Carlsson, Marie Hjälm, Lars Egevad and Pär Stattin who support the National Prostate Cancer Register (Stockholm Region).

Authors' contributions

Study design and conception: ME, MVH, NK, KB; acquisition of data: HO, ME; Statistical analysis of data: KB, interpretation of results: KB, NK, TN, MA, AWL, MVH, JA, ME; drafting manuscript KB; revision of manuscript: KB, HO, TN, MA, AWL, MVH, JA, ME. All authors approved the final manuscript.

Author details

[1]Translational Oncology & Urology Research, Comprehensive Cancer Centre, King's College London, 3rd Floor, Bermondsey Wing, Guy's Hospital, London SE1 9RT, UK. [2]University of South Australia, Centre for population Health Research Adelaide Australia, Adelaide, Australia. [3]Department of Urology, The Royal Marsden Hospital, London, UK. [4]Department of Medical Epidemiology and Biostatistics, Karolinska Institutet, Stockholm, Sweden. [5]Department of Molecular Medicine and Surgery, Karolinska Institutet, Stockholm, Sweden. [6]CLINTEC-Department, Karolinska Institutet, Stockholm, Sweden. [7]Unit of Epidemiology, Institute of Environmental Medicine, Karolinska Institutet, Stockholm, Sweden.

References

1. Baade PD, Youlden DR, Krnjacki LJ. International epidemiology of prostate cancer: geographical distribution and secular trends. Mol Nutr Food Res. 2009;53(2):171–84.
2. Hugosson J, Carlsson S. Overdetection in screening for prostate cancer. Curr Opin Urol. 2014;24(3):256–63.
3. Loeb S. Guideline of guidelines: prostate cancer screening. BJU Int. 2014; 114(3):323–5.
4. Ohmann EL, Loeb S, Robinson D, Bill-Axelson A, Berglund A, Stattin P. Nationwide, population-based study of prostate cancer stage migration between and within clinical risk categories. Scand J Urol. 2014;48(5):426–35.
5. Albertsen PC. Observational studies and the natural history of screen-detected prostate cancer. Curr Opin Urol. 2015;25(3):232–7.
6. Klotz L. Active surveillance for low-risk prostate cancer. Curr Opin Urol. 2017; 27(3):225–30.
7. Auffenberg GB, Lane BR, Linsell S, Cher ML, Miller DC. Practice- vs physician-level variation in use of active surveillance for men with low-risk prostate Cancer: implications for collaborative quality improvement. JAMA Surg. 2017;152(10):978–80.
8. Loeb S, Folkvaljon Y, Curnyn C, Robinson D, Bratt O, Stattin P. Uptake of active surveillance for very-low-risk prostate Cancer in Sweden. JAMA Oncol. 2017;3(10):1393–8.
9. Kinsella N, Stattin P, Cahill D, Brown C, Bill-Axelson A, Bratt O, Carlsson S, Van Hemelrijck M. Factors influencing Men's choice of and adherence to active surveillance for low-risk prostate Cancer: a mixed-method systematic review. Eur Urol. 2018.
10. Dall'Era MA. Patient and disease factors affecting the choice and adherence to active surveillance. Curr Opin Urol. 2015;25(3):272–6.
11. Dall'Era MA, Albertsen PC, Bangma C, Carroll PR, Carter HB, Cooperberg MR, Freedland SJ, Klotz LH, Parker C, Soloway MS. Active surveillance for prostate cancer: a systematic review of the literature. Eur Urol. 2012;62(6):976–83.
12. van den Bergh RC, Korfage IJ, Bangma CH. Psychological aspects of active surveillance. Curr Opin Urol. 2012;22(3):237–42.
13. Pickles T, Ruether JD, Weir L, Carlson L, Jakulj F, Team SC. Psychosocial barriers to active surveillance for the management of early prostate cancer and a strategy for increased acceptance. BJU Int. 2007;100(3):544–51.
14. Kotwal AA, Schumm P, Mohile SG, Dale W. The influence of stress, depression, and anxiety on PSA screening rates in a nationally representative sample. Med Care. 2012;50(12):1037–44.
15. Consedine NS. Are we worrying about the right men and are the right men feeling worried? Conscious but not unconscious prostate anxiety predicts screening among men from three ethnic groups. Am J Mens Health. 2012; 6(1):37–50.

16. Wade J, Rosario DJ, Howson J, Avery KN, Salter CE, Goodwin ML, Blazeby JM, Lane JA, Metcalfe C, Neal DE, et al. Role of information in preparing men for transrectal ultrasound guided prostate biopsy: a qualitative study embedded in the ProtecT trial. BMC Health Serv Res. 2015;15:80.
17. Wade J, Rosario DJ, Macefield RC, Avery KN, Salter CE, Goodwin ML, Blazeby JM, Lane JA, Metcalfe C, Neal DE, et al. Psychological impact of prostate biopsy: physical symptoms, anxiety, and depression. J Clin Oncol. 2013; 31(33):4235–41.
18. Macefield RC, Metcalfe C, Lane JA, Donovan JL, Avery KN, Blazeby JM, Down L, Neal DE, Hamdy FC, Vedhara K, et al. Impact of prostate cancer testing: an evaluation of the emotional consequences of a negative biopsy result. Br J Cancer. 2010;102(9):1335–40.
19. Mishra MV, Bennett M, Vincent A, Lee OT, Lallas CD, Trabulsi EJ, Gomella LG, Dicker AP, Showalter TN. Identifying barriers to patient acceptance of active surveillance: content analysis of online patient communications. PLoS One. 2013;8(9):e68563.
20. Volk RJ, McFall SL, Cantor SB, Byrd TL, Le YC, Kuban DA, Mullen PD. It's not like you just had a heart attack': decision-making about active surveillance by men with localized prostate cancer. Psychooncology. 2014;23(4):467–72.
21. Nordstrom T, Aly M, Clements MS, Weibull CE, Adolfsson J, Gronberg H. Prostate-specific antigen (PSA) testing is prevalent and increasing in Stockholm County, Sweden, despite no recommendations for PSA screening: results from a population-based study, 2003-2011. Eur Urol. 2013; 63(3):419–25.
22. Tomic K, Sandin F, Wigertz A, Robinson D, Lambe M, Stattin P. Evaluation of data quality in the National Prostate Cancer Register of Sweden. Eur J Cancer. 2015;51(1):101–11.
23. Nationellt vårdprogram för prostatacancer, Cancercentrum i samverkan [https://www.cancercentrum.se/samverkan/cancerdiagnoser/prostata/vardprogram/gallande-vardprogram-prostatacancer/].
24. Van Hemelrijck M, Garmo H, Wigertz A, Nilsson P, Stattin P. Cohort profile update: the National Prostate Cancer Register of Sweden and prostate Cancer data base--a refined prostate cancer trajectory. Int J Epidemiol. 2016; 45(1):73–82.
25. Charlson ME, Pompei P, Ales KL, MacKenzie CR. A new method of classifying prognostic comorbidity in longitudinal studies: development and validation. J Chronic Dis. 1987;40(5):373–83.
26. Cooperberg MR, Carroll PR. Trends in Management for Patients with Localized Prostate Cancer, 1990-2013. JAMA. 2015;314(1):80–2.
27. Weerakoon M, Papa N, Lawrentschuk N, Evans S, Millar J, Frydenberg M, Bolton D, Murphy DG. The current use of active surveillance in an Australian cohort of men: a pattern of care analysis from the Victorian prostate Cancer registry. BJU Int. 2015;115(Suppl 5):50–6.
28. Richard PO, Alibhai SM, Panzarella T, Klotz L, Komisarenko M, Fleshner NE, Urbach D, Finelli A. The uptake of active surveillance for the management of prostate cancer: a population-based analysis. Can Urol Assoc J. 2016; 10(9–10):333–8.
29. Taylor KL, Shelby R, Kerner J, Redd W, Lynch J. Impact of undergoing prostate carcinoma screening on prostate carcinoma-related knowledge and distress. Cancer. 2002;95(5):1037–44.
30. Roumier X, Azzouzi R, Valeri A, Guillemin F, Fournier G, Cussenot O, Mangin P, Cormier L. Adherence to an annual PSA screening program over 3 years for brothers and sons of men with prostate cancer. Eur Urol. 2004;45(3):280–5 author reply 285-286.
31. Consedine NS, Morgenstern AH, Kudadjie-Gyamfi E, Magai C, Neugut AI. Prostate cancer screening behavior in men from seven ethnic groups: the fear factor. Cancer Epidemiol Biomark Prev. 2006;15(2):228–37.
32. Fascelli M, George AK, Frye T, Turkbey B, Choyke PL, Pinto PA. The role of MRI in active surveillance for prostate cancer. Curr Urol Rep. 2015;16(6):42.

11

Electrical conductivity-based contrast imaging for characterizing prostatic tissues: In vivo animal feasibility study

Yong Soo Cho[1†], Young Hoe Hur[2†], Hyun Ju Seon[1], Jin Woong Kim[1*] and Hyung Joong Kim[3*]

Abstract

Background: Electrical conductivity-based magnetic resonance (MR) imaging may provide unique information on tissue condition because its contrast originates from the concentration and mobility of ions in the cellular space. We imaged the conductivity of normal canine prostate in vivo and evaluated tissue contrast in terms of both the conductivity distribution and anatomical significance.

Methods: Five healthy laboratory beagles were used. After clipping the pelvis hair, we attached electrodes and placed each dog inside the bore of an MRI scanner. During MR scanning, we injected imaging currents into two mutually orthogonal directions between two pairs of electrodes. A multi spin echo pulse sequence was used to obtain the MR magnitude and magnetic flux density images. The projected current density algorithm was used to reconstruct the conductivity image.

Results: Conductivity images showed unique contrast depending on the prostatic tissues. From the conductivity distribution, conductivity was highest in the center area and lower in the order of the middle and outer areas of prostatic tissues. The middle and outer areas were, respectively, 11.2 and 25.5% lower than the center area. Considering anatomical significance, conductivity was highest in the central zone and lower in the order of the transitional and peripheral zones in all prostates. The transitional and peripheral zones were, respectively, 7.5 and 17.8% lower than the central zone.

Conclusions: Current conductivity-based MR imaging can differentiate prostatic tissues without using any contrast media or additional MR scans. The electrical conductivity images with unique contrast to tissue condition can provide a prior information on tissues in situ to be used for human imaging.

Keywords: Electrical conductivity, Magnetic resonance imaging, Prostate, Central zone, Peripheral zone

Background

Prostate cancer and benign prostatic hyperplasia are the most common diseases and significant causes of death for older adult men [1]. The morphological and functional examinations are widely used to characterize the tissue properties of prostatic diseases [2, 3]. The prostate gland can be divided into the central area and peripheral area [4]. The central area consists of the central and transitional zones. The peripheral area consists of the peripheral zone and a small amount of anterior fibromuscular stroma without glandular tissue. There exist differences in volume, tissue composition, and incidence of prostatic diseases among the three zones [4, 5]. Specifically, the incidence of prostate cancers and prostatitis is higher in the peripheral zone than in the other zones. Therefore, image-based qualitative and quantitative information on prostatic tissues can provide a prior knowledge of the zonal information with prostatic diseases.

The prostate is an imaging area of growing concern related with aging. Although prostate cancer is a common cancer in older adult men, imaging diagnosis in detection

* Correspondence: jw4249@hanmail.net; bmekim@khu.ac.kr
†Yong Soo Cho and Young Hoe Hur contributed equally to this work.
[1]Department of Radiology, Chosun University Hospital and Chosun University College of Medicine, 365 Pilmun-daero, Dong-gu, Gwangju 61453, South Korea
[3]Department of Biomedical Engineering, Kyung Hee University, 23 Kyungheedaero, Dongdaemungu, Seoul 02447, South Korea
Full list of author information is available at the end of the article

and localization of prostate cancer remains challenging compared with other abdominopelvic cancers [6]. Among imaging modalities, magnetic resonance imaging (MRI) is a powerful tool for visualizing tissue conditions because of its excellent soft tissue contrast by various imaging parameters [7]. In general, T2-weighted MR imaging provides enough contrast on zonal information, but tumor localization is limited and prostate biopsy is mandatory to diagnose prostate cancer. Recently, the introduction of a multi-parametric MR imaging method, which is a combination of dynamic contrast-enhanced MRI and diffusion-weighted imaging and MR spectroscopy, has improved the diagnostic accuracy in prostatic diseases [6]. The multi-parametric MR imaging is used for assessing intraprostatic diseases, while positron emission tomography (PET) has advantage in the detection of extraprostatic diseases [8]. Despite these technical advances, there still exist difficulties in tumor diagnosis and the assessment of treatment response after hormonal or radiation therapy. Thus, prostate biopsy is performed in almost all patients with suspected prostate cancer [6, 9]. New imaging techniques are being studied to improve the diagnosis and monitor the treatment response in patients with prostate cancer.

MR-based tissue property mapping is an emerging technique that uses an MR scanner to obtain non-invasive information concerning electrical tissue properties such as conductivity and permittivity [10–12]. Such electrical tissue properties provide alternative information on tissue structure and function, and can serve as a good complement to the information provided by traditional MRI methods [13–15]. Several studies reported the electrical properties of the prostatic tissues by measuring its values in vitro or ex vivo [16], but no in vivo imaging study can non-invasively provide information on the tissue condition in situ. The recent magnetic resonance electrical impedance tomography (MREIT) method enables high-resolution imaging of electrical conductivity by the externally injected currents [12, 14, 17]. The electrical conductivity of biological tissues is primarily determined by the concentration and mobility of ions that exist in the intra- and extracellular structures [17, 18]. The electrical conductivity contrast is closely related to the structural and functional conditions of tissues and organs [11, 12, 17, 18]. Therefore, the electrical conductivity has potential to provide direct information on the microscopic structures that can be represented as a macroscopic images with novel contrast.

The purpose of this study was to show the feasibility of in vivo conductivity imaging of the prostate, which can provide novel contrast on the tissue condition relating to the zonal information. From the normal canine prostate, we imaged in vivo electrical conductivity of prostatic tissues and measured its values in terms of both the conductivity distribution and anatomical significance to quantitatively distinguish the tissue condition.

Methods

Animal preparation

Five healthy laboratory beagles (2–5 years old, weighing 5–13 kg; Harlan Interfauna, Huntingdon, Cambridgeshire, UK) were used for imaging experiments. All experimental protocols were performed in accordance with the regulations of the Institutional Animal Care and Use Committee (IACUC), and were approved by the Ethics Committee of Kyung Hee University, Korea (No. KHUASP-14-25). All were healthy without a history of any known disease or signs of metabolic and neurological problems. We injected 0.1 mg/kg of atropine sulfate to prevent the dog from salivating during the experiments. Ten minutes later, we anesthetized the dog with an intramuscular injection of 0.2 ml/kg Tiletamine and Zolazepam (Zoletil 50, Virbac, France). After clipping and shaving the hair at four locations on the pelvis, we attached four carbon-hydrogel electrodes (HUREV Co. Ltd., Korea) and placed the dog inside the bore of a 3 T MRI scanner (Achieva TX, Philips, Amsterdam, the Netherlands) (Fig. 1). Inside the MR scanner, we intubated the dog using an endotracheal tube and began general anesthesia using a veterinary anesthesia system (VME, MATRX, USA). We used 2% isoflurane mixed with oxygen at 800 ml/min flow rate. Ventilation was machine-controlled using a ventilator (M-2002, Hallowell EMC, USA) at a respiration rate of 15 bpm and tidal volume of 200 ml.

Imaging experiment

Anatomical T1-weighted, T2-weighted MR images were obtained to confirm the morphological information of the canine pelvis. For the electrical conductivity images of the in vivo prostate, a multi-echo spin echo pulse sequence was used to simultaneously obtain the MR magnitude and magnetic flux density (B_z) images [17]. The imaging parameters were as follows; TR/TE = 900/15, 30, 45 ms (3 echoes), FOV = 220 × 220 mm^2, slice thickness = 3 mm, NEX = 8, matrix size = 128 × 128, number of slices = 6, and total imaging time = 40 min. During MR scanning, the first current I_1 was injected between one opposing pair of electrodes using a constant current source. The injected current was 5 mA amplitude and a total pulse width of 81 ms. After acquiring the first magnetic flux density (B_z) dataset for I_1, the second injection current I_2 with the same amplitude and pulse width was injected through the other pair of opposing electrodes to obtain the second dataset. After imaging experiments, dogs were euthanized with sodium pentobarbital (80 mg/kg IV; Entobar Injection, Hanrim Pharm, Gyeonggi, South Korea) [19].

Conductivity image reconstruction and data analysis

The raw data was extracted from the MR spectrometer after finishing the imaging experiments. To reconstruct electrical

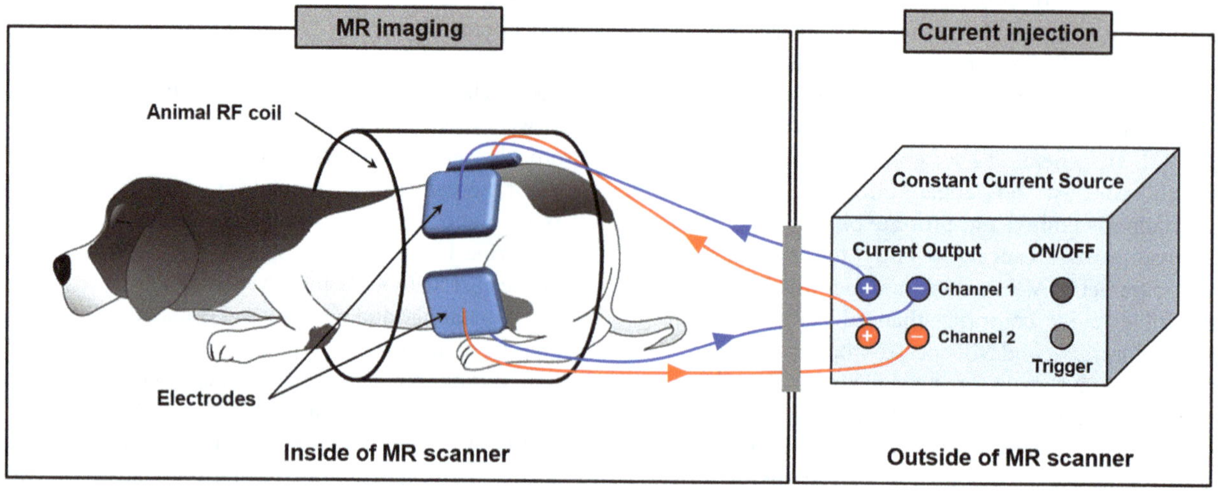

Fig. 1 Experimental setup for electrical conductivity-based MR imaging in a canine pelvis. The imaging objects are located inside the MR scanner and the imaging current is injected into the pelvis through the electrodes during MR scanning

conductivity images of the canine pelvis, the magnetic flux densities were generated by removing the effects of injected current at raw datasets. Specifically, the magnetic flux density information was determined by subtracting the two datasets with positive and negative currents. And the final low-frequency conductivity was reconstructed from the measured magnetic flux density by applying the projected current density method [20]. The detailed image reconstruction for conductivity was described in the work of Sajib et al [21]. The quantitative analysis was performed on the results from three dogs which covered the entire prostatic tissues such as the central, transitional, and peripheral zones. The regions-of-interest (ROIs) were positioned at several prostatic tissues by an experienced radiologist and their values were measured from both the signal change in conductivity distribution (Fig. 4a) and anatomical significance in T2-weighted MR images (Fig. 5a). All values were expressed as means ± standard deviations, and plotted as bar graphs to compare between different prostatic zones.

Results

Electrical conductivity images of prostate

Figure 2 shows typical results of electrical conductivity-based MR imaging from an in vivo canine pelvis. The

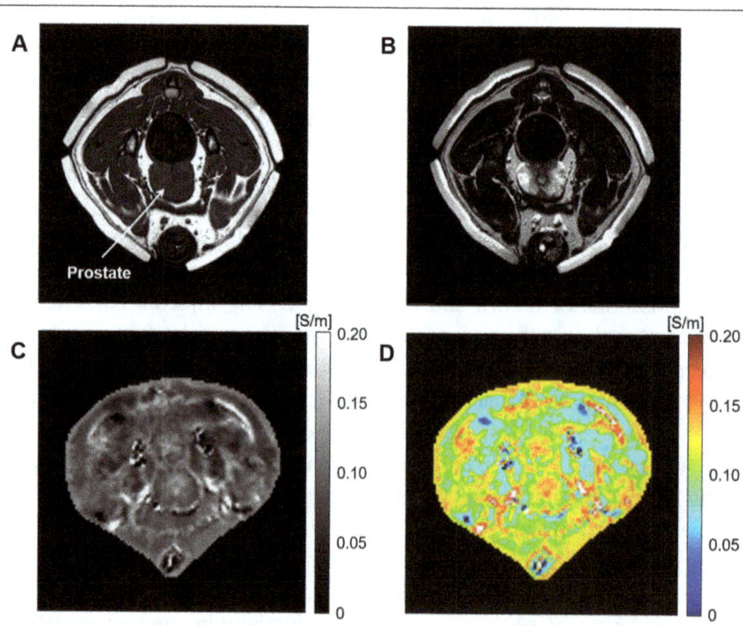

Fig. 2 Typical results of electrical conductivity imaging in a canine pelvis. **a** T1-weighted MR image, **b** T2-weighted MR image, **c** reconstructed conductivity image, and **d** pseudo color image of pelvis

T1- and T2-weighted MR images (Fig. 2a and b) indicate the anatomical structures and MR tissue contrast of the canine pelvis. The electrical conductivity and its pseudo color images (Fig. 2c and d) show different conductivity contrasts of pelvis regions, including muscles, bones, and adipose tissues. When we focused on the prostate, there was no tissue contrast in the T1-weighted image, but the T2-weighted and electrical conductivity images showed clear contrast between the prostatic tissues. Specifically, the signal intensity of the peripheral area was the highest in the T2-weighted image, but the lowest in the electrical conductivity image. On the contrary, the signal intensity of the central area was the lowest in the T2-weighted image, but the highest in the electrical conductivity image.

Figure 3 shows the electrical conductivity images with three continuous slices from two canine prostates. The anatomical structure and size of the prostate can be confirmed from the T2-weighted MR images (Fig. 3a). The electrical conductivity (Fig. 3b and d) and its pseudo color images (Fig. 3c and e) of two prostates showed the unique contrast between the prostatic tissues. The conductivity of the central area was higher than that of the peripheral area in all slices.

Prostatic tissue analysis by electrical conductivity

Figure 4 and Table 1 represent the quantitative analysis of prostatic tissues based on the contrast changes in electrical conductivity images. The regions-of-interest (ROIs) were located and confirmed by an experienced radiologist at three regions, indicating the urethra, ROI A, and ROI B, which are marked in Fig. 4a. Most of ROI A covered the central area, while ROI B was the peripheral area. From the results of three prostates, the conductivity was the highest in the urethra and lower in the order of ROI A and ROI B. Specifically, ROI A was

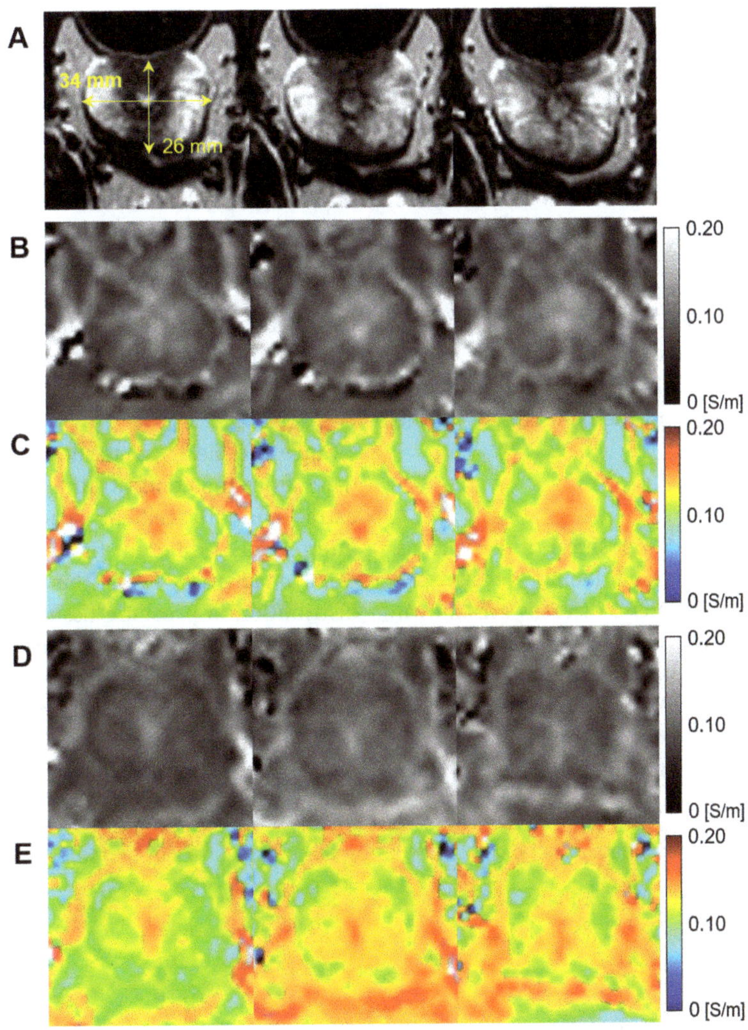

Fig. 3 Resulting conductivity images in three continuous slices from two canine prostates. **a** T2-weighted MR images, **b** and **c** reconstructed conductivity and pseudo color images of the first prostate, **d** and **e** images from the second prostate

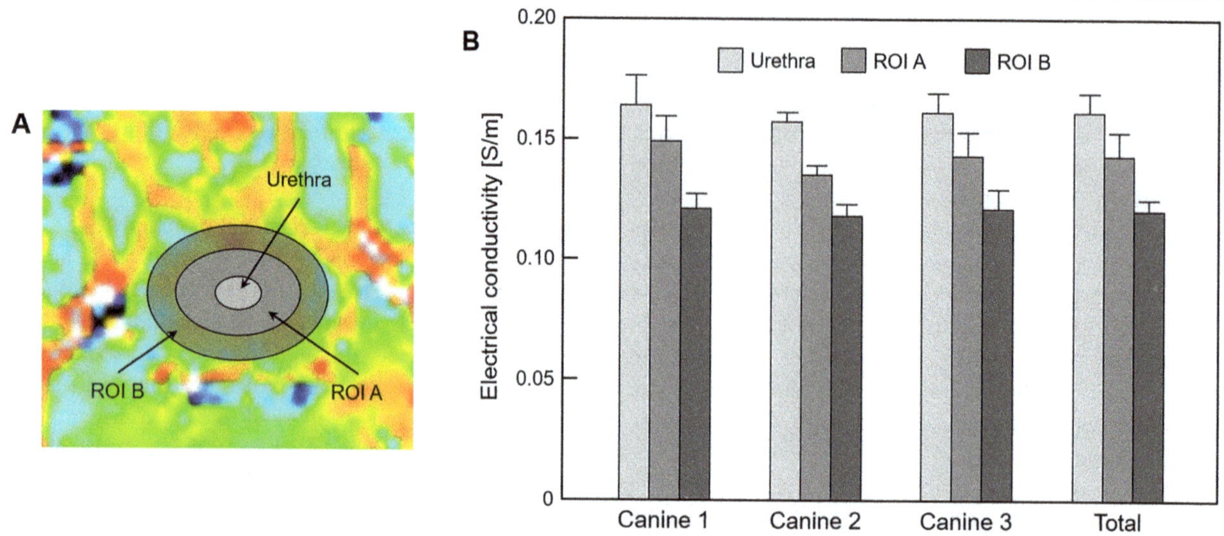

Fig. 4 Bar graph showing the comparison of prostatic tissues based on the contrast changes in electrical conductivity images. **a** ROIs are located in three prostatic tissues, **b** electrical conductivity is measured from the corresponding regions

about 11.2% and ROI B was about 25.5% lower than the conductivity of the urethra (Table 1).

Figure 5 and Table 2 represent the quantitative analysis of prostatic tissues based on the anatomical significance in the T2-weighted MR image. The ROIs were located and confirmed by an experienced radiologist at three zones, indicating the central, transitional, and peripheral zones, which are marked in Fig. 5a. The conductivity was the highest in the central zone, while it was the lowest in the peripheral zone in all prostates. Specifically, the transitional zone was about 7.5% and peripheral zone was about 17.8% lower than the conductivity of the central zone (Table 2).

Discussion

Differences exist in the tissue composition of the various prostate zones, such as the gland (acini) density per zone, and the incidence of prostatic diseases are known to have zonal predilections [5]. The water-rich duct and acini within the peripheral zone are similar to that of central zone. However, the peripheral zone has a larger extracellular space than the central zone because the density of the stroma, which connects between the duct and acini, is lower in the peripheral zone than in the central zone [4, 5]. Moreover, prostate cancer has a higher density of glandular elements and lesser space of mucin or fluid than a normal prostate gland and benign prostate hyperplasia. This difference in histologic composition makes prostate cancer different from a normal prostate gland and benign prostate hyperplasia in the prostate. The difference is even more pronounced in the peripheral zone. This cellular environment is one factor for determining electrical tissue conductivity that can be represented as a macroscopic image with novel contrast [18, 20, 21].

Since the electrical tissue conductivity basically originates from the concentration and mobility of ions in the extra- and intracellular space, image contrast can be interpreted as different tissue conditions in terms of bioelectromagnetics. From the results of the conductivity distribution in prostatic tissues, the conductivity was decreased in the order of the urethra, ROI A, and ROI B. The high conductivity of the urethra originates from the urethra itself and a certain amount of urine, which contains many electrolytes. ROI A and B roughly correspond to the central and peripheral areas of the prostate,

Table 1 Measurement of electrical conductivity of prostatic tissues based on the conductivity distribution

Conductivity [S/m]	Urethra	ROI A	ROI B
Canine 1	0.164 ± 0.012	0.149 ± 0.010, (9.1%)[a]	0.121 ± 0.006, (26.2%)[a]
Canine 2	0.157 ± 0.004	0.135 ± 0.004, (14.0%)	0.118 ± 0.005, (24.8%)
Canine 3	0.161 ± 0.008	0.143 ± 0.010, (11.2%)	0.121 ± 0.008, (24.8%)
Average	0.161 ± 0.008	0.143 ± 0.010, (11.2%)	0.120 ± 0.005, (25.5%)

Values are presented as mean ± standard deviation
[a]Parentheses indicate the percentage changes based on the conductivity of the urethra

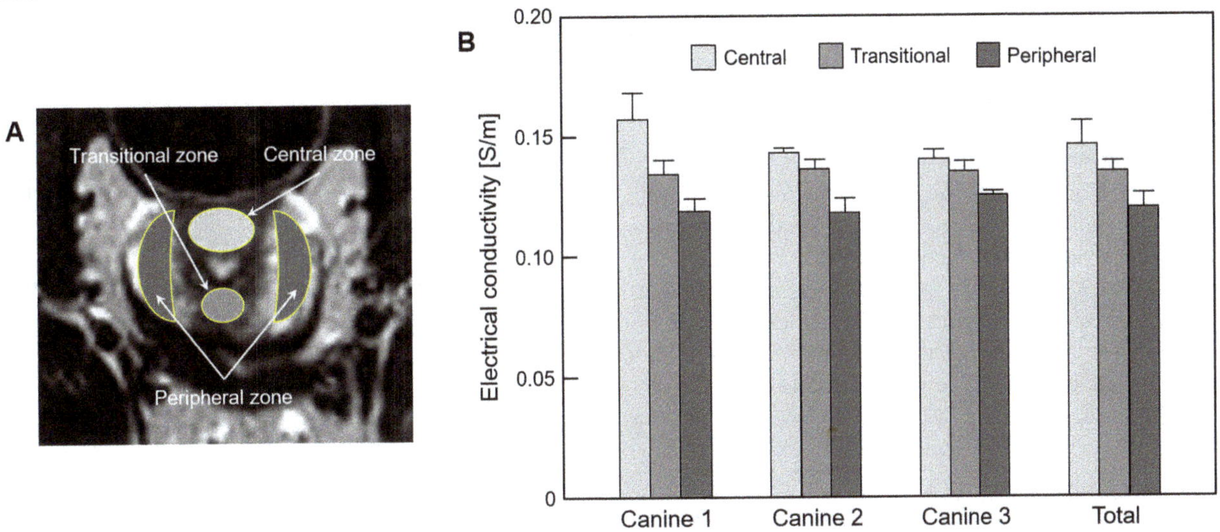

Fig. 5 Bar graph showing the comparison of prostatic tissues based on the anatomical significance in the T2-weighted MR image. **a** ROIs are located in three anatomical regions of the prostate, **b** electrical conductivity is measured from the corresponding regions

respectively. The conductivity of the central area, which consists of central and transition zones, was higher than that of the peripheral area, mostly including the peripheral zone. This is consistent with the difference in conductivity due to the anatomical significances.

From the anatomical zonal analysis, the conductivity was decreased in the order of the central, transitional, and peripheral zones. The major difference between the prostatic zones is the volume of glandular tissue and density of connective tissues, such as the stroma. The central and transitional zones occupy 25% of the volume of the glandular tissue and the peripheral zone occupies roughly 75% [22–24]. The density of the stroma is higher in the central and transitional zones than in the peripheral zone [22–24]. There has been no in vivo measurement study of prostate tissues, but the electrical conductivity of glandular tissue and the stroma have been reported as 0.097 and 0.120 S/m, respectively, at low-frequency by in vitro measurements [16, 25, 26]. Although there exists a difference between in vivo and in vitro measurements, the low conductivity of the peripheral zone can be explained from these results. The histological characteristics between the central and transitional zones are almost similar, with the only difference being the volume, location, and tissue composition ratio [5]. However, our results show that there was a difference in conductivity between the two zones. From the viewpoint of the bio-electromagnetism, the transitional zone may have an intermediate tissue condition between the central and peripheral zones, but a detailed comparison should be addressed in future studies.

In vivo electrical conductivity imaging (ECI) could provide alternative information on tissue structure and function using electrical tissue properties such as conductivity and permittivity. Electrical conductivity is an inherent physical property of living tissues and it provides absolute values [11, 17, 18]. Therefore, the tissue condition can be quantified and discriminated on the basis of absolute conductivity values. These preliminary results suggest the possibility of ECI as a new imaging biomarker for prostate disease. ECI may serve as a good complement to current prostate imaging in diagnosing prostate disease and assessing treatment response, especially for prostate cancer. Moreover, ECI can provide

Table 2 Measurement of electrical conductivity of prostatic tissues based on the anatomical significance

Conductivity [S/m]	Central zone	Transitional zone	Peripheral zone
Canine 1	0.157 ± 0.011	0.134 ± 0.006, (14.6%)[a]	0.119 ± 0.005, (24.2%)[a]
Canine 2	0.143 ± 0.002	0.136 ± 0.004, (4.9%)	0.118 ± 0.006, (17.5%)
Canine 3	0.140 ± 0.004	0.135 ± 0.004, (3.6%)	0.125 ± 0.002, (10.7%)
Average	0.146 ± 0.010	0.135 ± 0.004, (7.5%)	0.120 ± 0.006, (17.8%)

Values are presented as mean ± standard deviation
[a]Parentheses indicate the percentage changes based on the conductivity of the central zone

immediate information on tissue anisotropy. When ECI is used with current multiparametric MR imaging, it may be helpful in the diagnosis of prostatic cancer, such as in localization and characterization, and in the assessment of the treatment response in the early period.

We acknowledge that this study has several limitations. First, the relatively long acquisition time and poor spatial resolution should be addressed for clinical applications. Recent advances in ECI technique, such as conductivity tensor imaging (CTI), have demonstrated the potential to improve current conductivity imaging methods in terms of acquisition time and spatial resolution [27]. In addition, the high sensitivity of ECI to tissue response following radiation therapy (RT) may reveal the possibility of ECI for clinical application in prostate diseases [28]. Second, the current study was performed on a small number of normal animal prostates, thus, further study should be performed with large numbers of normal prostates for statistical analysis, animal disease models such as prostate cancer or benign prostate hyperplasia, and human prostates. Third, the lack of accurate correlation between tissue histology and the value of ECI according to ROI and zonal anatomy might be problematic. However, regarding the well established zonal anatomy on T2-weighted imaging in the current study, ECI could provide different values according to the zones and regions of the prostate.

Conclusion

In this feasibility study, we applied an in vivo electrical conductivity-based MR imaging method to image the differences in prostatic tissues. From the electrical conductivity images, we could quantify the tissue condition in terms of the conductivity distribution and anatomical significance. Conductivity images shown in this study indicated that the contrast between the prostatic tissues are distinguishable in a different way compared with conventional MR imaging techniques. Future studies will be focused on the verification and evaluation of conductivity differences between normal healthy men and patients with prostatic diseases.

Abbreviations

ECI: Electrical conductivity imaging; MR: Magnetic resonance;
MREIT: Magnetic resonance electrical impedance tomography; ROI: Region of Interest

Acknowledgements

Not applicable.

Authors' contributions

YSC and JWK were involved in animal imaging experiments, data collection, and manuscript writing. YHH and HJS were involved in data collection and analysis. HJK was involved in image processing, quantitative analysis, and manuscript editing. All authors read and approved the final manuscript.

University (2019). These foundations did not interfere in the design of the study and collection, analysis, and interpretation of data and in writing the manuscript.

Author details

[1]Department of Radiology, Chosun University Hospital and Chosun University College of Medicine, 365 Pilmun-daero, Dong-gu, Gwangju 61453, South Korea. [2]Department of Hepato-Biliary-Pancreas Surgery, Chonnam National University Hwasun Hospital and Chonnam National University Medical School, Gwangju 61469, South Korea. [3]Department of Biomedical Engineering, Kyung Hee University, 23 Kyungheedaero, Dongdaemungu, Seoul 02447, South Korea.

References

1. Jemal A, Siegel R, Ward E, Hao Y, Xu J, Murray T, Thun MJ. Cancer statistics, 2008. CA Cancer J Clin. 2008;58:71–96.
2. Catalona WJ. Prostate cancer screening. Med Clin North Am. 2018;102:199–214.
3. Price CP, Allard J, Davies G, Dawnay A, Duffy MJ, France M, Mandarino G, Ward AM, Patel B, Sibley P, Sturgeon C. Pre- and post-analytical factors that may influence use of serum prostate-specific antigen and its isoforms in a screening programme for prostate cancer. Ann Clin Biochem. 2001;38:188–216.
4. McNeal JE. The zonal anatomy of the prostate. Prostate. 1981;2:35–49.
5. McNeal JE. Normal histology of the prostate. Am J Surg Pathol. 1988;12: 619–33.
6. Hoeks CM, Barentsz JO, Hambrock T, Yakar D, Somford DM, Heijmink SW, Scheenen TW, Vos PC, Huisman H, van Oort IM, Witjes JA, Heerschap A, Fütterer JJ. Prostate cancer: multiparametric MR imaging for detection, localization, and staging. Radiology. 2011;261:46–66.
7. Metcalfe P, Liney GP, Holloway L, Walker A, Barton M, Delaney GP, Vinod S, Tome W. The potential for an enhanced role for MRI in radiation-therapy treatment planning. Technol Cancer Res Treat. 2013;12:429–46.
8. Wallitt KL, Khan SR, Dubash S, Tam HH, Khan S, Barwick TD. Clinical PET imaging in prostate cancer. Radiographics. 2017;37(5):1512–36.
9. Verma S, Rosenkrantz AB, Choyke P, Eberhardt SC, Eggener SE, Gaitonde K, Haider MA, Margolis DJ, Marks LS, Pinto P, Sonn GA, Taneja SS. Commentary regarding a recent collaborative consensus statement addressing prostate MRI and MRI-targeted biopsy in patients with a prior negative prostate biopsy. Abdom Radiol. 2017;42:346–9.
10. Katscher U, Voigt T, Findeklee C, Vernickel P, Nehrke K, Dössel O. Determination of electric conductivity and local SAR via B1 mapping. IEEE Trans Med Imaging. 2009;28:1365–74.
11. Seo JK, Kim MO, Lee J, Choi N, Woo EJ, Kim HJ, Kwon OI, Kim DH. Error analysis of non-constant admittivity for MR-based electric property imaging. IEEE Trans Med Imaging. 2012;31:430–7.
12. Kim HJ, Jeong WC, Sajib SZ, Kim MO, Kwon OI, Je Woo E, Kim DH. Simultaneous imaging of dual-frequency electrical conductivity using a combination of MREIT and MREPT. Magn Reson Med. 2014;71:200–8.
13. Haemmerich D, Staelin ST, Tsai JZ, Tungjitkusolmun S, Mahvi DM, Webster JG. In vivo electrical conductivity of hepatic tumours. Physiol Meas. 2003;24: 251–60.
14. Oh TI, Jeong WC, McEwan A, Park HM, Kim HJ, Kwon OI, Woo EJ. Feasibility of MREIT conductivity imaging to evaluate brain abscess lesion: in vivo canine model. J Magn Reson Imaging. 2013;38:189–97.
15. Lee SK, Bulumulla S, Wiesinger F, Sacolick L, Sun W, Hancu I. Tissue electrical property mapping from zero echo-time magnetic resonance imaging. IEEE Trans Med Imaging. 2015;34:541–50.
16. Halter RJ, Schned A, Heaney J, Hartov A, Paulsen KD. Electrical properties of prostatic tissues: I. single frequency admittivity properties. J Urol. 2009;182: 1600–7.
17. Seo JK, Woo EJ. Electrical tissue property imaging at low frequency using MREIT. IEEE Trans Biomed Eng. 2014;61:1390–9.
18. Sajib SZK, Kwon OI, Kim HJ, Woo EJ. Electrodeless conductivity tensor imaging (CTI) using MRI: basic theory and animal experiments. Biomed Eng Lett. 2018;8:273–82.

19. An D, Park J, Shin JI, Kim HJ, Jung DI, Kang JH, Kim G, Chang DW, Sur JH, Yang MP, Lee C, Kang BT. Temporal evolution of MRI characteristics in dogs with collagenase-induced intracerebral hemorrhage. Comp Med. 2015;65(6):517–25.
20. Jeong WC, Meng ZJ, Kim HJ, Kwon OI, Woo EJ. Experimental validations of in vivo human musculoskeletal tissue conductivity images using MR-based electrical impedance tomography. Bioelectromagnetics. 2014;35:363–72.
21. Sajib SZK, Kim HJ, Kwon OI, Woo EJ. Regional absolute conductivity reconstruction using projected current density in MREIT. Phys Med Biol. 2012;57:5841–59.
22. Lee JJ, Thomas IC, Nolley R, Ferrari M, Brooks JD, Leppert JT. Biologic differences between peripheral and transition zone prostate cancer. Prostate. 2015;75:183–90.
23. Noguchi M, Stamey TA, Neal J, Yemoto C. An analysis of 148 consecutive transition zone cancers: clinical and histological characteristics. J Urol. 2000;163:1751–5.
24. McNeal JE, Redwine EA, Freiha FS, Stamey TA. Zonal distribution of prostatic adenocarcinoma: correlation with histologic pattern and direction of spread. Am J Surg Pathol. 1988;12:897–906.
25. Halter RJ, Schned A, Heaney J, Hartov A, Paulsen KD. Electrical properties of prostatic tissues: II. Spectral admittivity properties. J Urol. 2009;182:1608–13.
26. Halter RJ, Schned A, Heaney J, Hartov A. Passive bioelectrical properties for assessing high- and low-grade prostate adenocarcinoma. Prostate. 2011;71:1759–67.
27. Katoch N, Choi BK, Sajib SZK, Lee EA, Kim HJ, Kwon OI, Woo EJ. Conductivity tensor imaging of in vivo human brain and experimental validation using giant vesicle suspension. IEEE Trans Med Imaging. 2019;38(7):1569–77.
28. Park JA, Kang KJ, Ko IO, Lee KC, Choi BK, Katoch N, Kim JW, Kim HJ, Kwon OI, Woo EJ. In vivo measurement of brain tissue response after irradiation: comparison of T2 relaxation, apparent diffusion coefficient, and electrical conductivity. IEEE Trans Med Imaging. https://doi.org/10.1109/TMI.2019.2913766.

12

Radiotherapy for prostate cancer: DISCERN quality assessment of patient-oriented websites in 2018

S. Janssen[1,4*†], F. B. Fahlbusch[2†], L. Käsmann[1], D. Rades[1] and D. Vordermark[3]

Abstract

Background: Prostate cancer is the most commonly diagnosed cancer in men. Radiotherapy represents one major treatment option in different therapeutic settings. As patients increasingly rely on internet-based medical information, we examined the quality of information on radiotherapy and prostate cancer in websites used by laypersons.

Methods: An Internet search from a patients` perspective was carried out using different search engines (Google, Yahoo and Bing, search terms: "prostate cancer" and "radiotherapy"). The quality of search results was analyzed with regard to the DISCERN score, HON code certification, the JAMA criteria and the ALEXA traffic rank.

Results: In general, websites were of good quality. The highest quality was found for websites operated by charity organizations. No significant differences in results obtained via the above-mentioned tools were seen for the examined search engines, but Google revealed the most stable search results in terms of temporal changes.

Conclusion: Patients with prostate cancer can sufficiently inform themselves on general treatment options including radiotherapy on websites directed at laypersons. However, no simple strategy could identify high quality websites in general. For treating physicians, it is important to support patients in interpreting and ranking the vast quantity of information.

Keywords: Prostate cancer, Radiotherapy, Internet, Health-related information, Online information

Background

Prostate cancer is the most commonly diagnosed cancer in the male population worldwide [1]. Radiotherapy for localized prostate cancer remains one of the mainstays among treatment approaches. Other fields of application are biochemical recurrences after prostatectomy, postoperative radiotherapy in high-risk situations and palliative settings e.g. painful bone metastases [2, 3]. As most patients do not have personal experiences with radiotherapy, a lack of information on risks and benefits is immanent. A recent Canadian survey revealed that more than 90% of men with newly diagnosed prostate cancer prefer to either play an active or collaborative role in treatment decision-making [4]. Thus, gaining valid medical information before initiating treatment seems essential for these patients to improve their decision-making.

Today, a significant number of patients with prostate cancer [5, 6] and radiation oncology patients [7, 8] utilize the Internet to obtain medical information. For cancer patients in general, Castleton et al. reported Internet utilization in approximately two thirds of patients [9]. However, the quality of online information for patients with prostate cancer is variable [6, 10–12]. For instance, Ilic et al. found the quality of websites on prostate cancer screening to be highly variable but mostly of poor standard [10]. Similarly, others found shortcomings in quality and accuracy of Internet health information for the special topic of prostate cancer and proton therapy [11]. Noteworthy, Shaverdian et al. showed that 39% of patients who selected the Internet as their primary information source reported their actual treatment experience to be worse than expected. Patients who had initially

* Correspondence: st-janssen@gmx.net
†S. Janssen and F. B. Fahlbusch contributed equally to this work.
[1]Department of Radiation Oncology, University of Luebeck, Luebeck, Germany
[4]Medical Practice for Radiotherapy and Radiation Oncology, Hannover, Germany
Full list of author information is available at the end of the article

gathered medical information by consulting their urologists, radiation oncologist or even other patients reported a significantly better treatment experience [6]. On the other hand, a recently published analysis revealed a high rating in quality, accessibility and usability of websites on prostate cancer in general [12].

To our knowledge, there is no current analysis of consumer health information on the Internet for patients with prostate cancer in need of a radiation therapy. In order to close that gap, our goal was to evaluate websites with the focus on prostate cancer and radiotherapy.

Methods

Website identification and selection

A complete list of analyzed and excluded websites is given in Additional file 1 of the appendix. Identification and selection of websites (English language) took place on August 22nd 2017 (9.00 a.m. CET). The keywords "prostate cancer" and "radiotherapy" were entered in the search-engines Google.com, Bing.com and Yahoo.com to emulate real user experience. A second search was carried out on September 9th 2017 (9.00 a.m. CET) to reveal possible temporal dynamics. The first 20 websites were subjected to further evaluation as it is known that patients rarely browse through further sites when searching the web [12–14]. To simulate a laypersons view, we excluded websites from further analysis when complete access was restricted by password, the websites only included personal experiences (e.g. blogs, videos) or contained limited information on radiotherapy (< one paragraph), as described by others [15, 16]. In detail, websites were excluded based on the following criteria: advertisement only ($n = 2$), a focus on clinical trials ($n = 4$), scientific articles ($n = 20$), newspaper articles (n = 2), video (n = 2), denied access (n = 2) and PowerPoint presentation ($n = 1$). The vast majority of excluded websites was found using the search engines Bing.com and Yahoo.com. For the Google search, only one website met the above exclusion criteria.

After the subtraction of duplicate websites (i.e. repeated appearance in different search engines and time points) a total number of 49 websites was subjected to further evaluation ($n = 39$ first search, $n = 10$ second search). Apart from HON code, JAMA benchmark criteria, ALEXA rank and DISCERN score, the country of origin and website operator were recorded for each website additionally. The quality of websites was evaluated by two investigators (SJ, LK) independently using the validated tools described below. Discrepancies were discussed and a consensus was reached.

The DISCERN tool was originally developed and validated in 1998 at the University of Oxford, UK. The aim was to analyze written medical information with 15 questions in terms of reliability and details on treatment (score of 1–5 for each question) [17, 18]. Overall quality was additionally rated by a 16th question in the DISCERN Plus score. As described by Nghiem et al. the results were rated from "excellent" to "very poor" [19]. This methodology was used in a similar way in a previous published work of our study group [20]. The individual DISCERN items used in our study are visualized in Table 1. Following DISCERN scoring, the respective websites were further analyzed by using HON code [21] and JAMA [22] (tools, as outlined by us in detail earlier [20]. With the ALEXA traffic tool (https://www.alexa.com/) popularity and engagement characteristics of websites can be assessed. It is a measure of how often a website is frequented relative to all other sites on the web over the past three months.

Statistical analyses

We performed statistical analysis using GraphPad Prism 7 (GraphPad Software Inc., La Jolla, CA, USA) employing Spearman correlation, linear regression analysis and two-tailed non-parametric Wilcoxon-Mann-Whitney test for group comparisons as described in a previous published work of our study group in detail [20].

Results

First, we analyzed the consistency of our data (i.e. exclusion rates, duplicate websites and temporal changes in search rank). Web search results obtained via Google seemed adequately directed at laypersons (one website excluded) and were highly consistent, as no duplicate results occurred and only a single new webpage was evident within the 20 hits in our second search after three weeks (Fig. 1A). In contrast, exclusion rates ($n = 8$ and

Table 1 DISCERN Plus instrument (modified according to Borgmann et al.)

Question 1: Aim clear?
Question 2: Aim achieved?
Question 3: Relevant?
Question 4: Sources clear?
Question 5: Dates of sources?
Question 6: Balanced and unbiased?
Question 7: Additional information?
Question 8: Areas of uncertainty?
Question 9: Describe treatment?
Question 10: Benefits of treatments?
Question 11: Risks of treatment?
Question 12: No treatment?
Question 13: Quality of life?
Question 14: Treatment choices?
Question 15: Shared decision-making?
Question 16: Overall quality?

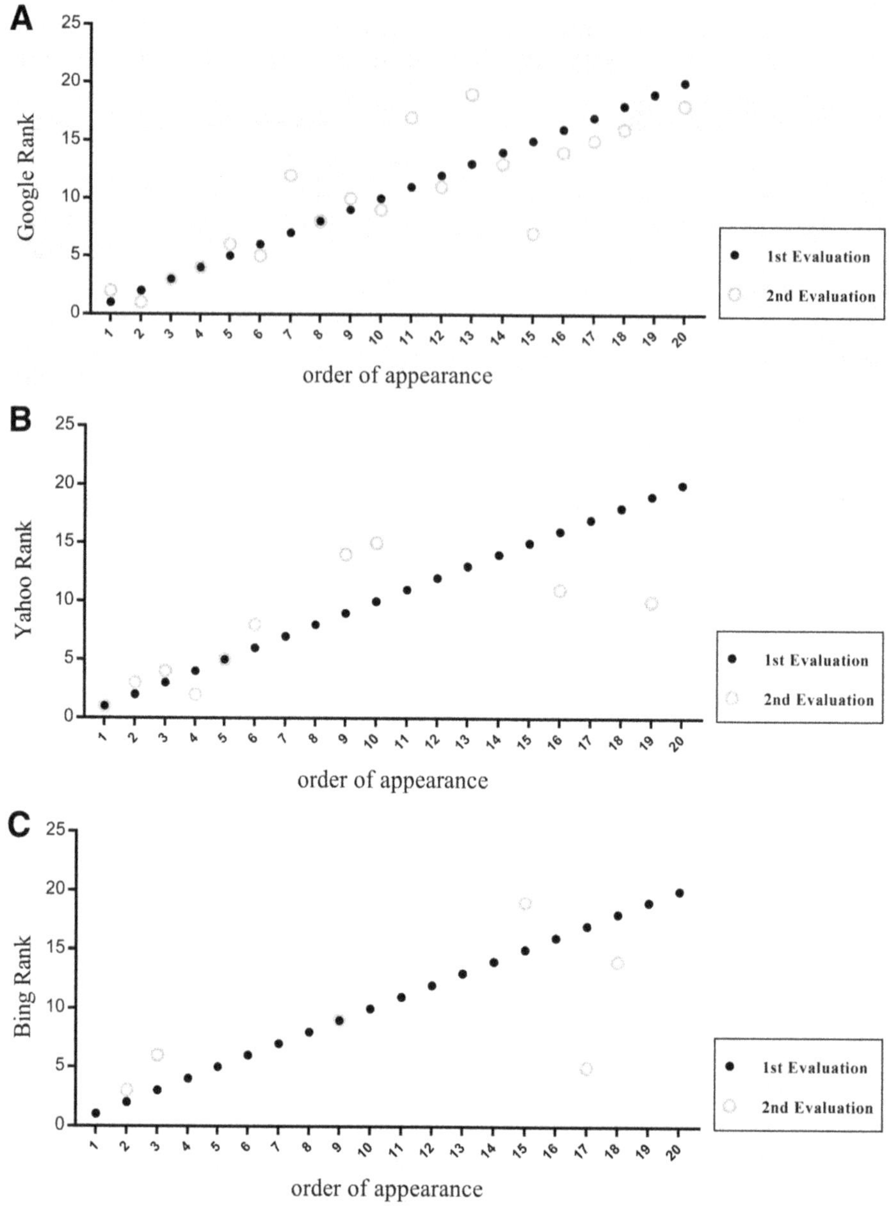

Fig. 1 a-c: Google, Bing and yahoo search ranking at two different time points (black dots: august 22nd 2017, Open circles: September 9th 2017)

25) and the incidence of double hits (n = 8 and 10) and of novel search results/ranks (*n* = 10 and 14, Fig. 1B, C) were higher when Bing and Yahoo were employed, respectively.

Overall, the quality of information on websites about prostate cancer and radiotherapy was good, with a mean DISCERN Plus score of 55.1 ± 10.0, 51.8 ± 10.3 and 50.7 ± 10.1 for Google, Yahoo and Bing, respectively. The scores ranged from a minimum of 34 to a maximum of 74. 13% of all websites were rated as excellent, 31, 48 and 8% as good, fair and poor, respectively. No website was rated as very poor. Figure 2 shows the item-based results of the DISCERN score for the first search results on August 22nd 2017 of all three search engines (*n* = 39 websites in total). The items with the lowest scores were related to website content concerning sources/references, up-to-dateness and quality of life issues (question 4–6 and 13, Table 1). The overall quality of websites (DISCERN Plus score) was neither dependent on the choice of search engines nor did we observe a significant temporal change in quality (Fig. 3). The main categories of websites retrieved from the first search were charity/NGO sites (46%), followed by sponsored medical news sites (28%), hospital/university sites (20%) and governmental sites (6%). Websites operated by charity organizations had significantly higher DISCERN Plus scores (mean score: 55.5 ± 9.3) compared to hospital sites

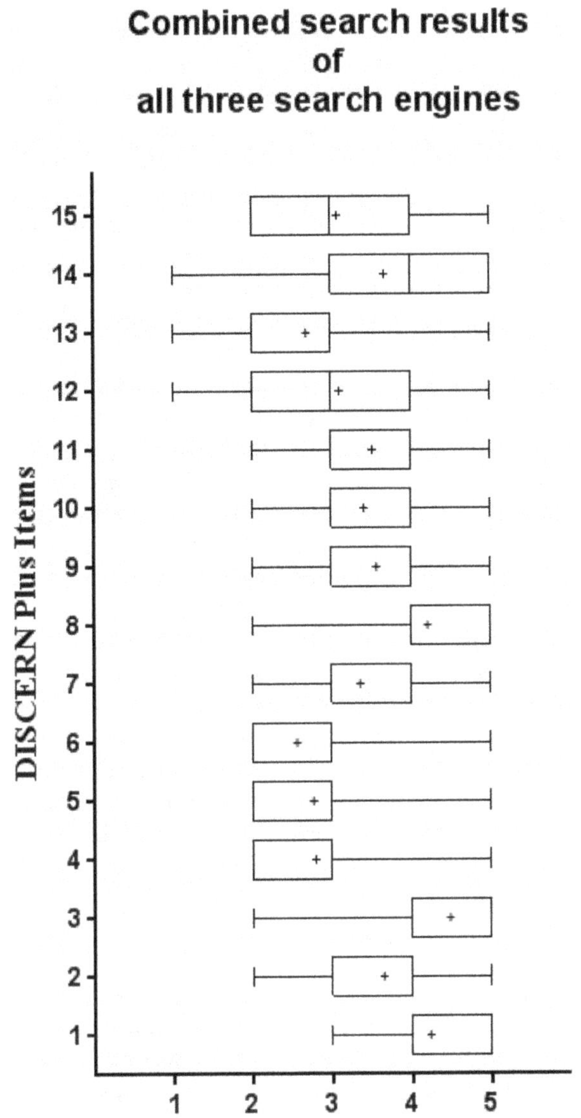

Fig. 2 Combined (n = 39 from Google, Bing and Yahoo) box and whiskers (min to max) analysis of the individual DISCERN Plus score items of the first search (mean indicated by +)

(mean score: 47.3 ± 9.6, $p < 0.042$) and medical news sites (mean score: 46.1 ± 6.1, $p < 0.009$), respectively. Most websites originated in the USA (46%) followed by the UK (33%), Australia/New Zealand (15%) and Canada (6%). The JAMA benchmark criteria were fulfilled for all four sections in 13%, for three, two and one section(s) in 13, 31 and 40%, respectively. One website did not fulfill any of the JAMA criteria. Only 13% of all websites were HON code certified. The median ALEXA global traffic rank was 62,375 with a minimum of five and a maximum of 4,710,605.

Neither the JAMA benchmark criteria, the HON code certification, the ALEXA traffic rank, the country of origin (except slightly superior DISCERN score for UK websites compared to USA websites, $p < 0.033$) nor the ranking within the search results showed a significant association with the respective DISCERN Plus score.

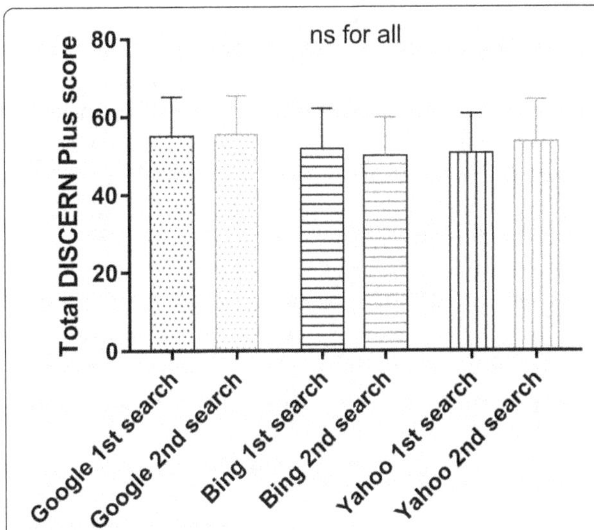

Fig. 3 Mean total DISCERN score for the three search engines at two different time points

Of all analyzed websites, the vast majority had a clear focus on radiotherapy for prostate cancer; four websites provided only information for radiotherapy in general. All analyzed websites had a focus on curative teletherapy (i.e. definitive radiotherapy to the prostate or to prostatic bed in a postoperative or salvage setting), 76, 51 and 22% of all websites mentioned brachytherapy, active surveillance and palliative radiotherapy (i.e. radiotherapy to other sites than the prostate or prostatic bed, e.g. bone metastases), respectively. In 57% the procedure of radiotherapy starting from first preparation, daily treatment and aftercare was described in detail. Special radiation techniques like "hypo-fractionation", "Intensity modulated Radiotherapy (IMRT)", "Image guided Radiotherapy (IGRT)" and "proton therapy" were mentioned in 37, 72, 27 and 31% of all analyzed websites, respectively.

Discussion

In recent years, the Internet has gained importance as a source for health-related information. Several study groups confirmed this fact in patients with oncological diseases in general [9, 23], as well as for patients with gynecologic cancers [24], breast cancer [19, 20], colorectal cancer [25], bladder cancer [26], laryngeal cancer [27] and prostate cancer [12] in particular. The increasing amount of data published within the last two years highlights its clinical relevance.

For prostate cancer in particular there is a high need for information because several treatment strategies exist. Radiotherapy represents a major component for the management of this oncologic entity. Thus, we performed an evaluation of websites addressing information on prostate cancer and radiotherapy. The first 20 websites were subjected to further evaluation as it is known that patients rarely browse through further sites when searching the web [13]. Ngyuen et al. showed that 72% of the patients even restricted their search to 1–5 websites only [14]. In a study of Borgmann et al. the list of evaluated websites was limited to 10 sites [12].

Overall, we found a good quality of information on analyzed websites according to the validated DISCERN Plus score (for Google search: mean DISCERN Plus score: 55.1 ± 10.0). Our results are in concordance with findings from studies analyzing website quality of other cancer entities, returning a mean DISCERN Plus score of 50 [27], 52 [25], 42 [28] and 42 [20], respectively. Notwithstanding, the only other comparable study evaluating websites with general information on prostate cancer, obtained higher DISCERN Plus scores (mean 77) [12]. Taken together, websites with information on prostate cancer seem to be of slightly better quality compared to websites covering other cancer entities. A potential reason why the web search by Borgmann et al. returned webpages of higher quality might be associated with the use of a more general and popular search term. This is reflected by a lower ALEXA traffic rank for prostate cancer sites in general (median ALEXA traffic rank in the study of Borgmann et al.: 2718) compared to our focus on radiotherapy and prostate cancer (median ALEXA traffic rank: 62375). In our study, webpage quality (DISCERN Plus score 2.14 ± 1.03) of less frequently visited websites ($n = 14$, ALEXA traffic rank < 62,375) was not significantly different from more frequently visited sites ($n = 15$, ALEXA traffic rank > 62,375, DISCERN Plus score 1.67 ± 0.98). We did not find an association of ALEXA traffic rank and superior DISCERN score (data not shown).

In our analysis only 13% of websites were HON code certified. Most other studies evaluating websites on cancer entities in general found higher certification rates ranging from 20 to 38% [12, 19, 20, 26, 29–31]. The vast majority of these studies showed that a higher HON code certification was not necessarily accompanied by a better content quality, as determined by the DISCERN Plus score. Borgmann et al. presumed a lower HON code certification frequency for websites on more specific topics, e.g. prostate cancer and radical prostatectomy. This phenomenon could also account for the low number of HON code certified websites in our study, which is in concordance with findings by the study group of Alkhateeb indicating 17% of HON code certification in their focused web search on prostate cancer and surgery [32].

The websites operated by charity organizations were of superior quality concerning the DISCERN score compared to hospital sites and sponsored medical news sites. In line with this finding, Liebl et al. also found websites of non-profit providers and self-help groups of superior quality compared with profit-driven websites for cancer patients in general [33]. Moreover, an earlier analysis of our study group also revealed better results for hospital and NGO websites compared to sponsored medical news sites for webpages with information on breast cancer [20]. Thus, currently non-commercial sites should be preferentially recommended to patients seeking information on prostate cancer and radiotherapy.

No significant differences in the DISCERN Plus score, JAMA benchmark criteria and HON code certification were found between the three search engines (data not shown). Search results obtained via Google were greatly directed at laypersons and showed a high grade of consistency (i.e. exclusion rates, duplicate websites and temporal changes in search rank), in contrast to the other search engines. These properties might render Google a reliable choice for laypersons searching for information on prostate cancer and radiotherapy.

Interestingly, a large percentage of analyzed websites provided information on modern radiotherapy techniques like IMRT (72%). Also, websites mentioned brachytherapy in the setting of curative treatment in 76% and the possibility of no treatment (active surveillance) in 51%. Despite the well-balanced information on modern treatment options for localized disease, we found a significant lack of information on palliative radiotherapy, which was only mentioned by 22% of websites.

Limitations

One has to be aware that besides the influence of temporal changes, internet search results may vary based on e.g. the choice of search engine, search term, search date and country of origin settings within the search engine. However, within Google.com, no substantial differences in search results were observed using different search terms (e.g. "radiation" or "radiation therapy" instead of "radiotherapy") or countries of origin (data not shown).

Websites with complete access restricted by password, websites with personal experiences only (e.g. blogs, videos) or with limited information on radiotherapy (< one paragraph), newspaper articles and PowerPoint presentations were excluded from further analysis. We are aware of the fact that those sources may also contain meaningful information for prostate cancer patients. However, the exclusion was executed to apply the above-mentioned tools in order to standardize evaluation and to preserve comparability. This was handled similar in other publications [15, 16].

Conclusion

Websites on radiotherapy and prostate cancer directed at laypersons have the potential to sufficiently inform patients about general treatment options. The fact that we were unable to find a simple strategy for the identification of high-quality websites (i.e. HON code certification, JAMA benchmark criteria, ALEXA ranking, different search engines or country of origin and DISCERN Plus score) emphasizes the responsibility of the treating physicians to interpret and rank the vast quantity of information.

Additional file

Additional file 1: web domains of the first google search (DOC 28 kb)

Abbreviation

HON: Health On the Net Foundation.; IMRT: Intensity modulated Radiotherapy.; IGRTA: Image guided Radiotherapy.; JAMA: Journal of the American Medical Association.; NGO: Non-governmental organizations.; SD: Standard deviation.

Acknowledgements

None.

Author details

[1]Department of Radiation Oncology, University of Luebeck, Luebeck, Germany. [2]Department of Pediatrics and Adolescent Medicine, Friedrich-Alexander-University Erlangen-Nuernberg, Erlangen, Germany. [3]Department of Radiation Oncology, University Hospital Halle (Saale), Halle, Germany. [4]Medical Practice for Radiotherapy and Radiation Oncology, Hannover, Germany.

References

1. Global Burden of Disease Cancer Collaboration, Fitzmaurice C, Allen C, Barber RM, Barregard L, Bhutta ZA, Brenner H, et al. Global, regional, and National Cancer Incidence, mortality, years of life lost, years lived with disability, and disability-adjusted life-years for 32 Cancer groups, 1990 to 2015: a systematic analysis for the global burden of disease study. JAMA Oncol. 2017 Apr 1;3(4):524–48.
2. Cornford P, Bellmunt J, Bolla M, Briers E, De Santis M, Gross T, et al. EAU-ESTRO-SIOG guidelines on prostate Cancer. Part II: treatment of relapsing, metastatic, and castration-resistant prostate Cancer. Eur Urol. 2017 Apr;71(4): 630–42.
3. Mottet N, Bellmunt J, Bolla M, Briers E, Cumberbatch MG, De Santis M, et al. EAU-ESTRO-SIOG guidelines on prostate Cancer. Part 1: screening, diagnosis, and local treatment with curative intent. Eur Urol. 2017 Apr;71(4):618–29.
4. Davison BJ, Breckon EN. Impact of health information-seeking behavior and personal factors on preferred role in treatment decision making in men with newly diagnosed prostate cancer. Cancer Nurs. 2012 Nov-Dec;35(6):411–8.
5. Smith RP, Devine P, Jones H, DeNittis A, Whittington R, Metz JM. Internet use by patients with prostate cancer undergoing radiotherapy. Urology. 2003 Aug;62(2):273–7.
6. Shaverdian N, Kishan AU, Veruttipong D, Demanes DJ, Kupelian P, McCloskey S, et al. Impact of the primary information source used for decision making on treatment perceptions and regret in prostate Cancer. Am J Clin Oncol. 2017 May 23.
7. Metz JM, Devine P, DeNittis A, Jones H, Hampshire M, Goldwein J, Whittington R. A multi-institutional study of internet utilization by radiation oncology patients. Int J Radiat Oncol Biol Phys. 2003 Jul 15;56(4):1201–5.
8. Adler J, Paelecke-Habermann Y, Jahn P, Landenberger M, Leplow B, Vordermark D. Patient information in radiation oncology: a cross-sectional pilot study using the EORTC QLQ-INFO26 module. Radiat Oncol. 2009;4:40.
9. Castleton K, Fong T, Wang-Gillam A, Waqar MA, Jeffe DB, Kehlenbrink L, Gao F, Govindan R. A survey of internet utilization among patients with cancer. Support Care Cancer. 2011 Aug;19(8):1183–90.
10. Ilic D, Risbridger G, Green S. Searching the internet for information on prostate cancer screening: an assessment of quality. Urology. 2004 Jul; 64(1):112–6.
11. Shah A, Paly JJ, Efstathiou JA, Bekelman JE. Physician evaluation of internet health information on proton therapy for prostate cancer. Int J Radiat Oncol Biol Phys. 2013 Mar 15;85(4):e173–7.
12. Borgmann H, Wölm JH, Vallo S, Mager R, Huber J, Breyer J, et al. Prostate Cancer on the web-expedient tool for Patients' decision-making? J Cancer Educ. 2017 Mar;32(1):135–40.
13. Sacchetti P, Zvara P, Plante MK. The internet and patient education--resources and their reliability: focus on a select urologic topic. Urology. 1999;53(6):1117–20.
14. Nguyen SK, Ingledew PA. Tangled in the breast cancer web: an evaluation of the usage of web-based information resources by breast cancer patients. J Cancer Educ. 2013;28(4):662–8.
15. Weissenberger C, Jonassen S, Beranek-Chiu J, Neumann M, Müller D, Bartelt S, et al. Breast cancer: patient information needs reflected in English and German web sites. Br J Cancer. 2004;91(8):1482–7.
16. Perzel S, Huebner H, Rascher W, Menendez-Castro C, Hartner A, Fahlbusch FB. Searching the web: a survey on the quality of advice on postnatal sequelae of intrauterine growth restriction and the implication of developmental origins of health and disease. J Dev Orig Health Dis. 2017;22:1–9.
17. Charnock D, Shepperd S, Needham G, Gann R. DISCERN: an instrument for judging the quality of written consumer health information on treatment choices. J Epidemiol Community Health. 1999;53(2):105–11.
18. Charnock D, Shepperd S. Learning to DISCERN online: applying an appraisal tool to health websites in a workshop setting. Health Educ Res. 2004;19(4):440–6.
19. Nghiem AZ, Mahmoud Y, Som R. Evaluating the quality of internet information for breast cancer. Breast. 2016;25:34–7.
20. Janssen S, Käsmann L, Fahlbusch FB, Rades D, Vordermark D. Side effects of radiotherapy in breast cancer patients : the internet as an information source. Strahlenther Onkol. 2017.
21. Boyer C, Selby M, Scherrer JR, Appel RD. The health on the net code of conduct for medical and health websites. Comput Biol Med. 1998;28(5):603–10.
22. Silberg WM, Lundberg GD, Musacchio RA. Assessing, controlling, and assuring the quality of medical information on the internet: Caveant lector et viewor--let the reader and viewer beware. JAMA. 1997;277(15):1244–5.
23. Mattsson S, Olsson EMG, Johansson B, Carlsson M. Health-related internet use in people with Cancer: results from a cross-sectional study in two outpatient clinics in Sweden. J Med Internet Res. 2017;19(5):e163.
24. McLeod J, Yu I, Ingledew PA. Peering into the deep: characterizing the internet search patterns of patients with gynecologic cancers. J Cancer Educ. 2017;32(1):85–90.
25. Grewal P, Alagaratnam S. The quality and readability of colorectal cancer information on the internet. Int J Surg. 2013;11(5):410–3.
26. Corfield JM, Lawrentschuk N. Health information quality on the internet for bladder cancer and urinary diversion: a multi-lingual analysis. Minerva Urol Nefrol. 2017.
27. Narwani V, Nalamada K, Lee M, Kothari P, Lakhani R. Readability and quality assessment of internet-based patient education materials related to laryngeal cancer. Head Neck. 2016;38(4):601–5.
28. Alsaiari A, Joury A, Aljuaid M, Wazzan M, Pines JM. The content and quality of health information on the internet for patients and families on adult kidney Cancer. J Cancer Educ. 2016.
29. Quinn EM, Corrigan MA, McHugh SM, Murphy D, O'Mullane J, Hill AD, Redmond HP. Breast cancer information on the internet: analysis of accessibility and accuracy. Breast. 2012;21(4):514–7.
30. Saeed F, Anderson I. Evaluating the quality and readability of internet information on Meningiomas. World Neurosurg. 2017 Jan;97:312–6.
31. Sobota A, Ozakinci G. The quality and readability of online consumer information about gynecologic cancer. Int J Gynecol Cancer. 2015;25(3): 537–41.
32. Alkhateeb S, Lawrentschuk N. Consumerism and its impact on robotic-assisted radical prostatectomy. BJU Int. 2011 Dec;108(11):1874–8.
33. Liebl P, Seilacher E, Koester MJ, Stellamanns J, Zell J, Hübner J. What cancer patients find in the internet: the visibility of evidence-based patient information - analysis of information on German websites. Oncol Res Treat. 2015;38(5):212–8.

13

Safety and efficacy of Holmium laser enucleation of the prostate (HoLEP) in patients with previous transperineal biopsy (TPB): Outcomes from a dual-centre case-control study

Chris Bell[1,2*†], Sacha L. Moore[1†], Amarit Gill[1,2], Obinna Obi-Njoku[2], Stephen F. Hughes[2], Asad Saleemi[3], Gidon Ellis[3], Farooq Khan[3] and Iqbal S. Shergill[1,2]

Abstract

Background: We investigated the surgical feasibility, safety and effectiveness of 50 W (low power) Holmium Laser enucleation of the prostate (HoLEP) in patients who have undergone previous template biopsy of the prostate (TPB).

Methods: Data encompassing pre-operative baseline characteristics, intra-operative measures and post-operative outcomes was collected for 109 patients undergoing HoLEP across two UK centres. Patients were stratified into two groups; group 1 ($n = 24$) had undergone previous TPB were compared with 'controls' (no previous TPB) in group 2 ($n = 85$). The primary outcome was successful HoLEP.

Results: There were no statistically significant differences in either key baseline characteristics or mass of prostate enucleated between groups 1 and 2. There was no statistically significant difference in enucleation or morcellation times parameters between the two groups other than enucleation efficiency in favour of group 1 ($p = 0.024$). Functional outcomes improved, without any statistically significant difference, in both groups.

Conclusions: In patients with a previous TPB, HoLEP is surgically feasible, safe and effective. TPB should not be considered a contraindication to HoLEP. Our work provides a strong foundation for further research in this area.

Keywords: Holmium laser Enucleation of the prostate (HoLEP), Benign prostatic enlargement (BPE), Transperineal template biopsy, Prostate, Lower urinary tract symptoms (LUTS), Urinary retention

Background

The advent of Holmium laser enucleation of the prostate (HoLEP) has triggered a paradigm shift in the surgical management of benign prostatic enlargement (BPE); with improved functional outcomes, lower complication rates and length of stay, and fewer repeat procedures required at 5–10 years versus transurethral resection of the prostate (TURP), open prostatectomy and other laser therapies. HoLEP is now regarded as the gold standard for BPE [1–3]. Evidence that HoLEP is safe and efficacious in a wider patient demographic with varying co-morbidities is necessary as its use spreads.

The use of transperineal prostate biopsy (TPB) is increasing as a result of improved accuracy in diagnosing (or excluding) clinically significant cancer coupled with negligible risk of sepsis [4, 5]. However, patients undergoing TPB may rarely suffer from refractory retention post-biopsy requiring surgical management, and in addition, there is a cohort of patients who develop unrelated retention or lower urinary

* Correspondence: christopher.bell@wales.nhs.uk
† Authors C Bell & S Moore are joint first authors.
[1] Chris Bell and Sacha L. Moore contributed equally to this work.
[2] Department of Urology, Wrexham Maelor Hospital, Wrexham, Wales, UK
North Wales Clinical Research Centre, Gwenfro, Wrexham Technology Park, Wrexham LL13 7YP, UK
Full list of author information is available at the end of the article

tract sy (LUTS) secondary to BPE after past TPB and require surgical intervention [6].

Trans-rectal ultrasound (TRUS) guided biopsies have been performed prior to HoLEP and have not been shown to affect the technical difficulty of the procedure [7–10]. However TPB has important differences including more extensive sampling of the transitional zone versus TRUS-guided biopsies. Due to this theoretical disruption of prostate architecture during TPB many surgeons feel that HoLEP may be more challenging in this cohort of patients and that operative and functional outcomes could be compromised.

Whilst recent literature has demonstrated HoLEP's use following previous prostate surgery such as TURP and prostatic urethral lift surgery without compromise, and in those undergoing active surveillance for prostate cancer or with very large prostates, to our knowledge no published data evaluating outcomes of HoLEP after TPB exists [11–13]. As such in this study, we aimed to assess the feasibility, safety, and efficacy of HoLEP in patients who had undergone previous TPB.

Methods

Data collection

Following local institution audit registration (reg no. 18/171) we conducted a dual centre analysis of men undergoing 50 W low-power HoLEP between January 2016 and October 2018. Patients were stratified into two groups; group 1 had undergone TPB prior to HoLEP, while group 2 men were biopsy-naïve ("controls"). Patients in group 1 were from two centres whereas "control" patients in group 2 were from the second centre only. This was due to the fact that group 2 patients were consecutive patients from early in the learning curve from one surgeon – hence this would serve as the baseline control. Both groups had several surgeons performing the procedure. Patients who had undergone any prostate surgery prior to HoLEP or TPB were excluded. Data was collected into an Excel database, with both electronic and paper notes retrospectively reviewed to address missing data where possible and to gather information on post-operative outcomes.

Collected data was categorised according to timepoint relative to HoLEP. Pre-HoLEP measures included indication for HoLEP, time from TPB to HoLEP, results of TPB, prostate specific antigen (PSA) level, prostate volume measured using trans-rectal ultrasound (TRUS), haemoglobin, and creatinine. International prostate symptoms scores (IPSS) including quality of life score (QoL) and uroflowmetry were recorded where possible and relevant. Intra-operative measures included lobes enucleated, mass enucleated, enucleation time, morcellation time, morcellation efficiency, and whether there was a conversion to TURP. Post-HoLEP measures included length of hospital stay, post-operative complications (indexed as per the Clavien-Dindo classification), and histological findings of enucleated tissue.

Procedure information

Template biopsies were taken as per the PROMIS trial method [14].All included patients underwent low-power HoLEP using 50 W Auriga XL laser (Boston Scientific Inc.), under general anaesthesia, according to previously well-described HoLEP technique [15]. Morcellation was performed with the Wolf Piranha Morcellator system, and the use of bipolar diathermy for haemostasis was performed according to the discretion of the operating surgeon.

Data analysis

The primary outcome measure was successful HoLEP. Success was defined according to outcome at follow-up depending on indication. For those undergoing HoLEP for LUTS, success was defined by improvement in post-operative IPSS of ≥6, or improvement in quality of life (QoL) score of ≥2 points. A similar improvement in IPSS has been considered successful in other studies [16]. In patients without a pre-operative IPSS+QoL for comparison, success was defined as a post-operative QoL of ≤2 at follow-up. In patients with LUTS but no documented IPSS pre- or post-operatively, success was defined as no need for further medication or intervention for LUTS by 6 months. In patients undergoing HoLEP for refractory retention, success was defined as ability to void spontaneously.

Data was analysed using SPSS version 25 for Windows (IBM Corp., Armonk, NY). Where data was normally distributed, parametric analysis was undertaken employing the student's T-test, while Mann-Whitney U testing was performed for non-parametric continuous data. Differences between categorical variables were calculated using chi-square tests. Confidence intervals were calculated using the Newcombe-Wilson method without continuity correction. Outcomes were reported in accordance with the STROBE statement [17].

Results

Demographic and baseline data

Over the 34-month period, 24 men were identified who had undergone TPB prior to HoLEP (group 1), and 85 men were identified in group 2. Table 1 demonstrates baseline demographic and pre-operative characteristics. The mean age of patients was 66.8 years in group 1 and 71.8 years in group 2 95% CI 1.2–8.9, $p = 0.012$). The median time from TPB to HoLEP was 38.6 weeks (range 7–163 weeks, IQR 17.6–79.4). In Group 1, 13 patients had undergone HoLEP for refractory urinary retention versus 51 in group 2 (not statistically significant), while 11 patients in group 1 underwent HoLEP for LUTS, as compared to 34 patients in Group 2 (not statistically significant). Mean length of hospital stay was 1.6 days

Table 1 pre-operative baseline data

	Group 1	Group 2	Difference (95% CI)	*p* value
Age (years)	66.8 (±8.2)	71.8 (±8.7)	5.0 (1.2, 8.9)	0.012
TRUS volume (cm^3)	76.1 (±35.0)	69.3 (±31.8)	8.5 (−24.1, 10.6)	0.402
PSA (ng/mL)	10.2 (±5.7)	5.0 (±3.9)	5.1 (2.5, 7.8)	< 0.001
Indication for HoLEP				
LUTS	11 (45.8%)	34 (40.0%)	5.8 (−15.0, 27.3)	0.644
Refractory retention	13 (54.2%)	51 (60.0%)		
Q_{max} (mL/sec)	9.9 (±4.3)	9.6 (±5.2)	0.4 (−3.0, 3.8)	0.817
PVR (mL)	181.4 (±99.6)	176.8 (±140.3)	4.6 (− 77.5, 86.8)	0.908
IPSS	22.4 (±4.7)	22.6 (±6.9)	0.2 (−3.7, 4.0)	0.923
Quality of life score	4.1 (±1.0)	4.4 (±1.2)	0.3 (−0.5, 1.1)	0.484
Serum creatinine (μmol/L)	81.0 (±16.0)	86.7 (±30.3)	5.7 (−3.5, 15.0)	0.219

CI Confidence intervals, *TRUS* Trans-rectal ultrasound, *PSA* Prostate specific antigen, *HoLEP* Holmium laser enucleation of the prostate, *LUTS* Lower urinary tract symptoms, Q_{max} maximum flow rate, *PVR* Post-void residual volume, *IPSS* International Prostate Symptom Score. Data presented as mean (SD) except *counts (%).

(range 1–8), and differed significantly between the two groups (1.3 days for group 1 versus 3.0 days for group 2, $p < 0.001$). Information on pre-operative medications is presented in Additional file 1: Table S1.

Of the 24 men in group 1 who underwent TPB, the mean number of biopsies per patient was 40.5 (IQR 32.5–58.75). 16/24 (67%) of patients had benign histology whilst 8/24 (33%) of patients had Gleason score ≥ 3 + 3 (3 + 3, $n = 7$; 3 + 4, $n = 1$), of which five were unilateral and three bilateral. Additional information on the template biopsy histology is presented in Additional file 2: Table S2.

Pre-operative IPSS scores were available for 11/24 (45.8%) patients in group 1 and 33/85 (38.8%) patients in group 2. Pre-operative maximum flow rate (Q_{max}) and post-void residual (PVR) was available for 10/24 (41.7%) patients in group 1 and 35/85 (41.2%) patients in group 2. There were no significant differences at baseline between the two groups in key pre-operative parameters including mean prostate volume, Q_{max}, PVR, and IPSS score. Baseline PSA was significantly different between the two groups (10.2 versus 5.7, $p < 0.001$).

Operative outcomes in biopsied versus biopsy-naive men

Table 2 displays intra-operative outcomes. There was no significant difference in the mass enucleated (mean 54.7 g in group 1 vs 44.2 g in group 2, 95% CI -4.8, 25.7, $p = 0.172$). Notably, enucleation and morcellation time were comparable between the two groups; enucleation time was 55.8 min in group 1 versus 59.7 min in group 2 (95% CI -7.6, 15.5, $p = 0.172$), while morcellation time was 12.7 min in group 2 versus 10.1 min in group 2 (95% CI -1.9, 7.2, $p = 0.248$). Enucleation efficiency was significantly improved in group 1 versus group 2 (1.05 g/min versus 0.76 g/min, 95% CI 0.04,0.54, $p = 0.024$), however there was no significant difference in morcellation efficiency (5.04 g/min versus 6.59 g/min, 95% CI -0.30, 3.39, $p = 0.100$). Use of bipolar diathermy was also comparable and minimal, and there were no conversions to TURP. Three surgeons operated on a similar number of patients each ($n = 43$, 34, 32 respectively), with no difference in enucleation efficiency ($p = 0.541$) or morcellation efficiency ($p = 0.581$) between surgeons.

Post-operative outcomes for both cohorts are described in Table 3. All HoLEPs in group 1 were deemed successful, while 91% of HoLEPs in group 2 were successful.

Post-operative IPSS and QoL scores were available for 14/24 (58.3%) patients in group 1 and 61/85 (71.8%) patients in group 2. Post-operative Q_{max} and PVR was available for 12/24 (50.0%) patients in group 1, whilst Q_{max} was available for 15/85 (17.6%) patients and PVR was available for 20/85 (23.5%) patients in group 2. There were no significant differences between groups 1 and 2 in post-operative Q_{max} (17.3 mL/sec vs 22.2 mL/sec, 95% CI -4.1, 14.1, $p = 0.264$), PVR

Table 2 intra-operative measures

	Group 1	Group 2	Difference (95% CI)	*p* value
Mass enucleated (g)	54.7 (±33.1)	44.2 (±29.6)	10.5 (− 4.8, 25.7)	0.172
Enucleation time (mins)	55.8 (±24.0)	59.7 (±24.4)	3.9 (−7.6, 15.5)	0.496
Enucleation efficiency (g/min)	1.05 (±0.50)	0.76 (±0.61)	0.29 (0.04, 0.54)	0.024
Morcellation time (mins)	12.7 (±9.5)	10.1 (±7.8)	2.6 (−1.9, 7.2)	0.248
Morcellation Efficiency (g/min)	5.04 (±1.45)	6.59 (±7.69)	1.55 (−0.30, 3.39)	0.100

CI Confidence intervals. Data presented as mean (SD) except *counts (%).

Table 3 post-operative measures

	Group 1	Group 2	Difference (95% CI)	*p* value
Q_{max} (mL/sec)	17.3 (±6.7)	22.2 (±15.1)	5.1 (− 4.1, 14.1)	0.264
PVR (mL)	70.9 (±121.6)	63.1 (±84.4)	7.8 (−76.1, 91.7)	0.847
IPSS	6.2 (±4.5)	6.2 (±5.8)	0.1 (−2.9, 2.9)	0.990
Quality of life score	1.0 (±0.8)	1.5 (±1.74)	0.5 (−0.1, 1.1)	0.116
Mean hospital stay (days)	1.3 (1.0)	3.0 (3.6)	1.7 (0.45, 0.77)	< 0.001

CI Confidence intervals, Q_{max} maximum flow rate, *PVR* Post-void residual volume, *IPSS* International Prostate Symptom Score. Data presented as mean (SD).

(70.9 mL versus 63.1 mL, 95% CI-76.1, 91.7, $p = 0.847$), IPSS (6.2 versus 6.2, 95% CI -2.9, 2.9, $p = 0.990$) or QoL score (1.0 versus 1.5, 95% CI -0.1, 1.1, $p = 0.116$). Additionally, pre-HoLEP TPB result was compared with each of these outcome measures. Although numbers are too small to be conclusive, there was no significant difference in post-operative Q_{max}, PVR, IPSS or QoL score in the eight patients with a previous positive biopsy compared with an age-matched representative sample of the cohort. Time to HoLEP had no effect on enucleation and morcellation efficiency on correlation analysis ($p = 0.326$ & 0.604 respectively).

24/109 (22.0%) patients were documented as having a complication post-HoLEP (4/24 in group 1 and 20/85 in group 2). All complications were Clavien-Dindo 1 or 2. 14/24 (58.3%) patients had temporary stress urinary incontinence as their sole complication. Seven patients (6.4% of total cohort) reported erectile dysfunction post-operatively in clinic. One patient required a blood transfusion. Four patients required a catheter on discharge, but these were all successfully removed with spontaneous voiding at 14, 22, 30, and 45 days. No patients required medications post-operatively.

All patients in both cohorts had samples sent from HoLEP for histology. 4/24 (16.7%) patients in group 1 had positive histology; seven patients had Gleason 3 + 3 disease with one patient having Gleason 3 + 4. 10/85 (11.8%) patients in group 2 had positive histology; eight patients had Gleason 3 + 3 disease, one patient had Gleason 3 + 4, and one patient had Gleason 5 + 4. One patient with Gleason 3 + 3 disease and the patient with Gleason 5 + 4 disease had a pre-existing diagnosis of prostate cancer and were on hormone therapy. There was no statistically significant difference between incidental detection of prostate cancer between the two groups ($p = 0.402$). Additional information on histological features in presented in Additional file 3: Table S3. Histology post-HoLEP was reviewed alongside complications; there was no significant difference in complication rate between benign and malignant groups. Additionally, pre-HoLEP TPB histology in group 1 was shown not to be significantly associated with complication rate.

Functional outcomes in biopsied versus biopsy-naive men

Pre- and post-operative IPSS were compared in both groups 1 and 2 (Fig. 1); mean IPSS significantly improved post-HoLEP in both groups (group 1 mean IPSS pre-operatively 22.4 vs 6.2 post-operatively, $p < 0.001$; group 2 mean IPSS pre-operatively 22.5 vs 6.2 post-operatively, $p < 0.001$). Pre- and post-operative QoL scores were also compared in both groups 1 and 2 (Fig. 2); mean QoL significantly improved post-HoLEP in both groups (group 1 mean QoL score pre-operatively 4.1 vs 1.0 post-operatively, $p < 0.001$; group 2 mean QoL score pre-operatively 4.4 vs 1.5 post-operatively, $p < 0.001$).

Pre- and post-operative Q_{max} was compared in both groups 1 and 2; mean Q_{max} significantly improved post-HoLEP in both groups (group 1 mean Q_{max} pre-operatively 9.9 mL/s vs 17.5 mL/s post-operatively, $p = 0.007$); group 2 mean Q_{max} pre-operatively 9.6 mL/s versus 22.1 mL/s post-operatively, $p < 0.001$). Pre- and post-operative PVR was also compared in both groups 1 and 2; mean PVR significantly improved post-HoLEP in both groups (group 1 mean PVR pre-operatively 181.4 mL vs 70.9 post-operatively, $p = 0.03$; group 2 mean PVR pre-operatively 176.8 mL vs 63.1 mL post-operatively, $p = 0.002$).

Discussion

Meaning of the study

As such, our study is the first to demonstrate that HoLEP is a safe and feasible option, following previous TPB. With increasing number of men undergoing TPB, the population we have studied represents a common cohort of prostate patients, and as such, is a vital addition to the HoLEP evidence base.

Crucially, there is a view by some that HoLEP could be more difficult in patients post-TPB due to altered architecture of prostatic tissue. Our study provides evidence to the contrary and confirms the safety and efficacy profile of HoLEP, to include men who have undergone TPB. Both groups in our study had comparable baseline characteristics, with no significant differences between key indicators including indication for HoLEP, prostate volume on TRUS, pre-operative Q_{max}, PVR, IPSS and QoL score ($p > 0.05$). PSA was significantly higher in group 1 ($p = < 0.001$) but this was expected given patients in group 1 likely underwent TPB for investigation of raised PSA originally.

As is shown in Table 2, there was no significant difference in key intra-operative markers. If, as hypothesized,

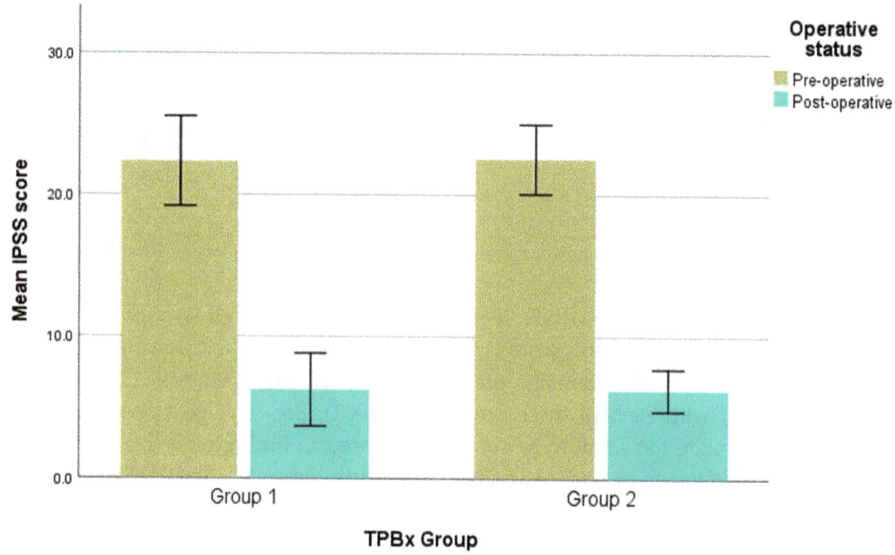

Fig. 1 Comparison of mean IPSS scores pre and post-HoLEP between those with previous template biopsy (group 1) and those without previous prostate intervention (group 2). Error bars denote 95% confidence intervals. IPSS: International Prostate Symptom Score; TPB: transperineal template biopsies

TPB led to an altered texture of prostate tissue and hence a more challenging HoLEP surgical procedure, it would be expected that in these cases enucleation and morcellation would take longer, which was not the case. Enucleation efficiency was, in fact, higher ($p = 0.024$) in the previous TPB group; we cannot provide evidence as to why this might be as to date there have not been any published studies in this area, however it is possible that there are physiological changes to prostate tissue post-biopsy and thus this is an area that warrants further research. The data therefore supports our assertion that is not made more technically challenging by a previous TPB.

Table 3 highlights no significant difference in key post-operative outcomes between the two groups, with marked improved pre- versus post-HoLEP in both groups. Additionally, all procedures in group 1 were deemed successful with a statistically significantly shorter length of hospital stay. Functionally, it is clear that HoLEP significantly improved both patient reported outcomes and objective outcomes regardless of previous TPB status, and thus is clearly an effective treatment option in both of these patient groups.

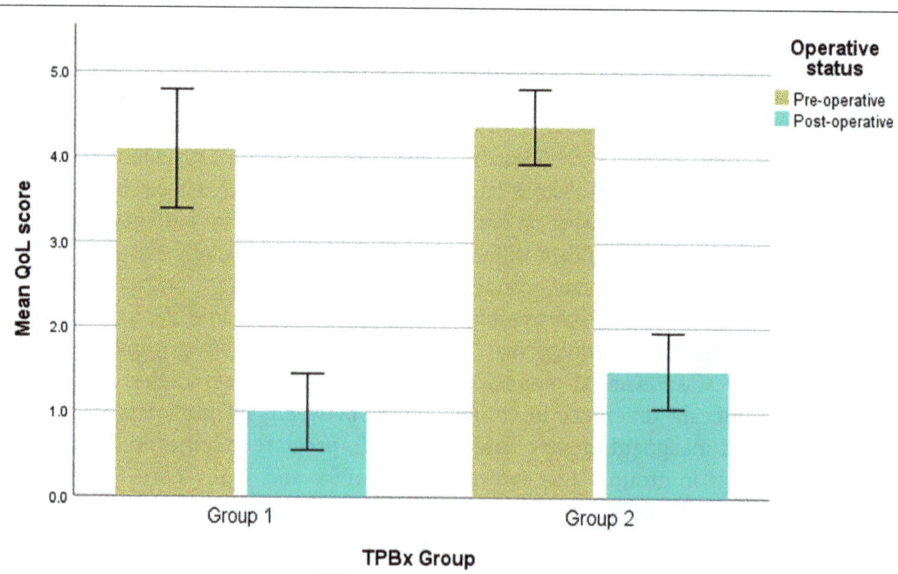

Fig. 2 Comparison of mean quality of life scores pre and post-HoLEP between those with previous template biopsy (group 1) and those without previous prostate intervention (group 2). QoL: quality of life score

Although complication rates were slightly higher than reported in the literature [18], it is worth noting that the majority of these were temporary stress urinary incontinence which resolved. It is also worth noting that patients in group 2 (where complication rate was higher compared to group 1) were all from one centre where the operating surgeon had just completed their learning curve [19]. Thus, this allowed for comparison between the potential challenge of patients post-biopsy in group 1 against control patients operated on by a surgeon with less experience in HoLEP.

Strengths and limitations

To our knowledge, this study provides the first evidence in the literature of the feasibility of HoLEP in those who have undergone TPB. The strength of our study lies in its provision of a breadth of data over two centres in two groups with comparable baseline characteristics. There were no significant differences between the groups recorded in key demographic and preoperative fields that might confound the results.

Nevertheless, we acknowledge that there are a number of limitations to our study. Although the data was largely collected from a prospectively-maintained database, some of the data (mainly post-operative measures) were retrospectively gathered and thus this opens up the possibility of misclassification bias. Likewise, data on IPSS/QoL scores in some patients with LUTS was missing either partially (i.e. only a pre-operative or post-operative score) or in its entirety. Consequently we were unable to quantify the degree of improvement in symptoms via this validated tool in a subgroup of patients. However, in this subgroup we used a pragmatic surrogate measure of success (no need for further medication or intervention for LUTS by 6 months) which we feel confers at least an acceptable level of accuracy.

Our study also focused on short-term post-operative outcome data and thus our study may miss long-term need for re-operation or longer term complications. There is also a large range of time from TPB to HoLEP, which could have an effect on patient expectations and therefore, potentially, outcomes.

Additionally, our study used 50 W low-power HoLEP, so application of these results to higher-power procedures has to be used with some degree of caution. The possible altered experience and adverse effect profile with higher-power lasers may mean differences in previously biopsied prostates become more prominent.

Recommendations for future research

Given this is the first study of its kind in this cohort of patients, there would be merit in building on this foundation further with fully-prospective multi-centre studies conducting an analysis of their patients in a similar way. Additionally, studies assessing long-term outcomes in patients that have undergone HoLEP post-TPB would be of value.

Conclusion

Our study demonstrates that 50 W low-power HoLEP is a feasible, safe and effective treatment modality for benign prostatic enlargement in patients with previous transperineal biopsy. Hence, transperineal prostate biopsy should not be considered a contraindication to HoLEP in men with benign prostatic enlargement. Further research building on this novel foundation is required to evaluate longer-term outcomes.

Supplementary information

Additional file 1: Table S1. Preoperative medications in patients undergoing HoLEP for lower urinary tract symptoms.

Additional file 2: Table S2. Histological detail of pre-HoLEP transperineal template biopsies of the prostate.

Additional file 3: Table S3. Histological features of post-transperineal template biopsy HoLEPs.

Abbreviations

BPE: Benign prostatic enlargement; HoLEP: Holmium laser enucleation of the prostate; IPSS: International prostate symptoms scores; LUTS: Lower urinary tract symptoms; PSA: Prostate specific antigen; PVR: Post-void residual volume; Q_{max}: Maximum flow rate; QoL: Quality of life score; TPB: Transperineal prostate biopsy; TRUS: Trans-rectal ultrasound; TURP: Transurethral resection of the prostate

Acknowledgements

The authors would like to thank Karen Kuschnir and the medical records department in Wrexham Maelor Hospital for their invaluable help with data collection for this project.

Authors' contributions

CB and SM contributed equally and therefore should be considered joint first authors of this work. CB & SM: analysis and interpretation of data, literature review, drafting, editing, and approval of manuscript; AG: drafting, editing, preparation, and approval of manuscript; OO: concept, study design, analysis and interpretation of data, editing and approval of manuscript; SFH, AS, GE, & FK: analysis and interpretation of data, editing and approval of manuscript; ISS: concept, study design, analysis and interpretation of data, literature review, drafting, editing and approval of manuscript.

Author details

[1]Department of Urology, Wrexham Maelor Hospital, Wrexham, Wales, UK. [2]North Wales Clinical Research Centre, Gwenfro, Wrexham Technology Park, Wrexham LL13 7YP, UK. [3]Department of Urology, Luton and Dunstable University Hospital, Lewsey Road, Luton LU4 0DZ, UK.

References

1. Michalak J, Tzou D, Funk J. HoLEP: the gold standard for the surgical management of BPH in the 21st century. Am J Clin Exp Urol. 2015;3(1):36.
2. Vincent MW, Gilling PJ. HoLEP has come of age. World J Urol. 2015;33(4):487–93.
3. Yin L, Teng J, Huang C-J, Zhang X, Xu D. Holmium laser Enucleation of the prostate versus transurethral resection of the prostate: a systematic review and meta-analysis of randomized controlled trials. J Endourol. 2013;27(5):604–11.
4. Grummet J, Pepdjonovic L, Huang S, Anderson E, Hadaschik B. Transperineal vs. transrectal biopsy in MRI targeting. Transl Androl Urol. 2017;6(3):368–75.

5. Abdulmajed MI, Hughes D, Shergill IS. The role of transperineal template biopsies of the prostate in the diagnosis of prostate cancer: a review. Expert Rev Med Devices. 2015;12(2):175–82.
6. Hannah M, Boam T, Bazo A. Complications post Transperineal template biopsy: a 3 year single-unit retrospective study. Int J Surg. 2017;47:S102.
7. Naspro R, Suardi N, Salonia A, Scattoni V, Guazzoni G, Colombo R, et al. Holmium laser enucleation of the prostate versus open prostatectomy for prostates >70 g: 24-month follow-up. Eur Urol. 2006;50(3):563–8.
8. Kuntz RM, Lehrich K. Transurethral holmium laser enucleation versus transvesical open enucleation for prostate adenoma greater than 100 gm.:: a randomized prospective trial of 120 patients. J Urol. 2002;168(4 Pt 1):1465–9.
9. Matlaga BR, Kim SC, Kuo RL, Watkins SL, Lingeman JE. Holmium laser enucleation of the prostate for prostates of >125 mL. BJU Int. 2006;97(1):81–4.
10. Kim M, Song SH, Ku JH, Oh S-J, Paick J-S. Prostate cancer detected after holmium laser enucleation of prostate (HoLEP): significance of transrectal ultrasonography. Int Urol Nephrol. 2014;46(11):2079–85.
11. Iqbal M, Jones R, Hughes S, Shergill I. Low power HOLEP after failed urolift: a case report using 50 watt laser. Urol case reports. 2018;16:114–5.
12. Jones P, Alzweri L, Rai BP, Somani BK, Bates C, Aboumarzouk OM. Holmium laser enucleation versus simple prostatectomy for treating large prostates: results of a systematic review and meta-analysis. Arab J Urol. 2016;14(1):50–8.
13. Kuebker JM, Miller NL. Holmium laser Enucleation of the prostate: patient selection and outcomes. Curr Urol Rep. 2017;18(12):96.
14. El-Shater Bosaily A, Parker C, Brown LC, Gabe R, Hindley RG, Kaplan R, et al. PROMIS — Prostate MR imaging study: A paired validating cohort study evaluating the role of multi-parametric MRI in men with clinical suspicion of prostate cancer. Contemp Clin Trials. 2015;42(11):26–40 Available from: http://www.ncbi.nlm.nih.gov/pubmed/15517144.
15. Gilling P. Holmium laser Enucleation of the prostate (HoLEP). BJU Int. 2007; 101(1):131–42.
16. Chuang FP, Lee SS, Wu ST, Yu DS, Chen HI, Chang SY, et al. Change in international prostate symptom score after transurethral prostatectomy in Taiwanese men with benign prostate hyperplasia: use of these changes to predict the outcome. Arch Androl. 2003;49(2):129–37 Available from: http://www.tandfonline.com/doi/full/10.1080/01480510390129250.
17. von Elm E, Altman DG, Egger M, Pocock SJ, Gøtzsche PC, Vandenbroucke JP, STROBE Initiative. Strengthening the reporting of observational studies in epidemiology (STROBE) statement: guidelines for reporting observational studies. BMJ. 2007;335(7626):806–8.
18. Shah HN, Mahajan AP, Hegde SS, Bansal MB. Peri-operative complications of holmium laser enucleation of the prostate: experience in the first 280 patients, and a review of literature. BJU Int. 2007;100(1):94–101.
19. Kampantais S, Dimopoulos P, Tasleem A, Acher P, Gordon K, Young A. Assessing the learning curve of holmium laser Enucleation of prostate (HoLEP). A Systematic Review. Urology. 2018;120:9–22.

Surface-projection-based transperineal cognitive fusion targeted biopsy of the prostate: An original technique with a good cancer detection rate

Lei Wang[1,2], Xiaofei Wang[1,2], Wenfeng Zhao[1,2], Zichen Zhao[1,2], Zhihu Li[1,2], Shengmin Fei[3], He Zhu[1,2], Xiang Ji[1,2], Bing Yang[1,2], Ningchen Li[1,2*] and Yanqun Na[1,2]

Abstract

Background: To report a new standardized cognitive fusion technique on transperineal targeted biopsy (TB) of prostate, and to evaluate its efficacy for cancer detection combined with systematic biopsy (SB) .

Methods: We present a retrospective review of consecutive patients undergoing multiparametric magnetic resonance (mpMRI) imaging of the prostate with subsequent transperineal prostate biopsy from January 2016 to December 2018. A free-hand 12-core SB was performed for each patient. PI-RADS 3–5 lesions were further targeted for biopsy with our TB technique. Firstly, a central point of suspicious lesion (B′) was registered cognitively on a transverse section of transrectal ultrasound (TRUS). Then, biopsy gun punctured vertically through a fixed pioneer site (A) on skin of perineum, and deep into the TRUS section to get A′. Next, targeted site (B), the surface-projection of B′, would be determined on skin of perineum by A and distance from B′ to A′. Finally, puncture through B to reach B′. Pathological findings of SB and TB were analyzed.

Results: A total of 126 patients underwent transperineal prostate biopsy (47 SB only, 79 SB + TB). The age of the patients was 68.7 ± 9.2 years. The median preoperative PSA value was 11.8 ng/mL. Preoperative prostate volume was 60.5 ± 50.0 mL. The numbers of patients with PI-RADS scores of 1 through 5 were 4, 43, 27, 21 and 31, respectively. The overall detection rate of cancer was 61/126 (48.4%), and it was significantly higher in the combination cohort (56/79, 70.9%) compared with the SB only cohort (5/47, 10.6%, $p<0.001$). When focused on the combination cohort, TB detected a similar overall rate of PCa (53/79, 67.1% vs 52/79, 65.8%; $p = 0.87$) compared with SB. The clinically significant PCa (csPC) detection rate was 52/79 (65.8%), while for TB and SB the csPC/PC rate was 51/53 (96.2%) and 48/52 (92.3%), respectively($p = 0.44$). TB demonstrated a better sampling performance (positive rate for each core) compared with SB (51.0% vs 31.3%, $p < 0.001$).

Conclusions: Surface-projection-based transperineal cognitive fusion targeted biopsy of the prostate has a good efficacy in detecting PCa.

Keywords: Clinically significant prostate cancer, Targeted biopsy, Cognitive fusion biopsy, PI-RADS version 2 score, Transperineal prostate biopsy

* Correspondence: wjpurologycenter@sina.com
[1]Department of urology, Peking University Shougang Hospital, Peking University Health Science Center, Beijing 100144, China
[2]Peking University Wu Jieping Urology Center, Peking University Shougang Hospital, Peking University Health Science Center, 9# Jinyuanzhuang Road, Shijingshan district, Beijing 100144, China
Full list of author information is available at the end of the article

Background

Prostate cancer (PCa) is one of the most frequently diagnosed malignant tumors worldwide [1]. In China, the incidence of PCa has increased rapidly in recent decades [2, 3]. Prostate biopsy is the gold standard for PCa diagnosis [4]. Hodge et al. [5]. first introduced the systematic sextant biopsy protocol under transrectal ultrasound (TRUS) guidance in 1989, and the technique of prostate biopsy has experienced a long evolution since then. Until recently, TRUS guided transperineal and transrectal biopsies are the two most frequently used approaches to obtain prostate tissue for diagnosis of PCa [6–8].

The conventional systematic method of prostate biopsy has been shown to have limited sensitivity for detecting prostate cancer in recent years [9], while multiparametric magnetic resonance imaging (mpMRI) of the prostate has become a very useful tool to improve the accuracy of prostate cancer detection. Suspicious lesions on mpMRI can guide targeted biopsies and allow for better detection of PCa, especially clinically significant PCa [10–12]. Targeted biopsy (TB) was introduced thereafter for sampling suspicious lesions shown by mpMRI. Currently, there are three primary modalities to perform a targeted biopsy: 1) MRI guided biopsy, in which biopsy is guided by real-time MRI images. This modality offers an increased sensitivity and specificity for prostate biopsy guidance; however, the disadvantages of being time-consuming and requiring specialized equipment has resulted in it not being widely used [13]. 2) MRI-TRUS fusion technique. This novel fusion technology can provide visualization of both recorded multiplanar reconstruction images on one monitor in real time, and it also produced encouraging results as reported by many researchers. However, the technology needs dedicated hardware and algorithm-based fusion software and their expense limits its widespread use [14, 15]. 3) Cognitive fusion technique, also called visual registration biopsy. This technique does not need any additional equipment but needs the operator to possess skills in reading both MRI and TURS images. It is convenient but usually requires a long learning curve [16, 17].

The cognitive fusion technique has been reported in many studies and has produced good results. However, the technique mainly relies on the operator's personal experience and is usually not standardized and thus not easy to learn. In the present study, we introduce a new method of cognitive fusion prostate biopsy and report our experience with using this standardized and easily learned technique.

Methods

Study design

This study was undertaken in a single university-affiliated hospital in Beijing, China. The ethics committee of the Peking University Shougang Hospital monitored, reviewed and approved the study protocol. All consecutive men who underwent prostate biopsy from January 2016 to December 2018 were retrospectively identified. Inclusion criteria for this study were an abnormal screening test with PSA or digital rectal examination (DRE). Exclusion criteria included those men (a) with transrectal biopsy (a traditional procedure performed by an ultrasonologist in our hospital); (b) did not have an mpMRI before biopsy; (c) with a previous history of PCa; (d) with prior negative biopsy; (e) unable to communicate effectively; (f) with symptoms of urinary tract infection, acute urinary retention, or (g) coagulation disorders.

Imaging

All of the enrolled patients underwent mpMRI on a GE Signa HDxt 3.0 T MR scanner with a 32-channel phased array coil, which included triplanar T2-weighted, axial dynamic contrast-enhanced and diffusion-weighted imaging. Image analyses were performed and supervised by two experienced uroradiologists. Suspicious lesions were assigned a likelihood score from 1 to 5 based on the standardized prostate imaging reporting and data system (PI-RADS) version 2 criteria scoring system.

Biopsy protocol

A transperineal systematic prostate biopsy was carried out for all of the enrolled patients under intravenous or intraspinal anesthesia. A single antibiotic was routinely given 30 min before the operation. After that, a targeted biopsy was performed for suspicious lesions with a PI-RADS score of 3 to 5. Informed consent was obtained preoperatively for every patient. Details of our systematic biopsy (SB) and TB procedures are described as follows:

Free hand 12-core transperineal systematic biopsy

The patient was placed in the lithotomy position. A transrectal ultrasound probe (BK Medical Aps, Mileparken 34, DK-2730 Herlev) was used to obtain TRUS transversal and sagittal images simultaneously with a bipolar model. The prostate gland was divided into 12 areas on transverse sections of the TRUS image (Fig. 1). First, a puncture guided needle is located at the right side of the perineum area, approximately 1.5 cm above the superior border of the anus, 1 cm to the right of the middle line of the perineum. We call this location the pioneer site (site A in Fig. 2).

When we make a vertical puncture through site A and deep into the prostate gland, we usually reach point 6 (Fig. 1). Site A is recorded as the surface projection of point 6 on the skin of perineum. Second, an 18-G Bard disposable biopsy gun (Bard Medical, Covington, GA, USA) punctures through the guide needle, reaches the prostate gland, and then percusses to collect tissue. Third, we change the direction of the guide needle tip upward and/or to the side to obtain other tissue samples

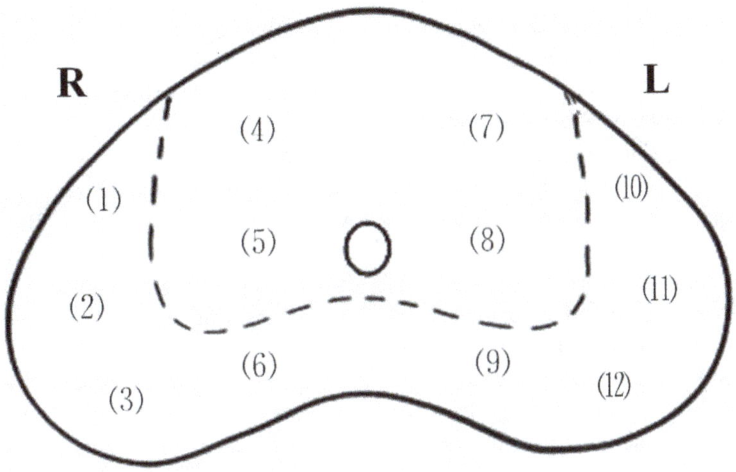

Fig. 1 Distribution of 12 cores on a TRUS transverse section in our free-hand transperineal systematic biopsy

one by one. Then, the guide needle will be moved to the left side to help collect another 6 tissue samples. If the prostate gland is larger than 60 ml, another 2–8 cores will be added to provide a better coverage of the entire gland. A deeper puncture may be necessary to cover the base of the enlarged gland.

Surface-projection-based cognitive fusion target biopsy

Before our targeted biopsy, the mpMRI image is read carefully by an urologist and a radiologist together. The cancer-suspicious lesion will be identified and marked on the transverse and sagittal T2 WI sequences. The ultrasound probe is moved back-and-forth to find the same section ("*target section*") on the TRUS transverse image as that on the MRI transverse image. After that step, four standardized steps will be performed:

Step 1: Make a vertical puncture through site A and deep into the prostate gland (the same step as that in systematic biopsy), then you will find a site representing the biopsy gun on the TRUS "target section". We call it site A' (Fig. 3). Site A' in our TB protocol is actually the point 6 in our SB protocol.

Step 2: Once the location of the suspicious lesion is confirmed on the mpMRI image, it can be registered over TRUS image through fusing images cognitively. We call the suspicious lesion site B′ (Fig. 3).

Step 3: This step is to locate site B, which is the surface projection of site B′ on the skin of perineum. After the above steps, the distance (d) and angle (a) between B

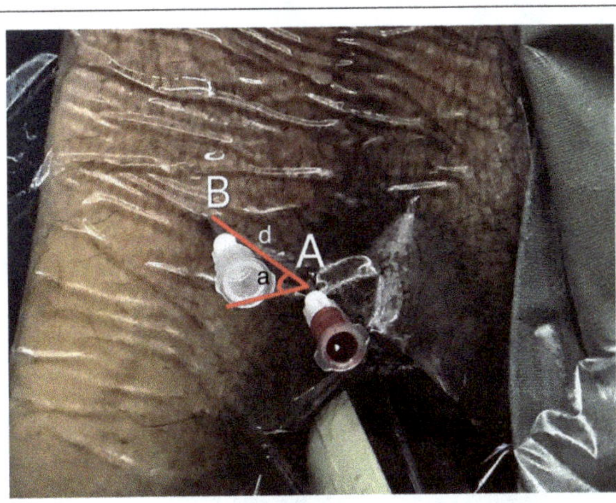

Fig. 2 Site A and B on the perineum skin. Site A is located 1.5 cm above and 1.0 cm to the side of the middle point of the superior border of the anus. It is usually a surface projection of the middle-right region of the peripheral zone (region 6 in Fig. 1). Site B should be the surface projection of the suspicious region of the prostate. Two guiding needles have been inserted through site A and B. d: distance from B to A; a: angle from B to A

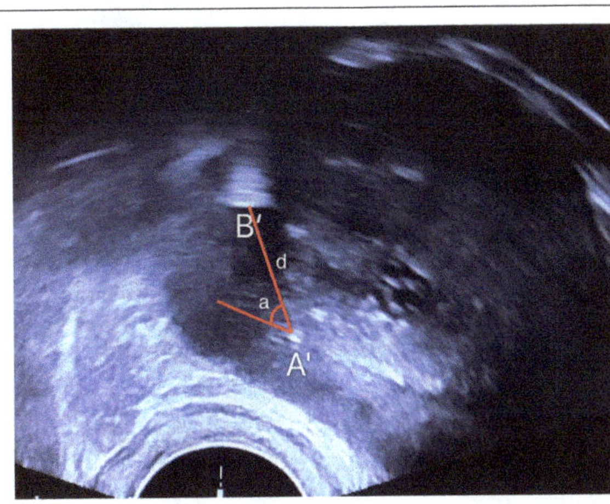

Fig. 3 Site A′ and B′ on the target transverse section of TRUS. When the biopsy gun punctured vertically through Site A and into this target section, we can get Site A′. Site B′ represents the central point of suspicious region on the target TRUS section and it is determined by cognitive fusion of the TRUS and mpMRI images. d: distance from B′ to A′; a: angle from B′ to A′

′ and A' can be measured in TRUS transverse section (Fig. 3). With the same relative distance and angle from A' to B′, we can locate site B (Fig. 2) from pioneer site A on the skin of perineum.

Step 4: The guide needle will be inserted through site B (Fig. 2). Then, our biopsy gun will puncture through the guide needle vertically into the prostate gland to make a targeted biopsy. If the biopsy needle cannot reach the suspicious lesion precisely, the deviation should be remembered, and a slight adjustment of insert direction should be made. The number of cores sampled is mainly determined by the quality of each core, which means whether or not the core could sample the central point of the lesion, two to three samples will usually be taken for each targeted lesion. A three-dimensional image is presented as Fig. 4 to make our technique clearer.

Clinical and pathological data

Clinical parameters involving age, DRE, PSA, prostate volume, pathological diagnosis, Gleason score, novel Gleason group, and numbers of positive cores were documented for each patient. Two pathologists independently evaluated the biopsy specimen and applied Gleason scores to the cases of PCa, and in cases of lack of consensus, a third senior pathologist evaluated the specimens. According to the novel prostate cancer grading system, we reclassified the patients by the new five grades based on the revised original Gleason score: group 1 (Gleason score ≤ 6), group 2 (Gleason score 3 + 4 = 7), group 3 (Gleason score 4 + 3 = 7), group 4 (Gleason score 8), and group 5 (Gleason score 9–10). Clinically significant cancer on biopsy was defined as a Gleason score 3 + 4 or higher or a Gleason score of 6 with positive cores ≥3.

Data analysis

Statistical analysis was performed using SPSS 21.0 Software (SPSS Inc., Chicago, IL, USA). The quantitative data were expressed as the mean ± standard deviation when they were normally distributed or were expressed as median (inter-quartile range) when they were distributed in a skewed way. Fisher's exact test was used to compare categorical variables. Pearson's chi-square test was used for comparing detection rates. A *P* value< 0.05 was considered to be statistically significant.

Results

There were 166 consecutive cases in total. Among these cases, 32 patients who underwent transrectal biopsy of the prostate, three who had no mpMRI before biopsy, and five who had prior negative biopsy were excluded. Thus, 126 cases met the criteria and were enrolled. The number of patients who underwent systematic biopsy only (SB only cohort) and who underwent systematic plus targeted biopsy (combination cohort) were 47 and 79, respectively. Among them, 42 patients had a positive DRE. The patients' demographics and summary of biopsy findings are shown in Table 1. The mean number of targeted biopsy cores per patient was 2.5 ± 0.7. The

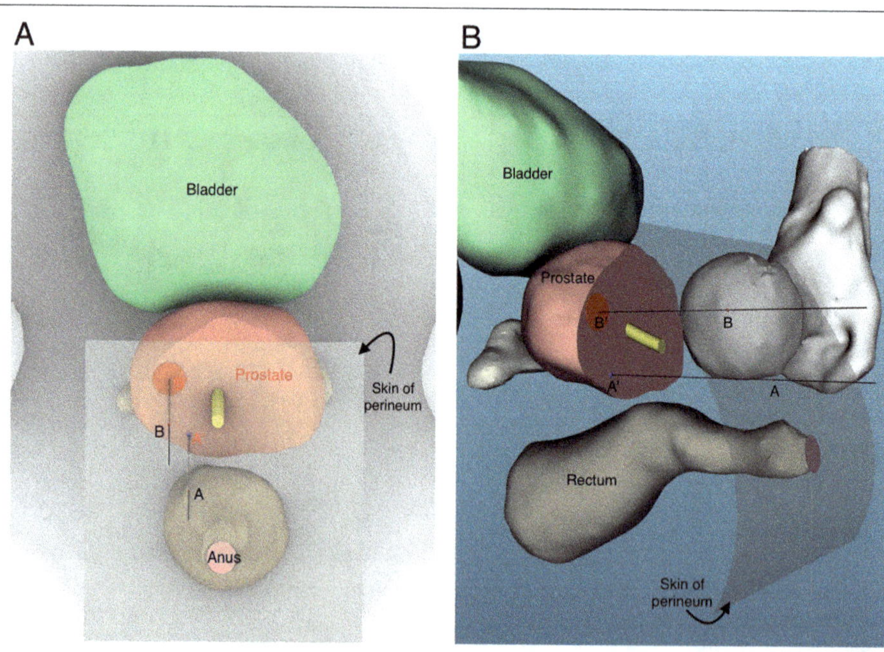

Fig. 4 Sketch map of our technique of surface-projection-based transperineal cognitive fusion targeted biopsy of the prostate (4A: Positive View, 4B: Side View). A: a pioneer site on skin of perineum, representing the surface projection of point A'; A': a pioneer point on transverse section of the prostate; B': the central point of suspicious lesion; B: a targeted site on skin of perineum, representing the surface projection of point B'

Table 1 Patient characteristic and positive biopsy rate by different biopsy approach and PSA level

	SB only	SB + TB	p	All
N	47	79		126
Age	66.9 ± 8.7	69.7 ± 9.3	0.09	68.7 ± 9.2
PSA	11.5 (5.2–16.3)	13.0 (6.7–33.6)	0.07	11.8 (6.5–25.2)
Volume	72.1 ± 64.1	53.6 ± 38.2	0.045	60.5 ± 50.0
PCa	5 (10.6%)	56 (70.9%)	<0.001	61 (48.4%)
csPC	2 (4.3%)	52 (65.8%)	<0.001	54 (42.9%)
PSA (pos./tot)				
<10	2/21 (9.5%)	17/31 (54.8%)	0.001	19/52 (36.5%)
10–20	3/17 (17.6%)	11/16 (68.8%)	0.005	14/33 (42.4%)
20–50	0/8 (0%)	12/16 (75.0%)	<0.001	12/24 (50.0%)
>50	0/1 (0%)	16/16 (100%)	0.006	16/17 (94.1%)
Bone meta	1/5 (20%)	19/56 (33.9%)	0.51	20/61 (32.8%)

SB: systematic biopsy; TB: targeted biopsy; csPC:clinically significant prostate cancer; pos.:positive; tot.: total; meta: metastasis

mean number of systematic biopsy cores per patient was 12.9 ± 1.7.

Of the total 126 patients, 61 (48.4%) were diagnosed with PCa, including 7 (11.5%) with clinically insignificant and 54 (88.5%) with significant cancers. Fourteen (23.0%) patients had a Gleason score of 3 + 3, 12 (19.7%) of 3 + 4, 13 (21.3%) of 4 + 3, 9 (14.8%) of 8 and 13 (21.3%) patients with a Gleason score of 9–10. According to the pathological and imaging results, patients who had localized, locally advanced and metastatic prostate cancer were 25 (41.0%), 16 (26.2%) and 20 (32.8%), respectively. Complications included blood in the urine in 6 patients (4.8%), difficulty urinating in 4 patients (3.2%) and epididymitis in one patient (0.8%). Twenty PCa patients (32.8%) accepted radical prostectomy subsequently.

As shown in Table 1, patients in the SB only cohort (PI-RADS 1–2) had similar ages (66.9 yrs. vs. 69.7 yrs., $p = 0.09$), a lower PSA level (11.5 ng/ml vs. 13.0 ng/ml, $p = 0.07$), a larger prostate volume (72.1 ml vs. 53.6 ml, $p = 0.045$) and a much lower PCa detection rate (10.6% vs. 70.9%, $p<0.001$) compared with the combination cohort (PI-RADS 3–5). When stratified by PSA level, the combination cohort also manifested a much better PCa detection rate in any of the subgroups than the SB only cohort.

From Table 2, we can see that the positive rate of targeted core biopsies can reach 51.0%, which is significantly higher than that of the systematic core biopsies (31.3%, $p<0.001$). In total, 4 patients were found to have clinically insignificant prostate cancer in the combination cohort, 2 were revealed from systematic cores only, and the other 2 from both systematic and targeted cores. In combination cohort, the use of TB alone would have led to 3 fewer cases of cancer, only 1 of which was clinically significant prostate cancer (csPC). The use of SB alone would have missed 4 cases of cancer, and all were clinically significant. For TB only vs. SB only, the total and csPC detection rate were 67.1% vs. 65.8% ($p = 0.87$) and 64.6% vs. 60.8% ($p = 0.62$) and the csPC/PC rate was 96.2% vs 92.3% ($p = 0.44$).

Discussion

TRUS guided biopsy has been proven to be an accurate method for diagnosis of prostate cancer. Additionally, with the application of mpMRI, targeted biopsy can be used to make a precise puncture. In the present study, we used an original cognitive fusion method to perform transperineal targeted prostate biopsies for patients with PI-RADS scores of 3 to 5, and this modality has been demonstrated to be easy to perform with a good PCa detection efficacy.

Targeted biopsies of the prostate under the guidance of TRUS have been widely reported with different modalities in different populations. Mischinger J and colleagues [18] reported a total and csPC detection rate of 61 and 51.9%, respectively, by using robot-assistant transperineal TB plus an SB technique in 202 patients with suspicious mpMRI. Hakozaki Y and colleagues [19] evaluated the effectiveness of MRI/US fusion TB on csPC detection and the positive rate was 57.1, 48.0, and 63.3% for SB, TB and the combination, respectively. H Lian et al. [14]. indicated that the PCa detection rates of TB, SB and combination were 30.7, 26.7 and 40.6%, respectively, by using free-hand transperineal MRI-TRUS fusion guided biopsy in Chinese men with repeated biopsy. Dekalo S et al. [20] reported their total and csPC detection rates of 52 and 35%, respectively, for 82 patients with suspicious prostate lesions on MRI by using cognitive fusion biopsy method. In our "TB + SB" cohort,

Table 2 Positive biopsy rate and positive core rate in patients with systematic plus targeted biopsy

PI-RADS score	No.	PCa	PCa. only by SB	PCa. only by TB	Positive rate of Systemic Core	Positive rate of Targeted Core	p
3	27	8 (29.6%)	2 (1 insig.)	1	17/339 (5.0%)	7/70 (10.0%)	0.16
4	21	17 (81.0%)	1 (1 insig.)	2	63/261 (24.1%)	24/49 (49.0)	<0.001
5	31	31 (100%)	0	1	227/380 (59.7%)	68/75 (90.7%)	<0.001
Total	79	56 (70.9%)	3 (2 insig.)	4 (0 insig.)	307/980 (31.3%)	99/194 (51.0%)	<0.001

SB Systematic biopsy, *TB* Targeted biopsy, insig.: clinically insignificant PCa the PCa detection rates of TB only, SB only and combination were 67.1, 65.8 and 70.9% respectively, while the csPC detection rate was 65.8% (Table 1). Our detection rate is higher than the results found in previous reports. The main reason for this is probably because we had more PCa patients with a higher risk and an advanced stage in this Chinese cohort. Similar to most of the previous reports, TB tended to find fewer or a similar number of overall PCas but have a higher csPC rate compared with SB in our combination cohort. For TB only, SB only and TB plus SB, the csPC/PC rates reached 96.2, 92.3 and 92.9%, respectively, in our combination cohort. However, the difference was statistically insignificant. The reason for this might be the small sample size as well as a lower rate of clinically insignificant PCa in our study. We also had a much better positive core rate for both TB and SB than in previous reports. This is mainly attributable to more advanced/high risk PCa patients in our Chinese cohort.

In the present study, as well as in other reports on Chinese patients [14, 21], there tends to be more PCa patients at high risk and in an advanced stage compared to data from western countries [15–18]. In Yang T's biopsy cohort [21], they had 34.6% patients with a PSA level ≥ 20 ng/ml, 33.6% PCa patients with a Gleason score ≥ 8, and a total PC detection rate of 45.6%, similar to the results found in our study (32.5, 37.5, and 48.4%, respectively). We also reported 41.3% patients with PI-RADS score ≥ 4 and 32.8% PCa patients had bone metastases at first diagnosis.

Cognitive fusion targeted biopsy [16, 20, 22] has previously been reported. This kind of modality is feasible and potentially able to identify cancerous regions for subsequent biopsy through analyzing mpMRI and real-time TRUS imaging cognitively during the operation without requiring a costly real-time MRI-TRUS fusion guided biopsy system [14]. However, it is usually not easy to learn how to perform this procedure and there might be different results because of operators with different experiences. In our method, there are four important sites—site A, A', B and B′. Site A is fixed and selected according to our previous experience in performing systematic biopsies. Site A' can be tracked on transverse section images of TRUS as the biopsy gun punctures vertically through site A. To locate site B′, the position of the suspicious lesion, precisely on the TRUS image is the key procedure in all cognitive fusion targeted biopsies. This requires a good understanding of MRI and TRUS images and for making a mental "registration" of mpMRI images to a corresponding section of TRUS through fusing images cognitively. Finally, site B, the surface projection of site B′ on the skin of perineum, is easily selected away from the pioneer site A based on the same relative distance from A' to B′. We believe the whole procedure is more standardized and easy to learn.

The learning curve of our technique is short and can be divided into three phases. In the first phase, the biopsy will be performed and the thought and protocol of this technique will be explained thoroughly. The trainees will visit 3–5 operations and learn how to observe the prostate gland through TURS during this period. In the second phase, the trainees will perform the biopsy by themselves under guidance. As the protocol is standardized and can be performed step by step, it is not hard to understand and operate. Most of the trainees could master this technique in 3–5 operations. After that, they will complete the biopsy independently in the last phase.

Although this method showed a good cancer detection rate in the present study, there are still several limitations. For one thing, it strictly relies on a good understanding of mpMRI and TRUS images by the operator; for another, if the suspicious lesion is smaller than 5 mm, it is hard to make a precise puncture, and more punctures should be made to increase the probability that your biopsy gun has punctured the target lesion.

For our study, there are also some shortcomings. This is a retrospective study with weak power to explain the difference of detection efficacy between the TB and SB techniques. In addition, the biopsy was performed by different operators, and there may exist an operator bias with regard to cancer detection. Finally, our study is relatively small and lacks comparisons with other methods of TB. Our data were only from one single medical center in Beijing, China, which can only partly represent the Chinese population, especially the population from northern China. A prospective and controlled study is expected to verify our new cognitive-fusion TB technique further.

Conclusions

In the present study, we introduced a new method of cognitive fusion targeted biopsy of prostate and confirmed that it had a good performance in cancer detection. We also revealed that our targeted biopsy had better efficacy in sampling, tended to find more csPC and less clinically insignificant PCa (although a statistically difference was not reached) compared with systematic biopsy. This modality is economical and practical, and is worth to be popularized.

Abbreviations

csPC: Clinically significant prostate cancer; DRE: Digital rectal examination; mpMRI: Multiparametric magnetic resonance; PCa: Prostate cancer; PI-RADS: Prostate Imaging, Reporting and Data System; PSA: Prostate specific antigen; SB: Systematic biopsy; TB: Targeted biopsy; TRUS: Transrectal ultrasound

Acknowledgements

We thank Miss Hui Ren and Mr. Kun Liu for helping us to draw and modify pictures. We also thank Miss Luxuan Zhang for helping us in improving English language within our manuscript.

Authors' contributions

LW: Project development, data analysis, manuscript writing; XW: Project development, data collection, data analysis; SF: MRI image analysis; ZL, WZ: Project development, data collection, manuscript writing; ZZ, HZ, XJ, BY: Data collection. NL: Project development, Manuscript Revision; YN: Manuscript Revision. All authors reviewed and approved the manuscript.

Author details

[1]Department of urology, Peking University Shougang Hospital, Peking University Health Science Center, Beijing 100144, China. [2]Peking University Wu Jieping Urology Center, Peking University Shougang Hospital, Peking University Health Science Center, 9# Jinyuanzhuang Road, Shijingshan district, Beijing 100144, China. [3]Department of medical imaging, Peking University Shougang Hospital, Peking University Health Science Center, Beijing 100144, China.

References

1. Siegel RL, Miller KD, Jemal A. Cancer statistics, 2018. CA Cancer J Clin. 2018; 68(1):7–30.
2. Chen W, Sun K, Zheng R, Zeng H, Zhang S, Xia C, et al. Cancer incidence and mortality in China, 2014. Chin J Cancer Res. 2018;30(1):1–12.
3. Chen W, Zheng R, Baade PD, Zhang S, Zeng H, Bray F, et al. Cancer statistics in China, 2015. CA Cancer J Clin. 2016;66(2):115–32.
4. Mottet N, Bellmunt J, Bolla M, Briers E, Cumberbatch MG, De Santis M, et al. EAU-ESTRO-SIOG guidelines on prostate cancer. Part 1: screening, diagnosis, and local treatment with curative intent. Eur Urol. 2017;71(4):618–29.
5. Hodge KK, McNeal JE, Terris MK, Stamey TA. Random systematic versus directed ultrasound guided transrectal core biopsies of the prostate. J Urol. 1989;142(1):71–4 discussion 74-75.
6. Chang DT, Challacombe B, Lawrentschuk N. Transperineal biopsy of the prostate-is this the future? Nat Rev Urol. 2013;10(12):690–702.
7. Ahallal Y, Sanchez-Salas R, Sivaraman A, Barret E, Secin FP, Validire P, et al. Clinical performance of transperineal template guided mapping biopsy for therapeutic decision making in low risk prostate cancer. Actas Urol Esp. 2016;40(10):615–20.
8. Grummet J. How to biopsy: transperineal versus transrectal, saturation versus targeted, what's the evidence? Urol Clin North Am. 2017;44(4):525–34.
9. Taira AV, Merrick GS, Galbreath RW, Andreini H, Taubenslag W, Curtis R, et al. Performance of transperineal template-guided mapping biopsy in detecting prostate cancer in the initial and repeat biopsy setting. Prostate Cancer Prostatic Dis. 2010;13(1):71–7.
10. Gayet M, van der Aa A, Beerlage HP, Schrier BP, Mulders PF, Wijkstra H. The value of magnetic resonance imaging and ultrasonography (MRI/US)-fusion biopsy platforms in prostate cancer detection: a systematic review. BJU Int. 2016;117(3):392–400.
11. Schoots IG, Roobol MJ, Nieboer D, Bangma CH, Steyerberg EW, Hunink MG. Magnetic resonance imaging-targeted biopsy may enhance the diagnostic accuracy of significant prostate cancer detection compared to standard transrectal ultrasound-guided biopsy: a systematic review and meta analysis. Eur Urol. 2015;68(3):438–50.
12. Marra G, Ploussard G, Futterer J, Valerio M. EAU-YAU Prostate Cancer Working Party. Controversies in MR targeted biopsy: alone or combined, cognitive versus software-based fusion, transrectal versus transperineal approach? World J Urol. 2019;37(2):277–87.
13. Sugano D, Sidana A, Calio B, Cobb K, Turkbey B, Pinto PA. MRI-targeted biopsy: is systematic biopsy obsolete? Can J Urol. 2017;24(4):8876–82.
14. Lian H, Zhuang J, Wang W, Zhang B, Shi J, Li D, et al. Assessment of free-hand transperineal targeted prostate biopsy using multiparametric magnetic resonance imaging-transrectal ultrasound fusion in Chinese men with prior negative biopsy and elevated prostate-specific antigen. BMC Urol. 2017;17(1):52.
15. Radtke JP, Schwab C, Wolf MB, Freitag MT, Alt CD, Kesch C, et al. Multiparametric magnetic resonance imaging (MRI) and MRI-transrectal ultrasound fusion biopsy for index tumor detection: correlation with radical prostatectomy specimen. Eur Urol. 2016;70(5):846–53.
16. Oberlin DT, Casalino DD, Miller FH, Matulewicz RS, Perry KT, Nadler RB, et al. Diagnostic value of guided biopsies: fusion and cognitive-registration magnetic resonance imaging versus conventional ultrasound biopsy of the prostate. Urology. 2016;92:75–9.
17. Hamid S, Donaldson IA, Hu Y, Rodell R, Villarini B, Bonmati E et al. The SmartTarget biopsy trial: a prospective, within-person randomised, blinded trial comparing the accuracy of visual-registration and magnetic resonance imaging/ultrasound image-fusion targeted biopsies for prostate cancer risk stratification. Eur Urol. 2018; epub ahead of print 2018 Nov 29; doi: https://doi.org/10.1016/j.eururo.2018.08.007.
18. Mischinger J, Kaufmann S, Russo GI, Harland N, Rausch S, Amend B, et al. Targeted vs systematic robot-assisted transperineal magnetic resonance imaging-transrectal ultrasonography fusion prostate biopsy. BJU Int. 2018; 121(5):791–8.
19. Hakozaki Y, Matsushima H, Kumagai J, Murata T, Masuda T, Hirai Y, et al. A prospective study of magnetic resonance imaging and ultrasonography (MRI/US)-fusion targeted biopsy and concurrent systematic transperineal biopsy with the average of 18-cores to detect clinically significant prostate cancer. BMC Urol. 2017;17(1):117.
20. Dekalo S, Matzkin H, Mabjeesh NJ. High cancer detection rate using cognitive fusion - targeted transperineal prostate biopsies. Int Braz J Urol. 2017;43(4):600–6.
21. Yang T, Zhang L, Chen Y, Cai Y, Jiang H, Ding Q. The predictive efficacy of hypoechoic lesion in ultrasound for prostate cancer in Chinese people: five-year experience in a moderated 10-core transperineal prostate biopsy procedure. Oncotarget. 2017;8(45):79433–40.
22. Galosi AB, Maselli G, Sbrollini G, Donatelli G, Montesi L, Tallè M, et al. Cognitive zonal fusion biopsy of the prostate: original technique between target and saturation. Arch Ital Urol Androl. 2016;88(4):292–5.

15

A meta-analysis and The Cancer Genome Atlas data of prostate cancer risk and prognosis using epithelial cell adhesion molecule (EpCAM) expression

Yu Hu[1†], Qiong Wu[1†], Jialin Gao[2], Yongrui Zhang[2] and Yuantao Wang[2*]

Abstract

Background: Epithelial cell adhesion molecule (EpCAM) expression has been reported in many types of cancer, including prostate cancer (PCa). However, the role of EpCAM expression remains inconsistent. We conducted a meta-analysis to assess the clinicopathological and prognostic significance of EpCAM expression in PCa.

Methods: Publications were searched online using electronic databases. The available data were obtained from The Cancer Genome Atlas (TCGA). The odds ratios (ORs) or hazard ratios (HRs) with their 95% confidence intervals (CIs) were calculated.

Results: We identified seven studies in which immunohistochemistry was used and that included 871 prostatic tissue samples. EpCAM expression was significantly higher in PCa samples than in benign and normal tissue samples (OR = 77.93, $P = 0.002$; OR = 161.61, $P < 0.001$; respectively). No correlation of EpCAM overexpression with pT stage and lymph node metastasis was observed; however, EpCAM overexpression showed a significant correlation with Gleason score (OR = 0.48, $P = 0.012$) and bone metastasis (OR = 145.80, $P < 0.001$). Furthermore, TCGA data showed that EpCAM overexpression was not closely correlated with age, pT stage, lymph node metastasis, number of lymph node, prostate-specific antigen level, Gleason score, biochemical recurrence, and overall survival. Based on multivariate Cox proportional-hazards regression analysis, a significant correlation was observed between EpCAM overexpression and 5-year worse biochemical recurrence free-survival.

Conclusions: EpCAM overexpression may be correlated with the development of bone metastasis and worse biochemical recurrence free-survival of PCa. Further studies are needed to verify these findings.

Keywords: EpCAM, Expression, Bone metastasis, Prognosis, Prostate cancer

Background

Prostate cancer (PCa) is the second commonest malignancy and the fifth leading cause of cancer-related deaths in men [1]. Based on GLOBOCAN estimates, approximately 1.3 million new cases were clinically diagnosed with PCa in 2018, leading to approximately 359, 000 PCa-related deaths worldwide [1]. Several therapeutic strategies, including radical prostatectomy and radiotherapy, have shown a better clinical outcome for patients with early-stage PCa [2, 3]. In contrast, patients with advanced stage PCa have distant metastases and consequently, worse prognosis because of the lack of the effective treatment options [4, 5]. Therefore, a novel molecular biomarker is required to improve the prognosis of patients with PCa.

Cancer stem cells (CSCs) are a small group of cells within tumors and are responsible for self-renewal, uncontrolled differentiation, and tumorigenicity [6, 7]. CSCs contribute to cancer development, progression, and metastasis [8–10]. Epithelial cell adhesion molecule (EpCAM), known as epithelial-specific antigen (ESA) or

* Correspondence: wangyuantaobs@163.com
[†]Yu Hu and Qiong Wu contributed equally to this work.
[2]Department of Urology, The First Hospital of Jilin University, No. 71 Xinmin Street, Changchun 130021, Jilin, China
Full list of author information is available at the end of the article

CD326, a membrane glycoprotein, plays an important role in Ca2+ independent hemophilic cell-to-cell adhesion, cell signaling, migration, proliferation, and differentiation [11, 12]. The presence of CSCs in PCa may partially play a role in cancer progression, metastasis, and chemoresistance [13, 14]. EpCAM is identified as a CSC marker and a potential therapeutic target for cancer [15]. EpCAM is expressed in many types of human cancer, such as breast cancer, gastric cancer, and colorectal cancer [16–18]. Recent studies also demonstrated that high EpCAM expression may predict poor clinical outcome in breast cancer [19], ovarian carcinoma [20], and hepatocellular carcinoma [21]. Some studies reported that EpCAM was frequently expressed and associated with worse prognosis of patients with PCa [22, 23].

The development of PCa develops involves the transition of normal epithelium to benign prostatic epithelium, and subsequent progression to malignant carcinoma through multiple sequences [24–26]. The role of EpCAM expression in PCa development and progression remains controversial. Ni 2013 et al. reported that the frequency of EpCAM expression was similar in PCa and benign prostatic tissue samples [22]. In contrast, Li et al. showed that EpCAM expression was notably higher in PCa than benign prostatic tissue samples [27]. Thus, the primary objective of this study was to identify the role of EpCAM in determining the risk of PCa development. The secondary objective was to perform a meta-analysis to assess the clinicopathological and prognostic value of EpCAM in PCa.

Methods

Search strategy from meta-analysis

This meta-analysis was conducted based on the preferred reporting items for systematic reviews and meta-analyses (PRISMA) statement criteria [28]. Articles published until December 1, 2018 were systematically searched in PubMed, EMBASE, Cochrane Library, EBSCO, Wanfang, and CNKI databases. The following keywords and search terms were used: "epithelial cell adhesion molecule OR EpCAM OR Ep-CAM OR CD326 OR 17-1A antigen OR GA733 OR CO17-1A OR EGP OR KS1-4 OR ESA OR MOC31 OR BerEP4 OR TACSTD1 OR TROP1," "prostate OR prostatic," "cancer OR carcinoma OR tumor OR neoplasm." We also manually screened the reference lists of the eligible studies to find other potential publications.

Selection criteria from meta-analysis

Studies that met the following criteria were selected: 1) patients were diagnosed with PCa by histopathological examination; 2) the immunohistochemical assessment of EpCAM using anti-EpCAM antibody was defined as a positive based on the publications; 3) studies provided the available data for the association of EpCAM expression between PCa and nonmalignant control groups; 3) studies provided the available data for the correlation of EpCAM expression with the clinicopathological features of patients with PCa; 4) studies provided sufficient data to evaluate the prognostic role of EpCAM expression using multivariate Cox proportional-hazards regression analysis. Only the latest or more accurate study was included when authors published several papers using duplicated sample data. The exclusion criteria were as follows: 1) letters, case reports, editorials, and studies conducted in animals and cell lines; 2) studies that lacked sufficient data.

Data extraction from meta-analysis

Data were extracted from all eligible studies independently by two authors. Discrepancies were resolved by a third author. The following information was extracted: name of the first author's names, year of publication, country, ethnicity and age of the patients, tumor stage, detection method, antibody, cut-off values, expression frequency, number of cancer patients and nonmalignant controls, clinicopathological characteristics, and survival data.

TCGA dataset

The RNA-sequencing PCa data and corresponding clinical information were downloaded from TCGA (https://cancergenome.nih.gov/). Finally, 495 PCa patients with the available clinical information and 52 normal prostatic samples were included.

Statistical analysis

Data were obtained from the original articles. The corresponding author of each study with an available email was also contacted to request useful information on missing or incomplete data. The pooled odds ratios (ORs) and the corresponding 95% confidence intervals (CIs) were used to estimate the difference in EpCAM expression between PCa and nonmalignant controls. The association of EpCAM expression with the clinicopathological parameters of PCa were also calculated using pooled ORs with 95% CIs. Based on multivariate Cox proportional-hazards regression analysis, the overall hazard ratios (HRs) with 95% CIs were used to determine the prognostic impact of EpCAM expression. The statistical heterogeneity between studies was estimated using the Cochran's Q statistic [29]. The random-effects model (DerSimonian and Laird method) was used to improve the reliability of the data [30]. When significant heterogeneity was present ($P < 0.1$), a sensitivity analysis was performed to evaluate the influence and stability of one study on the results by deleting a single study [31]. Publication bias was measured using Egger's linear regression test (≥ 10 studies) [32]. Meta-analysis was performed using Stata software (version 12.0, Stata Corporation, College Station, TX, US).

For TCGA dataset, the difference in EpCAM expression between PCa and normal prostatic tissues was determined using the t-test. The relationship between EpCAM expression and the clinical features was analyzed using the univariate logistic regression model. Survival curve were analyzed by Kaplan-Meier method and log-rank test. The univariate and multivariate Cox proportional-hazards regression analyses were used to determine the influence of EpCAM expression on survival. The patients were divided into high and low expression groups based on the median value of EpCAM expression. TCGA data were conducted using R version 3.5.1 (R Core Team, 2018).

Results

Characteristics of the eligible studies from meta-analysis

Figure 1 shows the detailed procedure of the selecting the publications. Based on the selection criteria, seven studies were finally selected; in these studies, immunohistochemistry (IHC) was performed to determine EpCAM expression in patients with PCa [22, 23, 27, 33–36], (PCa tissue samples, $n = 671$; normal prostatic tissue samples, $n = 30$; benign prostatic tissue samples, $n = 170$). Four studies involving 536 patients with PCa reported data related to EpCAM expression and clinicopathological characteristics [27, 33, 34, 36]. One study reported the prognostic information using multivariate Cox proportional-hazards regression analysis in patients with PCa. The basic characteristics of the included publications are listed in Table 1.

Association between EpCAM expression and PCa risk from meta-analysis

175 PCa tissue samples were compared with 170 benign prostatic tissue samples and 33 PCa tissue samples were compared with 30 normal prostatic tissue samples (Table 2). The results showed that EpCAM expression in PCa was significantly higher than in benign and normal tissue samples (OR = 77.93, 95% CI = 4.90–1238.45, $P = 0.002$; OR = 161.61, 95% CI = 17.65–1479.55, $P < 0.001$; respectively; Fig. 2).

Significant heterogeneity was detected between PCa and benign prostatic tissue samples ($P = 0.043 < 0.1$). To evaluate the change in pooled OR and heterogeneity based on the omission of an individual study, a sensitivity analysis was performed (PCa versus benign controls). When the study of Ni 2013 et al. [22] was removed, the re-calculated OR was 237.96 (95% CI = 32.59–1737.73, $P < 0.001$), resulting in a significantly decreased heterogeneity ($P = 0.242$).

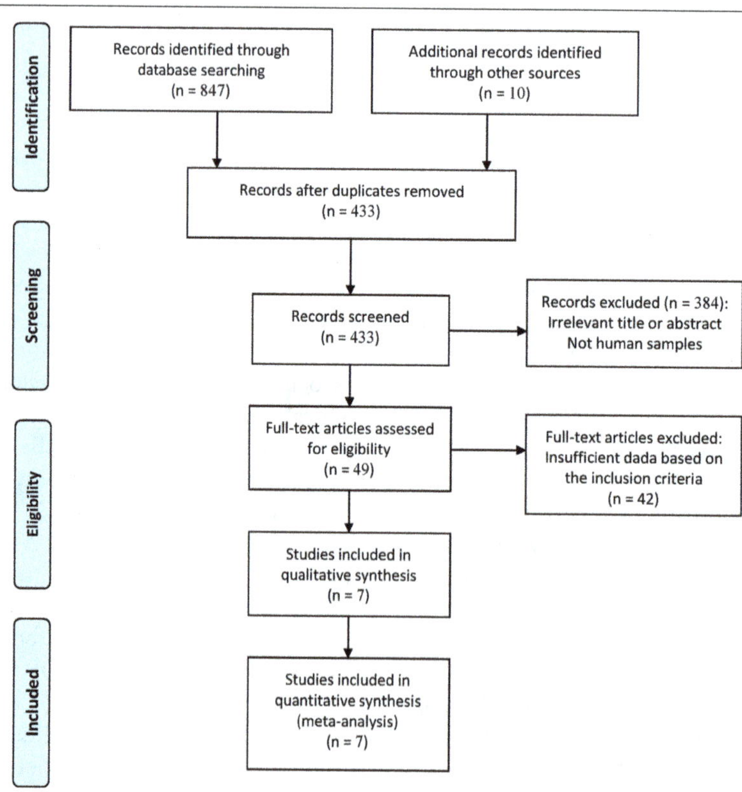

Fig. 1 Flow diagram of the study selection

Table 1 The basic characteristics of the eligible studies

First author	Country	Age	Stage	Antibodies	Positivity (IHC)	Control groups	Cancer	Control	GS (≥ 7)	GS (≤ 6)	T stage 3–4	T stage 1–2	Lymph node metastasis (Yes)	Lymph node metastasis (No)	Bone metastasis (Yes)	Bone metastasis (No)	Clinical outcome-MA
							N (%)	N (%)	E+/N	E+/N	E+/N	E+/N	E+/N	E+/N	E+/N	E+/N	
Went 2006 [36]	Switzerland	NA	T1-T4	ESA, clone VU-1D9, Novocastra, Newcastle upon Tyne, UK, dilution 1: 50	> 70%		414 (87.2%)		138/168	223/246	82/89	276/321	8/10	329/378			No
Mukherjee 2009 [35]	USA	NA	NA	Abcam, cat. #11294, dilution 1:200	≥ 20%	Normal	23 (91.3%)	20 (0%)									No
Benko 2013 [23]	Croatia	65	T2-T3	ab32392, ABCAM, Cambridge, MA, dilution 1:600	≥ 40%	Benign	102 (52%)	102 (1%)									Yes
Ni 2013 [22]	Australia	NA	NA	Epitomics, Inc.dilution 1:100	≥ 25%	Benign	10 (100%)	10 (90%)									No
Ni 2013 [22]	Australia	NA	NA	Epitomics, Inc.dilution 1:100	≥ 25%	Normal	10 (100%)	10 (20%)									No
Rybalov 2014 [34]	The Netherlands	NA	T2-T4	Clone VU-1D9, Leica Biosystems, Newcastle, UK, dilution 1:100	Weak-strong		17 (82.4%)		11/14	2/2	11/14	3/3					No
Li 2015 [27]	China	NA	NA	NA	1–9 scores	Benign	63 (88.9%)	58 (0%)							20/20	2/5	No
Campos 2016 [32]	Mexico	NA	NA	clone VU-1D9, Leica Biosystems, Newcastle, UK, dilution 1:100	TIS ≥ 1		42 (50%)						21/21	0/21	19/20	0/14	No

N number of the study population, E+ positive expression, *MA* multivariate analysis, *NA* not applicable, *TIS* total immunostaining score, *IHC* immunohistochemistry

Table 2 Summary of the pooled results from meta-analysis

Group	Studies	Cancer samples	Nonmalignant samples	OR with 95% CI	*P*	SE
Cancer vs. Benign	3	175	170	77.93 (4.90–1238.45)	0.002	1.411
Cancer vs. Normal	2	33	30	161.61 (17.65–1479.55)	< 0.001	1.13
Clinicopathological characteristics						
Gleason score (≥7 vs. ≤6)	2	430		0.48 (0.27–0.85)	0.012	0.293
T stage (T3–4 vs. T1–2)	2	427		1.75 (0.78–3.91)	0.175	0.411
Lymph node metastasis (Positive vs. Negative)	2	430		27.89 (0.004–1.7e+ 05)	0.455	4.481
Bone metastasis (Positive vs. Negative)	2	59		145.80 (14.58–1458.02)	< 0.001	1.175

OR odds ratio, *95% CI* 95% confidence interval, *SE* standard error

Association between EpCAM expression and clinicopathological characteristics from meta-analysis

Data from two studies with 427 patients with PCa showed that EpCAM overexpression was not linked to pT stage ($P = 0.175$). Data from two studies with 430 PCa cases demonstrated no relationship between EpCAM overexpression and lymph node metastasis ($P = 0.455$; Fig. 3).

Data from two studies with 430 PCa cases demonstrated that EpCAM overexpression was associated with Gleason score (≥7 vs. ≤6 scores: OR = 0.48, 95% CI = 0.27–0.85, $P = 0.012$; Fig. 3). Data from two studies with 59 patients with PCa showed that EpCAM overexpression was closely correlated to bone metastasis (OR = 145.80, 95% CI = 14.58–1458.02, $P < 0.001$; Fig. 3). Moreover, no heterogeneity was measured between EpCAM overexpression and the Gleason score and bone metastasis of PCa ($P > 0.1$).

Association between EpCAM expression and PCa prognosis from meta-analysis

A study reported that EpCAM overexpression was significantly correlated with 5-year worse biochemical recurrence free-survival using multivariate Cox proportional-hazards regression analysis (HR = 6.79, 95% CI = 2.38–19.45) in 102 patients with PCa [23].

TCGA

Four hundred ninety-five PCa cases with the available clinical information and 52 normal prostatic tissue samples were identified from TCGA. EpCAM expression level was notably higher in PCa than in normal prostatic tissues ($P < 0.001$; data not shown).

Univariate analysis using logistic regression showed that EpCAM overexpression was not significantly associated with the clinicopathological characteristics of PCa

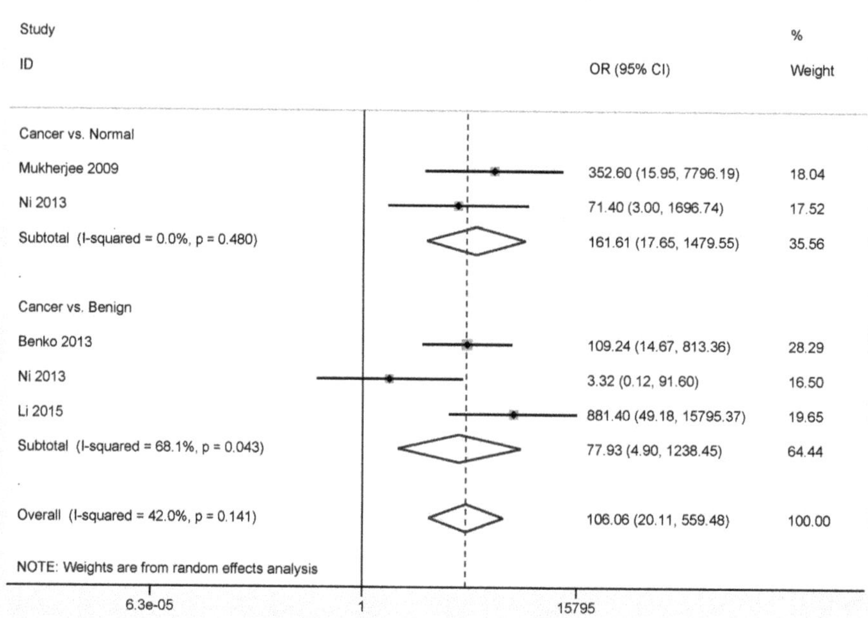

Fig. 2 Forest plot of the association between EpCAM immunoexpression and prostate cancer

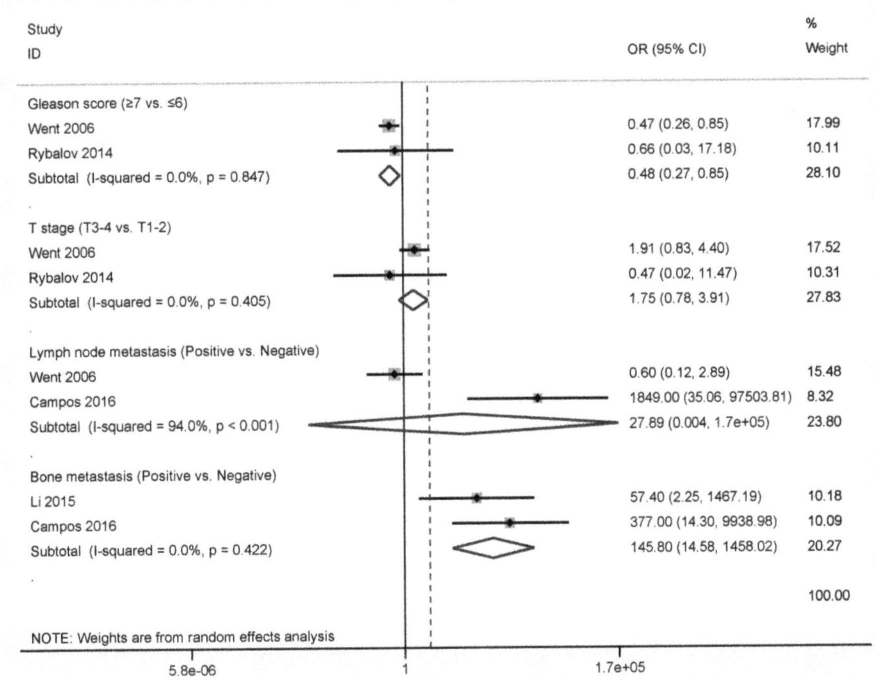

Fig. 3 Forest plot of the association of EpCAM immunoexpression with the clinicopathological features of patients with prostate cancer

(Table 3), including age ($P = 0.065$), pT stage (T3–4 vs. T1–2: $P = 0.78$), lymph node metastasis (positive vs. negative: $P = 0.889$), number of lymph node (> 10 vs. ≤ 10: $P = 0.39$), prostate-specific antigen (PSA) value (≥ 10 vs. < 10: $P = 0.288$), Gleason score (≥ 7 vs. ≤ 6: $P = 0.561$), and biochemical recurrence (yes vs. no: $P = 0.408$).

To further evaluate the prognostic value of EpCAM overexpression in patients with PCa, Kaplan-Meier survival analysis was performed. This revealed that EpCAM overexpression was not correlated with the prognosis of overall survival ($P = 0.25$; data not shown).

Table 3 Association of EpCAM overexpression with the clinicopathological characteristics from The Cancer Genome Atlas (TCGA)

Factors	Total (N)	OR with 95% CI	*P*
Age (≥61 vs. < 61)	495	0.72 (0.5–1.02)	0.065
T stage (T3–4 vs. T1–2)	488	0.95 (0.66–1.37)	0.78
Lymph node metastasis (Positive vs. Negative)	422	1.04 (0.63–1.69)	0.889
Number of lymph node (> 10 vs. ≤ 10)	420	1.18 (0.81–1.74)	0.39
Biochemical recurrence (Yes vs. No)	427	0.79 (0.45–1.38)	0.408
Gleason score (≥ 7 vs. ≤ 6)	483	1.19 (0.66–2.14)	0.561
PSA value (≥ 10 vs. < 10)	438	1.75 (0.62–4.89)	0.288

N number of the study population, *PSA* prostate-specific antigen, *OR* odds ratio, *95% CI* 95% confidence interval

Discussion

CSCs, a special subpopulation of tumor cells, have the ability to form the bulk of the tumor and contribute to tumor progression and relapse [9]. Therefore, eradication of CSCs is considered as a crucial challenge for a successful cancer therapy [37]. EpCAM is identified as a CSC marker that is closely linked to tumor progression [38]. EpCAM plays an important role in the cell-cell adhesion, cell signaling, migration, proliferation, and differentiation [39]. EpCAM also plays an important role in mediating migration of immune cells [38]. EpCAM in PCa is associated with tumor progression and metastasis and therapeutic resistance via the PI3K/Akt/mTOR signaling pathway [22]. EpCAM is frequently overexpressed across a wide range of human cancer, including pancreatic adenocarcinoma, breast cancer, ovarian cancer, and head and neck squamous cell cancer [40]. EpCAM overexpression is correlated with worse prognosis in some types of cancer [19, 41, 42]. Some studies reported that EpCAM is highly expressed in patients with PCa [22, 27, 33, 34]. However, the function of EpCAM and its clinical effect in PCa remains largely unclear. In this study, we analyzed the clinicopathological significance of EpCAM expression and its role in the prognosis of PCa.

The pooled data demonstrated that EpCAM expression was significantly higher in PCa than in benign and normal prostatic tissue samples, suggesting that EpCAM overexpression may be associated with the development of PCa. Our results were consistent with the previous studies that EpCAM was expressed more frequently in PCa than in benign [23, 27] and normal prostatic tissue samples [22, 35]. Moreover, TCGA data also showed that EpCAM expression was notably increased in PCa than in normal tissue samples.

We further analyzed whether EpCAM overexpression was correlated with the clinicopathological characteristics of patients with PCa. EpCAM overexpression was not linked to pT stage and lymph node metastasis, but was associated with Gleason score and bone metastasis. TCGA data revealed that EpCAM overexpression was not closely correlated with the clinicopathological characteristics in 495 patients with PCa, including age, pT stage, lymph node metastasis, number of lymph node, prostate-specific antigen (PSA) level, Gleason score, and biochemical recurrence. The pooled analyses suggested that EpCAM overexpression may predict bone metastasis. However, as the sample size was small, the relationship between EpCAM overexpression and bone metastasis requires further investigation.

EpCAM overexpression was reported to be closely associated with 5-year worse biochemical recurrence free-survival using multivariate Cox proportional-hazards regression analysis in 102 patients with PCa [23]; this suggests that EpCAM overexpression may be a potential prognostic biomarker for predicting poor biochemical recurrence free-survival. However, no association was found between EpCAM overexpression and overall survival of patients with PCa.

Our result showed no correlation between EpCAM overexpression and lymph node metastasis among two studies with 430 patients with PCa, which was consistent with the study of Went 2006 et al. [36] among a large cohort (388 patients). Heterogeneity was found in the correlation of PCa and benign prostatic tissue samples ($P = 0.043$). When we removed the study by Ni 2013 et al. [22], the re-calculated OR remained significant with no obvious evidence of heterogeneity. The analysis suggested that our results were reliable. The reasons of the heterogeneity were not very clear; the inappropriate conditions of IHC methods may cause the bias.

There were some limitations in the current study. First, as none of the present meta-analyses included ≥10 studies, we could not examine and rule out the risk of the potential publication bias. Although we systematically searched PubMed, EMBASE, Cochrane Library, EBSCO, Wanfang, and CNKI databases to minimize the potential bias, the eligible studies were restricted to papers published in English or Chinese. Moreover, studies published in language other than English and Chinese, unpublished papers, or conference abstracts were excluded based on incomplete information. Furthermore, studies with negative results are less likely to be published than papers with positive results. These reasons may cause potential bias. Second, the main ethnic population in this meta-analysis was European; other ethnic groups, such as Asians and Africans, were underrepresented. Third, the studies regarding the associations of EpCAM overexpression with bone metastasis and biochemical recurrence free-survival were relatively small. Further studies with large sample size are needed to further confirm these results. Finally, the cut-off values of EpCAM expression were different among some studies, which showed inconsistent definitions for "negative" and "positive," leading to the potential heterogeneity. Therefore, the results need to be interpreted with caution. EpCAM expression should be defined as positive or negative based on a uniform standard in the future.

Conclusions

In conclusion, the current meta-analysis suggested that EpCAM expression was significantly high in PCa than in benign and normal prostatic tissue samples. EpCAM overexpression was not associated with age, pT stage, lymph node metastasis, number of lymph node, prostate-specific antigen (PSA) level, biochemical recurrence, and overall survival. EpCAM overexpression may be related to the development of bone metastasis and worse biochemical recurrence free-survival of PCa. Our results should be interpreted with caution owing to the small sample size. Additional large-scale prospective studies are required to further validate our findings.

Abbreviations

CIs: Confidence intervals; CSCs: Cancer stem cells; EpCAM: Epithelial cell adhesion molecule; ESA: Epithelial-specific antigen; HRs: hazard ratios; IHC: Immunohistochemistry; ORs: The odds ratios; PCa: Prostate cancer; PSA: Prostate-specific antigen; TCGA: The Cancer Genome Atlas

Acknowledgments

None.

Authors' contributions

Study conception and design: WYT, HY, WQ. Manuscript writing and editing: HY and WQ. Data collection: HY, WQ, GJL, ZYR. Data management/analysis: HY, WQ, GJL, ZYR, WYT. All authors read and approved the final manuscript.

Author details

[1]Department of Pathology, China-Japan Union Hospital, Jilin University, Changchun, Jilin, China. [2]Department of Urology, The First Hospital of Jilin University, No. 71 Xinmin Street, Changchun 130021, Jilin, China.

References

1. Bray F, Ferlay J, Soerjomataram I, Siegel RL, Torre LA, Jemal A. Global cancer statistics 2018: GLOBOCAN estimates of incidence and mortality worldwide for 36 cancers in 185 countries. CA Cancer J Clin. 2018;68(6):394–424.
2. Hussein AA, Punnen S, Zhao S, Cowan JE, Leapman M, Tran TC, Washington SL, Truesdale MD, Carroll PR, Cooperberg MR. Current use of imaging after primary treatment of prostate Cancer. J Urol. 2015;194(1):98–104.
3. Fossa SD, Nilssen Y, Kvale R, Hernes E, Axcrona K, Moller B. Treatment and 5-year survival in patients with nonmetastatic prostate cancer: the Norwegian experience. Urology. 2014;83(1):146–52.

4. Norum J, Nieder C. Treatments for metastatic prostate Cancer (mPC): a review of costing evidence. Pharmacoeconomics. 2017;35(12):1223–36.
5. Crawford ED, Petrylak D, Sartor O. Navigating the evolving therapeutic landscape in advanced prostate cancer. Urol Oncol. 2017;35S:S1–S13.
6. Han S, Huang T, Li W, Wang X, Wu X, Liu S, Yang W, Shi Q, Li H, Hou F. Prognostic value of CD44 and its isoforms in advanced Cancer: a systematic meta-analysis with trial sequential analysis. Front Oncol. 2019;9:39.
7. Steinbichler TB, Dudas J, Skvortsov S, Ganswindt U, Riechelmann H, Skvortsova II. Therapy resistance mediated by cancer stem cells. Semin Cancer Biol. 2018;53:156–67.
8. Han S, Huang T, Wu X, Wang X, Liu S, Yang W, Shi Q, Li H, Hou F. Prognostic value of CD133 and SOX2 in advanced Cancer. J Oncol. 2019;2019:3905817.
9. Koren E, Fuchs Y. The bad seed: Cancer stem cells in tumor development and resistance. Drug Resist Updat. 2016;28:1–12.
10. Mueller MT, Hermann PC, Heeschen C. Cancer stem cells as new therapeutic target to prevent tumour progression and metastasis. Front Biosci (Elite Ed). 2010;2:602–13.
11. Balzar M, Winter MJ, de Boer CJ, Litvinov SV. The biology of the 17-1A antigen (ep-CAM). J Mol Med (Berl). 1999;77(10):699–712.
12. Litvinov SV, Bakker HA, Gourevitch MM, Velders MP, Warnaar SO. Evidence for a role of the epithelial glycoprotein 40 (ep-CAM) in epithelial cell-cell adhesion. Cell Adhes Commun. 1994;2(5):417–28.
13. Ni J, Cozzi PJ, Hao JL, Beretov J, Chang L, Duan W, Shigdar S, Delprado WJ, Graham PH, Bucci J, et al. CD44 variant 6 is associated with prostate cancer metastasis and chemo–/radioresistance. Prostate. 2014;74(6):602–17.
14. Chen X, Rycaj K, Liu X, Tang DG. New insights into prostate cancer stem cells. Cell Cycle. 2013;12(4):579–86.
15. Salnikov AV, Groth A, Apel A, Kallifatidis G, Beckermann BM, Khamidjanov A, Ryschich E, Buchler MW, Herr I, Moldenhauer G. Targeting of cancer stem cell marker EpCAM by bispecific antibody EpCAMxCD3 inhibits pancreatic carcinoma. J Cell Mol Med. 2009;13(9B):4023–33.
16. Han S, Zong S, Shi Q, Li H, Liu S, Yang W, Li W, Hou F. Is ep-CAM expression a diagnostic and prognostic biomarker for colorectal Cancer? A systematic meta-analysis. EBioMedicine. 2017;20:61–9.
17. Dai M, Yuan F, Fu C, Shen G, Hu S, Shen G. Relationship between epithelial cell adhesion molecule (EpCAM) overexpression and gastric cancer patients: a systematic review and meta-analysis. PLoS One. 2017;12(4):e0175357.
18. Cimino A, Halushka M, Illei P, Wu X, Sukumar S, Argani P. Epithelial cell adhesion molecule (EpCAM) is overexpressed in breast cancer metastases. Breast Cancer Res Treat. 2010;123(3):701–8.
19. Schmidt M, Hasenclever D, Schaeffer M, Boehm D, Cotarelo C, Steiner E, Lebrecht A, Siggelkow W, Weikel W, Schiffer-Petry I, et al. Prognostic effect of epithelial cell adhesion molecule overexpression in untreated node-negative breast cancer. Clin Cancer Res. 2008;14(18):5849–55.
20. Shim HS, Yoon BS, Cho NH. Prognostic significance of paired epithelial cell adhesion molecule and E-cadherin in ovarian serous carcinoma. Hum Pathol. 2009;40(5):693–8.
21. Zhou L, Zhu Y. The EpCAM overexpression is associated with clinicopathological significance and prognosis in hepatocellular carcinoma patients: a systematic review and meta-analysis. Int J Surg. 2018;56:274–80.
22. Ni J, Cozzi P, Hao J, Beretov J, Chang L, Duan W, Shigdar S, Delprado W, Graham P, Bucci J, et al. Epithelial cell adhesion molecule (EpCAM) is associated with prostate cancer metastasis and chemo/radioresistance via the PI3K/Akt/mTOR signaling pathway. Int J Biochem Cell Biol. 2013;45(12):2736–48.
23. Benko G, Spajic B, Kruslin B, Tomas D. Impact of the EpCAM expression on biochemical recurrence-free survival in clinically localized prostate cancer. Urol Oncol. 2013;31(4):468–74.
24. Elschot M, Selnaes KM, Sandsmark E, Kruger-Stokke B, Storkersen O, Giskeodegard GF, Tessem MB, Moestue SA, Bertilsson H, Bathen TF. Combined (18) F-Fluciclovine PET/MRI shows potential for detection and characterization of high-risk prostate Cancer. J Nucl Med. 2018;59(5):762–8.
25. Merseburger AS, Kramer MW, Hennenlotter J, Simon P, Knapp J, Hartmann JT, Stenzl A, Serth J, Kuczyk MA. Involvement of decreased Galectin-3 expression in the pathogenesis and progression of prostate cancer. Prostate. 2008;68(1):72–7.
26. Henshall SM, Afar DE, Rasiah KK, Horvath LG, Gish K, Caras I, Ramakrishnan V, Wong M, Jeffry U, Kench JG, et al. Expression of the zinc transporter ZnT4 is decreased in the progression from early prostate disease to invasive prostate cancer. Oncogene. 2003;22(38):6005–12.
27. Li ZL, Jin RS. Expression of the epithelial cell adhesion molecule in prostate cancer and its clinical significance. Zhonghua Nan Ke Xue. 2015;21(4):320–4.
28. Liberati A, Altman DG, Tetzlaff J, Mulrow C, Gotzsche PC, Ioannidis JP, Clarke M, Devereaux PJ, Kleijnen J, Moher D. The PRISMA statement for reporting systematic reviews and meta-analyses of studies that evaluate health care interventions: explanation and elaboration. PLoS Med. 2009;6(7):e1000100.
29. Zintzaras E, Ioannidis JP. HEGESMA: genome search meta-analysis and heterogeneity testing. Bioinformatics. 2005;21(18):3672–3.
30. Han S, Huang T, Wu X, Wang X, Li W, Liu S, Yang W, Shi Q, Li H, Shi K, et al. Prognostic value of ALDH1 and nestin in advanced cancer: a systematic meta-analysis with trial sequential analysis. Ther Adv Med Oncol. 2019;11:1758835919830831.
31. Higgins JP, Thompson SG, Deeks JJ, Altman DG. Measuring inconsistency in meta-analyses. BMJ. 2003;327(7414):557–60.
32. Egger M, Davey Smith G, Schneider M, Minder C. Bias in meta-analysis detected by a simple, graphical test. BMJ. 1997;315(7109):629–34.
33. Campos AK, Hoving HD, Rosati S, van Leenders GJ, de Jong IJ. EpCAM Expression in Lymph Node and Bone Metastases of Prostate Carcinoma: A Pilot Study. Int J Mol Sci. 2016;17(10):9.
34. Rybalov M, Ananias HJ, Hoving HD, van der Poel HG, Rosati S, de Jong IJ. PSMA, EpCAM, VEGF and GRPR as imaging targets in locally recurrent prostate cancer after radiotherapy. Int J Mol Sci. 2014;15(4):6046–61.
35. Mukherjee S, Richardson AM, Rodriguez-Canales J, Ylaya K, Erickson HS, Player A, Kawasaki ES, Pinto PA, Choyke PL, Merino MJ, et al. Identification of EpCAM as a molecular target of prostate cancer stroma. Am J Pathol. 2009;175(6):2277–87.
36. Went P, Vasei M, Bubendorf L, Terracciano L, Tornillo L, Riede U, Kononen J, Simon R, Sauter G, Baeuerle PA. Frequent high-level expression of the immunotherapeutic target ep-CAM in colon, stomach, prostate and lung cancers. Br J Cancer. 2006;94(1):128–35.
37. Kuhlmann JD, Hein L, Kurth I, Wimberger P, Dubrovska A. Targeting Cancer stem cells: promises and challenges. Anti Cancer Agents Med Chem. 2016;16(1):38–58.
38. Martowicz A, Seeber A, Untergasser G. The role of EpCAM in physiology and pathology of the epithelium. Histol Histopathol. 2016;31(4):349–55.
39. Ni J, Cozzi PJ, Duan W, Shigdar S, Graham PH, John KH, Li Y. Role of the EpCAM (CD326) in prostate cancer metastasis and progression. Cancer Metastasis Rev. 2012;31(3–4):779–91.
40. Moldenhauer G, Salnikov AV, Luttgau S, Herr I, Anderl J, Faulstich H. Therapeutic potential of amanitin-conjugated anti-epithelial cell adhesion molecule monoclonal antibody against pancreatic carcinoma. J Natl Cancer Inst. 2012;104(8):622–34.
41. Matsuda T, Takeuchi H, Matsuda S, Hiraiwa K, Miyasho T, Okamoto M, Kawasako K, Nakamura R, Takahashi T, Wada N, et al. EpCAM, a potential therapeutic target for esophageal squamous cell carcinoma. Ann Surg Oncol. 2014;21(Suppl 3):S356–64.
42. Prince S, Zeidman A, Dekel Y, Ram E, Koren R. Expression of epithelial cell adhesion molecule in gallbladder carcinoma and its correlation with clinicopathologic variables. Am J Clin Pathol. 2008;129(3):424–9.

16

Clinically significant Prostate Cancer diagnosed using a urinary molecular biomarker-based risk score

Pieter Minnee[1], Daphne Hessels[2], Jack A. Schalken[3] and Wim Van Criekinge[4*]

Abstract

Background: Identifying men for a repeat prostate biopsy is a conundrum to urologists. Risk calculators (RCs) such as the European Randomized Study of Screening for Prostate Cancer (ERSPC) RCs have been developed to predict the outcome of prostate biopsies and have been shown to improve diagnostic accuracy compared to PSA alone. However, it was recently shown that the outcome for high-grade prostate cancer (PCa) upon biopsy tended to be underestimated in men with previous negative biopsies using ERSPC RC model 4. For these men, an individualized approach combining the clinical information with the outcome of biomarker-related urine tests may help to make a more informed decision.

Case presentation: Two men, aged 66 and 69 respectively when presented in the clinic, show the typical dilemma of urologist and patient for electing repeat prostate biopsy. Both men had normal DRE findings, did not have a family history of PCa, presented with serum PSA values between 3 and 10 ng/ml and the first biopsies were negative for disease. The ERSPC RC4 did not indicate a biopsy in these men. The urinary molecular biomarker-based test for *HOXC6* and *DLX1*, combining biomarker-expression profiling with clinical risk factors, resulted in SelectMDx Risk scores for these men that were higher than the cut-off of the test. Based on this outcome, mpMRI was performed with an outcome of PI-RADS ≥4 in both men. Histopathological evaluation of TRUS-guided biopsies confirmed high-grade PCa.

Conclusions: The urinary molecular biomarker-based risk score played a pivotal role in the diagnosis of clinically significant PCa whereas ERSPC RC4 outcome would not have indicated further diagnostic follow-up in these two cases. The timely diagnosis was shown to be crucial for the curative treatment by radical retropubic prostatectomy and the potential life-years gained for these two vital males.

Keywords: Case report, Risk stratification, Prostate Cancer, Risk calculator, Biopsy, Urine, Biomarkers, HOXC6, DLX1

Background

Early detection of significant prostate cancer (PCa) increases the curative success rate. Histopathologic evaluation of transrectal ultrasound -guided systematic core needle biopsy (TRUS-Bx) tissue is the main method to diagnose the disease, and the decision to take a biopsy is made in case of serum prostate-specific antigen (PSA) > 3 ng/ml and/or an abnormal digital rectal examination (DRE). For more than 30 years, serum PSA has been considered the most valuable tool in early detection of the disease, but its low specificity for PCa has resulted in the detection and treatment of slow growing PCa's that will not cause harm in a man's lifetime and a negative biopsy rate of 70% in men with benign prostate diseases such as benign prostatic hyperplasia (BPH) or prostatitis. The chance of missing a cancer upon TRUS-Bx is ~ 25% because it is systematic, non-targeted, and directed towards the peripheral gland. Therefore, repeat biopsies are warranted in cases with persistent indication (abnormal

* Correspondence: Wim.Vancriekinge@gmail.com
[4]Department of Mathematical Modelling, Statistics and Bioinformatics, Ghent University, Ghent, Belgium
Full list of author information is available at the end of the article

DRE, elevated PSA value and/or histopathological findings suggestive of malignancy at the initial biopsy) [1, 2]. In the second set of biopsies, a detection rate of approximately 10–35% has been reported [2]. For a patient, these repeat biopsies will result in additional anxiety, physical discomfort and complication risk. The proportion of men undergoing biopsy who experienced non-sepsis infectious complications is ~ 18, and 3% of men experience sepsis that requires hospitalization [3, 4]. Hence a physician's and patient's decision to elect for prostate biopsy is guided by the fear of missing a clinically significant PCa that may become life-threatening when left untreated.

Currently, the decision to perform prostate biopsies is based on clinical judgement of the physician guided by European Association of Urology (EAU) recommendations which incorporates the results of PSA testing, DRE outcome and/or the additional diagnostic options such as a risk calculator (RC), an additional serum- or urine-based test or imaging [5].

Multiparametric MRI (mpMRI) is the most accurate imaging modality for localization of PCa. The use of mpMRI before biopsy could indicate whether the patient requires a biopsy because of a significant cancer identified on mpMRI or whether biopsy could be avoided. The EAU guideline committee recommends the use of mpMRI before repeat biopsy to allow targeted biopsies of suspicious lesions in addition to standard biopsies. However, the risk of missing 16.2 to 39.7% clinically significant prostate cancers using mpMRI targeted biopsy for mpMRI Prostate Imaging Reporting and Data System outcome (PI-RADS) ≥3 stresses the need to use RCs or biomarker-based tests for an improved risk stratification for a repeat biopsy [6].

The Rotterdam arm of the European Randomized Study of Screening for Prostate Cancer (ERSPC) developed several RCs, using the clinical data and prostate biopsy outcome from thousands of previously unscreened men and men with previous negative prostate biopsy, calculating the chance of finding PCa on a TRUS-guided biopsy. The ERSPC RC4 is designed and used by urologists to determine the likelihood of cancer in repeat biopsy. Recently, external validation of the ERSPC RC3 and ERSPC RC4 in a contemporary Dutch clinical cohort using a biopsy scheme showed that the RCs performed well, but that in the repeat biopsy setting the outcomes for PCa risk and clinically significant PCa tended to be underestimated for ERSPC RC4 [7]. For men with a previous negative biopsy, an individualized approach combining the clinical information with the outcome of biomarker-related urine tests may help to make a more informed decision.

Recently, gene expression profiling was used to identify diagnostic and predictive biomarkers for high grade PCa followed by a stepwise biomarker selection and testing of a gene panel consisting of Homeobox C6 (*HOXC6*), Tudor domain containing 1 (*TDRD1*) and Distal-less homeobox 1 (*DLX1*) in post-DRE urine sediments for the diagnosis of biopsy Gleason score ≥ 7 PCa [8]. Using whole urine as a substrate, the combination of *HOXC6* and *DLX1* had the best performance to predict high-grade PCa on biopsy which was successfully validated in an independent cohort [9]. *DLX1* and *HOXC6* are involved in prostate cancer progression and are associated with high-grade PCa [10, 11]. When this patient-specific biomarker expression profile is combined with traditional clinical risk factors, a likelihood risk score is obtained to detect clinically significant PCa (Gleason score (GS) ≥7) upon biopsy [9]. It was shown that SelectMDx risk score correlates with PI-RADS ≥3 and can contribute to the stratification of patients for mpMRI [12].

Clinical utility of this urinary molecular biomarker-based test, SelectMDx® for Prostate Cancer (hereafter SelectMDx), was evaluated in 34 men with a previous negative biopsy identified in routine clinical practice, with no study-specific visits or interventions. In five men, both the ERSPC RC4 and the SelectMDx test indicated the need for biopsy. Three men (60%) underwent prostate biopsies and in two significant PCa was found. Of the 14 men who were low risk for both the ERSPC RC4 and SelectMDx test, two (14%) underwent negative biopsies. The SelectMDx test indicated a risk for high-grade PCa upon biopsy in 15 ERSPC RC4 low risk men. Six of these men (40%) underwent prostate biopsy and in three men significant PCa was confirmed (see Table 1).

This report describes two cases, identified in the latter group, in which the SelectMDx test was pivotal in the early diagnosis of clinically significant PCa.

Case presentation 1

In January 2015, a 66-year-old male presented at the Urology ward of the LangeLand Hospital with a serum PSA of 6.4 ng/ml which was elevated compared to the upper limit of normal serum PSA of 4.5 ng/ml of men of his age. The patient had no paternal history of PCa and had no urinary complaints. The physical examination of the prostate gland (DRE) by the physician was normal. Prostate volume by TRUS was 35 cm^3 and TRUS findings were normal. TRUS-Bx was performed (5 left and 5 right). Biopsies were negative for malignancy.

In June 2015, the serum PSA increased to 7.2 ng/ml and there was no sign of a urinary tract infection. Therefore, the physician used ERSPC RC4 with TRUS or DRE (www.

Table 1 Concordance table urine biomarker test versus ERSPC R4

Previous Negative Biopsy Cohort	ERSPC R4 (+)	ERSPC R4 (−)	Total
SelectMDx test (+)	5	15	20
SelectMDx test (−)	0	14	14
Total	5	29	34

prostatecancer-riskcalculator.com) containing PSA, DRE (normal/abnormal), TRUS (normal/abnormal), TRUS-assessed volume and biopsy history. This model can be used for biopsy-naïve men and for men that have had a previous biopsy with a benign result. After entering the available data, the risk of having PCa or high-grade PCa is displayed. The ERSPC RC4 showed that this man's risk for PCa and high-grade PCa was 17 and 3%, respectively. Prostate biopsy is indicated when the ERSPC RC4 risk for PCa is > 20% and if the risk for PCa is between 12.5 and 20%, in combination with a risk for high-grade disease of > 4%. Biopsy is not indicated when the risk for PCa on biopsy is < 12.5%. Based on this outcome, patient and physician elected for PSA follow-up.

Six months later, serum PSA increased to 10.8 ng/ml. At that time the physician used the urine biomarker test, SelectMDx test (MDxHealth B.V.). After DRE, 16 ml of first void urine was collected from the patient using the urine sample collection kit (Catalogue number UrNCSE1, MDxHealth B.V.). Using this kit, the urinary RNA was immediately preserved in 4 ml of preservative. On the day of collection, samples were shipped at room temperature to the clinical diagnostic laboratory (Nijmegen, the Netherlands), after which the samples were stored at −20 °C prior to analysis. Reverse transcriptase PCR (RT-PCR) was used to determine the amount of *HOXC6* and *DLX1* mRNA in the patient's urine. The patient-specific biomarker expression profile was then combined with the patient's traditional clinical risk factors, including PSA, DRE, prostate volume, age and family history using a dedicated algorithm [9]. The outcome is a patient-specific SelectMDx Risk score. If the SelectMDx Risk Score is below the cut-off point of − 2.8 a very low risk report will be generated with a negative predictive value (NPV) of 98% for Gleason score ≥ 7 PCa. A Risk Score higher or equal to this cut-off point is converted into the likelihood that subsequent biopsy will detect prostate cancer or high-grade prostate cancer. For this man, the likelihood for having PCa was 49% and the chance of having high-grade disease was 22%.

Based on this outcome, a prostate MRI was done in January 2016 (see Fig. 1). The outcome was PI-RADS 5 in the left peripheral zone of the prostate. TRUS-Bx revealed Gleason score 3 + 4 = 7 PCa in 4 of 5 biopsies taken from the left peripheral zone.

In May 2016, the patient underwent a robot-assisted radical retropubic prostatectomy (RRP). The prostate specimen was found to contain extensive carcinoma with a Gleason score 3 + 4 = 7 in both lobes (pT2c), margins and lymph nodes were clear. As part of the follow-up, the PSA is still < 0.01 ng/ml.

Case presentation 2

In September 2012, a 69-year-old male with an unknown paternal history for PCa came to the Urology ward of the LangeLand hospital with an increased serum PSA level of 8.7 ng/ml. He had a prostate volume of 43.5 cm^3, a normal DRE outcome and normal TRUS findings. TRUS-Bx (5 left and 5 right) were negative for malignancy. In October 2013, his PSA increased to 26.6 ng/ml. This marked elevation in serum PSA was likely caused by acute prostatitis for which the urologist prescribed antibiotics. Under antibiotics his PSA decreased to 4.3 ng/ml at the beginning of 2014.

In December 2015, the PSA was 15.4 ng/ml. The ERSPC RC4 showed that the man's risk for PCa and high-grade PCa was 16 and 4% respectively. Based on this outcome there was no clear biopsy indication. The SelectMDx test was performed and for this man the likelihood for having PCa was 39% and the chance of having high-grade PCa was 14%. Based on this outcome, a prostate MRI was performed indicating a PI-RADS 4 in the right peripheral zone of the prostate. However, the three MRI-guided biopsies were negative for PCa.

In August 2016, the PSA increased to 20 ng/ml. Based on the prostatitis history and the negative prostate biopsies antibiotics was prescribed, but under treatment the PSA increased to 21.4 ng/ml. Since the SelectMDx test indicated an elevated risk for high-grade PCa for this patient, the urologist decided to repeat TRUS-Bx in October 2016. This resulted in the diagnosis of Gleason score 3 + 4 = 7 and 10% cribriform intraductal carcinoma in 2 out of 5 biopsies in the right peripheral zone of the prostate. The presence of intraductal carcinoma is usually associated with adverse prognostic parameters (e.g. high-grade Gleason score, large tumour volume, extra-prostatic extension and seminal vesicle invasion) and correlates with worse disease outcomes.

In December 2016, the patient underwent robot-assisted RRP. The prostate specimen was found to contain 2 tumours in the right peripheral zone of the prostate: one Gleason score 4 + 4 = 8 and one Gleason score 3 + 3 = 6 PCa (pT2a), margins and lymph nodes were clear and PSA nadir was < 0.01 ng/ml.

Discussion and conclusions

Identifying men for a repeat prostate biopsy is a conundrum to urologists. Following negative biopsy, men frequently exhibit persistently elevated PSA, raising concerns for missed diagnosis of an aggressive PCa. Decision making regarding repeat biopsies is a balance between avoiding anxiety and risk of complications associated with the procedure and the fear for missing a clinically significant cancer. Furthermore, there is the risk with repeat biopsy of detecting and treating low-grade and low volume PCa that is not life-threatening. In this report, two cases are described that show the typical dilemma of urologist and patient within daily clinical practice for electing repeat prostate biopsy. Here the SelectMDx test played a pivotal

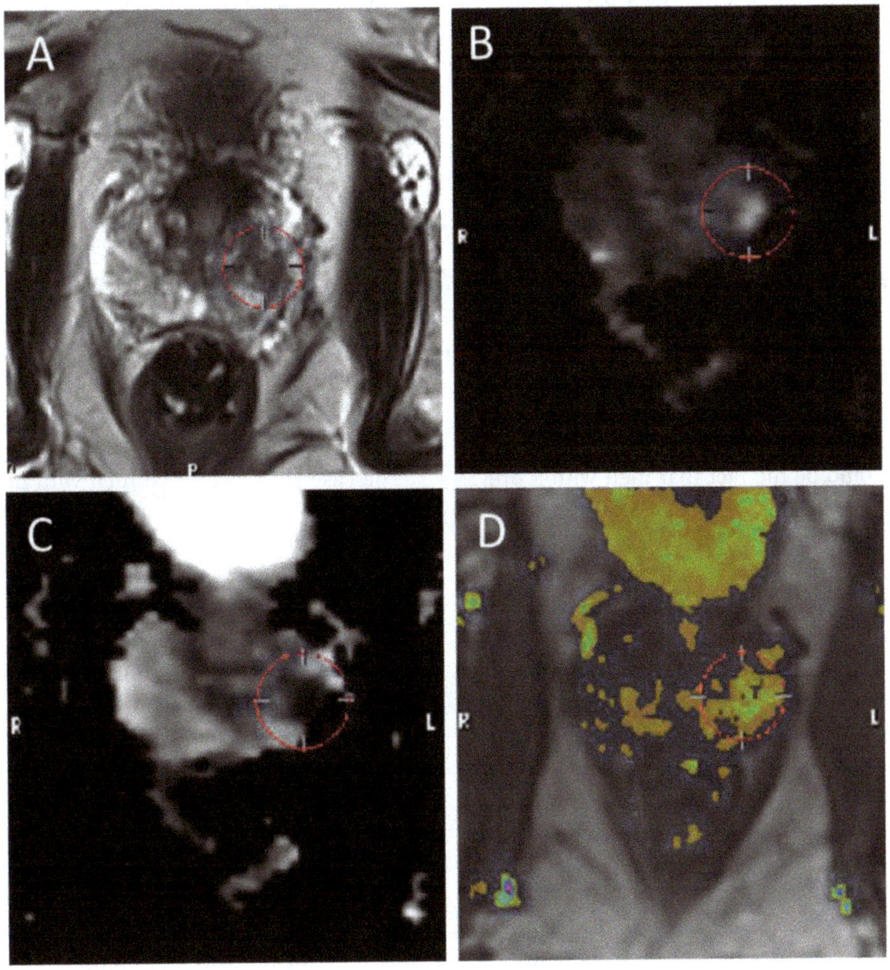

Fig. 1 In November 2015, the patient of case 1 had a PSA level of 10.8 ng/ml and was referred for multiparametric prostate 3 T MRI for diagnostic purposes because the urinary biomarker-based risk score was 22% for high-grade PCa indicating the need for prostate biopsy. **a** An axial T2-weighted image shows a lesion on the left peripheral zone at the prostate base anterior side (red circle). **b** An axial diffusion-weighted image (DWI) shows an area of increased signal at the left peripheral zone. **c** An axial apparent diffusion coefficient (ADC) map shows a corresponding area of low ADC value (red circle). **d** A colorized perfusion map created from dynamic contrast-enhanced MRI (DCE-MRI) acquisition shows corresponding abnormal enhancement kinetics at the same location. All sequences identified the same region in the left anterior peripheral zone. The PI-RADS 5 outcome confirmed the biopsy indication of the urinary biomarker-based test outcome. TRUS-guided biopsies from that region confirmed high-grade Gleason 3 + 4 = 7 PCa

role in the timely diagnosis of clinically significant PCa which was crucial for the curative treatment by RPP and the potential life-years gained for these vital males.

The decision to perform prostate biopsies is guided by EAU recommendations which incorporates mpMRI, RC and/or an additional serum- or urine-based test (e.g. based on *HOXC6* and *DLX1*) to individualize the need for a repeat biopsy [5]. In the second case, mpMRI targeted biopsies were performed that did not find the tumour. Recently, Pepe and collegues showed that if only targeted biopsy was performed when mpMRI showed a suspicious lesion (PI-RADS≥3), the number of biopsies could potentially have been reduced by 50%. However, 16.2–39.7% of the clinically significant prostate cancers would be missed using this approach [6]. Therefore, targeted biopsies should be done together with mapping biopsies and for risk-stratification mpMRI should be combined with an RC or biomarker-based test as the EAU guideline committee recommends.

Risk calculators are models, which take a patient's risk factors, combines them all into an equation and assigns a level of risk for having a disease. Several RCs were developed based on the Rotterdam arm of the ERSPC, using the clinical data and prostate biopsy outcome from 3624 previously unscreened men and 2896 men with previous negative prostate biopsy [13]. For the men described in the presented cases, the physicians used ERSPC RC4 containing PSA, DRE (normal/abnormal), TRUS (normal/abnormal), TRUS-assessed volume and biopsy history. For both men, the ERSPC RC4 indicated not to perform a prostate biopsy.

Recently, in a contemporary Dutch cohort, the ERSPC PCa probability threshold of ≥20% was shown to be acceptable for the biopsy-naïve men, missing only 2% of significant cases while saving 20% of prostate biopsies [7]. However, in men with previous negative biopsies, the ERSPC RC4 underestimated the outcomes for PCa and significant PCa. At this threshold, the RC4 would have missed 23% of significant cases while saving 47% of prostate biopsies. Gayet et al. showed that a threshold of ≥10% for PCa and > 2% for significant PCa would have been most optimal for men with previous negative biopsies, missing only 2% of significant cases and saving 21% of prostate biopsies. A possible factor attributing to the underestimation could be the fact that men with a previous negative biopsy were a higher risk cohort compared with the ERSPC cohort in which every man with an elevated serum PSA > 3 ng/ml at repeat screening was biopsied again within 4 years after initial biopsy [7].

An improvement of RCs would be the inclusion of biomarkers that are measured in body fluids of a patient. Prostate cells, cancerous or benign, shed cellular content such as cell-free nucleic acid in the urine. Therefore, urine as liquid biopsy offers an attractive alternative for tissue biopsies due to the direct contact of the urinary flow with draining of the genitourinary organs such as the prostate [14]. By combining the patient-specific biomarker expression profile with the clinical information of the patient, the resulting individualized risk score will allow the physician and patient to make the most informed choice about undergoing or delaying a prostate biopsy. Van Neste et al. already showed that this newly developed risk score outperformed the Prostate Cancer Prevention Trial Risk Calculator (PCPTRC) resulting in an improved patient risk stratification for high-grade PCa and biopsy decision-making [9].

The two cases presented here were identified in routine clinical practice in a Dutch hospital, with no study-specific visits or interventions. The novel urine biomarker test led to the use of prostate MRI prior to prostate biopsy. A recent systematic review on the NPV of mpMRI in excluding PCa at biopsy showed that the NPV depends on the prevalence of PCa [15]. At an overall PCa prevalence of 30% the NPV of mpMRI could be 88%, but when compared to the prevalence of 40% in the Van Neste et al study, the NPV of mpMRi would decrease to 82% [15]. Recently, it was shown that there is a correlation between the urine biomarker risk score and mpMRI outcomes [12]. Since the NPV of the urine-based genetic test is 98% and the risk score correlates with mpMRI outcomes, this urine biomarker test may become an important decision tool, not just for biopsy, but to risk stratify patients for mpMRI as well.

Recently, Cucchiara et al. showed that genomic biomarkers in combination with clinical and pathological variables have improved the detection, prognosis, and risk evaluation of PCa [16]. The SelectMDx test is a useful tool to reduce the number of unnecessary biopsies and stratify low-risk from high-risk tumors. Cost effectiveness studies have shown that quality-adjusted survival can be improved using this test by decreasing the number of biopsies performed and by not treating indolent tumors [17–19]. We acknowledge that the here described data only represents two cases and that no firm claims can be made based on these results. Large-scale case-controlled studies should confirm the applicability and reliability of using the SelectMDx test over the ERSPC RC4 in risk stratification for repeat biopsy.

The case reports on two men with persistent suspicion of PCa but negative prostate biopsy stress the need to use all the tools that EAU guidelines propose (mpMRI, RCs, biomarker-based tests) to individualize the need for biopsy. Although RCs are recommended and commonly used by urologists to predict repeat biopsy outcome, the fact that there may be an underestimate of the outcomes for high-grade PCa stresses the need to use multivariate risk stratification tools (e.g. combine the clinical information with biomarkers for high-grade disease) in order to make a more informed repeat biopsy decision. These two routine clinical practice examples demonstrate that the urine biomarker test for *HOXC6* and *DLX1*, combining clinical data with biomarkers detected in urine from a patient, offers an easy and individualized tool for stratifying men for mpMRI and biopsy.

Abbreviations

ADC: Apparent Diffusion Coefficient; BPH: Benign Prostatic Hyperplasia; DCE-MRI: Dynamic Contrast-Enhanced MRI; DLX1: Distal-less homeobox 1; DRE: Digital Rectal Examination; DWI: diffusion-weighted image; EAU: European Association of Urology; ERSPC: European Randomized Study of Screening for Prostate Cancer; GS: Gleason Score; HOXC6: Homeobox C6; NPV: Negative Predictive Value; PCa: Prostate Cancer; PI-RADS: Prostate Imaging Reporting and Data System; PSA: Prostate Specific Antigen; RC: Risk Calculator; RC4: Risk Calculator Model 4; RRP: radical retropubic prostatectomy; TDRD1: Tudor domain containing 1; TRUS-Bx: Transrectal ultrasound guided biopsies

Acknowledgements

The authors would like to thank the patients for their consent to participate to these case reports.

Authors' contributions

PM was the urologist of the patients and participated in the design and writing of this manuscript. DH was instrumental in the design, development and writing of this manuscript. JS participated in design and writing of the paper. WC participated in design, writing of the paper. All authors read and approved the final manuscript.

Author details

[1]Department of Urology, LangeLand Ziekenhuis, Zoetermeer, The Netherlands. [2]MDxHealth BV, Nijmegen, The Netherlands. [3]Department of

Urology, Radboud University Nijmegen Medical Centre, Nijmegen, The Netherlands. [4]Department of Mathematical Modelling, Statistics and Bioinformatics, Ghent University, Ghent, Belgium.

References

1. Daneshgari F, Taylor GD, Miller GJ, Crawford ED. Computer simulation of the probability of detecting low volume carcinoma of the prostate with six random systematic core biopsies. Urology. 1995;45:604–9.
2. Shariat SF, Roehrborn CG. Using biopsy to detect prostate cancer. Rev Urol. 2009;10:262–80.
3. Gershman B, Van Houten HK, Herrin J, Moreira DM, Kim SP, Shah ND, et al. Impact of prostate-specific antigen (PSA) screening trials and revised PSA screening Guidelines on rates of prostate biopsy and Postbiopsy complications. Eur Urol. 2016;71:55–65.
4. Loeb S, Vellekoop A, Ahmed HU, Catto J, Emberton M, Nam R, et al. Systematic review of complications of prostate biopsy. Eur Urol. 2013; 64:876–92.
5. EAU. EAU Guidelines. Copenhagen: Edn. presented at the EAU Annual Congress; 2018. ISBN 978-94-92671-01-1
6. Pepe P, Garufi A, Priolo GD, Galia A, Fraggetta F, Pennisi M. Is it time to perform only magnetic resonance imaging targeted cores? Our experience with 1032 men who underwent prostate biopsy. J Urol. 2018;200:774–8.
7. Gayet M, Mannaerts CK, Nieboer D, Beerlage HP, Wijkstra H, Mulders PFA, et al. Prediction of prostate Cancer: external validation of the ERSPC risk calculator in a contemporary Dutch clinical cohort. Eur Urol Focus. 2016; S2405-4569(16):30107–9. https://doi.org/10.1016/j.euf.2016.07.007.
8. Leyten GHJM, Hessels D, Smit FP, Jannink SA, de Jong H, Melchers WJG, et al. Identification of a candidate gene panel for the early diagnosis of prostate Cancer. Clin Cancer Res. 2015;21:3061–70.
9. Van Neste L, Hendriks RJ, Dijkstra S, Trooskens G, Cornel EB, Jannink SA, et al. Detection of high-grade prostate Cancer using a urinary molecular biomarker-based risk score. Eur Urol. 2016;70(5):740–8. https://doi.org/10.1016/j.eururo.2016.04.012.
10. Zhou J, Yang X, Song P, Wang H, Wang X. HOXC6 in the prognosis of prostate cancer. Artif Cells Nanomed Biotechnol. 2019;47(1):2715–20.
11. Liang M, Sun Y, Yang H-L, Wen J, Shi B-K. DLX1, a binding protein of beta-catenin, promoted the growth and migration of prostate cancer cells. Exp Cell Res. 2018;363(1):26–32.
12. Hendriks RJ, Van der Leest MMG, Dijkstra S, Barentsz JO, Van Criekinge W, Hulsbergen-van de Kaa CA, Schalken JA, Mulders PFA, Van Oort IM. A urinary biomarker-based risk score correlates with multiparametric MRI for prostate cancer detection. Prostate. 2017;77:1401–7. https://doi.org/10.1002/pros.23401.
13. Roobol MJ, van Vugt HA, Loeb S, Zhu X, Bul M, Bangma CH, et al. Prediction of prostate cancer risk: the role of prostate volume and digital rectal examination in the ERSPC risk calculators. Eur Urol. 2011;61:577–83.
14. Lin SY, Linehan JA, Wilson TG, Hoon DSB. Emerging utility of urinary cell-free nucleic acid biomarkers for prostate, bladder, and renal cancers. Eur Urol Focus. 2017;S2405-4569(17):30077–9. https://doi.org/10.1016/j.euf.2017.03.009.
15. Moldovan PC, Van den Broeck T, Sylvester R, Marconi L, Bellmunt J, van den Bergh RCN, et al. What is the negative predictive value of multiparametric magnetic resonance imaging in excluding prostate Cancer at biopsy? A systematic review and meta-analysis from the European Association of Urology prostate Cancer Guidelines panel. Eur Urol. 2017;72:250–66.
16. Cucchiara V, Cooperberg MR, Dall'Era M, Lin DW, Montorsi F, Schalken JA, Evans CP. Genomic markers in prostate Cancer decision making. Eur Urol. 2018;73:572–82.
17. Dijkstra S, Govers TM, Hendriks RJ, Schalken JA, Van Criekinge W, Van Neste L, Grutters JPC, Sedelaar JPM, van Oort IM. Cost-effectiveness of a new urinary biomarker-based risk score compared to standard of care in prostate cancer diagnostics - a decision analytical model. BJU Int. 2017;120(5):659–65.
18. Sathianathen NJ, Kuntz KM, Alarid-Escudero F, Lawrentschuk NL, Bolton DM, Murphy DG, Weight CJ, Konety BR. Incorporating biomarkers into the primary prostate biopsy setting: a cost-effectiveness analysis. J Urol. 2018. https://doi.org/10.1016/j.juro.2018.06.016.
19. Govers T, Hessels D, Vlaeminck-Guillem V, Schmitz-Dräger BJ, Stief CG, Martinez-Ballesteros C, et al. Cost-effectiveness of SelectMDx for prostate cancer in four European countries: a comparative modeling study. Prostate Cancer Prostatic Dis. 2018. https://doi.org/10.1038/s41391-018-0076-3.

17

Three-dimensional grayscale transrectal ultrasound-guidance and biopsy core preembedding for detection of prostate cancer: Dutch clinical cohort study

Anouk Anna Maria Arnoldus van der Aa[1,4*†], Christophe Koenraad Mannaerts[5†], Maudy C. W. Gayet[1,4], Johannes Cornelis van der Linden[2], Barthold Philip Schrier[1], J. P. Michiel Sedelaar[3], Massimo Mischi[4], Harrie P. Beerlage[4,5] and Hessel Wijkstra[4,5]

Abstract

Background: To overcome the limitations regarding two dimensional (2D) greyscale (GS) transrectal ultrasound (TRUS)-guided biopsy in prostate cancer (PCa) detection and tissue packaging in biopsy processing, there is an ongoing focus on new imaging and pathology techniques. A three-dimensional (3D) model of the prostate with biopsy needle guidance can be generate by the Navigo™ workstation (UC-care, Israel). The SmartBX™ system (UC-care, Israel) provides a prostate biopsy core preembedding method. The aim of this study was to compare cancer detection rates between the 3D TRUS-guidance and preembedding method with conventional 2D GS TRUS-guidance among patients undergoing prostate biopsies.

Methods: We retrospectively analyzed the records of all patients who underwent prostate biopsies for PCa detection at our institution from 2007 to 2016. The cohort was divided into a 2D GS TRUS-guidance cohort (from 2007 to 2013, $n = 1149$) and a 3D GS TRUS-guidance with preembedding cohort (from 2013 to 2016, $n = 469$). Effect of 3D GS TRUS-guidance with preembedding on detection rate of PCa and clinically significant PCa (Gleason score ≥ 7 or > 2 biopsy cores with a Gleason score 6) was compared to 2D GS TRUS-guidance using regression models.

Results: Detection rate of PCa and clinically significant PCa was 39.0 and 24.9% in the 3D GS TRUS cohort compared to 33.5 and 19.0% in the 2D GS TRUS cohort, respectively. On multivariate regression analysis the use of 3D GS TRUS-guidance with preembedding was associated with a significant increase in detection rate of PCa (aOR = 1.33; 95% CI: 1.03–1.72) and clinically significant PCa (aOR = 1.47; 95% CI: 1.09–1.98).

Conclusion: Our results suggest that 3D GS TRUS-guidance with biopsy core preembedding improves PCa and clinically significant PCa detection compared to 2D GS TRUS-guidance. Additional studies are needed to justify the application of these systems in clinical practice.

Keywords: Prostatic neoplasms, Biopsy, Three-dimensional imaging, Tissue embedding, Diagnosis

* Correspondence: A.v.d.Aa@jbz.nl
†Anouk Anna Maria Arnoldus van der Aa and Christophe Koenraad Mannaerts contributed equally to this work.
[1]Department of Urology, Jeroen Bosch Hospital, Post office box 90153, 's-Hertogenbosch 5200 ME, The Netherlands
[4]Electrical Engineering, Eindhoven University of Technology, Eindhoven, The Netherlands
Full list of author information is available at the end of the article

Background

Prostate cancer (PCa) is the most common malignancy among Western males [1]. Early detection of PCa reduces PCa-related mortality and reduces the risk of being diagnosed and developing advanced or metastatic disease [2].

PCa detection with systematic prostate biopsies under ultrasound guidance, in men identified with elevated serum prostate-specific antigen (PSA) and / or abnormal digital rectal examination (DRE), is considered as the preferred diagnostic method by guidelines from leading organizations [3, 4]. Although standard two dimensional (2D) greyscale (GS) transrectal ultrasound (TRUS)--guided biopsy is able to detect PCa, it has well known limitations. 2D GS TRUS has low sensitivity and specificity for detection of PCa and is therefore used to guide prostate biopsies rather than used as a diagnostic modality. Even in TRUS-guided biopsy there is still a 20–30% risk of sampling error with underdiagnosis of PCa that requires definitive treatment as a result [5, 6]. There is also poor correlation with final pathology [7–9]. Unfortunately, imaging is not the only part with influence on PCa detection as inadequate tissue packaging in biopsy processing also tends to reduce PCa detection outcomes [10].

To overcome these limitations and improve PCa detection, there is an ongoing focus on new imaging and pathology techniques.

3D GS TRUS is an imaging method that allows simultaneous imaging of the prostate in axial and sagittal plane, followed by a computer reconstructed third coronal plane as well as a 3D image [5]. Effectiveness of 3D GS TRUS in detection and local staging of PCa is controversial as limited studies reported different outcomes [5, 11–13]. However, the feasibility of 3D TRUS in assisting biopsy needle guidance was recognised in phantom and patient studies [14–16]. More recently, Peltier et al. reported significant higher detection rates of clinically significant PCa using a 3D TRUS-guided biopsy system in clinical practice [17].

Biopsy processing with preembedding methods of prostate biopsy cores result in optimal tissue presentation with preservation of shape and avoidance of artefacts and deformation, and have shown to improve histologic yield [18, 19]. Moreover, Rogatsch et al. demonstrated that the improvement of histologic yield using an optimized preembedding method led to a higher frequency of PCa diagnosis [20].

Based on these findings, prostate biopsy sessions in our institution are performed since September 2013 with a phantom validated 3D GS TRUS-guided biopsy system (Navigo™ workstation, UC-care Medical Systems Israel) and a semi-automated prostate biopsy core preembedding method proven to improve histologic yield (the SmartBX™ system, UC-care Medical Systems Israel) [15, 21]. The purpose of the present study was to investigate the value of 3D GS TRUS-guidance and biopsy core preembedding in the detection of (clinically significant) PCa compared to conventional 2D GS TRUS-guidance in a consecutive cohort of men undergoing systematic prostate biopsies due to a clinical suspicion of PCa.

Methods

In this retrospective cohort study, all consecutive men who underwent prostate biopsies between January 2007 and January 2016 in the Urology Department at the Jeroen Bosch Hospital in 's Hertogenbosch, the Netherlands, were included. Patient files were consulted for relevant information. Prostate biopsy sessions performed in patients with no prior history of PCa and a serum PSA level between 4.0 and 10.0 µg/L or PSA < 4.0 µg/L and a suspicious DRE were included in the study. We divided the eligible prostate biopsy sessions into two cohorts. From January 2007 up to September 2013 consecutive biopsy sessions were performed in the 2D TRUS cohort. The 3D TRUS cohort consisted of the consecutive biopsy sessions with preembedding from September 2013 up to January 2016.

2D TRUS cohort protocol

All prostate biopsy sessions were performed with prophylactic antibiotics in the lateral decubitus position. The prostate gland was assessed and scanned and prostate volume measurements were done using the ellipsoid formula, using a BK medical ultrasound machine (type 2202) and BK medical sidefire probe (type 8808, 6–10 MHz). A 12-core biopsy protocol, under periprostatic local anaesthesia, was then performed consisting of biopsies on both sides in the peripheral zone, 2 biopsies of each base, mid and apex. The biopsy was performed using a spring-loaded gun with 18-gauge needles (Bard Magnum biopsy gun). Biopsy cores were placed in two vials, each vial containing 6 cores of one prostate lobe. Prostate cores were processed and examined in the hospital pathology laboratory. Number of cores per vial, length of biopsy cores, number of positive biopsy cores, ISUP 2005 Gleason score and tumour volume% of biopsy cores (since 2012) were reported.

3D TRUS cohort protocol

The 3D GS TRUS protocol is basically similar to the 2D TRUS protocol. The 3D GS TRUS system (Navigo™ workstation) was incorporated side by side in the room with 2D ultrasound images transferred and displayed on the 3D TRUS screen. A 3D model of the prostate was built after prostate volume measurements and planimetry was done. The outline of the prostate border was manually traced and recorded on a slice-by-slice basis. In real time using an electromagnetic system (Fig. 1), the 12-core biopsy protocol was performed with tracking, displaying and recording of biopsy needle trajectory locations. Previously marked regions of interest were shown with colour indications on screen and sampled. Biopsy cores were fixed separately on six different cassettes (two cores of apex, mid and base on both sides) using the Smart-Bx device (Additional file 2). SmartBx™ device is a semi-automated prostate biopsy core preembedding method, with a designed membrane to which the cores stay attached throughout pathology lab processing, and placed in two formalin-filled vials (3 cassettes in each vial with two cores of apex, mid and base of one prostate lobe).

In both cohorts, biopsy sessions were performed by different operators. Operator was recorded for analysis and split into experienced (> 100 procedures/year and > 10 years of experience using TRUS guided biopsies) and less experienced (< 100 procedures/year). The following primary outcomes were compared: detection rate of PCa and detection rate of clinically significant (Gleason score ≥ 7 or Gleason score 6 with at least 3 positive biopsy cores). The following secondary outcomes were compared in patients with PCa at biopsy: amount of positive biopsy cores; ratio positive biopsy cores per total biopsy cores; tumour volume% of biopsy cores and Gleason score.

Statistical

Statistical analyses were performed using SPSS Statistics 23.0®. Descriptive statistics were used to summarize baseline characteristics. Continuous variables were presented with means and standard deviations (SD) or median and interquartile ranges (IQR) based on symmetrical distribution with the independent two sample t-test or Mann-Whitney U test used to assess differences, respectively. Percentage scores were presented for categorical variables with differences assessed using the Pearson Chi-Square test. To determine association between (clinically significant) PCa and the 3D GS TRUS-guided system with preembedding we calculated the crude and adjusted odds ratio with their 95% confidence intervals (CI) for each outcome compared to the 2D GS TRUS cohort using univariate and multivariate logistic regression analyses. Covariables were entered on multivariate analysis, selected based on literature and/or performance: inclusion in the adjusted model when addition of the variable resulted in at least 10% change in the regression coefficient. A $P < 0.05$ was considered statistically significant in all analyses [3, 22–24].

Results

Between January 2007 and January 2016 we performed 2917 prostate biopsy sessions in 2171 different patients (Fig. 2). 2D TRUS biopsies were performed from 2007 to 2013 and 3D TRUS biopsies were performed from 2013

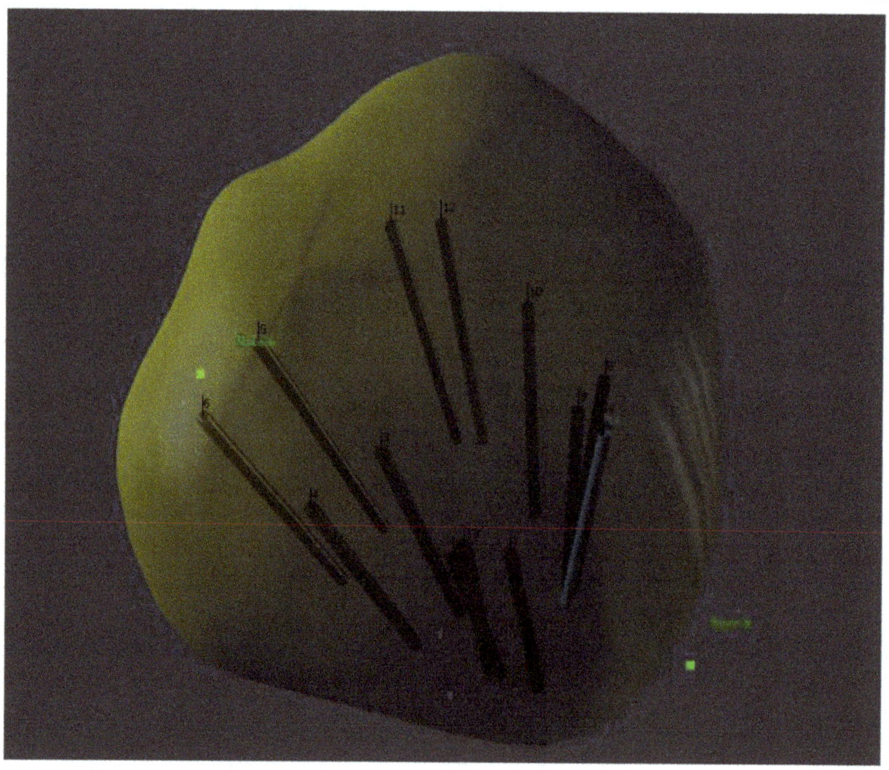

Fig. 1 Navigo™ 3D model with biopsy locations

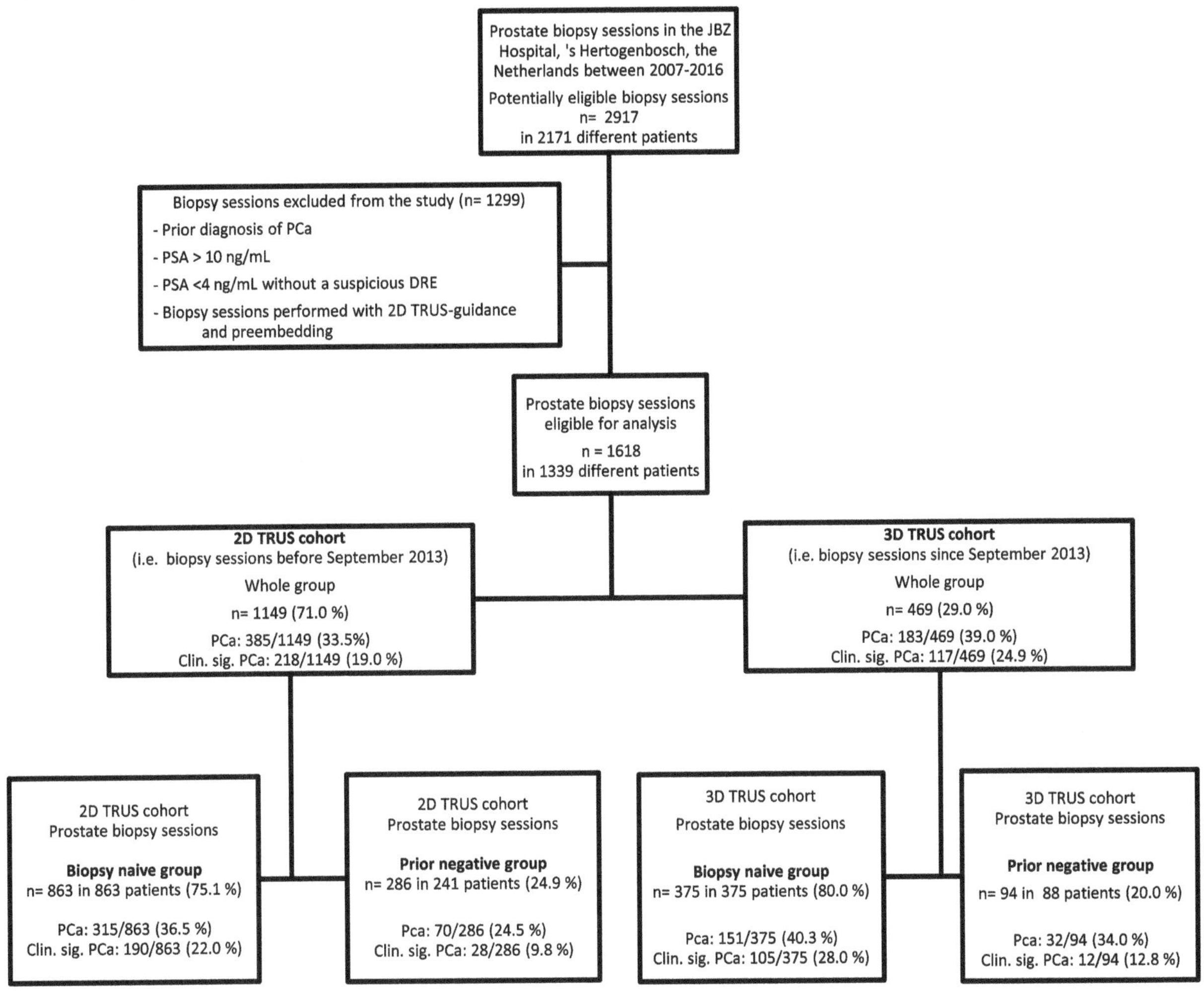

Fig. 2 Study population

to 2016. A total of 1618 prostate biopsy sessions in 1339 different patients met inclusion criteria. 469 (29.0%) and 1149 (71.0%) biopsy sessions were performed in the 3D TRUS and 2D TRUS cohort respectively. Patients with missing data on clinical, biopsy and pathology variables (PSA $n = 4$, DRE $n = 112$, prostate volume $n = 13$, length of cores $n = 20$) were excluded for multivariate analyses. Additionally, information on primary outcome was inadequate for 45 biopsy sessions and therefore these sessions were revised by one uropathologist.

Patient and biopsy characteristics

Several characteristics differed among the two cohorts for whole group and subgroups (biopsy naive and prior negative biopsy sessions only) analyses (Table 1). For whole group analysis, prostate biopsy sessions in the 3D TRUS cohort were more likely done in older patients (mean age in years; 64.6 vs. 63.0, $p < 0.001$), in patients with larger prostate volumes (median volume in cc; 46 vs. 40, $p < 0.001$), in a biopsy naive setting (80.0% vs. 75.1%, $p < 0.05$) and by the experienced operator (73.6% vs. 43.3%, $p < 0.001$) compared to the 2D TRUS cohort. The amount of biopsy cores taken per session was comparable in both cohorts (mean cores 12.3 vs. 12.3, $p = 0.555$), while fragmentation of biopsy cores occurred significantly less often in the 3D TRUS cohort (37.7% vs. 1.9%, $p < 0.001$). The length of biopsy cores in millimetres was significantly larger in the 3D TRUS cohort (mean length in mm; 16.08 vs. 12.38, $p < 0.001$).

Detection rate

In the 3D TRUS cohort, a total of 183 out of 469 (39.0%) and 117 out of 469 (24.9%) were found positive for PCa and clinically significant PCa compared to 335 out of 1149 (33.5%) and 218 out of 1149 (19.0%) in the 2D TRUS cohort, respectively (Table 2). On univariate analysis the 3D TRUS cohort was significantly associated with detection of PCa (OR = 1.27, 95% CI 1.02–1.59) and clinically significant PCa (OR 1.42, 95% CI 1.10–1.83). On multivariate regression analysis with age, DRE,

Table 1 Patient and biopsy characteristics

	Total	2D TRUS	3D TRUS	*P* value
Whole group (1339 patients)				
Number of biopsy sessions	*N* = 1618	N = 1149 (71.0%)	*N* = 469 (29.0%)	
Age in years, mean (SD)	63.4 (SD: 6.30)	63.0 (SD: 6.27)	64.6 (SD: 6.24)	< 0.001
PSA in ng/mL, mean (SD)	6.92 (SD: 1.84)	6.95 (SD: 1.85)	6.84 (SD: 1.84)	0.248
DRE:				
• benign, n (%)	1028 (68.3%)	739 (69.3%)	289 (65.7%)	0.167
• suspicious, n (%)	478 (31.7%)	327 (30.7%)	151 (34.3%)	
Prostate volume in ml, median (IQR)	41 (30–56)	40 (30–54)	46 (33–63)	< 0.001
Type of biopsy sessions:				
• Biopsy naive, n (%)	1238 (76.5%)	863 (75.1%)	375 (80.0%)	0.037
• Prior negative, n (%)	380 (23.5%)	286 (24.9%)	94 (20.0%)	
Type of operator:				
• Experienced, n (%)	843 (52.1%)	498 (43.3%)	345 (73.6%)	< 0.001
• Less experienced, n (%)	775 (47.9%)	651 (56.7%)	124 (26.4%)	
Biopsy cores per session, mean (SD)	12.3 (SD 1.04)	12.3 (SD 1.05)	12.3 (SD 1.02)	0.555
Biopsy sessions with fragmentation, n (%)	442 (27.3%)	433 (37.7%)	9 (1.9%)	< 0.001
Length of biopsy cores in mm, mean (SD)[a]	13.84 (SD: 2.98)	12.38 (SD: 2.82)	16.08 (SD: 1.41)	< 0.001
Biopsy naïve group (1238 patients)				
Number of biopsy sessions	*N* = 1238	*N* = 863 (69.7%)	*N* = 375 (30.3%)	
Age in years, mean (SD)	63.5 (SD: 6.46)	63.0 (SD: 6.43)	64.7 (SD: 6.35)	< 0.001
PSA in ng/mL, mean (SD)	6.73 (SD: 1.87)	6.72 (SD: 1.87)	6.74 (SD: 1.86)	0.877
DRE:				
• benign, n (%)	777 (66.9%)	556 (68.6%)	221 (63.0%)	0.063
• suspicious, n (%)	385 (33.1%)	255 (31.4%)	130 (37.0%)	
Prostate volume in ml, median (IQR)	40 (30–55)	40 (29–52)	44 (32–60)	< 0.001
Type of operator:				
• Experienced, n (%)	643 (51.9%)	368 (42.6%)	275 (73.3%)	< 0.001
• Less experienced, n (%)	595 (48.1%)	495 (57.4%)	100 (26.7%)	
Biopsy cores per session, mean (SD)	12.2 (SD 0.79)	12.2 (SD 0.80)	12.2 (SD 0.77)	0.779
Biopsy sessions with fragmentation, n (%)	334 (27.0%)	325 (37.7%)	9 (2.4%)	< 0.001
Length of biopsy cores in mm, mean (SD)[a]	13.84 (SD: 2.96)	12.33 (SD: 2.78)	16.07 (SD: 1.40)	< 0.001
Prior negative group (321 patients)				
Number of biopsy sessions	*N* = 380	*N* = 286 (75.3%)	*N* = 94 (24.7%)	
Prior negative sessions specified:				
• Second session	300 (78.9%)	225 (78.7%)	75 (79.8%)	0.658
• Third session	64 (16.8%)	47 (16.4%)	17 (18.1%)	
• Fourth session	14 (3.7%)	12 (4.2%)	2 (2.1%)	
• Fifth session	2 (0.5%)	2 (0.7%)	0	
Age in years, mean (SD)	63.1 (SD: 5.79)	62.8 (SD: 5.80)	63.9 (SD: 5.73)	0.135
PSA in ng/mL, mean (SD)	7.54 (SD: 1.60)	7.65 (SD: 1.54)	7.20 (SD: 1.73)	0.023
DRE:				
• benign, n (%)	251 (73.0%)	183 (71.8%)	68 (76.4%)	0.396
• suspicious, n (%)	93 (27.0%)	72 (28.2%)	21 (23.6%)	
Prostate volume in ml, median (IQR)	46 (32–62)	44 (31–58)	54 (39–70)	< 0.001

Table 1 Patient and biopsy characteristics *(Continued)*

	Total	2D TRUS	3D TRUS	*P* value
Type of operator:				
• Experienced, n (%)	200 (52.6%)	130 (45.5%)	70 (74.5%)	< 0.001
• Less experienced, n (%)	180 (47.4%)	156 (54.5%)	24 (25.5%)	
Biopsy cores per session, mean (SD)	12.6 (SD 1.56)	12.7 (SD 1.53)	12.6 (SD 1.67)	0.519
Biopsy sessions with fragmentation, n (%)	113 (29.7%)	113 (39.2%)	0	< 0.001
Length of biopsy cores in mm, mean (SD)[a]	13.81 (SD: 3.05)	12.54 (SD: 2.96)	16.10 (SD: 1.48)	< 0.001

[a]Biopsy sessions with fragmentation were excluded for these analyses

prostate volume and type of operator included as covariates, the 3D TRUS cohort remained significantly associated with detection of PCa (aOR 1.33, 95% CI 1.03–1.72) and clinically significant PCa (aOR 1.47, 95% CI 1.09–1.98). The association between 3D TRUS and detection of (clinically significant) PCa on multivariate regression analysis for the subgroups demonstrated significance for clinically significant PCa in the biopsy naive group (aOR 1.41, 95% CI 1.02–1.96) and for PCa in the prior negative group (aOR 1.78, 95% CI (1.04–3.04) (Table 2).

PCa positive biopsies: biopsy characteristics and Gleason score

Tumour biopsy characteristics between the 3D GS TRUS cohort and the 2D GS TRUS cohort in patients with positive PCa biopsies were not statistically different as the amount of positive biopsy cores, the ratio positive biopsy cores out of the total biopsy cores and the percentage of tumour volume per PCa biopsy session did not differ between both groups (Additional file 3). The biopsy Gleason score among patients with PCa positive biopsies was significantly different between the 3D TRUS and 2D TRUS cohort in the whole group and biopsy naive subgroup analyses as more clinically significant and Gleason score ≥ 7 PCa was found in the 3D TRUS cohort ($P < 0.05$) (Additional file 4).

Discussion

Limited studies with small sample sizes have been performed to assess the value of 3D GS TRUS in guiding prostate biopsies. Peltier et al. published the first cohort study into 3D TRUS-guided prostate biopsy and detection rate of PCa. In 220 consecutive biopsy naive men, detection rate of PCa was significantly higher in the 3D TRUS group using the Urostation (Koelis®) compared with 2D TRUS (50.0% versus 33.6%, $p < 0.05$) [17]. In contrary, a previous study carried out in our institution with 325 men showed no added value of 3D TRUS guidance compared to 2D with all biopsy cores preembedded (aOR 0.79, 95% CI 0.47–1.34) [25].

This present study, covering a period of 9 full years with 1618 prostate biopsy sessions, demonstrated higher detection rates of PCa and clinically significant PCa with the use of 3D TRUS-guidance and preembedding compared to conventional 2D GS TRUS-guidance. These findings may be explained by different hypotheses. On one side, 3D TRUS could have improved detection as it offers the ability to accurately register the location of the biopsy needle tract within the gland, possibly leading to better distribution of biopsy cores; instead needle placement with 2D-guidance is not always homogeneously distributed and tends to cluster.[15, 26–28] Besides, length of biopsy cores was significantly larger and fragmentation occurred significantly less in the 3D GS TRUS cohort possibly also aiding detection of PCa as Iczkowski et al. and Rogatsch et al. demonstrated in their studies that length of biopsy tissue significantly correlates with PCa detection rate and higher frequency of PCa diagnosis was found with an improved preembedding method, respectively [19, 20, 25].

Multiparametric MRI (mpMRI) of the prostate is increasingly used in the diagnostic pathway of PCa and three large studies, evaluating the detection rates of an MRI-targeted biopsy approach and TRUS guided systematic biopsy approach, have recently been performed in biopsy-naïve men [30–32].

While the PRECISION trial demonstrated that an MRI targeted biopsy approach detected significantly more clinically significant PCa in comparison with a TRUS systematic biopsy approach both the MRI First and 4 M Study demonstrated comparable detection rates of clinically significant PCa between the standard TRUS systematic biopsy and MRI targeted biopsy approach.

Obtaining an mpMRI before biopsy improves the detection of clinically significant PCa but at present does not avoid the need for systematic biopsy as shown in the systematic review from Moldovan et al. and the MRI FIRST study where 10 to 15% of clinically significant PCa were still missed in men with a negative mpMRI [31, 33]. Even in the Dutch 4 M study with high-quality MRI standards, 7% (21/317) of all men with a suspicious mpMRI scan had clinically significant PCa only on systematic biopsy [32]. A high-quality TRUS systematic biopsy, possibly with the use of 3D TRUS-guidance and preembedding, could therefore still be important in the current diagnostic setting where mpMRI is also included.

Table 2 Detection rate of all prostate cancer and clinically significant prostate cancer

Whole group			
Detection rate of PCa			
Biopsy cohort:	n/N (%)	Crude OR (95% CI)	aOR[a] (95% CI)
Total	568/1618 (35.1%)		
3D TRUS	183/469 (39.0%)	1.27 (1.02–1.59)	1.33 (1.03–1.72)
2D TRUS	385/1149 (33.5%)	Reference	Reference
Detection rate of clinically significant PCa			
	n/N (%)	Crude OR (95% CI)	aOR[a] (95% CI)
Total	335/1618 (20.7%)		
3D TRUS	117/469 (24.9%)	1.42 (1.10–1.83)	1.47 (1.09–1.98)
2D TRUS	218/1149 (19.0%)	Reference	Reference
Biopsy naive group			
Detection rate of PCa			
	n/N (%)	Crude OR (95% CI)	aOR[b] (95% CI)
Total	466/1238 (37.6%)		
3D TRUS	151/375 (40.3%)	1.17 (0.92–1.50)	1.20 (0.90–1.60)
2D TRUS	315/863 (36.5%)	Reference	Reference
Detection rate of clinically significant PCa			
	n/N (%)	Crude OR (95% CI)	aOR[b] (95% CI)
Total	295/1238 (23.8%)		
3D TRUS	105/375 (28.0%)	1.38 (1.04–1.82)	1.41 (1.02–1.96)
2D TRUS	190/863 (22.0%)	Reference	Reference
Prior negative group			
Detection rate of PCa			
	n/N (%)	Crude OR (95% CI)	aOR[c] (95% CI)
Total	102/380 (26.8%)		
3D TRUS	32/94 (34.0%)	1.59 (0.96–2.64)	1.78 (1.04–3.04)
2D TRUS	70/286 (24.5%)	Reference	Reference
Detection rate of clinically significant PCa			
	n/N (%)	Crude OR (95% CI)	aOR[d] (95% CI)
Total	40/380 (10.5%)		
3D TRUS	12/94 (12.8%)	1.35 (0.66–2.77)	–
2D TRUS	28/286 (9.8%)	Reference	Reference

[a]adjusted Odds Ratio: adjusted for age, DRE, prostate volume and physician (PSA and Type of biopsy session resulted in < 10% change in β)
[b] adjusted Odds Ratio: adjusted for age, DRE and prostate volume and physician (PSA resulted in < 10% change in the β)
[c] adjusted Odds Ratio: adjusted for age and Log (prostate volume), (age, PSA, DRE and physician resulted in < 10% change in the β)
[d] the number of events per variable are too low to be analyzed in multivariable logistic regression analysis

On the other side, as a retrospective study, our analysis has important limitations that could have influenced the outcome. First of all, biopsy sessions after September 2013 were performed with 3D TRUS guidance and the preembedding method; as a consequence, their independent influence on the detection rate of PCa cannot be assessed. However as both procedures act on different aspects of PCa diagnosis, a joint positive effect was hypothesized over masking of independent results. Secondly, difference in study time period could have had an impact on PCa detection rate as different unidentified factors influencing PCa detection rate could have changed during these time periods. Prostate biopsy selection in both cohorts however was not based on important pre-biopsy tests such as mpMRI and/or novel biomarkers. Both cohorts differed in baseline characteristics with older age, lower prostate volume and a biopsy naive setting all associated with higher odds of PCa and significant PCa on univariate and multivariate analysis in our study (Additional file 1: Table S1). Beside this, we decided in our study to include the Large Grade Group 1 (GS 3 + 3) as clinically significant PCa. Recent EAU guidelines use the definition of GG ≥ 2 (GS ≥3 + 4) for clinical significant PCa. This matches with the newly introduced ISUP scoring system, where no separation is made between large and small GG 1 (GS 3 + 3) PCa [29]. We decided to include large GS 3 + 3 = 6 PCa as clinically significant as this is currently still used as a criteria for active surveillance versus radical treatment in low-risk PCa patients.

In addition, experience level of operators was various. Although a correction strategy was implemented, residual confounding could still be possible. Last, 32.4% (944/2917) of all our prostate biopsy sessions were excluded on the basis of PSA inclusion criteria. In line with the literature we excluded men with high PSA levels as improved detection of significant PCa cancer is most necessary in the PSA grayzone from 4 to 10 ng/mL, while men with higher PSA levels tend to be diagnosed accurately with TRUS-guided systematic biopsies [30–32].

As a result, association between 3D TRUS-guidance with preembedding and detection of PCa could be partially biased on the basis of confounding and selection.

Despite these limitations in relation to the detection of PCa, there are other possible clinical applications for our approach. The 3D TRUS system is not only developed for direct imaging and navigation, but also for procedure planning with recording and integration of exact locations of biopsy cores and updating of pathology results. With the possibility to assess the exact spatial coordinates of each previous needle trajectory, a 'biopsy map' can be built based on (positive) previous core taken and adequate sample sites can potentially be chosen in prior negative patients or in patients in active surveillance. Additionally, in our study biopsy core length and Gleason score were significantly higher in the cohort with 3D GS TRUS-guidance and preembedding. As more biopsy core length from a presumably spatial better biopsied prostate gland can be pathologically examined, correlation with prostatectomy specimens could possibly be improved and thereby prevent men with unfavourable disease to be placed in active surveillance or less aggressive treatments. However caution should be exercised for interpretation of Gleason score differences between both cohorts as Gleason grading of PCa was updated at the end of 2014 during an ISUP Consensus Conference [29].

As a consequence, higher Gleason scores in the 3D TRUS cohort could be partially the result of these new grading pattern definitions. We will therefore investigate these potential applications in future prospective studies and pathology concordance studies. These findings highlight the need for future research regarding the complementary value of 3D TRUS guidance and preembedding in the combination with mpMRI and other new diagnostic applications.

Conclusion

The current study suggests an added value of 3D TRUS-guidance and preembedding compared to conventional 2D GS TRUS-guidance regarding detection rate of PCa and clinically significant PCa among patients undergoing prostate biopsies. At the same time, 3D TRUS-guidance and preembedding provided significant more biopsy core tissue length and higher biopsy Gleason scores. Additional prospective studies and studies concerning pathology correlation are needed to justify the routine application of 3D GS TRUS-guidance and biopsy core preembedding.

Additional files

Additional file 1: Table S1. Univariate and multivariate logistic regression analyses of individual risk factors for detection of prostate cancer and clinically significant prostate cancer. (DOCX 14 kb)

Additional file 2: SmartBx™ device prostate biopsy core preembedding. (PPTX 95 kb)

Additional file 3: Tumour biopsy characteristics among patients with positive biopsies. (XLSX 12 kb)

Additional file 4: Biopsy Gleason score among patients with positive biopsies. (XLSX 13 kb)

Abbreviations

2D: Two-dimensional; 3D: Three-dimensional; CI: Confidence interval; DRE: Digital rectal examination; GS: Greyscale; IQR: Interquartile range; mpMRI: Multiparametric Magnetic Resonance Imaging; OR: Odds ratio; PCa: Prostate cancer; PSA: prostate-specific antigen; SD: Standard deviation; TRUS: Transrectal ultrasound

Acknowledgements

Not applicable.

Author details

[1]Department of Urology, Jeroen Bosch Hospital, Post office box 90153, 's-Hertogenbosch 5200 ME, The Netherlands. [2]Department of Pathology, Jeroen Bosch Hospital, 's-Hertogenbosch, The Netherlands. [3]Department of Urology, Radboud University Medical Centre, Nijmegen, The Netherlands. [4]Electrical Engineering, Eindhoven University of Technology, Eindhoven, The Netherlands. [5]Department of Urology, AMC University Hospital, Amsterdam, The Netherlands.

References

1. Arnold M, Karim-Kos HE, Coebergh JW, Byrnes G, Antilla A, Ferlay J, et al. Recent trends in incidence of five common cancers in 26 European countries since 1988: analysis of the European Cancer observatory. Eur J Cancer. 2015;51(9):1164–87.
2. Schröder FH, Hugosson J, Carlsson S, Tammela TL, Määttänen L, Auvinen A, et al. Screening for prostate Cancer decreases the risk of developing metastatic disease: findings from the European randomized study of screening for prostate Cancer. Eur Urol. 2012;62(5):745–52.
3. Schröder FH, Hugosson J, Roobol MJ, Tammela TL, Zappa M, Nelen V, et al. Screening and prostate cancer mortality: results of the European randomised study of screening for prostate Cancer (ERSPC) at 13 years of follow-up. Lancet. 2014;384(9959):2027–35.
4. Wolf AM, Wender RC, Etzioni RB, Thompson IM, D'Amico AV, Volk RJ, et al. American Cancer Society guideline for the early detection of prostate cancer: update 2010. CA Cancer J Clin. 2010;60(2):70–98.
5. Smeenge M, de la Rosette JJ, Wijkstra H. Current status of transrectal ultrasound techniques in prostate cancer. Curr Opin Urol. 2012;22(4): 297–302.
6. Ukimura O, Coleman JA, de la Taille A, Emberton M, Epstein JI, Freedland SJ, et al. Contemporary role of systematic prostate biopsies: indications, techniques and implications for patient care. Eur Urol. 2013;63(2):214–30.
7. Wilkinson BA, Hamdy FC. State-of-the-art staging in prostate cancer. BJU Int. 2001;87(5):423–31.
8. Ploussard G, Salomon L, Xylinas E, Allory Y, Vordos D, Hoznek A, et al. Pathological findings and prostate specific antigen outcomes after radical prostatectomy in men eligible for active surveillance--does the risk of misclassification vary according to biopsy criteria? J Urol. 2010; 183(2):539–44.
9. Bul M, Zhu X, Rannikko A, Staerman F, Valdagni R, Pickles T, et al. Radical prostatectomy for low-risk prostate cancer following initial active surveillance: results from a prospective observational study. Eur Urol. 2012; 62(2):195–200.
10. Bjurlin MA, Carter HB, Schellhammer P, Cookson MS, Gomella LG, Troyer D, et al. Optimization of initial prostate biopsy in clinical practice: sampling, labeling and specimen processing. J Urol. 2013;189(6):2039–46.
11. Sedelaar JP, van Roermund JG, van Leenders GL, van de Kaa CA H, Wijkstra H, de la Rosette JJ. Three-dimensional grayscale ultrasound: evaluation of prostate cancer compared with benign prostatic hyperplasia. Urology. 2001; 57(5):914–20.
12. Mehta SS, Azzouzi AR, Hamdy FC. Three dimensional ultrasound and prostate cancer. World J Urol. 2004 Nov;22(5):339–45.
13. Mitterberger M, Pinggera GM, Pallwein L, Gradl J, Frauscher F, Bartsch G, et al. The value of three-dimensional transrectal ultrasonography in staging prostate cancer. BJU Int. 2007 Jul;100(1):47–50.
14. Cool D, Sherebrin S, Izawa J, Chin J, Fenster A. Design and evaluation of a 3D transrectal ultrasound prostate biopsy system. Medical physics. 2008; 35(10):4695–707.
15. Cohen M, Cytron S, Nativ O, Shmitz A, Yudkevich B, Shental J. 816 3D TRUS prostate biopsy recording and guidance - the Navigo system. Eur Urol Suppl. 2012;11(1):e816,e816a.
16. Chin JL, Downey DB, Mulligan M, Fenster A. Three-dimensional transrectal ultrasound guided cryoablation for localized prostate cancer in nonsurgical candidates: a feasibility study and report of early results. J Urol. 1998;159(3): 910–4.
17. Peltier A, Aoun F, El-Khoury F, Hawaux E, Limani K, Narahari K, et al. 3D versus 2D systematic Transrectal ultrasound-guided prostate biopsy: higher Cancer detection rate in clinical practice. Prostate cancer. 2013; 2013:783243.
18. Pryaluhkin AE, Vandromme A, Dellmann A, Donhuijsen K, Hammerer PG. Prostate biopsy core handling: comparison of contemporary preembedding methods. Urol Int. 2015;95(2):203–8.
19. Rogatsch H, Mairinger T, Horninger W, Gschwendtner A, Bartsch G, Mikuz G. Optimized preembedding method improves the histologic yield of prostate core needle biopsies. Prostate. 2000;42(2):124–9.
20. Rogatsch H, Moser P, Volgger H, Horninger W, Bartsch G, Mikuz G, et al. Diagnostic effect of an improved preembedding method of prostate needle biopsy specimens. Hum Pathol. 2000;31(9):1102–7.
21. Cohen M, Shefler A, Patsiansky S, Shapira-Schweitzer K, Nativ O, Bejar J. The SmartBx™ – initial experience with a semi-automated prostate biopsy core download system. Poster presented at the 6th international symposium on

focal therapy and imaging in prostate and kidney Cancer, Amsterdam. Poster retrieved from: https://www.focaltherapy.org/2013/Poster_Abstracts/Focal_2013_PP-22a.pdf.

22. Bokhorst LP, Zhu X, Bul M, Bangma CH, Schröder FH, Roobol MJ. Positive predictive value of prostate biopsy indicated by prostate-specific-antigen-based prostate cancer screening: trends over time in a European randomized trial*. BJU Int. 2012;110(11):1654–60.
23. Roobol MJ, van Vugt HA, Loeb S, Zhu X, Bul M, Bangma CH, et al. Prediction of prostate cancer risk: the role of prostate volume and digital rectal examination in the ERSPC risk calculators. Eur Urol. 2012;61(3):577–83. https://doi.org/10.1016/j.eururo.2011.11.012
24. Lawrentschuk N, Toi A, Lockwood GA, Evans A, Finelli A, O'Malley M, et al. Operator is an independent predictor of detecting prostate cancer at transrectal ultrasound guided prostate biopsy. J Urol. 2009;182(6):2659–63.
25. Gayet M, van der Aa A, Schmitz P, Beerlage HP, Schrier BP, Mulders PF, et al. 3D Navigo™ versus TRUS-guided prostate biopsy in prostate cancer detection. World J Urol. 2016;34(9):1255–60.
26. Cool DW, Connolly MJ, Sherebrin S, Eagleson R, Izawa JI, Amann J, et al. Repeat prostate biopsy accuracy: simulator-based comparison of two- and three dimensional transrectal USmodalities. Radiology. 2010;254(2):587–94.
27. Wan G, Wei Z, Gardi L, Downey DB, Fenster A. Brachytherapy needle deflection evaluation and correction. Med Phys. 2005;32:902–9.
28. Iczkowski KA, Casella G, Seppala RJ, Jones GL, Mishler BA, Qian J, et al. Needle core length in sextant biopsy influences prostate cancer detection rate. Urology. 2002;59(5):698–703.
29. Epstein JI, Egevad L, Amin MB, Delahunt B, Srigley JR, Humphrey PA, et al. The 2014 International Society of Urological Pathology (ISUP) consensus conference on Gleason grading of prostatic carcinoma: definition of grading patterns and proposal for a new grading system. Am J Surg Pathol. 2016;40(2):244–52.
30. Kasivisvanathan V, Rannikko AS, Borghi M, Panebianco V, Mynderse LA, Vaarala MH, et al. MRI-targeted or standard biopsy for prostate-Cancer diagnosis. N Engl J Med. 2018;378(19):1767–77. https://doi.org/10.1056/NEJMoa1801993
31. Rouvière O, Puech P, Renard-Penna R, Claudon M, Roy C, Mège-Lechevallier F. Use of prostate systematic and targeted biopsy on the basis of multiparametric MRI in biopsy-naive patients (MRI-FIRST): a prospective, multicentre, paired diagnostic study. Lancet Oncol. 2019;20(1):100–9.
32. van der Leest M, Cornel E, Israel B, Hendriks R, Padhani AR, Hoogenboom M, et al. Head-to-head comparison of Transrectal ultrasound-guided prostate biopsy versus multiparametric prostate resonance imaging with subsequent magnetic resonance-guided biopsy in biopsy-naïve men with elevated prostate-specific antigen: a large prospective multicenter clinical study. Eur Urol. 2018; In Press.
33. Moldovan PC, van den Broeck T, Sylvester R, Marconi L, Bellmunt J, van den Bergh RCN, et al. What is the negative predictive value of multiparametric magnetic resonance imaging in excluding prostate Cancer at biopsy? A systematic review and meta-analysis from the European Association of Urology prostate Cancer guidelines panel. Eur Urol. 2017;72(2):250–66.

18

A phosphodiesterase 5 inhibitor, tadalafil, suppresses stromal predominance and inflammation in a rat model of nonbacterial prostatitis

Mikio Sugimoto*, Xia Zhang, Nobufumi Ueda, Hiroyuki Tsunemori, Rikiya Taoka, Yusi Hayashida, Hiromi Hirama, Yasuyuki Miyauchi, Yuki Matsuoka, Hirohito Naito, Yu Osaki and Yosiyuki Kekehi

Abstract

Background: Chronic inflammation is thought to be a major causative factor for the development of benign prostatic hyperplasia (BPH) and lower urinary tract symptoms (LUTS). Tadalafil, a phosphodiesterase type 5 inhibitor (PDE5-I), which has been used for the treatment of BPH-LUTS in daily practice, is known to act at several urinary organs. In this study, focused on the prostate, we examined the effect of tadalafil on the pathological changes and inflammatory factors in a rat nonbacterial prostatitis (NBP) model.

Methods: Forty ten-month-old male Wistar rats were divided into nonbacterial prostatitis (NBP), NBP with tadalafil treatment (NBP-tadalafil), control, and control treated with tadalafil (control-tadalafil) groups ($n = 10$ per group). The NBP and NBP-tadalafil groups were castrated and then received daily subcutaneous 17β-estradiol for 30 days. The control-tadalafil and NBP-tadalafil groups were administered daily oral tadalafil for 30 days. All rats were then sacrificed and pathological changes and inflammatory factors were assessed in the prostatic tissues.

Results: In the NBP group, the stroma-to-epithelium (S/E) ratio in the ventral prostate was significantly higher than in the control group ($P < 0.001$). In the NBP-tadalafil group, the S/E ratio was significantly lower than in the NBP group ($P < 0.001$). The macrophage levels and the extent of T-cell infiltration in the NBP-tadalafil group were significantly lower than in the NBP group ($P < 0.005$; $P < 0.001$, respectively). Compared with the NBP group, tissue concentrations of inflammatory cytokines, such as tumor necrosis factor-α, interleukin-8, and interleukin-1β, were significantly downregulated in the NBP-tadalafil group ($P < 0.01$; $P < 0.05$; $P < 0.005$, respectively).

Conclusions: Tadalafil suppressed stromal predominance and showed anti-inflammatory effects in a rat NBP model in association with downregulation of inflammatory cytokines.

Keywords: Benign prostatic hyperplasia, Inflammatory cytokines, Lower urinary tract symptoms, Nonbacterial prostatitis, Tadalafil

* Correspondence: micsugi@med.kagawa-u.ac.jp
Department of Urology, Kagawa University Faculty of Medicine, 1750-1 Ikenobe, Miki-cho, Kita-gun, Kagawa 761-0793, Japan

Background

Lower urinary tract symptoms (LUTS) associated with benign prostatic hyperplasia (BPH) is common in aging males worldwide. Because LUTS/BPH often interferes with activities of daily living, many patients seek definitive treatment to improve their quality of life [1–3].

The etiology of LUTS is highly complex and is likely to be multifactorial, and several processes may contribute to the development of LUTS in BPH. Chronic inflammation in the prostate may contribute to prostate growth, tissue damage, and prostate enlargement [4]. The Medical Therapies of Prostate Symptoms (MTOPS) study, the largest study to examine chronic prostatic inflammation, suggests that the risk of serious BPH-related outcomes, including acute urinary retention and the need for BPH-related surgery, is increased. Therefore it is important to study the action of clinically used drugs on prostatic inflammation.

Phosphodiesterase type 5 inhibitors (PDE5-Is), such as tadalafil, are effective for the treatment of LUTS/BPH [5, 6], and have been acknowledged in the recent guidelines published by the Japanese Urological Association [7] and the European Association of Urology [8], with Level 1 evidence. Several LUT tissues—prostate, urethra, and bladder, as well as their vasculatures—are thought to be potential targets for tadalafil [9]. There are several reports focused on prostate inflammation regarding the mechanism of tadalafil in several animal models. Single or repeated dosing with tadalafil improves prostate hypoxia in spontaneously hypertensive rats [10]. In the prostate of rabbits fed a high-fat diet, chronic tadalafil treatment produces inhibition of inflammation, fibrosis, and hypoxia [11]. More recently, repeated treatment with tadalafil was found to suppress tactile allodynia in rat non-bacterial prostatitis induced by 17β-estradiol treatment combined with castration [12]. Although inflammatory changes, including histopathological changes and increases in several cytokine/chemokine levels, were demonstrated in this model in the absence of tadalafil treatment, whether tadalafil affects these kinds of pathological conditions in this hormone/castration-induced prostatitis model was not investigated [12].

This study aimed to elucidate the effect of the repeated administration of tadalafil on the inflammatory changes in a rat model of hormone/castration-induced prostatitis as a model of nonbacterial prostatitis (NBP) as indicated by changes in prostate histology and inflammatory factors.

Methods

Animals

Forty adult male 40-week-old Wistar rats (580–720 g) were purchased from Charles River Laboratories (Yokohama, Japan). Rats were housed in a climate-controlled room and allowed free access to food and water according to the Guide for the Care and Use of Laboratory Animals of Kagawa University.

Preparation of tadalafil

Tadalafil (Cayman Chemical; Ann Arbor, MI, USA) was suspended in 0.5% methylcellulose solution (Wako, Japan) to yield a concentration of 2 mg/ml for oral administration.

Experimental design

The 40 rats were numbered and randomly divided into 4 groups of 10 each by means of a random digits table, i.e., NBP, NBP with tadalafil treatment (NPB-tadalafil), control, and control treated with tadalafil (control-tadalafil) groups. NBP was induced according to the method of Kamijo et al. [13]. Briefly, the rats in the NBP and NBP-tadalafil groups underwent castration and then were injected subcutaneously with a daily dose of 0.25 mg/kg 17β-estradiol in 0.1 ml sesame oil for 30 days. Meanwhile, the control-tadalafil and NBP-tadalafil groups received once-daily oral tadalafil at a dose 5 ml/kg. After 30 days of tadalafil treatment, the rats were deeply anesthetized with an intraperitoneal injection of sodium pentobarbital at 200 mg/kg. Ventral prostate tissue was obtained from all rats. Some tissue samples were stored at − 80 °C for cytokine assay and the remaining tissue was fixed in 10% neutral buffered formalin and embedded in paraffin, after which 3–4 μm serial sections were made and examined histologically.

Immunohistochemical staining

After deparaffinization, immunohistochemical staining was performed using the avidin-biotin-peroxidase complex method (SAB-PO Kit; Vector Laboratories Inc., Burlingame, CA, USA) and microwave antigen retrieval. The primary antibodies were antimacrophage rat monoclonal antibody ab56297 (Abcam, Cambridge, UK) and anti-CD3 rabbit monoclonal antibody ab16669 (Abcam). The anti-CD3 antibody was an anti-rat T-cell antibody used to identify infiltrating T-cells. The macrophages and T-cells in the sections were counted in five randomly selected fields under 400× magnification and the average was calculated.

Evaluation of stroma-to-epithelium ratio

To evaluate the stroma-to-epithelium (S/E) ratio in the rat ventral prostate, Masson trichrome staining was performed and a computerized image-analysis system was used, as previously reported [14]. The slides were photographed using a BX51 light microscope (Olympus, Tokyo, Japan) and then analyzed with WinRoof image-analysis software (Ver. 3.6, Mitani Corporation, Japan).

Determination of cytokines

The levels of cytokines in the supernatant of the prostate homogenate was measured as described previously [14]. Tumor necrosis factor-α (TNF-α) and interleukin-1β (IL-1β) enzyme-linked immunosorbent assay kits from R&D Systems (Minneapolis, MN, USA), and an interleukin-8 (IL-8) kit from LifeSpan BioSciences (Seattle, WA, USA) were used for the assays. Each assay was performed three times.

Statistical analysis

Data analysis was performed using IBM SPSS software (Ver. 20; IBM, Armonk, NY, USA). The number of macrophages and T-cells, the S/E ratio in the rat prostate, and the tissue concentration of cytokines were all presented as the mean ± SD. One-way analysis of variance (ANOVA) followed by Tukey's HSD test was used for comparison of groups. A result was considered statistically significant when the P-value was ≤0.05.

Results

Effect of tadalafil on rat body and prostate weights

After 30 days of treatment, the mean rat body weights (BW) and prostate weights (PW) in the NBP and NBP-tadalafil groups were significantly lower than in the control group (BW: $P < 0.001$, $P < 0.001$; PW: $P < 0.001$, $P < 0.001$, respectively). The mean PW and BW were not significantly different between the control and control-tadalafil groups. Toxicity associated with tadalafil treatment was not apparent throughout the study (Table 1).

Effect of tadalafil on histopathological features in the prostate

The S/E ratios in NBP rats were higher than in the non-prostatitis control rats. The administration of tadalafil significantly suppressed stromal predominance ($P < 0.001$; Fig. 1). High macrophage levels and extent of T-cell infiltration surrounding the gland were observed in rats with prostatitis. The numbers of macrophages and T-cells in the ventral prostate of control rats with prostatitis were greater than in non-prostatitis control rats ($P < 0.005$, $P < 0.001$, respectively; Figs. 2 and 3).

Table 1 Body and prostate weight in NBP, NBP-tadalafil, control and control-tadalafil groups

Group	No. Rats	Mean ± SD (g) Body weight	Prostate weight
NBP	10	561.9 ± 32.4**	0.45 ± 0.11**
NBP-tadalafil	10	581.4 ± 30.9**	0.65 ± 0.14**
Control	9	730.1 ± 52.4	1.34 ± 0.36
Control-tadalafil	10	694.8 ± 27.3	1.18 ± 0.43

NBP nonbacterial prostatitis, *NBP-tadalafil* NBP with tadalafil treatment, *Control-tadalafil* Control with tadalafil treatment. Significant differences compared with control group, ** $P < 0.01$

Tadalafil treatment resulted in significantly reduced macrophage and T-cell infiltration in the NBP rats ($P < 0.001$, $P < 0.001$, respectively; Figs. 2 and 3), but had no effect in non-prostatitis rats.

Effect of tadalafil on proinflammatory cytokine levels

The tissue concentrations of three representative proinflammatory cytokines, TNF-α, IL-8, and IL-1β, were determined. These cytokines are considered to be induced by macrophage infiltration, and they were significantly higher in the prostatitis group. Oral administration of tadalafil markedly suppressed the concentrations of all three cytokines in the NBP rat prostate ($P < 0.01$, $P < 0.05$, $P < 0.005$, respectively; Fig. 4). There was no significant effect of tadalafil on the concentrations of these cytokines in non-prostatitis rats.

Discussion

Chronic inflammation (mostly nonbacterial and asymptomatic) is associated with symptom development in BPH [4]. To investigate the underlying mechanisms of chronic inflammation in the prostate that are responsible for symptomatic BPH, experimental animal models with inflammatory prostatitis are needed. Kamijo et al. [13] and our group [14–16] used 10-month-old rats treated with 17β-estradiol for 30 days after castration to investigate the effects of therapeutic agents such as cernitin pollen extract and Eviprostat. Therefore, this was an appropriate model to use for evaluation of the effects of drugs on inflammatory changes in the prostate. Although this animal model does not match human BPH in prostate size or glandular hyperplasia, it demonstrates certain characteristics, including severe acinar gland atrophy and stromal predominance, in addition to inflammatory infiltrates, which mimic symptom progression in BPH.

Recently Yamaguchi et al. [12] found that an increase in pelvic pain is induced in this NBP model and that this pain is suppressed by repeated treatment with tadalafil. However, they did not investigate the effects of tadalafil on inflammatory changes. In the present study, we demonstrated for the first time that the administration of tadalafil showed a reduction in macrophage levels and the extent of T-cell infiltration in the same NBP model. Meanwhile, the increased concentrations of TNF-α, IL-8, and IL-1β in the prostate tissue of NBP rats were also suppressed in the tadalafil administration group. We assume that the attenuation of pelvic pain shown by Yamaguchi et al. [12] is partly due to these effects of tadalafil. IL-1β and TNF-α are both pro-inflammatory cytokines and reported to be up-regulated in prostatic sections of prostatitis, suggesting that these are the key markers in inflammatory prostate [17]. IL-8 also seems to be a key mediator in human BPH: its concentrations

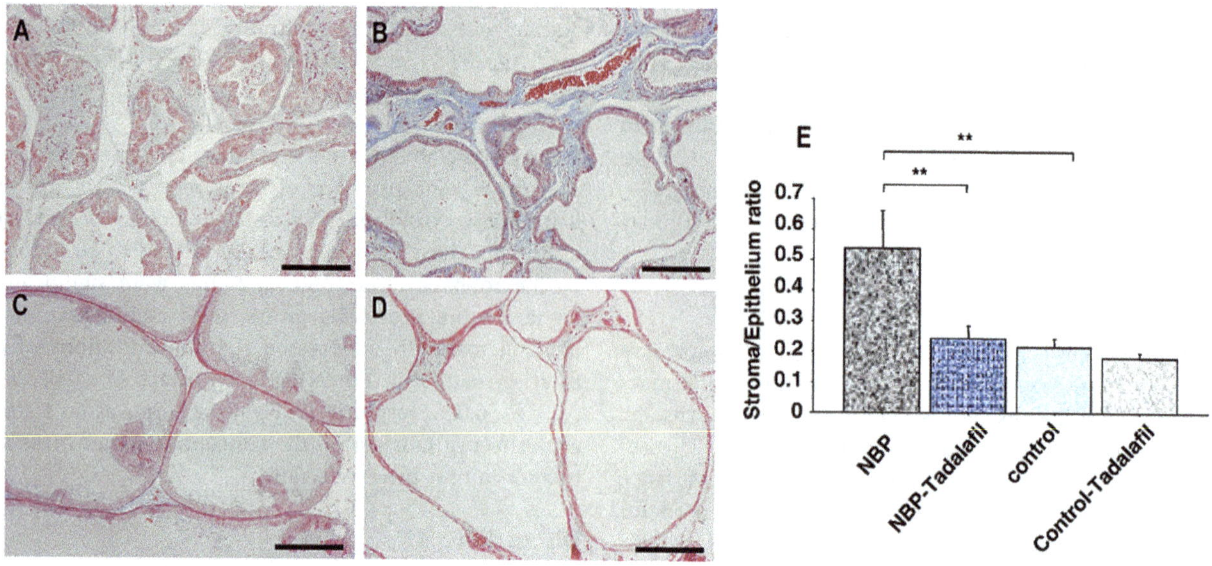

Fig. 1 Masson trichrome staining of prostate tissue sections in NBP (**a**), NPB-tadalafil (**b**), control (**c**), and control-tadalafil (**d**) groups. Scale bars represent 100 μm. Effect of tadalafil on mean stroma-to-epithelium ratio in the prostate of NBP and non-NBP rats (**e**). Each bar represents the mean ± SD. * $P < 0.05$, ** $P < 0.01$

in prostatic secretions from patients with BPH accompanied by inflammation are higher than in patients with BPH alone [18].

This study is consistent with other available evidence that PDE5-Is reduce chronic inflammation in the prostate, because several investigators have reported their anti-inflammatory effects in different animal models such as metabolic syndrome-induced prostatitis in the rabbit [11] and spontaneously hypertensive rats [10], as well as in human BPH cells [19]. In addition, tadalafil has protective effects on prostatic structural and functional changes induced by chronic pelvic ischemia [20]. Moreover, in a rat model of experimental autoimmune prostatitis, tadalafil reduces prostatic inflammation [21].

The latest evidence on the pathophysiology of LUTS/BPH has provided the rationale for use of PDE5-Is, which bring about improvement of LUT oxygenation, smooth muscle relaxation, negative regulation of proliferation, transdifferentiation of LUT stroma, and reduction of bladder afferent nerve activity [22]. Besides protection of the prostate by tadalafil, several investigators have shown the effect of tadalafil on chronic ischemia-related bladder dysfunction in animal models, including a rat model of chronic pelvic ischemia [23]

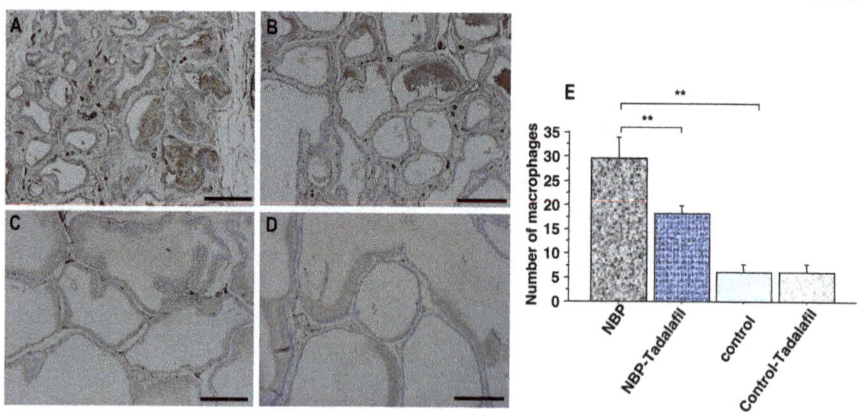

Fig. 2 Immunohistochemical staining of paraffin-embedded prostate tissue sections with anti-macrophage antibody in NBP (**a**), NPB-tadalafil (**b**), control (**c**), and control-tadalafil (**d**) groups. Scale bars represent 100 μm. Effect of tadalafil on macrophage infiltration in the prostate of NBP and non-NBP rats (**e**). Each bar represents the mean ± SD. * $P < 0.05$, ** $P < 0.01$

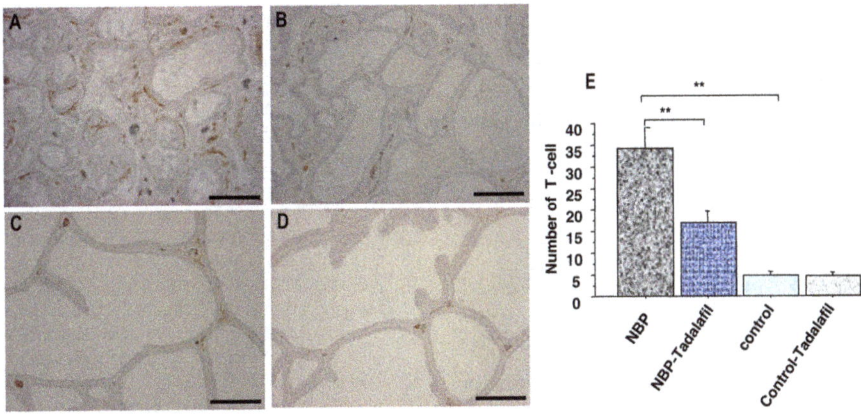

Fig. 3 Immunohistochemical staining of paraffin-embedded prostate tissue sections with anti-CD3 antibody in NBP (**a**), NPB-tadalafil (**b**), control (**c**), and control-tadalafil (**d**) groups. Scale bars represent 100 μm. Effect of tadalafil on T-cell infiltration in the prostate of NBP and non-NBP groups (**e**). Each bar represents the mean ± SD. * $P < 0.05$, ** $P < 0.01$

and bladder outlet obstruction [24]. It has been hypothesized that PDE5-Is could reduce inflammation and the associated fibrosis and improve oxygenation in the human prostate and bladder, with normalization of prostatic and bladder structural anatomy and physiologic activity. All of these effects of tadalafil may contribute to the amelioration of bladder dysfunction.

Previous studies have evaluated the pharmacological effects of tadalafil in animal models, almost all of which used oral administration of tadalafil at doses of 2 or 10 mg/kg. For example, Morelli et al. [10] demonstrated an improvement in prostate gland oxygenation by tadalafil at 2 mg/kg/day for 1, 7 or 28 days. Nomiya et al. [23] have described the protective effects of tadalafil on bladder function at 2 mg/kg/day for 8 weeks in a rat model of chronic bladder ischemia induced by iliac arterial endothelial injury. Kawai et al. [24] reported that the repeated administration of tadalafil at 10 mg/kg/day for 14 days ameliorated the bladder function in a rat model of bladder outlet obstruction. According to these reports, in this study we used tadalafil at 10 mg/kg/day for 30 days. Recently Yoshinaga et al. [25] reported that C_{max} values of 68.5 and 460 ng/ml in rats after single oral doses of tadalafil of 2 and 10 mg/kg, respectively are physiologically relevant with the clinical plasma concentration of tadalafil is 95.6 ng/ml when the drug is administered at 5 mg/person (for BPH patients) and 446 ng/ml when it is administered at 40 mg/person (for PAH patients). Since the doses of tadalafil used in current studies are similar to the plasma concentrations in humans being treated for BPH and PAH, the results we showed in the paper partly may explain the protective mechanisms of Tadalafil in BPH patients.

In the present study, the anti-inflammatory effect of tadalafil was demonstrated in the NBP rat model. However, this model is hormone-induced, and there is are anatomic differences between the rat and the human prostate. The effect of tadalafil on the relief of LUTS

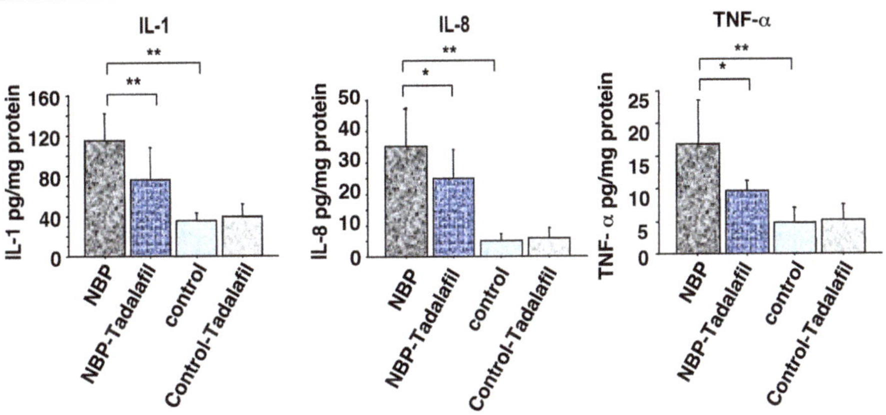

Fig. 4 Effect of tadalafil on IL-1β, IL-8, and TNF-α levels in the prostate of NBP and non-NBP rats. Each assay was performed three times and each bar represents the mean ± SD ($n = 10$). * $P < 0.05$, ** $P < 0.01$

cannot therefore be assessed in this model. Despite this experimental limitation, the results obtained in the present study partially clarify the mechanism by which tadalafil prevents the development of BPH through the suppression of nonbacterial inflammation. To elucidate the mechanism of the effect of tadalafil in more detail, further study is needed.

Conclusion

The phosphodiesterase 5 inhibitor tadalafil suppressed the increase in inflammatory factors and stromal proliferation in a rat model of nonbacterial prostatitis, providing evidence for anti-inflammatory effects of tadalafil in this model.

Abbreviations

BPH: Benign prostatic hyperplasia; BW: Body weights; control-tadalafil: control treated with tadalafil; IL-1β: Interleukin-1β; IL-8: Interleukin-8; LUTS: Lower urinary tract symptoms; MTOPS: Medical Therapy of Prostate Symptoms; NBP: Nonbacterial prostatitis; NBP-tadalafil: NBP with tadalafil treatment; NO/cGMP: Nitric oxide cyclic-guanine monophosphate; PDE5-I: Phosphodiesterase type 5 inhibitor; PW: Prostate weights; S/E: Stroma-to-epithelium; TNF-α: Tumor necrosis factor-α

Acknowledgements

Not applicable

Authors' contributions

(MS, XZ, NU, HT, RT, YH, HH, YM[1], YM[2], HN, YO, YK) Conception and design: MS and YK; MS, XZ, NU, HT, RT, YH, HH, YM[1], YM[2], HN and YO carried out the experiments; data analysis: MS, XZ, NU, RT, HH, YH, YM[1], YM[2], and YO; drafting of the manuscript: MS, XZ, HT, HH, HN, YK; statistical analysis: XZ, HH and HT; interpretation of data: MS, XZ, HT and YK. We confirm that all authors read and approved the final manuscript. All authors read and approved the final manuscript.

References

1. Irwin DE, Milsom I, Hunskaar S, Reilly K, Kopp Z, Herschorn S, Coyne K, Kelleher C, Hampel C, Artibani W, et al. Population-based survey of urinary incontinence, overactive bladder, and other lower urinary tract symptoms in five countries: results of the EPIC study. Eur Urol. 2006;50(6):1306-14 discussion S1314-1305.
2. Coyne KS, Sexton CC, Thompson CL, Milsom I, Irwin D, Kopp ZS, Chapple CR, Kaplan S, Tubaro A, Aiyer LP, et al. The prevalence of lower urinary tract symptoms (LUTS) in the USA, the UK and Sweden: results from the epidemiology of LUTS (EpiLUTS) study. BJU Int. 2009;104(3):352–60.
3. Li MK, Garcia LA, Rosen R. Lower urinary tract symptoms and male sexual dysfunction in Asia: a survey of ageing men from five Asian countries. BJU Int. 2005;96(9):1339–54.
4. Kramer G, Mitteregger D, Marberger M. Is benign prostatic hyperplasia (BPH) an immune inflammatory disease? Eur Urol. 2007;51(5):1202–16.
5. Uckert S, Oelke M. Phosphodiesterase (PDE) inhibitors in the treatment of lower urinary tract dysfunction. Br J Clin Pharmacol. 2011;72(2):197–204.
6. Cantrell MA, Baye J, Vouri SM. Tadalafil: a phosphodiesterase-5 inhibitor for benign prostatic hyperplasia. Pharmacotherapy. 2013;33(6):639–49.
7. Homma Y, Gotoh M, AKawauchi A, Kojima Y, Maeda K, Masumori N, Nagai A, Saitoh T, Sakai H, Takahashi S, et al. Clinical guidelines for male lower urinary tract symptoms and benign prostatic hyperplasia. Tokyo: RichHill Medical Inc.; 2017.
8. Oelke M, Bachmann A, Descazeaud A, Emberton M, Gravas S, Michel MC, N'Dow J, Nordling J, de la Rosette JJ. European Association of U: EAU guidelines on the treatment and follow-up of non-neurogenic male lower urinary tract symptoms including benign prostatic obstruction. Eur Urol. 2013;64(1):118–40.
9. Giuliano F, Uckert S, Maggi M, Birder L, Kissel J, Viktrup L. The mechanism of action of phosphodiesterase type 5 inhibitors in the treatment of lower urinary tract symptoms related to benign prostatic hyperplasia. Eur Urol. 2013;63(3):506–16.
10. Morelli A, Sarchielli E, Comeglio P, Filippi S, Mancina R, Gacci M, Vignozzi L, Carini M, Vannelli GB, Maggi M. Phosphodiesterase type 5 expression in human and rat lower urinary tract tissues and the effect of tadalafil on prostate gland oxygenation in spontaneously hypertensive rats. J Sex Med. 2011;8(10):2746–60.
11. Morelli A, Comeglio P, Filippi S, Sarchielli E, Vignozzi L, Maneschi E, Cellai I, Gacci M, Lenzi A, Vannelli GB, et al. Mechanism of action of phosphodiesterase type 5 inhibition in metabolic syndrome-associated prostate alterations: an experimental study in the rabbit. Prostate. 2013;73(4):428–41.
12. Yamaguchi H, Kurita M, Okamoto K, Kotera T, Oka M. Voiding behavior and chronic pelvic pain in two types of rat nonbacterial prostatitis models: attenuation of chronic pelvic pain by repeated administration of tadalafil. Prostate. 2019;79(5):446–53.
13. Kamijo T, Sato S, Kitamura T. Effect of cernitin pollen-extract on experimental nonbacterial prostatitis in rats. Prostate. 2001;49(2):122–31.
14. Tsunemori H, Sugimoto M, Xia Z, Taoka R, Oka M, Kakehi Y. Effect of the phytotherapeutic agent Eviprostat on inflammatory changes and cytokine production in a rat model of nonbacterial prostatitis. Urology. 2011;77(6): 1507 e1515–20.
15. Sugimoto M, Oka M, Tsunemori H, Yamashita M, Kakehi Y. Effect of a phytotherapeutic agent, Eviprostat (R), on prostatic and urinary cytokines/chemokines in a rat model of nonbacterial prostatitis. Prostate. 2011;71(4):438–44.
16. Shibuya S, Xia Z, Sugimoto M, Ueda N, Haba R, Kakehi Y. The phytotherapeutic agent, eviprostat, suppresses stromal proliferation and inflammation even after establishment of nonbacterial prostatitis in the rat prostate. Urology. 2014;83(3):528–34.
17. Nadler RB, Koch AE, Calhoun EA, Campbell PL, Pruden DL, Bennett CL, Yarnold PR, Schaeffer A. IL-1beta and TNF-alpha in prostatic secretions are indicators in the evaluation of men with chronic prostatitis. J Urol. 2000; 164(1):214–8.
18. Liu L, Li Q, Han P, Li X, Zeng H, Zhu Y, Wei Q. Evaluation of interleukin-8 in expressed prostatic secretion as a reliable biomarker of inflammation in benign prostatic hyperplasia. Urology. 2009;74(2):340–4.
19. Vignozzi L, Gacci M, Cellai I, Morelli A, Maneschi E, Comeglio P, Santi R, Filippi S, Sebastianelli A, Nesi G, et al. PDE5 inhibitors blunt inflammation in human BPH: a potential mechanism of action for PDE5 inhibitors in LUTS. Prostate. 2013;73(13):1391–402.
20. Zarifpour M, Nomiya M, Sawada N, Andersson KE. Protective effect of tadalafil on the functional and structural changes of the rat ventral prostate caused by chronic pelvic ischemia. Prostate. 2015;75(3):233–41.
21. Okamoto K, Kurita M, Yamaguchi H, Numakura Y, Oka M. Effect of tadalafil on chronic pelvic pain and prostatic inflammation in a rat model of experimental autoimmune prostatitis. Prostate. 2018;78(10):707–13.
22. Gacci M, Andersson KE, Chapple C, Maggi M, Mirone V, Oelke M, Porst H, Roehrborn C, Stief C, Giuliano F. Latest evidence on the use of Phosphodiesterase type 5 inhibitors for the treatment of lower urinary tract symptoms secondary to benign prostatic hyperplasia. Eur Urol. 2016;70(1): 124–33.
23. Nomiya M, Burmeister DM, Sawada N, Campeau L, Zarifpour M, Keys T, Peyton C, Yamaguchi O, Andersson KE. Prophylactic effect of tadalafil on bladder function in a rat model of chronic bladder ischemia. J Urol. 2013; 189(2):754–61.
24. Kawai Y, Oka M, Yoshinaga R, Fuchikami C, Oyama T. Effects of the phosphodiesterase 5 inhibitor Tadalafil on bladder function in a rat model of partial bladder outlet obstruction. Neurourol Urodyn. 2016;35(4):444–9.
25. Yoshinaga R, Fukui T, Yoshifuji M, Fujimura M, Oyama T, Oka M. Comparison of the effects of Tadalafil and α_1-Adrenoceptor antagonists on spontaneous seminal emission and electrical field stimulation-induced seminal vesicle contraction in rats. J Sex Med. 2019;16(5):680–90.

19

Dysuria due to benign prostatic hyperplasia of the median lobe with ketamine-associated uropathy in a young male

Zhangcheng Liao[1,2], Zhao Wang[1], Zhongyuan Jin[3] and Zhengyan Tang[1,2,4*]

Abstract

Background: Benign prostatic hyperplasia (BPH) rarely occurs in children or young males. In this case report, a 29-year-old male patient diagnosed with BPH coexisting with ketamine-associated uropathy was reported to investigate the possible relationship between BPH and ketamine-associated uropathy as well as therapeutic strategies.

Case presentation: A 29-year-old male patient with a 3-year history of ketamine inhalation, complaining of dysuria with frequency and urgency, was admitted. Hydronephrosis, hydroureters, uneven bladder wall thickening and a tumour located in the outlet of the bladder were detected with computed tomography (CT). The patient agreed to cystoscopy under general anaesthesia. A spherical tumour with a diameter of approximately 2 cm was found to originate from the median lobe of the prostate and follicular lesions were diffusely distributed on the right bladder wall. The tumour and follicular lesions in the bladder were resected successfully, and pathology demonstrated BPH and chronic inflammation of the mucous membranes separately. The patient quit ketamine completely during the one-year follow-up. Dysuria was relieved completely and no tumour or follicular neoplasm recurrence was found.

Contribution: Inflammation in the urothelium, as a direct or indirect consequence of ketamine, may contribute to the development of BPH. Both surgical interventions to remove obstruction and ketamine cessation are necessary approaches.

Keywords: Dysuria, Young male, Benign prostatic median lobe hyperplasia, Ketamine-associated uropathy

Background

Benign prostatic hyperplasia (BPH) is a common disease that usually develops in middle-aged and older men. The occurrence of BPH in children or young men seems to be very rare. This report presents a case of BPH with ketamine-associated uropathy in a young patient which, to our knowledge, has never been reported before.

Case presentation

A 29-year-old male patient was admitted on April 2017 because of dysuria with frequency and urgency. The patient began quitting ketamine for one year after 3 years of ketamine inhalation (once weekly at first and then once every 2–3 days up to a maximum of approximately 10 g/day). Duplex ultrasonography of the urinary system showed bilateral hydronephrosis and hydroureters, a thick-walled bladder and a post-void residual volume of approximately 100 ml. Computed tomography (CT) showed moderate bilateral hydronephrosis and hydroureters (Fig. 1a) as well as uneven bladder wall thickening with bladder diverticulum (Fig. 1b and c). A round, vague shadow approximately 2 cm in diameter near the bladder outlet (Fig. 1d) was detected after the CT image had been analysed carefully, but it was hard to distinguish its origin. The patient agreed to cystoscopy under general anaesthesia. A spherical tumour with a diameter of approximately 2 cm was found to originate from the median lobe of the prostate, obstructing the

* Correspondence: xytzyan@163.com
[1]Department of Urology, Xiangya Hospital, Central South University, Changsha, Hunan, China
[2]Provincial Laboratory for Diagnosis and Treatment of Genitourinary System Disease, Changsha, China
Full list of author information is available at the end of the article

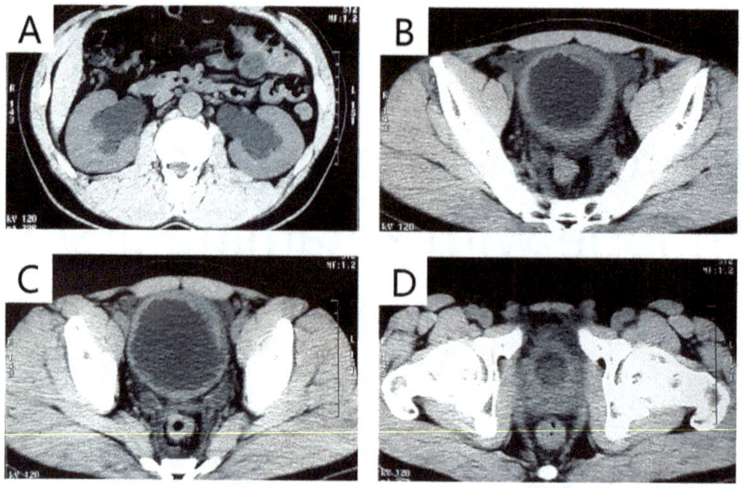

Fig. 1 **a** Bilateral hydronephrosis. **b** and **c** Uneven bladder wall thickening with bladder diverticulum. **d** A round vague shadow near the bladder outlet

prostatic urethra (Fig. 2a), which impeded further progress with cystoscopy. The enlarged median lobe of the prostate was removed with transurethral resection of the prostate (TURP) completely and successfully (Fig. 2b). The bladder capacity was measured to be 200 ml (average of three measurements). Trabeculation and multiple bladder diverticula were visible on the rough mucosal surface of the bladder. On the right wall of the bladder, there was a significant amount of follicular neoplasm (Fig. 2c and d). Follicular lesions were resected completely. The pathology of the enlarged median lobe of the prostate demonstrated benign prostatic hyperplasia (Fig. 3a), and the pathology of the follicular lesions demonstrated chronic inflammation with denudation or loss of epithelium and marked inflammatory infiltration (Fig. 3b). During the one-year follow-up, the patient quit ketamine completely and did not report any complaints except mild frequency which did not trouble him much, and there were no voiding or sexual complaints. Additionally, hydronephrosis and hydroureter were alleviated.

Discussion and conclusions

Prior to 2018, there were approximately 8 reported cases of male patients aged 30 or younger diagnosed with BPH in the literature, as listed in Table 1 [1–8].

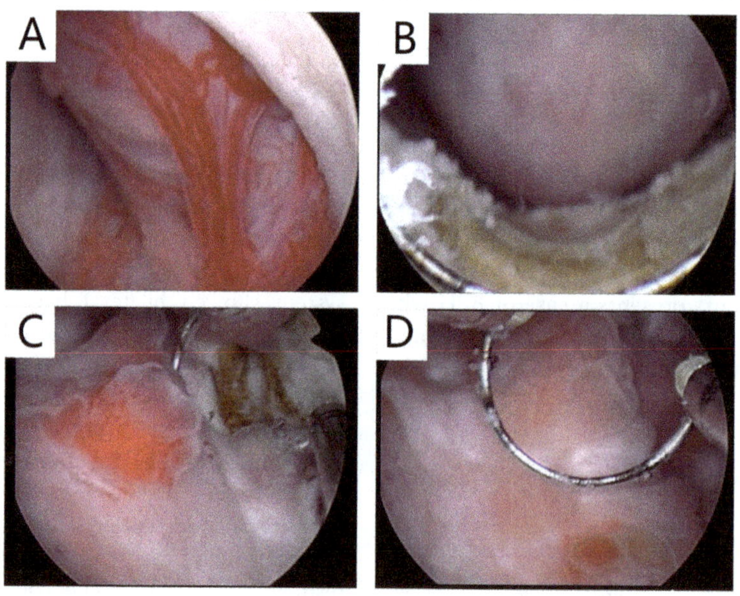

Fig. 2 **a** The enlarged median lobe of the prostate protruding into the urethra and cyst. **b** The enlarged median lobe of the prostate and the surgical wound after TURP. **c** and **d** A fair amount of follicular neoplasm located on the right wall of the bladder

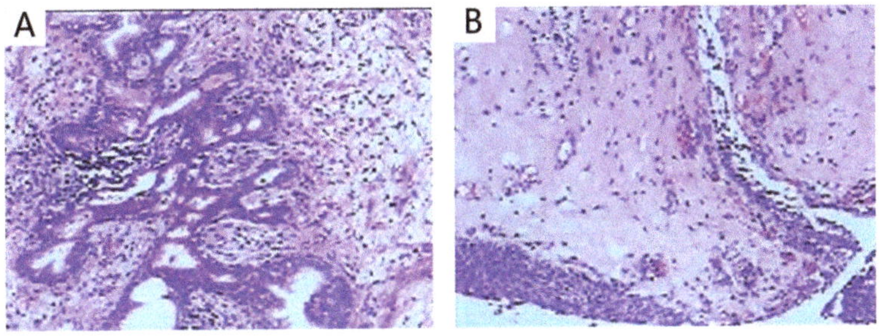

Fig. 3 a Pathology of prostate tissues showing benign prostatic hyperplasia involving both the gland and stroma. The hyperplasic glands are well-differentiated with eosinophilic crystals in the lumen. **b** Pathology of follicular lesions showing chronic inflammation with denudation or loss of epithelium and marked inflammatory infiltration

Of these cases, the youngest was 10 years old, while the oldest was 29 years old. In most cases, the cause was not described. However, some authors illuminated possible pathogenic factors as causes in their cases as follows: Powell [1] reported a man aged 17 years old who developed benign prostatic hyperplasia after gonadotrophin therapy due to cryptorchidism. A case of a 23-year-old man who was admitted with acute urinary retention indicating BPH was reported by Romano et al. [4], who investigated the possible relationship between BPH and acromegaly due to the 2.03-m height of the patient. Zouari et al. [8] reported a 22-year-old man with acute urinary retention caused by BPH whose biopsy during examination indicated glandular cystitis. Unexpectedly, the pathological examination after transurethral resection of the median lobe of the prostate showed BPH. The author concluded that further research was needed to determine the correlation between BPH and cystitis glandularis. Eight patients underwent surgery for open suprapubic transvesical prostatectomy or transurethral resection of the prostate (TURP). Only one patient underwent nonoperative treatment who ever accepted treatment with gonadotropic hormones due to cryptorchidism before the occurrence of BPH [1]. The patient in our case had no history of endocrinological disease or other possible relevant factors except 3-year ketamine inhalation.

Prostate specific antigen (PSA) seems to represent a prominent difference in BPH between elderly men and young males. According to the cases listed in Table 1, all young BPH patients were characterized by a normal PSA range except those who did not have reported PSA levels, and in our case, the PSA level was 1.80 g/ml. Elderly patients usually have a PSA level that is higher than the normal range.

To our knowledge, there has been no case of BPH with ketamine-associated uropathy ever reported in young patients. The exact pathophysiology of ketamine-associated cystitis remains greatly unknown. An important theory is that ketamine and/or its metabolites accumulates at a high concentration in urine, leading to a direct toxic effect on the urothelium and resulting in significant inflammation. The nuclear factor-kappa B (NF-κB) pathway was found to be activated during inflammatory signalling of ketamine-induced cystitis in the bladder in a rat model [9]. Furthermore, there exists a significant increase in pro-inflammatory cytokines, such as IL-1β, IL-2, IL-4, IL-6, IFN-γ, NGF, and COX-2, in bladder tissue in ketamine-associated cystitis [10, 11]. Similarly, although ageing and androgens are the two established risk factors in the progression of benign prostatic hyperplasia (BPH), the pathogenesis of BPH is still largely unresolved. Currently, increasing evidence indicates that inflammation is strongly involved in the aetiology and progression of BPH. Particularly, it has been identified that inflammatory cytokines, IL2, IL4, IL7, IL17, IFN-γ and their relevant receptors are upregulated in and that inflammatory cells infiltrate into BPH tissues [12–14]. Anti-inflammatory agent was proved to produce an antiproliferative effect during BPH by markedly decreased BPH-related upregulation of COX-2 protein expression [15]. It is possible that inflammation in the urinary tract due to the direct and indirect effects of ketamine stimulates the enlargement of the prostate. However, few studies have investigated the direct effect of ketamine or its metabolites on the prostate, and their relationship needs to be confirmed with further research.

Ketamine-induced upper urinary tract lesions seem not to be paid enough attention due to a greater incidence of apparent lower urinary tract syndromes [16]. Hydronephrosis and ureteral wall thickening were reported most frequently in ketamine-induced upper urinary tract damage. According to clinical case summaries, the incidence of hydronephrosis (bilateral or unilateral) can be as high as 44.4% [17] or 51% [18]. Huang LK et al. [17] reported three patients with unilateral hydronephrosis and nine with bilateral hydronephrosis among twelve ketamine-induced uropathy patients with hydronephrosis. In addition, nine patients had ureteral wall thickening, and two had ureterovesical junction involvement.

Table 1 BPH in children or young men < 30 years old

author	time	age	symptoms	PSA	treatment	comments
Powell	1939	17	dysuria	not mentioned	conservative treatments	gonadotrophin administration for the treatment of cryptorchidism.
Sumiya	1987	20	Dysuria, pain in the perineal area	not mentioned	suprapubic prostatectomy, excisional tissues 380 g	
Harada	1989	28	Dysuria, haematuria	not mentioned	suprapubic prostatectomy, excisional tissues 31 g	
Romano	2001	23	Dysuria, acute urinary retention, urinary incontinence, enuresis	not mentioned	TURP, excisional tissues approximately 38 g	Combined with acromegaly, height 2.03 m.
Choi	2005	10	Dysuria, uroschesis, haematuria	0.02 ng/ml.	TURP, excisional tissues approximately 33 g	The same patient was diagnosed with BPH at 10 and 13 years old.
		13	Dysuria, fever, weakness	0.04 ng/ml	suprapubic prostatectomy, excisional tissues 55 g	
Georgiades	2014	27	LUTS, haemospermia	0.33 ng/ml	TURP, excisional tissues 181 g	with spermatocystitis, retrograde ejaculation after TURP.
Yagmur	2016	17	Dysuria, acute urinary retention, haematuria	not mentioned	TURP	prostatic hyperplasia of the middle lobe.
Zouari	2018	22	Dysuria, acute urinary retention	1.6 ng/ml	TURP, excisional tissues approximately 60 g	biopsy indicated glandular cystitis, but pathological examination after operation demonstrated BPH.

BPH: benign prostatic hyperplasia
PSA: prostate-specific antigen
TURP: transurethral resection of the prostate
LUTS: lower urinary tract symptoms

Bilateral upper ureteric narrow and mild bilateral hydronephrosis were detected in 3 patients in a 6-patients cases report [19]. Misra S et al. [20] reported that two of 34 patients had bilateral hydronephrosis with hydroureters to the vesicoureteral junction. In another case of A 26-year-old man with ketamine abuse, bilateral hydronephrosis, obstructive nephropathy and kidney injury were detected in spite of no obstruction at the ureteric orifices [21]. Many other studies referred to bilateral or unilateral hydronephrosis in ketamine-related uropathy but did not report the ureteric or renal lesions [18, 22]. In our case, bilateral moderate hydronephrosis with hydroureters to the vesicoureteral junction was detected, but ureteral wall thickening or ureteric narrow was not found. Therefore, obstruction due to BPH and bladder damage in anatomy and function may be the primary causes of hydronephrosis and hydroureters in our case.

The general treatment of BPH in elderly men includes medical and surgical approaches. Medical approaches may not work due to the indefinite aetiology of BPH in young men. For ketamine-associated uropathy, the aims of management of ketamine-associated urinary symptoms are symptom control and preservation of renal function and are ultimately to prevent irreversible damage to the urinary tract [23]. Due to the small number of cases of BPH in young people, there has been no consensus established on treatment. However, as shown in Table 1, most cases of children or young adults with BPH underwent surgery therapy, and surgical intervention may be necessary in most cases. Meanwhile, avoiding potential or possible pathogenic factors (ketamine in our case) are also necessary during the following treatment.

The simultaneous occurrence of BPH and ketamine-associated uropathy in young males has never been reported before. Inflammation in the urinary system, as a consequence of ketamine, may contribute to the development of BPH. Both surgical interventions and ketamine cessation are important approaches for relieving symptoms. This case may deserve significant attention as ketamine addiction among young population increases globally.

Abbreviations

BPH: Benign prostate hyperplasia; CT: Computed tomography; PSA: Prostate specific antigen; TURP: Transurethral resection of the prostate

Acknowledgements

Not applicable.

Authors' contributions

ZCL made contributions to data collection, literature search and manuscript writing. ZW was involved in data collection and literature search. ZYJ carried out the pathology part interpretation and description. ZYT was responsible for the patient's diagnosis and treatment. All authors have read and approved the manuscript, and ensure that this is the case.

Author details

Department of Urology, Xiangya Hospital, Central South University, Changsha, Hunan, China. [2]Provincial Laboratory for Diagnosis and Treatment of Genitourinary System Disease, Changsha, China. [3]Department of Pathology, Xiangya Hospital, Central South University, Changsha, Hunan, China. [4]National Clinical Research Center for Geriatric Disorders, Changsha, Hunan, China.

References

1. Powell TO. Precocious hypertrophy of prostate following persistent treatment with gonadotropic hormone. Urol. 1939;2(41):206–9.
2. Sumiya H, Fuse H, Matsuzaki O, Shimazaki J. Benign prostatic hypertrophy in a young male. Eur Urol. 1987;13(5):355–7.
3. Harada M, Kase T, Tajima M, Sawamura Y, Matsushima M. Shibuya K: [a case of prostatic hyperplasia in a young male]. Hinyokika kiyo Acta urologica Japonica. 1991;37(7):769–73.
4. Romano SV, Bechara A, Casabe A, Castillo EC, Cobreros C, Fredotovich N. Acute urinary retention due to benign prostatic hyperplasia in a 23-year-old patient. J Urol. 2001;166(1):217–8.
5. Choi YD, Cho NH, Kwon DH, Yang WJ, Oh YT, Choi SK. Juvenile prostatic hyperplasia. Urology. 2005;66(4):881.
6. Georgiades F, Demosthenous S, Antoniades G, Kouriefs C. Giant benign prostatic hyperplasia in a young adult male. Urology. 2014;84(2):e4–5.
7. Yagmur I, Turna B, Tekin A, Akincioglu E, Sarsik B, Ulman I: Benign prostatic hyperplasia: Case report of a 17-year-old. J Pediatr Urol. 2016;12(4).
8. Zouari S, Bouassida K, Ben Ahmed K, Thabet AB, Krichene MA, Jebali C. Acute urinary retention due to benign prostatic hyperplasia associated with cystitis glandularis in a 22-year-old patient. Pan Afr Med J. 2018;30.
9. Juan YS, Lee YL, Long CY, Wong JH, Jang MY, Lu JH, Wu WJ, Huang YS, Chang WC, Chuang SM. Translocation of NF-kappaB and expression of cyclooxygenase-2 are enhanced by ketamine-induced ulcerative cystitis in rat bladder. Am J Pathol. 2015;185(8):2269–85.
10. Wang Q, Wu Q, Wang J, Chen Y, Zhang G, Chen J, Zhao J, Wu P: Ketamine Analog Methoxetamine Induced Inflammation and Dysfunction of Bladder in Rats. International journal of molecular sciences. 2017;18(1).
11. Fan GY. Cherng JH. Chang SJ: The Immunomodulatory Imbalance in Patients with Ketamine Cystitis. 2017;20172329868.
12. Kramer G, Mitteregger D, Marberger M. Is benign prostatic hyperplasia (BPH) an immune inflammatory disease? Eur Urol. 2007;51(5):1202–16.
13. Kramer G, Steiner GE, Handisurya A, Stix U, Haitel A, Knerer B, Gessl A, Lee C, Marberger M. Increased expression of lymphocyte-derived cytokines in benign hyperplastic prostate tissue, identification of the producing cell types, and effect of differentially expressed cytokines on stromal cell proliferation. Prostate. 2002;52(1):43–58.
14. Steiner GE, Stix U, Handisurya A, Willheim M, Haitel A, Reithmayr F, Paikl D, Ecker RC, Hrachowitz K, Kramer G. Cytokine expression pattern in benign prostatic hyperplasia infiltrating T cells and impact of lymphocytic infiltration on cytokine mRNA profile in prostatic tissue. Lab Investig. 2003; 83(8):1131.
15. Chung K-S, Cheon S-Y, An H-J. Effects of resveratrol on benign prostatic hyperplasia by the regulation of inflammatory and apoptotic proteins. J Nat Prod. 2015;78(4):689–94.
16. Wang Z, Tang ZY, Huang L, Zhu Q. Ketamine-induced upper urinary tract lesions deserve more attention. Neurourol Urodyn. 2017;36(3):824–5.
17. Huang LK, Wang JH, Shen SH, Lin AT, Chang CY. Evaluation of the extent of ketamine-induced uropathy: the role of CT urography. Postgrad Med J. 2014;90(1062):185–90.
18. Chu PS, Ma WK, Wong SC, Chu RW, Cheng CH, Wong S, Tse JM, Lau FL, Yiu MK, Man CW. The destruction of the lower urinary tract by ketamine abuse: a new syndrome? BJU Int. 2008;102(11):1616–22.
19. Lai Y, Wu S, Ni L, Chen Z, Li X, Yang S, Gui Y, Guan Z, Cai Z, Ye J. Ketamine-associated urinary tract dysfunction: an underrecognized clinical entity. Urol Int. 2012;89(1):93–6.
20. Misra S, Chetwood A, Coker C, Thomas P. Ketamine cystitis: practical considerations in management. Scandinavian journal of urology. 2014;48(5): 482–8.
21. Selby NM, Anderson J, Bungay P, Chesterton LJ, Kolhe NV. Obstructive nephropathy and kidney injury associated with ketamine abuse. NDT plus. 2008;1(5):310–2.

22. Chung SD, Wang CC, Kuo HC. Augmentation enterocystoplasty is effective in relieving refractory ketamine-related bladder pain. Neurourol Urodyn. 2014;33(8):1207–11.
23. Tsai TH, Cha TL, Lin CM, Tsao CW, Tang SH, Chuang FP, Wu ST, Sun GH, Yu DS, Chang SY. Ketamine-associated bladder dysfunction. International journal of urology : official journal of the Japanese Urological Association. 2009;16(10):826–9.

20

Similar incidence of DNA damage response pathway alterations between clinically localized and metastatic prostate cancer

Isaac E. Kim Jr[1], Sinae Kim[2], Arnav Srivastava[3], Biren Saraiya[4], Tina Mayer[4], Wun-Jae Kim[5] and Isaac Yi Kim[3*]

Abstract

Background: In this era of precision medicine, the DNA damage response (DDR) pathway has been shown to be a viable target of intervention in metastatic castration-resistant prostate cancer (CRPC) as approximately one-third of CRPC patients harbor DDR pathway mutations. To determine whether DDR pathway is a potential therapeutic target in localized disease, we analyzed The Cancer Genome Atlas (TCGA) in the present study.

Methods: TCGA is a publically available cancer genome database that is sponsored by the United States National Cancer Institute. Total of 455 cases were available in the database at the time of this analysis.

Results: DDR pathway gene mutations or copy number alterations were present in 136 (29.9%) of the 455 cases. On a univariate analysis, DDR pathway status did not correlate with serum prostate specific antigen, tumor stage or grade. However, among patients with high-risk features post-operatively (pathologic stage ≥ T3, Gleason score ≥ 8, or PSA > 20 ng/ml), DDR pathway alteration was associated with a lower overall survival ($p = 0.0291$).

Conclusions: Collectively these results suggest that DDR pathway alterations may also be significant in localized prostate cancer and agents such as PARP inhibitors should be considered in patients with a high-risk disease.

Background

Prostate cancer (PCa) remains the most common malignancy among men in the United States [1]. Due to the heterogeneity of the disease, recent studies have utilized next-generation sequencing to identify predictive biomarkers and provide molecular stratification. Identifying driver mutations which contribute to tumorigenesis and disease progression can lead to development and implementation of targeted therapy. High rates of genomic mutations in DNA damage repair (DDR) genes, such as breast cancer 2, early onset (BRCA2) and ataxia telangiectasia mutated (ATM) genes, have been detected in multiple malignancies [2–4]. More recently, it has been suggested that tumors with such homologous recombination defects may be sensitive to poly (adenosine diphosphate-ribose) polymerase (PARP) 1 inhibitors, such as olaparib [5, 6].

With regards to PCa specifically, approximately 30% of metastatic castration-resistant prostate cancer (CRPC) have been reported to contain an aberrant DDR pathway [7]. However, the full extent and prevalence of DDR pathway alterations has not been extensively analyzed in localized disease. Thus far two prior studies suggested the incidence to range 8–20% [8, 9]. Therefore, in the present study, we analyzed the largest publically available version of The Cancer Genome Atlas (TCGA) to assess the rate of altered DNA damage repair machinery in localized prostate cancer. We report that the incidence of DDR pathway alterations is significantly higher than previously thought and approaches 30%.

Methods

Both the Provisional and Cell 2015 TCGA data were initially extracted as TSV files. At the time of this analysis, there were 455 patients in the Provisional TCGA database (http://www.cbioportal.org/index.do?session_id=5b8fc998498eb8b3d567b2ac). Three sets of data

* Correspondence: kimiy@cinj.rutgers.edu
[3]Section of Urologic Oncology, Division of Urology, Rutgers Cancer Institute of New Jersey and Rutgers Robert Wood Johnson Medical School, Rutgers, The State University of New Jersey, 195 Little Albany Street, #4565, New Brunswick, NJ 08903, USA
Full list of author information is available at the end of the article

were extracted and compiled based on the following criteria: pathologic Gleason score and stage, pre-operative PSA, and survival. The Provisional data was used for the pathologic Gleason score and stage, the Cell 2015 data was used for pre-operative PSA, and both the Provisional and Cell 2015 data were merged for the survival.

The programming language Python was used to extract the samples in which the Neoplasm American Joint Committee on Cancer Clinical Distant Metastasis M Stage was M0. These samples were first separated into two categories, the first being normal (unaffected) and the second being altered (affected; include mutations and copy number alterations). Within these categories, the samples were then placed into sets based on three factors:

1. Pathologic Gleason score, divided into less than or equal to 6, equal to 7, and greater than or equal to 8, which was computed by summing the Gleason pattern primary and the Gleason pattern secondary.
2. Pathologic stage, divided into organ confined (T2) vs non-organ confined (≥ T3a).
3. Pre-operative PSA, divided into ranges [0–10], [10–20], and greater than or equal to 20, which was extracted by cross-referencing the given sample ID from the Provisional data to the Cell 2015 data.

The attributes that were recorded and placed into the respective Excel files that included the sample ID, the months that the patient was disease free, months of overall survival, and overall survival status.

Baseline patient and clinical characteristics were summarized using descriptive statistics. Fisher's exact test was performed to test the association between two categorical variables. Student's t-test was used to compare mean age between the affected and unaffected group. The association of DDR mutation status with time from diagnosis to death from any cause was evaluated using log-rank tests and Kaplan-Meier curve estimates were plotted. All statistical tests were two-sided and $p < 0.05$ was considered to indicate statistical significance. All analyses were performed by Python and SAS 9.4 (Cary, NC).

Results

The overall incidence of DDR pathway alterations in localized prostate cancer approaches 30%. To assess the potential pathologic significance of DDR pathway in localized prostate cancer, we analyzed the TCGA prostate cancer database for mutations or copy number alterations of the following twelve genes (CHEK1, CHEK2, RAD51, BRCA1, BRCA2, MLH1, MSH2, ATM, ATR, MDC1, PARP1, and FANCF). The results revealed that 136 of the 455 cases were affected (29.9%), with 54 containing mutations and 92 copy number alterations (CNAs) (11.9 and 20.2%, respectively). The summary statistics of the patients with DDR pathway alterations are shown in Table 1. In men with DDR pathway alterations, an organ confined (pT2) and non-organ confined disease (pT3/4) comprised 34.6 and 65.4%, respectively ($p = 0.57$). With respect to pathologic Gleason score 6, 7, and ≥ 8, the proportion affected was 6.6, 49.3, and 44.1% ($p = 0.61$).

Figure 1 illustrates the breakdown of the affected genes from the data base analysis. As a comparison, similar analysis was carried out for the metastatic castration resistant prostate cancer (mCRPC) cases by pooling three databases within the cbioportal website [10–12]. The overall rate of DDR pathway alteration in this pooled dataset was 33% (91 of 272 patients). The proportion of altered cases between mutations and CNAs was similar to that of the localized cases (14 and 24%, respectively) (Fig. 2).

Table 1 Summary statistics on DNA Damage Response pathway alterations in clinically localized prostate cancer

Parameters	Normal (unaffected)	Mutated (affected)	*p*-value
Total sample size, *N*	319	136	
Age (years), median (range)	61 (41–77)	62 (43–78)	0.034
PSA pre-operative, median (ng/ml), (range), *n*	6.8 (2.2–56.4), 125	9.7 (2.2–87.0), 39	Not significant
Stage, pathologic American Joint Committee on Cancer Tumor Stage Code, *N* (%)			Not significant
pT2	127 (39.8)	47 (34.6)	
pT3	186 (58.3)	86 (63.2)	
pT4	6 (1.9)	3 (2.2)	
Gleason score, pathologic, *N* (%)			Not significant
6	28 (8.8)	9 (6.6)	
7	163 (51.1)	67 (49.3)	
8–10	128 (40.1)	60 (44.1)	

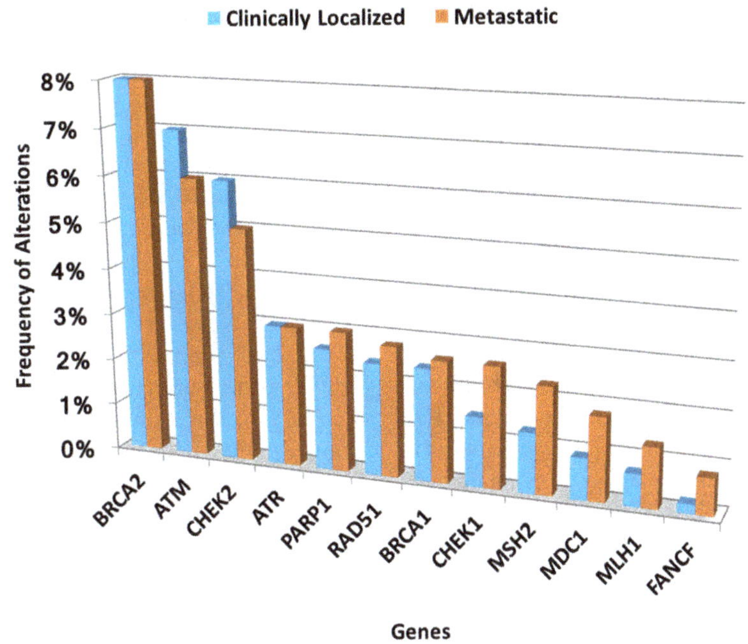

Fig. 1 Breakdown of DDR pathway alterations in localized and metastatic prostate cancer. Most frequent DDR pathway alterations were BRCA2 and ATM for both localized and metastatic prostate cancer

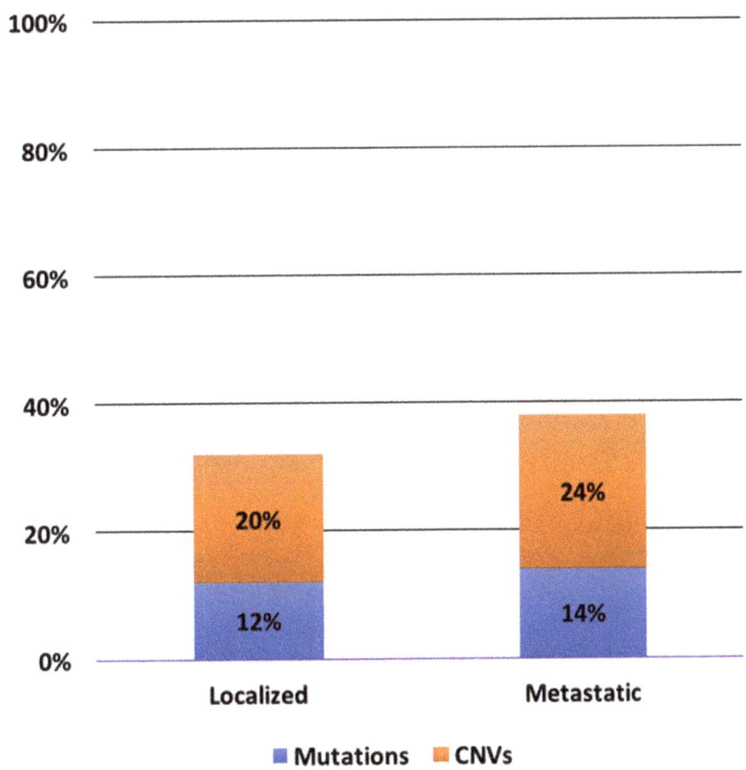

Fig. 2 Breakdown of mutations and copy number alterations in DDR pathways. The overall proportion of mutations and copy number alterations were similar for localized and metastatic prostate cancer

DDR pathway alterations associated with poor prognosis in men with high-risk prostate cancer. Next, we stratified the data based on pre-operative PSA and pathologic Gleason score and stage and investigated the potential prognostic value of DDR pathway alterations. Of the 455 cases in the database, survival data was available in 371 while pre-operative PSA in 164. The results were not significant for pre-operative PSA and pathologic Gleason score. However, in patients with pT3 or higher disease, DDR pathway alterations was associated with a lower overall survival (OS) (Fig. 3, $p = 0.0046$). In addition, in men with features of high-risk of recurrence following radical prostatectomy (pathologic Gleason score 8 or higher, pathologic stage T3 or higher, or pre-operative PSA ≥ 20 ng/ml), DDR pathway alterations again correlated with a shorter OS (Fig. 4, $p = 0.0291$).

Discussion

In the present study, we investigated DDR pathway alterations in localized prostate cancer using the TCGA database. We found that DDR pathway alteration rate is surprisingly high and occurred in approximately 30% of the cases. In addition, DDR pathway alteration was associated with a shorter OS in men with high-risk features post-operatively. These results suggest that a dysregulated DDR pathway may occur earlier during prostate cancer progression than previously thought and that available inhibitors of DDR pathway may have a therapeutic role in localized prostate cancer.

The observed DDR pathway alterations rate in localized prostate cancer was significantly higher than expected based on the reported range of 8–20% [8, 9]. Previously, DDR pathway has been reported to be altered in the 30% range in men with mCRPC. For example, in the landmark clinical trial that investigated the role of the PARP inhibitor olaparib [7], DDR pathway mutations were seen in 33% of mCRPC. Consistent with such result, we have also observed that the percentage of metastatic prostate cancer patients with DDR pathway mutations or copy number alterations was 33% in three publically available databases. In this context, the present observation that 30% of the TCGA's prostate cancer cases contain DDR pathway alterations is significantly higher than expected because the database represents entirely a non-metastatic, clinically localized prostate cancer. Accordingly, alterations in DDR pathway may occur earlier during prostate carcinogenesis.

The present finding also has therapeutic implications. Currently, there are multiple agents such as olaparib, niraparib, and rucaparib [5, 13, 14] that target the DDR pathway. Among these PARP inhibitors, olaparib has been shown to be effective in men with mCRPC as a monotherapy and in combination with abiraterone [7, 15]. Since DDR pathway alterations were seen at similar rate between localized and metastatic prostate cancer, it is

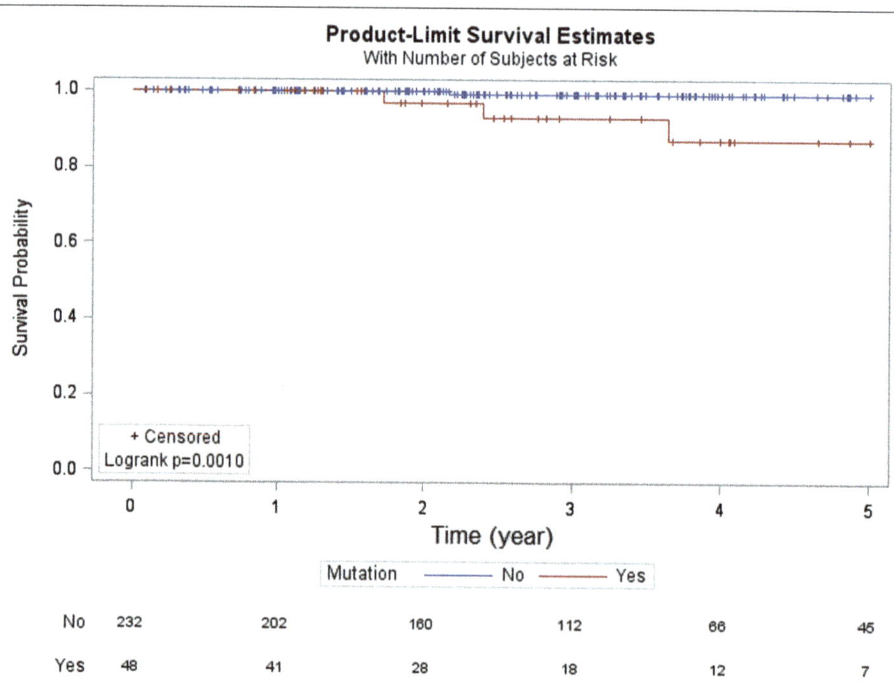

Fig. 3 Overall survival in pT3 or higher stage prostate cancer. DDR pathway alteration was associated with a shorter overall survival in patients with pT3 or higher stage prostate cancer

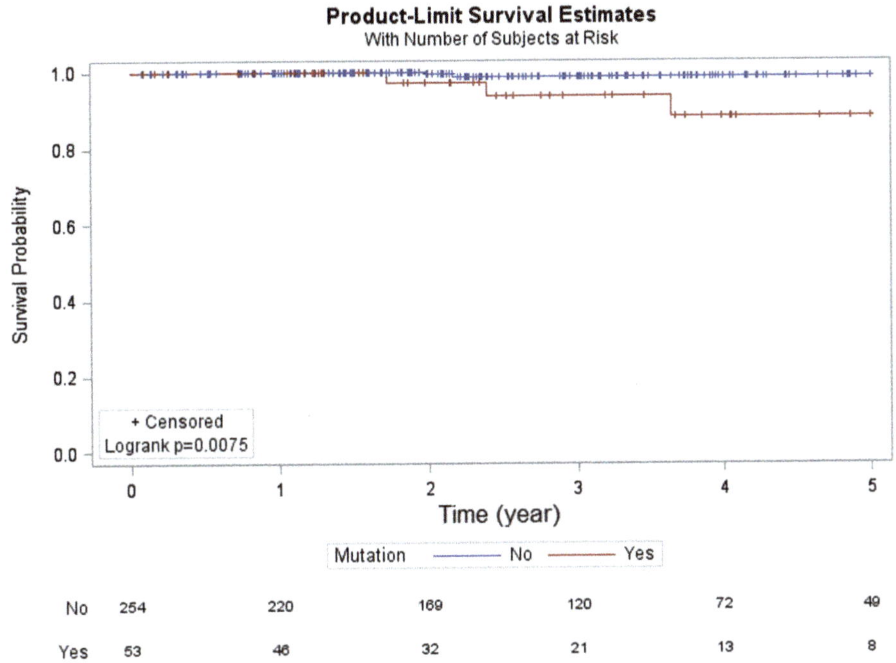

Fig. 4 Overall survival in high risk prostate cancer. In men with high risk prostate cancer (pT3 or higher, Gleason score 8 or higher, or pre-operative PSA greater than or equal to 20), DDR pathway alteration was associated with a shorter overall survival

plausible that PARP inhibitors may also have a therapeutic effect in localized prostate cancer. To test this possibility we are currently designing an adjuvant trial that will assess the effect of a PARP inhibitor in prostate cancer patients with high-risk features post-operatively.

It should be noted that a recent manuscript also investigated the DDR pathway in localized prostate cancer using the same TCGA database [9]. However, there were two significant differences between the present and the aforementioned study. First, the sample size analyzed is significantly larger with the current study as TCGA provisional data was used as compared to the TCGA Cell 2015 [8]. Second, as indicators of pathway alterations, we included both mutations and CNAs while the published study limited the investigation to mutations. Although the precise biological differences between mutations and CNAs is not clear, CNAs likely also represent a dysregulated pathway and should be analyzed in any therapies that target the DDR pathway.

This study has limitations. First, TCGA database does not contain all the relevant clinical information. Second, the biological significance of DDR pathway alterations cannot be assessed. Indeed, as indicators of altered DDR pathway, both mutations and CNAs were included. It is entirely possible that these various types of genetic changes may have different pathologic implications. Nevertheless, the present results suggest that DDR pathway alterations in localized prostate cancer is similar to that of heavily treated mCRPC, which supports further investigations into therapeutic strategies in this population.

Conclusions

DDR pathway alterations in localized prostate cancer in the TCGA database was approximately 30%. Such high rate suggests that agents such as PARP inhibitors may be an effective part of the treatment armamentarium in localized prostate cancer.

Abbreviations

CRPC: Castration-resistant prostate cancer; DDR: DNA Damage Response; mCRPC: Metastatic castration-resistant prostate cancer; OS: Overall survival; PARP: Poly (adenosine diphosphate-ribose) polymerase; PCa: Prostate cancer; TCGA: The Cancer Genome Atlas

Authors' contributions

All authors have read and approved the manuscript. Specific author contributions are as below. Programming and extracting the data: IEK. Statistical analysis: IEK and SK. Data analysis: AS, BS, TM, WJK, and IYK. Manuscript writing: IEK, SK, AS, BS, TM, WJK, and IYK. Supervision of the entire project: WJK and IYK.

Author details

[1]The Warren Alpert Medical School of Brown University, Providence, RI, USA. [2]Department of Biostatistics, Rutgers School of Public Health, The State University of New Jersey, New Brunswick, NJ, USA. [3]Section of Urologic

Oncology, Division of Urology, Rutgers Cancer Institute of New Jersey and Rutgers Robert Wood Johnson Medical School, Rutgers, The State University of New Jersey, 195 Little Albany Street, #4565, New Brunswick, NJ 08903, USA. [4]Department of Internal Medicine, Rutgers Robert Wood Johnson Medical School, Rutgers, The State University of New Jersey, New Brunswick, NJ, USA. [5]Department of Urology, Chungbuk National University College of Medicine, Cheongju, South Korea.

References

1. Siegel RL, Miller KD, Jemal A. Cancer statistics, 2017. CA Cancer J Clin 2017; 67(1):7–30. Epub 2017/01/06. doi: https://doi.org/10.3322/caac.21387. PubMed PMID: 28055103.
2. van Gent DC, Kanaar R. Exploiting DNA repair defects for novel cancer therapies. Mol Biol Cell 2016;27(14):2145–2148. Epub 2016/07/16. doi: https://doi.org/10.1091/mbc.E15-10-0698. PubMed PMID: 27418635; PubMed Central PMCID: PMCPMC4945134.
3. Oda K, Tanikawa M, Sone K, Mori-Uchino M, Osuga Y, Fujii T. Recent advances in targeting DNA repair pathways for the treatment of ovarian cancer and their clinical relevance. Int J Clin Oncol 2017;22(4):611–618. Epub 2017/05/17. doi: https://doi.org/10.1007/s10147-017-1137-7. PubMed PMID: 28508305.
4. O'Connor MJ. Targeting the DNA damage response in Cancer. Mol Cell 2015;60(4):547–560. Epub 2015/11/23. doi: https://doi.org/10.1016/j.molcel.2015.10.040. PubMed PMID: 26590714.
5. Lorusso D, Tripodi E, Maltese G, Lepori S, Sabatucci I, Bogani G, et al. Spotlight on olaparib in the treatment of BRCA-mutated ovarian cancer: design, development and place in therapy. Drug Des Devel Ther 2018;12: 1501–1509. Epub 2018/06/09. doi: https://doi.org/10.2147/DDDT.S124447. PubMed PMID: 29881257; PubMed Central PMCID: PMCPMC5983012.
6. Gavande NS, VanderVere-Carozza PS, Hinshaw HD, Jalal SI, Sears CR, Pawelczak KS, et al. DNA repair targeted therapy: the past or future of cancer treatment? Pharmacol Ther 2016;160:65–83. Epub 2016/02/21. doi: https://doi.org/10.1016/j.pharmthera.2016.02.003. PubMed PMID: 26896565; PubMed Central PMCID: PMCPMC4811676.
7. Mateo J, Carreira S, Sandhu S, Miranda S, Mossop H, Perez-Lopez R, et al. DNA-repair defects and Olaparib in metastatic prostate Cancer. N Engl J Med 2015;373(18):1697–1708. Epub 2015/10/29. doi: https://doi.org/10.1056/NEJMoa1506859. PubMed PMID: 26510020; PubMed Central PMCID: PMCPMC5228595.
8. Cancer Genome Atlas Research N. The Molecular Taxonomy of Primary Prostate Cancer. Cell. 2015;163(4):1011–1025. Epub 2015/11/07. doi: https://doi.org/10.1016/j.cell.2015.10.025. PubMed PMID: 26544944; PubMed Central PMCID: PMCPMC4695400.
9. Marshall CH, Fu W, Wang H, Baras AS, Lotan TL, Antonarakis ES. Prevalence of DNA repair gene mutations in localized prostate cancer according to clinical and pathologic features: association of Gleason score and tumor stage Prostate Cancer Prostatic Dis 2018. Epub 2018/09/02. doi: https://doi.org/10.1038/s41391-018-0086-1. PubMed PMID: 30171229.
10. Grasso CS, Wu YM, Robinson DR, Cao X, Dhanasekaran SM, Khan AP, et al. The mutational landscape of lethal castration-resistant prostate cancer. Nature. 2012;487(7406):239–243. Epub 2012/06/23. doi: https://doi.org/10.1038/nature11125. PubMed PMID: 22722839; PubMed Central PMCID: PMCPMC3396711.
11. Robinson D, Van Allen EM, Wu YM, Schultz N, Lonigro RJ, Mosquera JM, et al. Integrative clinical genomics of advanced prostate Cancer. Cell. 2015; 162(2):454. Epub 2015/07/16. doi: https://doi.org/10.1016/j.cell.2015.06.053. PubMed PMID: 28843286.
12. Kumar A, Coleman I, Morrissey C, Zhang X, True LD, Gulati R, et al. Substantial interindividual and limited intraindividual genomic diversity among tumors from men with metastatic prostate cancer. Nat Med 2016; 22(4):369–378. Epub 2016/03/02. doi: https://doi.org/10.1038/nm.4053. PubMed PMID: 26928463; PubMed Central PMCID: PMCPMC5045679.
13. Berek JS, Matulonis UA, Peen U, Ghatage P, Mahner S, Redondo A, et al. Safety and dose modification for patients receiving niraparib. Ann Oncol 2018;29(8):1784–1792. Epub 2018/05/17. doi: https://doi.org/10.1093/annonc/mdy181. PubMed PMID: 29767688.
14. Dal Molin GZ, Omatsu K, Sood AK, Coleman RL. Rucaparib in ovarian cancer: an update on safety, efficacy and place in therapy. Ther Adv Med Oncol 2018;10:1758835918778483. Epub 2018/07/07. doi: https://doi.org/10.1177/1758835918778483. PubMed PMID: 29977351; PubMed Central PMCID: PMCPMC6024342.
15. Clarke N, Wiechno P, Alekseev B, Sala N, Jones R, Kocak I, et al. Olaparib combined with abiraterone in patients with metastatic castration-resistant prostate cancer: a randomised, double-blind, placebo-controlled, phase 2 trial. Lancet Oncol 2018;19(7):975–986. Epub 2018/06/09. doi: https://doi.org/10.1016/S1470-2045(18)30365-6. PubMed PMID: 29880291.

21

Anterior gland focal cryoablation: Proof-of-concept primary prostate cancer treatment in select men with localized anterior cancers detected by multi-parametric magnetic resonance imaging

Christina Sze[1,2*], Efrat Tsivian[1], Kae Jack Tay[1,3], Ariel A. Schulman[1], Leah G. Davis[1], Rajan T. Gupta[1,4] and Thomas J. Polascik[1]

Abstract

Background: Due to their location away from the nerve bundles, anterior prostate cancers (APC) represent a rational target for image-guided cryoablation. This report describes the feasibility and short-term outcomes of anterior focal cryosurgery.

Methods: A retrospective review between 2012 and 2016 of patients with clinically localized APC treated with anterior gland cryoablation was performed. Descriptive statistics were used to report: age, PSA, prostate volume, prostate cancer grade group (PGG), median time to follow-up, and changes in functional status measured with the International Prostate Symptom Score (IPSS) and the International Index of Erectile Function (IIEF-5) score.

Results: A total of 17 patients underwent anterior focal cryoablation with a median follow-up of 15 months. Median age and PSA at diagnosis were 67 years and 8.7 ng/mL. Pre-operative PGG1 was identified in 12 (71%) men and PGG2 in 5 (29%) men. Median (IQR) lesion volume was 2 mL(0.86, 3.1). Preoperative median IIEF-5 and IPSS scores were 19.5 and 5, and decreased to 19 and 4, post-operatively. All patients remained continent with no change in sexual function. All post-procedure targeted biopsies of the treated cancers were negative.

Conclusion: Our pilot study demonstrates the feasibility of treating APCs with image-guided targeted focal cryoablation as a good balance between short-term oncologic control and near complete preservation of genitourinary function. Further follow-up is necessary to examine the potential benefits long-term.

Keywords: Focal cryoablation, Anterior gland, Prostate cancer, Erectile function, Continence

Background

Prostate Cancer (PCa) is the second leading cause of cancer-related deaths among men in the United States with the American Cancer Society estimating 164,699 new cases and 29,430 deaths in 2018 [1]. Conventional methods for treating PCa, such as radical prostatectomy or radiation therapy, although effective, often cause inadvertent but significant damage to surrounding structures leading to erectile dysfunction (ED), incontinence, or bowel irritation to a variable degree [2]. Many men report complete social withdraw from sexual contact and intimacy leading to relationship discord, frustration, and depression [3].

Advances in techniques and associated technologies, such as nerve-sparing focal therapy (FT), have proven to be effective in treating patients with localized prostate cancer in the short and intermediate term, and when applied in a targeted manner provide excellent preservation

* Correspondence: christina.sze89@gmail.com
[1]Urologic Surgery, Duke University Medical Center and the Duke Cancer Institute, Durham, NC, USA
[2]Division of Urology, Department of Surgery, Duke University Medical Center, Box 2804, Yellow Zone, Durham, NC 27710, USA
Full list of author information is available at the end of the article

of sexual and urinary function [4, 5]. One such therapy, focal cryotherapy, uses small needles to deliver lethal cold energy that causes direct cellular damage, tissue necrosis, and resultant apoptosis through the formation of ice crystals and other mechanisms [4]. Reported potency rates from this procedure can range from 60 to 90% and depend on preoperative erectile function and tumor location in relationship to the neurovascular bundles (NVB) [4]. Even with these advancements, a large disparity in post-surgical potency exists, making it challenging to predict sexual function outcomes.

Anterior prostate cancer (APC) accounts for 10–30% of PCa [6]. Due to its location, APCs represent a good therapeutic target for focal cryoablation. APCs are located far from the neurovascular bundles (NVBs), allowing for adequate surgical margins while preserving nerve integrity. However, their location is also a diagnostic blind spot and is often missed with systematic biopsies and the digital rectal examination [7]. Consequently, patients frequently present with higher PSA levels, larger tumor volumes, and often have histories of multiple biopsies [8]. The development and widespread adoption of multi-parametric MRI (mpMRI) for clinical use have improved the earlier detection and localization of these previously occult tumors [9].

This study describes the feasibility and short-term outcomes of anterior focal cryoablation as a new technique applied to a mpMRI-characterized disease entity.

Methods

Patient selection

After receiving institutional review board approval, a retrospective review was performed between 2012 to 2016 of patients who were treated with anterior gland cryoablation for clinically localized cancer. All patients had a prostate mpMRI. If a suspicious lesion was described on mpMRI, patients underwent image-targeted mpMRI-TRUS fusion biopsy to confirm the malignant nature of the lesion. At least 2 cores were obtained from the target lesion followed by a systematic biopsy sampling of 6–12 cores, depending on the prostate volume. Patients without lesions seen on mpMRI ($n = 1$), discordance between mpMRI and previous biopsy ($n = 2$), or due to patient preference (n = 2) underwent 3D transperineal template-guided prostate mapping biopsy (TTMB). Our 3D TTMB technique has been previously described [10]. Erectile and urinary functional outcomes were assessed by self-reported standardized instruments using the International Index of Erectile Function (IIEF-5) and the International Prostate Symptom Score (IPSS), respectively. No patient had received any other primary treatment for their prostate cancer. An smaller cohort was expected given the novelty of the technique. Cryoablation was performed by a single provider.

Multi-parametric MRI technique

Our mpMRI technique is similar as described previously in our work [11]. Briefly, mpMRI scans were obtained utilizing 3.0 Tesla scanners (Signa HDx, GE Healthcare, Waukesha, WI and Skyra, Siemens Healthcare, Erlangen, Germany) with a single-channel endorectal coil as well as multichannel surface coils. The imaging protocol includes multiplanar fast spin-echo T2-weighted imaging (T2WI), diffusion-weighted imaging (DWI) using multiple b values and calculation of apparent diffusion coefficient (ADC) maps. Dynamic contrast-enhanced imaging sequences were obtained after administration of a weight-based dose of extracellular MRI contrast agent with a 4- to 5-s temporal resolution for 5–6 min. All image interpretation lesion and segmentation was carried out on by a third party analysis software (DynaCAD, Invivo Corp.,Gainesville, FL) by a single board-certified, fellowship-trained radiologist with 5 years of experience in interpreting prostate mpMRI.

Surgical technique

Our anterior gland focal cryotherapy technique has been previously published [12]. Briefly, freezing the entire prostate generally involves the placement of three horizontal rows of 2–4 cryoprobes from the anterior to posterior gland. Each probe is placed within 2 cm of one another beginning with the most anterior row. Anterior gland ablation is defined as using up to only the first two anteriorly positioned horizontal rows of the standard probe template. The traditional posterior row of cryoprobes are not placed, thereby allowing a bilateral nerve sparing procedure. Temperature thermocouples are positioned to monitor the temperature of the following structures: urethral sphincter, Denonvillier's fascia, and the NVBs on both sides (Fig. 1). Cystoscopy is then performed to ensure no

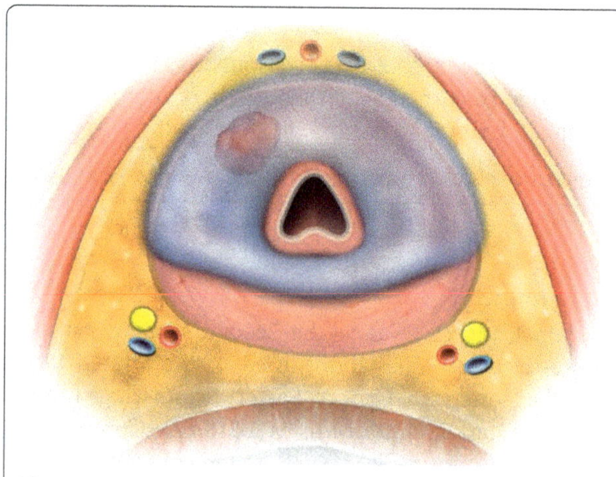

Fig. 1 Transaxial view of the prostate illustrating anterior cryoablation template. Ice, depicted in transparent blue, can be run posteriorly all the way to the peripheral zone leaving the neurovascular bundles [yellow/red/blue circles] untouched. Tumor depicted anteriorly in red, urethra in center of schematic

probe violates the urethra. Two freeze-thaw cycles are performed. At no time is the ice edge enabled to come close to the NVBs nor is the temperature around those structures allowed to go below 35C. This is an outpatient procedure and the patient is discharged with a short-term urethral catheter, an alpha-blocker and belladonna/opium suppositories.

Follow-up

The 2015 International Consultation on Urological Disease consensus on follow-up after focal therapy was used as a reference [13]. Patients are advised to follow-up 3 months post-operatively and then every 6 months for the next 5 years. At every visit, PSA, DRE, continence status, IIEF-5 and IPSS scores were recorded. At approximately 12 months post-operatively, patients underwent a mpMRI with targeted biopsy of the treated area, and any new suspicious lesions. A systematic biopsy (6–12 cores) of the untreated area was also performed for purposes of active surveillance due to the multifocal nature of PCa. Those patients without lesions on mpMRI or negative biopsies are to be re-evaluated with biopsy and mpMRI imaging at 5 years post-operatively. MpMRI surveillance continues annually otherwise through 5 years.

Statistical analysis

Descriptive statistics have been generated using median and interquartile range for continuous data (limited sample size) and counts and percentages for binary, ordinal and categorical endpoints. Clinically significant changes in IIEF-5 scores prior to and post procedure was defined by a difference of 4 points [14]. All analyses were performed using R 3.3.3 software.

Results

Between 2012 to 2016, 17 patients with complete follow-up were identified with APC and elected treatment with anterior gland prostate cryotherapy. The median serum PSA, and prostate volume at cryoablation were 8.7 ng/ml (6.7–11.76), and 35 cc (24–47.7), respectively. At the time of ablation, the median number of biopsy sessions a patient had undergone was 3 [2, 3]. Pre-ablation mpMRI identified anterior gland lesions in 16/17 (94%) of subjects with a median tumor volume of 2 cc (0.86, 3.1) (Table 1). To confirm the mpMRI detected lesion, the majority (71%) underwent a pre-treatment mpMRI-TRUS fusion biopsy of whom 25% chose to have only the mpMRI detected lesions sampled while 75% had a sextant biopsy in addition. A total of 5 (29%) patients elected TTMB incorporating targeted biopsy of the lesion along with detailed mapping comprising at least 50 cores. No patients had both types of biopsies (e.g. transrectal fusion plus TTMB) prior to cryoablation. One patient was found to have anterior prostate cancer by TTMB alone. A 3-D volume of the tumor was calculated based on mapped location of the cancer in X-Y-Z coordinates along with needle core cancer length. PGG1 disease was present in 12 (71%) patients while the remaining patients (29%) had PGG2 disease. Those with PGG1 or PGG2 disease had similar median lesion volumes on mpMRI, 2 cc (0.74, 2.94) and 2.04 cc (0.98, 4.5), respectively.

Post-ablation PSA data was available for 15/17 (88%) patients. The median PSA nadir and time to nadir were 0.82 ng/ml (0.55, 1.75) and 4 months (3, 7.5), respectively (Table 2). Follow-up mpMRI was performed in 9/17 (53%) patients at a median time of 14 months [13, 15] after ablation. mpMRI did not identify any lesions in all patients. Post ablation biopsy was performed in 10/17

Table 1 Patient and disease characteristics pre-ablation

Characteristic	Value
PSA (ng/ml), median (IQR)	8.7 (6.7, 11.76)
TRUS Prostate Volume (cc), median (IQR)	35 (24.3, 47.7)
No. prior biopsy sessions[†], median (IQR)	3 (2,3)
MRI lesion volume (mL), median (IQR):	
Overall	2 (0.86, 3.1)
PGG 1	2 (0.74, 2.94)
PGG 2	2.04 (0.98, 4.5)
Biopsy type[‡]:	
Fusion, No. (%)	12 (71)
TTMB, No. (%)	5 (29)
No. cores[‡], mean (range)	24.8 (1, 68)
No. positive cores [b] (%):	
1	11 (64.7)
2	4 (23.5)
4	2 (11.8)
PGG, No. (%)	
1	12 (71)
2	5 (29)

PGG prognostic grade group, *TTMB* transperineal template-guided prostate mapping biopsy

[†]Includes most recent biopsy performed at Duke

[‡]Most recent biopsy performed at Duke prior to cryoablation

Table 2 Post-ablation imaging, biochemical and pathological data

Characteristic	Value
Follow-up (mos.), median (IQR)	15 (13,17)
PSA nadir (ng/ml), median (IQR)	0.82 (0.55, 1.75)
Time to nadir (mos.), median (IQR)	4 (3, 7.5)
Time to MRI (mos.), median (IQR)	14 (13, 15)
No. positive biopsy (%):	
PGG 1	2 (100)

PGG prognostic grade group

(59%) patients. Biopsies of all ablated areas were negative for cancer (Fig. 2).

However, random surveillance biopsy in 2 patients revealed 1 mm or less of clinically insignificant or PGG1 disease in an untreated area of the prostate (Table 3). These two patients had PSA elevation at 6 and 13 months and PSA nadir of 2 ng/ml and 3.7 ng/ml respectively. IPSS scores were available for all 17 subjects. Median (IQR) pre- and 12-month post-ablation IPSS scores were 5 (2, 0) and 4 (2,4), respectively with a median difference between pre- and post-ablation scores of – 2 (– 3,0). IIEF-5 scores were available for 16/17 patients. Median pre- and 12-month post-ablation IIEF-5 scores were 19.5 [16, 17] and 19 [14, 18], respectively with a median difference between pre- and post-ablation scores of – 1 (– 3.25, 0). Eight subjects (47%) had a pre-operative IPSS score < 5 and 13 subjects had an IPSS score < 5 (76%) at > 12 months post-operatively. Three subjects (19%) had a pre-operative IIEF-5 score > 21 and 3 (19%) subjects had an IIEF-5 score > 21 at > 12 months post-operatively. Median time

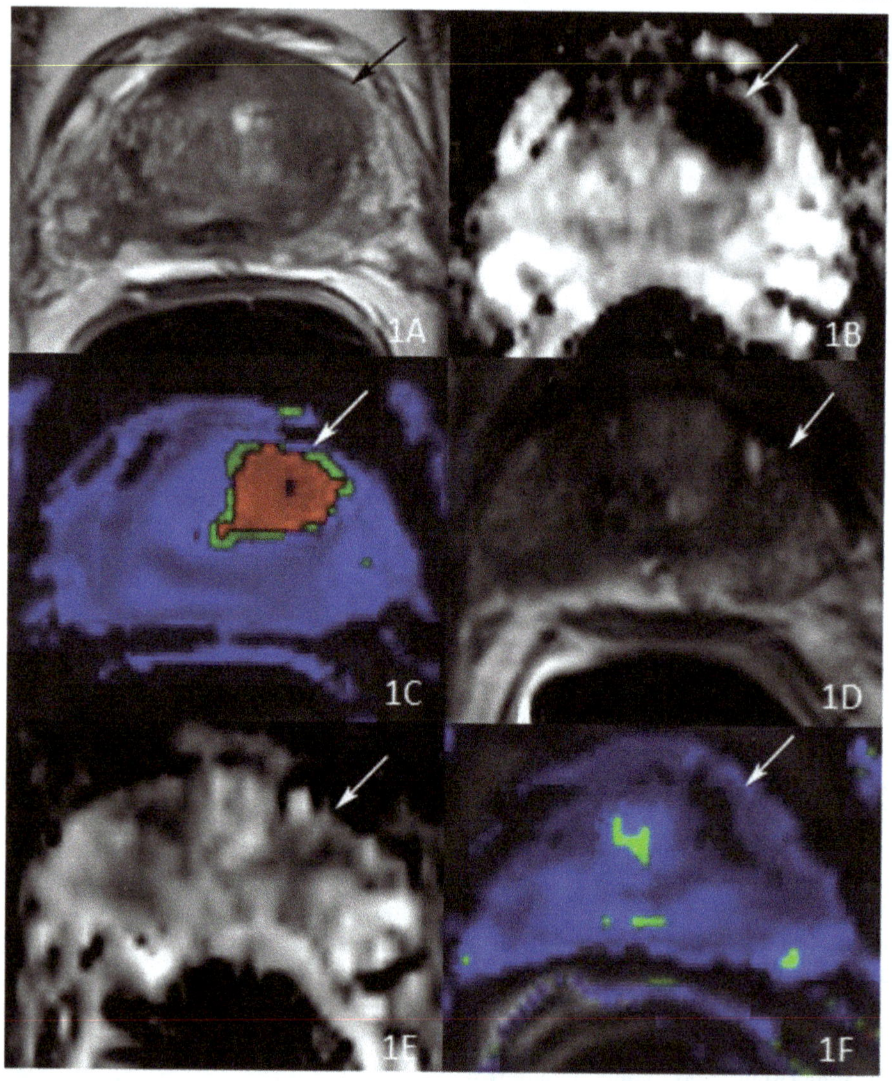

Fig. 2 a Axial T2-weighted (T2W) image reveals ill-defined decreased T2 signal at the level of the left anterior transition zone at the level of the base (arrow). **b** Axial apparent diffusion coefficient (ADC) map demonstrates markedly restricted diffusion in this region (arrow). **c** Colored perfusion map created using post-processing software from dynamic contrast-enhanced MRI (DCE-MRI) acquisition demonstrates suspicious perfusion kinetics for prostate cancer (arrow), corresponding to the findings seen on T2W and DWI. This lesion was scored as a PI-RADS 4 and patient underwent MRI-US fusion biopsy which revealed Gleason 3 + 3 = 6 prostate cancer at the targeted area. Based on these findings, patient elected to undergo anterior focal cryoablation of this lesion. **d,e,f** Axial T2W image, ADC map and colored perfusion map created using post-processing software from DCE-MRI acquisition in the post-ablation setting reveals ablation defect with no suspicious findings in the area of treatment and specifically, no abnormal perfusion kinetics. Patient's PSA continued to decrease with a nadir at 0.6 ng/mL confirming successful targeted anterior cryoablation

Table 3 Details of two recurrences detected on follow-up

Patient	Ablated anterior gland location	Pre ablation MRI lesion volume (cc)	Pos biopsy location Location	PGG	CCL (mm)	% CCL
1	Left medial apex TZ	3	Left lateral apex & Left lateral mid	1	Core 1: < 1 Core 2: < 1	Core 1: 5% Core 2: 2%
2	Left medial apex TZ	0.73	left lateral apex	1	1	7.7%

PGG prognostic grade group, *CCL* core cancer length, *TZ* anterior transition zone, *Pos* positive

from surgical intervention to follow-up IIEF-5 and IPSS scores were 15 months. No Clavien-Dindo complications or incontinence requiring absorbent pads were reported.

Discussion

This proof-of-concept study describes the feasibility of a new image-guided focal therapy application for appropriate candidates with APC aimed to achieve good oncological outcomes with preserved continence and erectile function [15]. Treatment of early PCa diagnosed in younger or sexually active patients deserves consideration as post-treatment sexual dysfunction can often lead to psychosocial consequences. Patient selection is one of the hallmarks of any FT application. Patients with PGG1 disease opted for anterior ablation due to large median lesion size of 2 mL, high suspicion score on mpMRI (lesions were either PIRADS 4 or 5) despite PGG1 by targeted biopsy, or not ideal candidates for active surveillance but considered over-treated if radical therapy was selected. High-volume Gleason pattern 3 has an increased risk of harboring higher grade cancer and has a one-in-ten chance of capsular invasion [19].

The anatomical and biological behavior of APCs are unique, and its definition varies. Villers defined the anterior borders of the prostate as the region of parenchyma at least 2.1 cm anterior to the posterior capsule that represents an area the transrectal biopsy needle characteristically fails to reach [20]. Anatomically, this is a portion of the prostate anterior to the urethra which includes areas of McNeal's transition zone, the anterior fibromuscular stroma and the anterior horns of the peripheral zone [16]. APCs can be derived from any of these tissue origins making it heterogenous as a group. Our study emphasizes the significance of APCs from a therapeutic perspective in that the defined target area is both located anteriorly and sufficiently away from the NVBs, and the treatment of which would foster a true bilateral nerve-preserving ablation without potentially sacrificing oncological outcomes in well-selected men.

Recently, a case series of patients with low- and intermediate-risk APCs treated with robotic partial prostatectomy demonstrated high continence rates of 100% and potency rates of 83% at 3 months post-operatively [20]. Procedures were completed without intraoperative complications however perioperative complications included anastomotic leak (12%), urinary tract infection (6%) and transient intestinal ileus (6%). These are risks not usually encountered when utilizing FT especially since targeted ablation is commonly performed as an outpatient procedure given its low perioperative morbidity. In cryotherapy, preventive measures such as use of a warming catheter are employed to prevent injury to the external striated sphincter and urethra when treating APCs. Thus, in anterior cryoablation, indirect injury to these structures are rarely seen. Additionally, temperature thermocouples are placed to monitor any potential changes to surrounding tissue, particularly the NVBs. Therefore, focal ablation is a viable option with minimal to no significant morbidity for treating APCs.

Although the concept of APC is not new, the role of mpMRI in detecting and staging APCs is one that has gained recent interest. The conventional tool to diagnose PCa, relying on random TRUS-guided biopsies (10–12 cores), is more adept at detecting posterior PCa. On average, detection of APCs requires more repeat biopsies compared to posteriorly located PCa and require inserting the biopsy needle deeper into the parenchyma [21]. In our series, patients typically have a history of at least 2 rounds of biopsies prior to APC detection. mpMRI-TRUS guided fusion biopsy increases the detection of APC and have been shown to significantly detect more APCs than TRUS-guided biopsy especially in those who have histories of previous negative TRUS-guided biopsies [17, 18]. This superior performance is due to the superior anatomic resolution of of T2 weighted-images (T2WI) combined with functional techniques such as apparent diffusion coefficient (ADC) mapping of mpMRI [22]. Given the increased incorporation of mpMRI into clinical decision-making, it is expected APCs will be increasingly detected in the future, possibly enabling more men to be considered candidates for anterior gland ablation. mpMRI is an additional diagnostic modality that has value in the initial clinical staging nomograms and may lead to fewer cores being taken and potentially be cost effective [23].

In this series, the median pre-operative IPSS scores decreased by 2 at 12 months post-operatively suggesting an improvement in urinary symptoms although not a significant change in this cohort as these men were not very symptomatic at onset. However, 5 additional men had a 1-year post-ablation IPSS < 5, suggesting further improvement in urinary function post-treatment as measured by this self-reported QOL instrument. The use of anterior gland FT seems to have little adverse impact on urinary function which is consistent with other reports on FT [24]. The very high rate of preserving urinary continence appears unique to FT in general and anterior gland ablation in particular. Previous studies have shown urinary incontinence rates ranging from 0 to 3.6% after FT [25]. Regarding erectile function, we allowed patients to self-report their scores before and after anterior gland cryoablation utilizing the validated IIEF-5 instrument. The median difference in IIEF-5 between pre- and post-ablation scores was − 1 following anterior gland ablation suggesting minimal change in sexual performance. Conceptually this is logical as the energy field is located far from the NVBs.

In terms of oncological outcomes, patients were free of clinically significant PCa on follow-up biopsy in the short term in those undergoing evaluation. Prostates were subjected to intense scrutiny with mpMRI, targeted biopsy of the ablated tumor and random, conventional biopsy of the untreated parenchyma on active surveillance. Two subjects demonstrated biopsy-proven low volume, ≤ 1 mm in each core, PGG1 disease in the untreated region at the apex. The apex is not uncommonly an area where recurrences or cancer persistence may occur post ablation largely due to conservative freezing of the area to avoid potential damage to the external sphincter [26]. mpMRI is the recommended imaging modality after FT because of its high negative predicative value (NPV) and sensitivity to detect clinically significant cancer, particularly high volume or high grade disease [27]. Previously, Radtke et al. showed that there is value in the use of systematic biopsy with the image-targeted biopsy as the combination of the two identified more clinically significant PCa than mpMRI alone [28]. The combination of extended biopsies along with targeted fusion biopsy augments the NPV of mpMRI to maximize the likelihood to detect persistent cancer or new occult tumors as PCa is typically multifocal.

We recognize certain limitations of this study. First, this is a retrospective extended case series with a smaller sample size therefore only descriptive analyses were completed. It is also worth mentioning that though each patient underwent anterior cryoablation, the procedures were customized according to the location of the tumor(s) and shape of the prostate. However, customization reflects a real-world application of FT whereby treatments should be individualized according to tumor location, size and focality. This series also consisted of a group of men having a relatively small mean prostate volume that has been shown to impact oncologic outcomes as larger prostate provides a surgeon a greater margin of error when performing FT [29]. Additionally, the study relies on patient reported measures to assess urogenital function using validated instruments that has its own merits and limitations regarding patient-reported data. This series was restricted to a short timeframe of median follow-up time 15 months. However, although this is a very short time frame to judge oncologic outcomes, it is of sufficient time to make determinations regarding functional outcomes. Due to the excellent functional profile that FT offers for maintaining potency and continence, many patients often feel they are back to baseline health relatively quickly. The disadvantage of such rapid recovery is that the patient may no longer feel the need to follow-up medically, therefore making acquisition of longer-term follow-up data even more challenging to accumulate. Of note, no peri-operative complications such as urinary tract infections or uncontrolled bleeding were recorded.

Conclusions

This extended cohort series describes the feasibility and short-term outcomes of anterior gland focal cryoablation as a new technique applied to a mpMRI-characterized disease entity, the APC. These findings provide clinicians and patients with data that could inform expectations regarding functional outcomes and short-term cancer control following this procedure. Ultimately, patients must weigh the relative value of cancer control and preservation of genitourinary function. Additional follow-up is needed to evaluate long-term outcomes of FT for APCs and better define those patients who may benefit most from this technique.

Abbreviations

APC: Anterior prostate cancers; FT: Focal therapy; IIEF-5: International Index of Erectile Function; IPSS: International Prostate Symptom Score; mpMRI: Multiparametric magnetic resonance imaging; NVBs: neurovascular bundles; PCa: Prostate cancer; PGG: prostate cancer grade group; TRUS: Transrectal ultrasound; TTMB: Transperineal template-guided prostate mapping biopsy

Acknowledgements

N/A

Authors' contributions

Study conception and design: C.S., E.T., K.T., T.P. Acquisition of data: C.S., E.T. Analysis and interpretation of data: C.S., E.T., L.D. Drafting of manuscript: C.S., E.T. Critical revision: C.S., E.T., K.T., A.S., R.G., T.P. All authors have read and approve this version.

Author details

[1]Urologic Surgery, Duke University Medical Center and the Duke Cancer Institute, Durham, NC, USA. [2]Division of Urology, Department of Surgery, Duke University Medical Center, Box 2804, Yellow Zone, Durham, NC 27710, USA. [3]Singapore General Hospital, Singapore, Singapore. [4]Department of Radiology, Duke University Medical Center, Durham, NC, USA.

References

1. Society AC. Key Statistics for Prostate Cancer 2018 [Available from: https://www.cancer.org/cancer/prostate-cancer/about/key-statistics.html.
2. McCullough AR. Sexual dysfunction after radical prostatectomy. Rev Urol. 2005;7(Suppl 2):S3–S10.

3. De Sousa A, Sonavane S, Mehta J. Psychological aspects of prostate cancer: a clinical review. Prostate Cancer Prostatic Dis. 2012;15(2):120–7.
4. Tay KJ, Polascik TJ. Focal Cryotherapy for localized prostate Cancer. Arch Esp Urol. 2016;69(6):317–26.
5. Mendez MH, Passoni NM, Pow-Sang J, Jones JS, Polascik TJ. Comparison of outcomes between preoperatively potent men treated with focal versus whole gland Cryotherapy in a matched population. J Endourol. 2015;29(10):1193–8.
6. Al-Ahmadie HA, Tickoo SK, Olgac S, Gopalan A, Scardino PT, Reuter VE, et al. Anterior-predominant prostatic tumors: zone of origin and pathologic outcomes at radical prostatectomy. Am J Surg Pathol. 2008;32(2):229–35.
7. Ouzzane A, Puech P, Lemaitre L, Leroy X, Nevoux P, Betrouni N, et al. Combined multiparametric MRI and targeted biopsies improve anterior prostate cancer detection, staging, and grading. Urology. 2011;78(6): 1356–62.
8. Mygatt J, Sesterhenn I, Rosner I, Chen Y, Cullen J, Morris-Gore T, et al. Anterior tumors of the prostate: clinicopathological features and outcomes. Prostate Cancer Prostatic Dis. 2014;17(1):75–80.
9. Tay KJ, Villers A, Polascik TJ. Targeted anterior gland focal therapy-a novel treatment option for a better defined disease. Curr Urol Rep. 2016;17(10):69.
10. Tsivian M, Abern MR, Qi P, Polascik TJ. Short-term functional outcomes and complications associated with transperineal template prostate mapping biopsy. Urology. 2013;82(1):166–70.
11. Gupta RT, Spilseth B, Patel N, Brown AF, Yu J. Multiparametric prostate MRI: focus on T2-weighted imaging and role in staging of prostate cancer. Abdom Radiol (NY). 2016;41(5):831–43.
12. Jack TK, T.J. Polascik Anterior Prostate Cancer Cryoablation: A Technique in Prostate Focal Therapy. Videourology. 2017;31(2):null.
13. Image-guided therapies for Prostate and Kidney Cancers. Melbourne, Australia: Société Internationale d'Urologie and International Consultation on Urological Diseases; 2015 October 15–18.
14. Rosen RC, Allen KR, Ni X, Araujo AB. Minimal clinically important differences in the erectile function domain of the international index of erectile function scale. Eur Urol. 2011;60(5):1010–6.
15. Mendez MH, Joh DY, Gupta R, Polascik TJ. Current trends and new frontiers in focal therapy for localized prostate cancer. Curr Urol Rep. 2015;16(6):35.
16. McNeal JE, Redwine EA, Freiha FS, Stamey TA. Zonal distribution of prostatic adenocarcinoma. Correlation with histologic pattern and direction of spread. Am J Surg Pathol. 1988;12(12):897–906.
17. Radtke JP, Boxler S, Kuru TH, Wolf MB, Alt CD, Popeneciu IV, et al. Improved detection of anterior fibromuscular stroma and transition zone prostate cancer using biparametric and multiparametric MRI with MRI-targeted biopsy and MRI-US fusion guidance. Prostate Cancer Prostatic Dis. 2015; 18(3):288–96.
18. Wright JL, Ellis WJ. Improved prostate cancer detection with anterior apical prostate biopsies. Urol Oncol. 2006;24(6):492–5.
19. Stamey TA, Freiha FS, McNeal JE, Redwine EA, Whittemore AS, Schmid HP. Localized prostate cancer. Relationship of tumor volume to clinical significance for treatment of prostate cancer. Cancer. 1993;71(3 Suppl): 933–8.
20. Villers A, Puech P, Flamand V, Haber GP, Desai MM, Crouzet S, et al. Partial prostatectomy for anterior Cancer: short-term oncologic and functional outcomes. Eur Urol. 2017;72(3):333–42.
21. Bott SR, Young MP, Kellett MJ, Parkinson MC. Contributors to the UCLHTRPD. Anterior prostate cancer: is it more difficult to diagnose? BJU Int. 2002;89(9):886–9.
22. Shinmoto H, Tamura C, Soga S, Okamura T, Horiguchi A, Asano T, et al. Anterior prostate Cancer: diagnostic performance of T2-weighted MRI and an apparent diffusion coefficient map. AJR Am J Roentgenol. 2015;205(2): W185–92.
23. de Rooij M, Crienen S, Witjes JA, Barentsz JO, Rovers MM, Grutters JP. Cost-effectiveness of magnetic resonance (MR) imaging and MR-guided targeted biopsy versus systematic transrectal ultrasound-guided biopsy in diagnosing prostate cancer: a modelling study from a health care perspective. Eur Urol. 2014;66(3):430–6.
24. Shah TT, Ahmed H, Kanthabalan A, Lau B, Ghei M, Maraj B, et al. Focal cryotherapy of localized prostate cancer: a systematic review of the literature. Expert Rev Anticancer Ther. 2014;14(11):1337–47.
25. Tay KJ, Polascik TJ, Elshafei A, Tsivian E, Jones JS. Propensity score-matched comparison of partial to whole-gland Cryotherapy for intermediate-risk prostate Cancer: an analysis of the Cryo on-line data registry data. J Endourol. 2017;31(6):564–71.
26. Shinohara K, Rhee B, Presti JC Jr, Carroll PR. Cryosurgical ablation of prostate cancer: patterns of cancer recurrence. J Urol. 1997;158(6):2206–9 discussion 9-10.
27. Tsivian M, Gupta RT, Tsivian E, Qi P, Mendez MH, Abern MR, et al. Assessing clinically significant prostate cancer: diagnostic properties of multiparametric magnetic resonance imaging compared to three-dimensional transperineal template mapping histopathology. Int J Urol. 2017;24(2):137–43.
28. Radtke JP, Schwab C, Wolf MB, Freitag MT, Alt CD, Kesch C, et al. Multiparametric magnetic resonance imaging (MRI) and MRI-Transrectal ultrasound fusion biopsy for index tumor detection: correlation with radical prostatectomy specimen. Eur Urol. 2016;70(5):846–53.
29. Elshafei A, Tay KJ, Kara O, Malkoc E, Nyame Y, Arora H, et al. Associations Between Prostate Volume and Oncologic Outcomes in Men Undergoing Focal Cryoablation of the Prostate. Clin Genitourin Cancer. 2017.

22

A retrospective feasibility study of biweekly docetaxel in patients with high-risk metastatic castration-naïve prostate cancer

Sang Eun Yoon[1], Youjin Kim[1], Jangho Cho[1], Minyong Kang[2], Hyun Hwan Sung[2], Hwang Gyun Jeon[2], Byoung Chang Jeong[2], Seong Il Seo[2], Seong Soo Jeon[2], Hyun Moo Lee[2], Han Yong Choi[2,3], Su Jin Lee[1] and Se Hoon Park[1*]

Abstract

Background: Results from randomized phase III trials have shown that thrice-weekly docetaxel added to androgen-deprivation therapy (ADT) has a significant impact on the survival of patients with metastatic castration-naïve prostate cancer (mCNPC) and established early chemotherapy as part of the standard of care for high-risk disease. Controversy remains, however, because some patients experience critical toxicities related to docetaxel. The purpose of the current study was to evaluate the feasibility and adverse events of biweekly-administered docetaxel in patients with previously-untreated, high-risk mCNPC.

Methods: The study included 35 consecutive patients with high-risk mCNPC who received ADT plus docetaxel 40 mg/m^2. Oral prednisone 5 mg twice daily was also given. Treatment was repeated every two weeks for up to 12 cycles or until disease progression or unacceptable toxicity occurred. High-risk was defined as bone metastases beyond axial skeleton and/or visceral disease.

Results: The included patients' median age was 68 years (range: 31–86 years) and 17 (49%) had visceral metastases. Biweekly docetaxel was generally well-tolerated; the most commonly observed adverse events, considering those of all grades, included alopecia (74%), nail changes (42%), and constipation (31%). Hematologic adverse events were infrequent, and no patient received hematopoietic growth factors. One patient died after the fourth cycle due to respiratory failure, which occurred as a complication of pneumonia. Among the 35 patients, 28 completed the planned 12 cycles of biweekly docetaxel. Prostate-specific antigen response (> 50% decrease from baseline) was recorded in 33 patients (94%), and the radiologic response rate was 49%. Median progression-free survival was 13.6 months (95% confidence interval: 6.7–20.4).

Conclusion: ADT plus biweekly-administered docetaxel appeared to be tolerated and effective in patients with high-risk mCNPC.

Keywords: Castration-naïve prostate cancer, Docetaxel, Biweekly

* Correspondence: hematoma@skku.edu
[1]Division of Hematology-Oncology, Department of Medicine, Samsung Medical Center, Sungkyunkwan University School of Medicine, 81 Irwon-ro, Gangnam-gu, Seoul 06351, South Korea
Full list of author information is available at the end of the article

Background

Prostate cancer is one of the greatest growing cancers in Korea, with an estimated 9785 new cases and 1667 deaths occurring in Korea in 2014 [1]. For patients with metastatic or advanced disease, androgen-deprivation therapy (ADT), which includes bilateral orchiectomy or medical castration with gonadotropin-releasing hormone (GNRH) agonists, can provide palliation of symptoms and prolong survival [2]. If a patient develops castration-resistant prostate cancer (CRPC), docetaxel is regarded as the standard first-line chemotherapy regimen from the results of two randomized clinical trials [3, 4].

Docetaxel is commonly administered at a dose of 75 mg/m^2 every 3 weeks established by the results from the TAX-327 study [5, 6], in which once every 3 weeks docetaxel (median: 19.2 months, 95% CI, 17.5 to 21.3 months) conferred a definite survival benefit over weekly docetaxel for 3 weeks (median: 17.8 months, 95% CI, 16.2 to 19.2 months).

In Asian countries, there was better survival benefit in every 3 weeks administration(12.5 months) than every week administration (8.0 months). No grade 3 or 4 neutropenia was showed in once weekly for 3 weeks, but Gr 3/4 neutropenia was observed more frequently about 75% of patients with CRPC who were treated with once every 3 weeks docetaxel [7]. Based on previous studies, a pharmacokinetics study conducted in Japan [8] and consideration of efficacy and toxicities in the management of solid tumors in a palliative setting [9], docetaxel is most commonly administered in Korea and Japan at a lower dose (i.e., 60 mg/m^2 every 3 weeks).

An additional option to prevent docetaxel-related hematologic toxicity is to use other administration schedules, such as weekly or biweekly regimens. On the side of this approach, biweekly administration of docetaxel 50 mg/m^2 showed a better time-to-failure (TTF; median: 5.6 months vs. 4.9 months; $P = 0.014$) than thrice-weekly docetaxel [10]. As expected, the biweekly regimen was better tolerated than the thrice-weekly docetaxel regimen, and importantly, efficacy was not compromised. In our own retrospective study [11], we showed that a docetaxel 40 mg/m^2 biweekly regimen was appropriate and well-tolerated in Korean patients with CRPC.

Although surgical or medical castration is considered standard treatment in castrate-naïve prostate cancer (CNPC), some patients with extensive metastatic (i.e., high-risk) disease at diagnosis, including visceral or bone involvement beyond the axial skeleton, have shorter survival times [12]. It is not enough to start standard hormone castration treatment alone to high tumor volume at CNPC diagnosis. The previous randomized phase III trials were conducted using either six or nine cycles of docetaxel 75 mg/m^2 every 3 weeks in the CNPC setting [13–15]. Their results led to early change to ADT in high-risk CNPC in most guidelines published by the oncology societies [16, 17]. Supposedly, the new standard therapy should only be applied in patients fit enough to receive docetaxel and tolerate the associated side effects. Based on these considerations, from October 2013, we adopted a biweekly low-dose docetaxel regimen (40 mg/m^2 every 2 weeks) as an institutional standard chemotherapy regimen for patients with chemotherapy-naïve CNPC. The present study was conducted to evaluate the tolerability of the regimen and to obtain feasibility data in anticipation of performing a prospective, formal phase II study.

Methods

We retrospectively collected and reviewed the medical records of 35 men with metastatic CNPC who were consecutively treated with biweekly docetaxel and ADT as first-line therapy between October 2015 and December 2016. In the present study, we included the patients with histologically-confirmed adenocarcinoma of the prostate and naïve to both ADT and chemotherapy. The other eligibility criteria consisted of an Eastern Cooperative Oncology Group (ECOG) performance status of 0 or 1, radiologic and clinical evidence of high-risk metastatic disease for which there was no curative treatment available, and acceptable major organ functioning to receive chemotherapy. High-risk was defined as bone metastases beyond the axial skeleton and/or visceral disease, regardless of prostate-specific antigen (PSA) level.

The choice of early docetaxel was determined by a multidisciplinary urologic oncology team composed of urologists, radiologists, pathologists, radiation oncologists, and medical oncologists. The study protocol was approved by the Samsung Medical Center (Seoul, Korea) Institutional Review Board, and all patients provided written informed consent prior to undergoing docetaxel chemotherapy.

Treatment

Our medical center standard chemotherapy for CRPC has been a biweekly docetaxel 40 mg/m^2 regimen [11], corresponding to a dose intensity of 20 mg/m^2/week (equivalent to 60 mg/m^2 every 3 weeks). Docetaxel was administered intravenously over 1 hour on day 1 with dexamethasone and antiemetics. Oral prednisolone 5 mg was administered twice daily from day 1 and continued throughout treatment. Supportive care, including the administration of blood products, bisphosphonates, and the use of analgesics, was given if judged appropriate by the treating physicians. Prior to initiation of the first dose of docetaxel, a complete history was taken from each patient. In addition, complete blood counts, serum chemistry analyses, chest X-rays, bone scans, and computed tomography (CT) scans of all involved sites were performed. Patients were seen every 2 weeks; during these visits, a brief history was taken; a physical examination was performed; and adverse events, blood counts, and PSA level were assessed. Treatment was repeated on an outpatient basis and continued until objective disease progression, unacceptable toxicity, patient refusal, or up to 12 cycles. Throughout the treatment period, ADT with GNRH agonists was given to all participants, except those who underwent surgical castration. Radiologic responses were evaluated every 8 weeks by bone scan, chest and abdomino-pelvic CT, or the same tests that were used for initial tumor staging. Adverse events were collected and graded according to the National Cancer Institute's Common Terminology Criteria for Adverse Events version 4.

Statistical analysis

The evaluation of toxicity was the primary endpoint for the study, and myelosuppression, specifically grade 3 or 4 neutropenia and febrile neutropenia, was considered to be the dose-limiting toxicity. Other endpoints included a PSA response, defined as a ≥ 50% decline in PSA level from baseline with no clinical or radiologic evidence of disease progression, overall survival (OS), and progression-free survival (PFS). PFS was defined as the time from the first administration of docetaxel to the date of disease progression (PSA or radiologic progression) or death. PSA progression was defined as an increase ≥25% and ≥ 2 ng/mL after 12 weeks according to the Prostate Cancer Working Group 2 criteria [18]. PFS and OS were calculated using the Kaplan–Meier method. All analyses were performed using R for Windows, version 2.11.1 (http://www.r-project.org; R Core Team, Vienna, Austria).

Results

The baseline patient characteristics of 35 patients who were registered between October 2015 and December 2016 are listed in Table 1. Their median age was 68 years (range: 31–86 years), and 71% had symptomatic (i.e., ECOG performance status of 1) disease. The most commonly involved metastatic sites were bone (97%) and lymph nodes (91%), and 17 participants (49%) had visceral metastases. ADT was initiated within 1 month of starting docetaxel in all patients in combination with leuprolide (57%), goserelin (40%), or degarelix (3%).

The included patients received a total of 1483 cycles of biweekly docetaxel (median: 12, range: 1–12). Three patients discontinued treatment after the first cycle, two due to toxicity or withdrawal and one due to disease progression. Docetaxel was delayed in 17 cycles (1%), and dose reduction was required in five patients (14%). As a dose intensity of docetaxel 20 mg/m^2/week was planned, the relative dose intensity was 98% [95% confidence interval (CI): 86–104]. Biweekly docetaxel showed manageable toxicities including all grades (Table 2). The most ordinary adverse events were alopecia (74%), nail changes (42%), and constipation (31%). Hematologic adverse events presented rarely. There were five patients required blood transfusion due to anemia and/or thrombocytopenia, but they did not receive hematopoietic growth factors. One patient died of respiratory failure induced pneumonia complication after completing the fourth cycle chemotherapy.

Table 1 Patient characteristics

	No.	%
Age, years		
Median (range)	68 (31–86)	
Disease status		
Metastatic at diagnosis	31	89
Recurrent	4	11
Gleason score		
6	1	3
7	5	14
8	13	37
9	12	34
10	4	11
Initial PSA, ng/mL		
Median (range)	330.08 (4–50,000)	
Type of metastases		
Bone and/or lymph nodes only	18	51
Visceral	17	49
Metastatic site		
Lymph node	32	91
Bone	34	97
Lung	16	46
Liver	4	11
ECOG performance status		
0	10	29
1	25	71

PSA prostate-specific antigen, *ECOG* Eastern Cooperative Oncology Group
Because the patients could have metastases at multiple sites, the total number of metastases cases is greater than the number of patients

There was no complete clinical response in the current study. 31 patients evaluated for radiologic responses and 17 patients (55, 95% CI: 46–64) presented partial responses. and 10 patients achieved stable disease. Finally, 87% of the overall patients obtained adequate disease control.

Thirty-three patients (94%) demonstrated PSA response (> 50% decrease from baseline), and 49% patients appeared radiologic response. Median PFS was 13.6 months (95% CI: 6.7–20.4). Median OS was not reached, but the OS rate at 1 year was identified as 75% (Fig. 1).

Table 2 Maximum grade of toxicities per patient

	Grades 1/2 N (%)	Grades 3/4 N (%)
Anemia	8 (22.9)	4 (11.4)
Neutropenia	6 (17.1)	0
Thrombocytopenia	4 (11.4)	1 (2.9)
Alopecia	26 (74.3)	0
Fatigue	6 (17.1)	0
Nausea	4 (11.4)	0
Anorexia	5 (14.3)	0
Peripheral neuropathy	8 (22.9)	0
Stomatitis	7 (20)	0
Diarrhea	3 (8.6)	1 (2.9)
Constipation	11 (31.4)	0
Skin	9 (25.7)	0
Nail changes	15 (42.9)	0

Discussion

There are newly developed numerous treatment options for advanced prostate cancer, but it is not yet possible to replace all of the docetaxel [17]. The standard docetaxel regimen (75 mg/m^2 every 3 weeks plus prednisone) should significantly improve overall survival for long time in metastatic CRPC, but more often grade 3–4 adverse events. In the current study, we reported that docetaxel 40 mg/m^2 every 2 weeks plus prednisolone was similar in efficacy and manageable toxicities compared to previous studies.

Docetaxel administrated 75 mg/m2 every 3 weeks is mostly used at the standard of chemotherapy of mCRPC. However, therapy-related adverse effects and treatment related mortality were prevalent in elderly and fragile patients to receive standard regimen. Although the response of docetaxel 75 mg/m2 every 3 weeks schedule was favorable, it did not show the good overall survival for these patients. [19].

In a retrospective study, we evaluated the feasibility of biweekly docetaxel 40 mg/m2 and compared with 75 mg/m2 every 3 weeks for mCRPC. Their median age was 68 years (range, 52–84). The patients received biweekly docetaxel 40 mg/m2 presented similar TTP (5.0 months vs 4.2 months, p-value = 0.530) and minor incidence of Gr 3/4 adverse events. This result exhibited one of the treatment schedule options for mCRPC [11].

There were no comparable studies of biweekly docetaxel 40 mg/m2 and 75 mg/m2 every 3 weeks for mCNPC. In the CHAARTED study, the researchers compared the efficacy and toxicity of docetaxel (at a dose of 75 mg/m^2 every 3 weeks for 6 cycles) plus ADT and ADT alone of 790 mCNPC patients. The docetaxel plus ADT regimen demonstrated better outcomes than ADT alone (57.6 months vs. 44.0 months; $P < 0.001$) in patient with mCNPC. The current outcome was not equally comparable with the CHAARTED due to the follow-up period was shorter, as so we need a long-term follow-up period to present the outcome including OS. However, adequate response rate reached 87% even in the short observation period, we considered one of the treatment options.

We already know that the high tumor burden is a poor prognostic factor. Each clinical study had also dealt with the correlation survival and high tumor burden. In the subgroup analysis from the CHAARTED study, a high volume of metastases was defined by the presence of visceral metastases or four or more bone lesions with at least one beyond the vertebral bodies and pelvis. There were 57 (14.4%) patients with visceral metastasis who had poor median OS (49.2 months) than in all CNPC patients (57.6 months) [13, 14]. In the GETUG-AFU15 study, the median OS was approximately 62.1 months

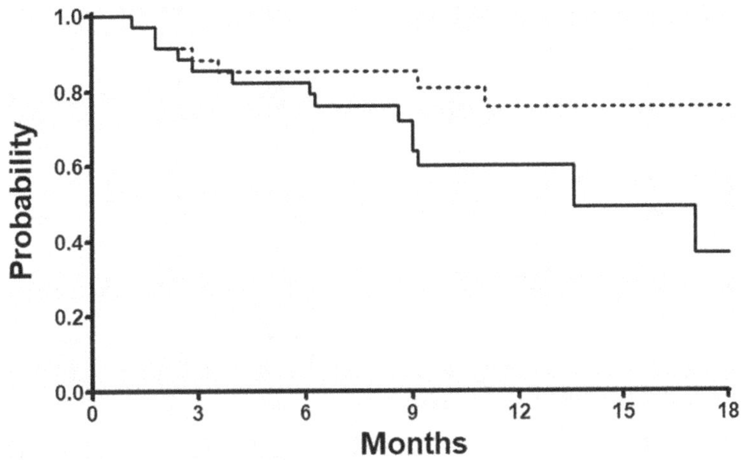

Fig. 1 Kaplan–Meier curve for PFS (solid line) and OS (dotted line)

in the mCNPC patients, and less than 36 months in the mCNPC patient with high-volume, high-risk disease [14].

In current study, we included that all patients had high-volume CNPC such as visceral metastasis (49%) and bone metastasis (51%). The result (median PFS: 13.6 months, 95% CI: 6.7–20.4) was not as bad as expected from high risk. However, it is limited in interpretation of the PFS because of small sample size and short follow up period. Based on recent randomized trials [13–15] and our data, the addition of docetaxel to ADT is recommended for patients with high-risk, metastatic CNPC who are medically-fit enough to tolerate docetaxel.

In the CHAARTED, the total dosage of docetaxel 75 mg/m^2 every 3 weeks for 6 cycles was 450 mg, and the period of administration was 18 weeks. Similarly, the total dosage of the 40 mg/m^2 every two-week regimen was 480 mg, and the period of administration was 24 weeks. There was a little difference in docetaxel dosage or administration period between the two regimens. Nevertheless, it showed a different pattern of drug toxicities between the two studies. Approximately 12.1% of patients in the CHAARTED had grade 3 or 4 neutropenia and 6.1% had grade 3 or 4 febrile neutropenia. [13, 14]. In present study, the most common hematologic toxicity of any grade was anemia ($n = 12$), and grade 3 or 4 hematological adverse events occurred infrequently. There was no big distinctness in the dose and the toxicity was lower in 40 mg/m^2 every two-week regimen. So, we could suggest A as other administration schedules on these results.

The major limitations of our retrospective study include small sample size and lack of a control arm to better define differences between biweekly dosing and standard dosing in this population. Further accumulation of cases with longer follow-up periods is necessary. Within the limitations of our study, we demonstrated that early chemotherapy with biweekly docetaxel regimen resulted in tolerability and activity in patients with high-risk CNPC.

ADT plus biweekly-administered docetaxel appeared to be tolerated and effective in patients with high-risk mCNPC comparable with CRPC. Our results suggest that a biweekly docetaxel chemotherapy regimen is considered to have manageable toxicities and to yield acceptable results compared to a thrice-weekly docetaxel regimen.

Conclusion

In conclusion, ADT plus biweekly-administered docetaxel appeared tolerable toxicities and similar efficacy compared with standard thrice-weekly docetaxel. From this result, we could suggest that docetaxel 40 mg/m2 biweekly regimen is an additional treatment option for mCNPC.

Abbreviations

ADT: Androgen-deprivation therapy; CNPC: Castration-naïve prostate cancer; CRPC: Castration-resistant prostate cancer; GNRH: Gonadotropin-releasing hormone

Acknowledgements

Abstract of this manuscript is presented in annual meeting of ASCO 2018

Authors' contributions

SHP conceived and designated the study; SEY, SEP, YJK and JJC participated in its design and coordination and helped to draft the manuscript. HGJ, HYC and SJL performed relevant operations and collected patients' data; MYK and HHS helped acquisition and interpretation of data; SEP and SHP participated in the statistical analysis; BCJ, SLS, SSJ and HML critically revised the manuscript; All authors read and approved the final manuscript.

Author details

[1]Division of Hematology-Oncology, Department of Medicine, Samsung Medical Center, Sungkyunkwan University School of Medicine, 81 Irwon-ro, Gangnam-gu, Seoul 06351, South Korea. [2]Department of Urology, Samsung Medical Center, Sungkyunkwan University School of Medicine, Seoul, South Korea. [3]Department of Urology, Kangbuk Samsung Hospital, Sungkyunkwan University School of Medicine, Seoul, South Korea.

References

1. Jung KW, Won YJ, Oh CM, Kong HJ, Lee DH, Lee KH, et al. Cancer statistics in Korea: incidence, mortality, survival, and prevalence in 2014. Cancer Res Treat. 2017;49(2):292–305.
2. Prostate Cancer Trialists' Collaborative Group. Maximum androgen blockade in advanced prostate cancer: an overview of the randomised trials. Lancet. 2000;355(9214):1491–8.
3. Petrylak DP, Tangen CM, Hussain MH, Lara PN Jr, Jones JA, Taplin ME, et al. Docetaxel and estramustine compared with mitoxantrone and prednisone for advanced refractory prostate cancer. N Engl J Med. 2004;351(15):1513–20.
4. Tannock IF, de Wit R, Berry WR, Horti J, Pluzanska A, Chi KN, et al. Docetaxel plus prednisone or mitoxantrone plus prednisone for advanced prostate cancer. N Engl J Med. 2004;351(15):1502–12.
5. Joly F, Tannock IF. Chemotherapy for patients with hormone-refractory prostate cancer. Ann Oncol. 2004;15(11):1582–4.
6. Berthold DR, Pond GR, Soban F, de Wit R, Eisenberger M, Tannock IF. Docetaxel plus prednisone or mitoxantrone plus prednisone for advanced prostate cancer: updated survival in the TAX 327 study. J Clin Oncol. 2008; 26(2):242–5.
7. Shimazui T, Kawai K, Miyanaga N, Kojima T, Sekido N, Hinotsu S, et al. Three-weekly docetaxel with prednisone is feasible for Japanese patients with hormone-refractory prostate cancer: a retrospective comparative study with weekly docetaxel alone. Jpn J Clin Oncol. 2007;37(8):603–8.
8. Taguchi T, Furue H, Niitani H, Ishitani K, Kanamaru R, Hasegawa K, et al. Phase I clinical trial of RP 56976 (docetaxel) a new anticancer drug. Gan To Kagaku Ryoho. 1994;21(12):1997–2005.
9. Lee JL, Kim JE, Ahn JH, Lee DH, Lee J, Kim CS, et al. Efficacy and safety of docetaxel plus prednisolone chemotherapy for metastatic hormone-refractory prostate adenocarcinoma: single institutional study in Korea. Cancer Res Treat. 2010;42(1):12–7.
10. Kellokumpu-Lehtinen PL, Harmenberg U, Joensuu T, McDermott R, Hervonen P, Ginman C, et al. 2-weekly versus 3-weekly docetaxel to treat castration-resistant advanced prostate cancer: a randomised, phase 3 trial. Lancet Oncol. 2013;14(2):117–24.
11. Kim HS, Lee JY, Lee SJ, Lim HY, Sung HH, Jeon HG, et al. A retrospective feasibility study of biweekly, reduced-dose docetaxel in Asian patients with castrate-resistant, metastatic prostate cancer. BMC Urol. 2017;17(1):63.
12. Millikan RE, Wen S, Pagliaro LC, Brown MA, Moomey B, Do KA, et al. Phase III trial of androgen ablation with or without three cycles of systemic chemotherapy for advanced prostate cancer. J Clin Oncol. 2008;26(36): 5936–42.

13. Sweeney CJ, Chen YH, Carducci M, Liu G, Jarrard DF, Eisenberger M, et al. Chemohormonal therapy in metastatic hormone-sensitive prostate Cancer. N Engl J Med. 2015;373(8):737–46.
14. Gravis G, Boher JM, Joly F, Soulie M, Albiges L, Priou F, et al. Androgen deprivation therapy (ADT) plus docetaxel versus ADT alone in metastatic non castrate prostate Cancer: impact of metastatic burden and long-term survival analysis of the randomized phase 3 GETUG-AFU15 trial. Eur Urol. 2016;70(2):256–62.
15. James ND, Sydes MR, Clarke NW, Mason MD, Dearnaley DP, Spears MR, et al. Addition of docetaxel, zoledronic acid, or both to first-line long-term hormone therapy in prostate cancer (STAMPEDE): survival results from an adaptive, multiarm, multistage, platform randomised controlled trial. Lancet. 2016;387(10024):1163–77.
16. Parker C, Gillessen S, Heidenreich A, Horwich A, Committee EG. Cancer of the prostate: ESMO clinical practice guidelines for diagnosis, treatment and follow-up. Ann Oncol. 2015;26(Suppl 5):v69–77.
17. Gillessen S, Attard G, Beer TM, Beltran H, Bossi A, Bristow R, et al. Management of Patients with advanced prostate Cancer: the report of the advanced prostate Cancer consensus conference APCCC 2017. Eur Urol. 2018;73(2): 178–211.
18. Scher HI, Halabi S, Tannock I, Morris M, Sternberg CN, Carducci MA, et al. Design and end points of clinical trials for patients with progressive prostate cancer and castrate levels of testosterone: recommendations of the prostate Cancer clinical trials working group. J Clin Oncol. 2008;26(7):1148–59.
19. Droz JP, Aapro M, Balducci L, Boyle H, Van den Broeck T, Cathcart P, et al. Management of prostate cancer in older patients: updated recommendations of a working group of the International Society of Geriatric Oncology. Lancet Oncol. 2014;15:e404–14.

23

Literature review of the burden of prostate cancer in Germany, France, the United Kingdom and Canada

J. Smith-Palmer[1*], C. Takizawa[2] and W. Valentine[1]

Abstract

Background: Prostate cancer is the most frequently reported cancer in males in Europe, and is associated with substantial morbidity and mortality. The aim of the current review was to characterize the clinical, economic and humanistic burden of disease associated with prostate cancer in France, Germany, the UK and Canada.

Methods: Literature searches were conducted using the PubMed, EMBASE and Cochrane Library databases to identify studies reporting incidence and/or mortality rates, costs and health state utilities associated with prostate cancer in the settings of interest. For inclusion, studies were required to be published in English in full-text form from 2006 onwards.

Results: Incidence studies showed that in all settings the incidence of prostate cancer has increased substantially over the past two decades, driven in part by increased uptake of prostate specific antigen (PSA) screening leading to earlier identification of tumors, but which has also led to over-treatment, compounding the economic burden of disease. Mortality rates have declined over the same time frame, driven by earlier detection and improvements in treatment. Both prostate cancer itself, as well as treatment and treatment-related complications, are associated with reduced quality of life.

Conclusions: Prostate cancer is associated with a significant clinical and economic burden, whilst earlier detection and aggressive treatment is associated with improved survival, over-treatment of men with indolent tumors compounds the already significant burden of disease and treatment can lead to long-term side effects including impotence and impaired urinary and/or bowel function. There is currently an unmet clinical need for diagnostic and/or prognostic tools that facilitate personalized prostate cancer treatment, and potentially reduce the clinical, economic and humanistic burden of invasive cancer treatment.

Keywords: Prostate cancer, Cost of illness, France, Germany, United Kingdom, Canada

Background

In Europe, prostate cancer is now the most common cancer in men, accounting for 23% of all male cancers (n = 417,000 cases) and 10% of cancer-related deaths in males (n = 92,000 deaths) in 2012 [1]. Prostate cancers are heterogeneous in terms of presentation and morphology but nearly all are classified as adenocarcinomas and in many instances remain asymptomatic until locally advanced or metastatic. The incidence of prostate cancer is strongly related to age, and in the UK it is estimated that 1 in 8 men will be diagnosed with prostate cancer during their lifetime [2]. However, in a large proportion of men, prostate cancer is indolent or slow growing so may not become clinically significant during the lifetime of the patient, such that the number of men who die with prostate cancer by far exceeds the number of men who die due to prostate cancer. Indeed, autopsy studies in men who died from causes other than prostate cancer report an incidental prostate cancer prevalence at the time of death ranging from 5% at age < 30 years to 59% at age > 79 years [3].

* Correspondence: smith-palmer@ossianconsulting.com
[1]Ossian Health Economics and Communications GmbH, Bäumleingasse 20, 4051 Basel, Switzerland
Full list of author information is available at the end of the article

In Western Europe and North America opportunistic screening for elevated prostate specific antigen (PSA) levels is commonly performed in middle-aged and elderly men. PSA is a serine protease that is expressed almost exclusively in the epithelial cells of the prostate gland and elevated PSA levels are a key indicator of prostate cancer. However, increased PSA levels can also occur as a result of several other conditions including, most notably, benign prostatic hyperplasia and prostatitis. Men with elevated PSA levels are therefore commonly referred for digital rectal examination (DRE) and/or biopsy to confirm the presence of cancer. In many settings PSA screening has contributed to enhanced detection, diagnosis and treatment of prostate cancer, but it is a contentious issue owing to the potential for over-diagnosis and over-treatment of prostate cancers that may not become clinically significant during the lifetime of the patient. Screening remains opportunistic rather than routine in many settings. In the United States, in 2008 the Preventative Services Task Force (USPSTF) recommended against routine screening due to its psychological harms and uncertainty around its clinical benefits [4]. However, the USPSTF recently updated its recommendations for men aged 55–69 years, stating that men should be informed of the potential benefits and harms of PSA screening and that the final decision should rest with the individual [5]. Other investigators have also suggested that population-based screening could lead to over-treatment [6].

In addition to the psychological harms cited by the US Preventative Services Task Force over-treatment may place an unnecessary burden on already overstretched health systems, and on an individual patient level increases the potential for treatment-related side-effects including impotence, impaired bowel function and incontinence, which can have a significant detrimental impact on quality of life. In particular, radical prostatectomy, the use of which has increased substantially in recent years, is generally advocated in men with localized disease with life expectancy > 10 years and who are willing to accept the risk of complications. Radical prostatectomy is associated with high medical resource use with reported median length of stay ranging from two to eight days in studies from the US and Europe [7–9]. A high proportion of men who undergo radical prostatectomy experience post-operative complications including erectile dysfunction and urinary incontinence, which can lead to impaired quality of life in terms of sexual and urinary function [10]. There is also a risk of complications for men who undergo radiation treatments, which can include painful urination, urinary incontinence, urethral stricture, rectal bleeding and/or leaking, erectile dysfunction and lymphedema. Moreover, such symptoms can negatively impact quality of life not only in men undergoing radical prostatectomy, but also in the partners of patients, who may also act as informal care givers in many instances.

The phenomenon of over-treatment is becoming increasingly recognized by physicians and consequently the strategies of watchful waiting and active surveillance are now recommended in several guidelines for men with low risk/early stage prostate cancer [11, 12]. Moreover, an increased uptake in active surveillance in recent years likely reflects efforts to reduce the over-treatment of low risk prostate cancer. The recently published ProtecT trial compared 10-year outcomes with active monitoring compared with surgery or radiotherapy in men with localized prostate cancer detected during PSA testing. Overall, 10-year prostate cancer-specific mortality rates were low in all trial arms and not significantly different between arms. However, significantly higher rates of disease progression and development of metastases were reported in the active monitoring group compared with either immediate surgery or radiotherapy [13]. As illustrated by the findings of ProtecT, as well as other trials, a key challenge in managing over-treatment is identifying and distinguishing between men with tumors that are likely to progress to clinically significant disease and those whose disease is likely to remain indolent for the remainder of their lifetime. Prostate cancer is a heterogeneous disease and current staging methods such as Gleason grade, whilst a powerful prognostic indicator, are associated with limitations. In particular, there may be inter-observer variability in determining Gleason grade and tumor tissue may be heterogeneous and may be multifocal in origin, which biopsy may not detect [14, 15]. Additionally, reported sensitivity rates for transrectal ultrasound-guided biopsy range from 49 to 87%, whilst specificity ranges from 38 to 93% [16]. There is currently a significant research effort directed towards characterizing and better understanding biomarkers that can aid prognosis and predict risk of recurrence and several genomic profiling tools have recently been developed, although the use of such tools in clinical practice is not currently widespread. Future research efforts in this area may help to identify to better distinguish between those patients whose disease is likely to progress versus those whose disease is likely to remain indolent or not clinically significant and therefore help to reduce over-treatment.

The high incidence of men with prostate cancer requiring treatment, as well as those with elevated PSA levels or low risk prostate cancer undergoing watchful waiting or active surveillance, means that the economic burden of prostate cancer is also substantial. In the UK alone, total annual costs for treatment in the first year following diagnosis have been estimated at approximately EUR 117 million and in France and Germany this figure is two- to three-fold higher [17]. Additionally, in the UK the active surveillance approach advocates repeat biopsy at 12 months after an observed elevation in PSA levels as well as regular follow up PSA tests and DREs. This approach is therefore also associated with notable medical resource utilization, although direct medical costs for these patients are likely to be substantially lower than for those patients undergoing treatment. In some settings, MRI is being increasingly used in to help guide biopsies and can improve the detection of clinically significant tumors relative to standard biopsy approaches alone, as well as providing the potential to exclude clinically insignificant tumors and reduce the requirement for subsequent biopsies [18]. Indeed, findings from the recently published PRECISION trial showed that a strategy of MRI prior to MRI-targeted biopsy (if required) was superior to standard transrectal ultrasonography-guided biopsy in terms of detecting clinically significant cancer [19]. MRI can also be used following negative transrectal ultrasound biopsy in high risk patients where it can be used to guide subsequent biopsies [18, 20], MRI also has an emerging role in active surveillance and detection of local recurrence following treatment, all of which have implications in terms of medical resource utilization [20].

Several factors contribute to the overall burden of disease of prostate cancer, these include the incidence and mortality rates as well as direct and indirect costs, the humanistic burden associated with the impact of a diagnosis of prostate cancer on quality of life as well as the burden placed on the caregivers of men with prostate cancer. To characterize the burden of prostate cancer in Europe and North America (using the specific examples of Germany, France, the United Kingdom and Canada) in terms of incidence, cost and impact on quality of life of prostate cancer, a literature review of recently published articles was undertaken.

Methods

Literature search strategies were designed to capture recently published data relating to the clinical, economic and humanistic burden of prostate cancer in France, Germany, the United Kingdom and Canada. Search strategies were designed using high level Medical Subject Heading (MeSH) terms supplemented with free text terms with the search syntax adapted as required for use in the PubMed, EMBASE and Cochrane Library database (full details of the search strategies used are available in the Additional file 1). Searches were limited to full text articles published in English since 2006. The scope of the search was limited to articles conducted in populations in France, Germany, the United Kingdom or Canada, or presenting data according to country-based subgroups including either France, Germany, the United Kingdom or Canada. For inclusion, epidemiologic studies were also required to report incidence and/or mortality rates for the overall or general population, consequently, studies presenting data only within or according to population subgroups (e.g. only reporting data from one age group, ethnic group or socioeconomic group) were excluded, secondary sources of data were also excluded. All searches were performed on 7 April, 2016.

Results

Literature searches

Literature searches across the PubMed, EMBASE and Cochrane Library identified a total of 2966 articles. After removal of duplicates a total of 2772 unique articles were screened. An initial first round screen of title and abstracts was performed to identify potentially relevant articles for full text screening. A total of 163 articles were identified for full text screening and a total of 49 articles were included in the final review.

Incidence, mortality and survival

A total of 16 articles reported the incidence of prostate cancer either in the overall population or in a representative sample of the overall population in France, Germany, the UK or Canada [21–36]. Although the searches required articles to be published from 2006 onwards, several articles published incidence data from before this cut off point. In both France and Germany, annual age-standardized incidence figures from 2005 onwards were consistently in the region of approximately 100–130 per 100,000 (Table 1). In terms of absolute numbers of cases, in both France and Germany, more than 50,000 incident cases were reported annually from 2004 onwards.

For the UK, the range of reported incidence figures from 2007 onwards showed greater variation from a low of 75 per 100,000 in 2007 in a study conducted in the West of Scotland using data from the Scottish Cancer Registry [32] to a high of 417 per 100,000 in a study utilizing data from the Anglican Cancer Network [29]. Only one UK-based study presented the absolute number of incident cases, here Mistry et al. reported that in 2007 there were > 36,000 incident cases of prostate cancer as well as projecting that by 2030 this figure will increase to > 61,000 [30].

One of the studies included in the review was a European-wide study of prostate cancer incidence and mortality over the past two decades [23]. This study showed a geographic gradient in prostate cancer incidence with the highest incidence rates reported in Northern Europe and the lowest in Eastern Europe. Analysis of incidence trends over the last two decades showed annual increases in prostate cancer of between 3 and 7% in most countries, which concurs with the findings of other studies included in the current review. However, in the final years of the multinational study by Bray et al. decreases in incidence were reported in several high incidence countries.

Table 1 Incidence of prostate cancer in France, Germany, the United Kingdom and Canada

Study (year)	Year of data	Age standardized incidence per 100,000	Incident number of cases, n
France			
Binder-Foucard et al. (2014) [21]	1980	24.8	—
	2005	127.1	—
	2012	—	53,465 (95% CI: 46,840 to 60,090)
Crocetti et al. (2013) [22]	1998–2002	122	183,136
Bray et al. (2010) [23]	1988–2002	115.0	—
Belot et al. (2008) [24]	1980	23	10,756
	1985	33	14,190
	1990	42.2	18,979
	1995	56.5	26,760
	2000	80.4	39,636
	2005	121.2	62,245
Germany			
Haberland et al. (2010) [25]	2004	112.0	58,574
	2015	—	70,904 (projected)
	2020	—	76,034 (projected)
Dorr et al. (2015) [26]	1990–1992	55.2	—
	2008–2010	106.0	—
Becker et al. (2007) [27]	2002	147.9 (crude)	—
Rohde et al. (2009) [28]	2001–2002	101.9	—
	2002–2003	125.6	—
	2004–2005	101.9	—
Bray et al. (2010) [23]	1975–2002	109.8	—
United Kingdom			
Greenberg et al. (2013) [29]	2000–2005 (total cases)	365.11	—
	2000–2005 (metastasis)	58.2	—
	2006–2010 (total cases)	416.73	—
	2006–2010 (metastasis)	51.13	—
Mistry et al. (2011) [30]	1984	40.5	11,714
	2007	97.2	36,083
	2030	104.8	61,089
Pashayan et al. (2006) [31]	1971	32	—
	2000	89	—
Shafique et al. (2012) [32]	1991	44	—
	2007	75	—
Feletto et al. (2015) [33]	2011	107.4	—
Westlake (2009) [34]	2004–2006	98.3	—
Bray et al. (2010) [23] (England and wales)	1980–2006	87.5	—
Canada			—
Kachuri et al. (2013) [35]	1970	53.8	—
	2007	124.7	—
Feletto et al. (2015) [33]	2007	133	—
Louchini et al. (2008) [36]	1988–2004	67.1 (66.5–67.7)	—

Only two studies reported age-standardized incidence in Canada from 2007 onwards, both of which were broadly consistent with incidence figures ranging from 125 to 133 per 100,000 in 2007 [33, 35]. Additionally, one of the Canada-based studies examined incidence rates over time, reporting that in 1970 age-standardized prostate cancer incidence was 54 per 100,000, showing that as in Western European settings the incidence of prostate cancer in Canada has increased steadily over time [35].

A total of 11 studies reported mortality rates in men with prostate cancer in France, Germany the UK and Canada [21, 23–25, 27, 28, 33–37]. The lowest mortality rates were reported in French studies, where the mortality rate for post-2005 studies ranged from 10 to 14 per 100,000 population [21, 24]. Two French studies also reported the absolute number of deaths attributable to prostate cancer; in France from 1995 onwards there were approximately 9000 prostate cancer deaths per year [21, 24], whilst in Germany in 2004 approximately 11,000 men died due to prostate cancer [25]. In the UK, Germany and Canada mortality rates from 2003 were broadly similar across all three settings ranging from 17 to 28 per 100,000 (Table 2). Studies that examined mortality rates over time consistently reported declining mortality over time [21, 24, 28, 35]. In particular, in Germany mortality rates decreased by 20% over the period 1999–2005 [28].

In addition to mortality figures, a total of six studies reported 5-year relative survival rates. One study was multinational [38] and the remaining five were conducted in Germany [26, 39–42]. In Germany, 5-year relative survival rates ranged from 81%, reported over the period 1995–2003 [42] to 95%, reported over the period 2005–2010 [26]. The multinational study by Trama et al. reported a 5-year survival rate over the period 2000–2007 of 89% for men in both France and Germany; however, for the UK, the corresponding figure was lower at 81% [38]. Additionally, UK-based evidence from Cancer Research UK, demonstrate the strength of the relationship between stage at diagnosis and 5-year relative survival. For men diagnosed with stage I prostate cancer, 5-year relative survival in the UK is 112% (implying that these men live longer than the general population), which decreases to 93% for men diagnosed with stage III disease and 30% for men diagnosed with stage IV disease [43].

A multinational study by Bray et al. also noted declining mortality rates were seen in a total of 13 countries, which were primarily high-income countries in Western Europe. The decreases in mortality that were seen over time in several studies have been attributed to increased uptake of opportunistic PSA screening from the early 1990s onwards leading to detection of prostate cancer at earlier stages as well as changes in treatment uptake and continual improvements in treatment modalities. However, the evidence for the reduced mortality due to increased PSA screening is not conclusive. For example, one study from the Munich Cancer Registry showed that treatment modalities have changed over time and that use of radical prostatectomy increased from approximately 20 to 50% over the last two decades, whilst the use of hormone therapy has decreased over this period [26]. A "stage shift" towards earlier detection of tumors was also evident in the UK; Greenberg et al. reported a significant increase in overall prostate cancer incidence, but a significant decrease in the incidence of metastatic prostate cancer in the period 2006–2010 compared with 2000–2005 [29]. The existence of a stage shift is however not universally supported as other studies including a UK-based study by Shafique et al. reported no evidence of a stage shift [32].

Economic burden of prostate cancer

The consensus among studies that investigated temporal trends in prostate cancer incidence is one of increasing incidence over time. This, together with high rates of over-treatment in many settings mean that the economic burden associated with the treatment and monitoring of men is both substantial and growing.

Only one study identified in the literature review examined the overall burden of prostate cancer on a national level [17], however, nine other study reported direct or indirect costs on a per patient level [44–52]. Fourcade et al. examined per patient and total costs for men with prostate cancer in the first year after diagnosis in five European countries (France, Germany, Italy, Spain and the UK) [17]. In the countries of interest, the total overall burden in the first year after diagnosis was highest in France at EUR 385 million, followed by Germany at EUR 244 million and then the UK at EUR 117 million per year (2006 EUR). Further, another study (identified by supplementary hand-searches) reported that in the EU the overall cost (including direct and indirect costs) of prostate cancer in 2009 was EUR 8.43 billion, which constitutes 7% of the overall economic burden of cancer in the EU and of which, EUR 5.43 billion were healthcare costs, EUR 0.73 billion was due to lost productivity and EUR 1.88 billion was attributable to costs associated with informal care [53]. The study by Fourcade et al. also reported per patient costs (excluding follow-up and adverse event costs), which were highest in France at EUR 5851 per patient, followed by Germany at EUR 3698 then the UK at EUR 3682 per patient. In a similar study from Canada, De Oliveria reported that the total healthcare costs in the first 12 months after diagnosis in men aged ≥45 years were CAD 15,170 per patient [47].

Two cost studies included in the review examined direct costs according to cancer stage and/or treatment [44, 50]. In the first of these, Molinier et al. report overall costs of EUR 12,731 per patient (2008 EUR), but when broken down according to stage, in France, patients with regional

Table 2 Prostate cancer-related mortality in France, Germany, the United Kingdom and Canada

Study (year)	Year of data	Age standardized mortality per 100,000	Number of deaths, n
France			
Binder-Foucard et al. (2014) [21]	1980	16.3	—
	2012	10.2	8876
Bray et al. (2010) [23]	1975–2007	24.9	—
Belot et al. (2008) [24]	1980	16.9	7001
	1985	17.8	8090
	1990	17.7	8875
	1995	16.7	9279
	2000	15.3	9295
	2005	13.5	9202
Germany			
Haberland et al. (2010) [25]	2004	22.2	11,135
Becker et al. (2007) [27]	2002	28.3 (crude)	—
Rohde et al. (2009) [28]	2001–2002	29.3	—
	2002–2003	28.9	—
	2004–2005	27.9	—
Bray et al. (2010) [23]	1975–2006	23.3	—
United Kingdom			
Feletto et al. (2015) [33]	2010	23.8	—
Westlake (2009) [34]	2004–2006	25.7	—
Bray et al. (2010) [23] (England and Wales)	1975–2007	26.8	—
Marshall et al. (2016) [37]	2003–2007	25.7	—
Canada			
Kachuri et al. (2013) [35]	1970	25.4	—
	2007	20.4	—
Feletto et al. (2015) [33]	2011	16.7	—
Louchini et al. (2008) [36]	1988–2004	16.8(16.5–17.1)	—

prostate cancer had the highest total costs at EUR 16,608 per patient, whilst those with metastatic disease had the lowest overall costs at EUR 9994 per patient [44]. Additionally, in terms of costs for specific treatment modalities, Molinier et al. also reported that external beam radiotherapy was consistently associated with the highest direct costs, followed by radical prostatectomy then androgen deprivation therapy. Notably, costs associated with a watchful waiting approach ranged from EUR 4730–9355. Similarly, in a Canadian study direct medical costs (per 100 days in health state) were highest for patients with advanced disease (Table 3).

The majority of cost studies identified reported direct or total costs, with only two studies reporting indirect costs in terms of patient time costs and also patient out--of-pocket costs. In one Canadian study mean (95% CI) annual patient time costs were CAD 838 (442–1233) (2006 CAD) and annual patient out of pocket costs were CAD 200 (109–290) [49]. However, both patient time and out-of-pocket costs were influenced by several parameters, including age. In particular, men aged ≤60 years had higher patient time and out-of-pocket costs compared with those aged > 60 years, with the difference in out-of-pocket costs being statistically significant ($p = 0.03$) [49]. In the UK, annual mean (95% CI) out-of-pocket costs were GBP 86 (28–144) and mean annual costs for informal care were GBP 197 (– 66–460) [46]. The Canadian study also examined patient time and out-of-pocket costs according to urinary function, bowel function and sexual function according to the Prostate Cancer Index (PCI) score. Patients with the lowest scores for urinary function (score = 0–25) had mean total (patient time and out-of-pocket) costs of CAD 4186 per year, which was almost ten-fold higher than for patients with the highest (75–100) PCI urinary function scores (CAD 444 per year). Similarly, total patient time and out-of-pocket costs for patients with the lowest PCI sexual function scores were almost two-fold higher than those with the highest scores (CAD 1401 versus CAD 728) [49].

Table 3 Per patient cost of prostate cancer in France, Germany, United Kingdom and Canada

Study (year)	Description of cost	Cost year	Currency	Mean cost
France				
Fourcade et al. (2010) [17]	Total direct cost of treatment in 12 months after diagnosis, excluding follow up and adverse event costs, for all diagnosed patients	2006	EUR	5851
Molinier et al. (2011) [44]	Mean total cost (all prostate cancer)	2008	EUR	12,731
	Mean total cost localized	2008	EUR	12,259
	Mean total cost regional	2008	EUR	16,608
	Mean total cost metastatic	2008	EUR	9994
Germany				
Fourcade et al. (2010) [17]	Total direct cost of treatment in 12 months after diagnosis, excluding follow up and AE costs, for all diagnosed patients	2006	EUR	3698
UK				
Hall et al. (2015) [45]	Cumulative hospital-based costs of care over 15 months following initial diagnosis in patients treated with curative intent	2011/12	GBP	3722 (95% CI, 3263–4208)
Fourcade et al. (2010) [17]	Total direct cost of treatment in 12 months after diagnosis, excluding follow up and AE costs, for all diagnosed patients	2006	EUR	3682
Marti et al. (2016) [46]	Total societal (and component costs) in prostate cancer survivors treated with curative intent over 12–15 months post-diagnosis period			
	Total societal cost (per month)	2012	GBP	117.9 (95% CI: 68.9–167.0)
	NHS costs (per month)	2012	GBP	92.1 (49.3–134.9)
	Patient OOP costs (per month)	2012	GBP	7.2 (2.3–12.0)
	Informal care costs (per month)	2012	GBP	16.4 (−5.5–38.3)
Canada				
De Oliveira et al. (2013) [47]	Total healthcare costs in 12 months after diagnosis in patients aged ≥45 years	2009[a]	CAD	15,170
Krahn et al. (2010) [48]	Direct medical costs for men diagnosed 1995–2002 according to phase	2004	CAD	
	Phase Ib (costs incurred in 6 months prior to prostate cancer diagnosis)	2004	CAD	1904
	Phase IIb (costs incurred in first 12 months after prostate cancer diagnosis)	2004	CAD	12,005
	Phase IIIb ("continued care" phase, costs per 100 days)	2004	CAD	1495
	Phase IVb (pre-terminal care in 18 to 6 months before death)	2004	CAD	20,543
	Phase Vb (terminal care, 6 months before death)	2004	CAD	28,834
De Oliveira et al. (2014) [49]	Patient time costs per year (all)	2006	CAD	838 (442–1233)
	Out of pocket costs per year (all)	2006	CAD	200 (109–290)
Krahn et al. (2014) [50]	Early health states: non-treated, non-metastatic[a]	2008	CAD	3440
	Early health states: radiation therapy[a]	2008	CAD	2160
	Early health states: radical prostatectomy[a]	2008	CAD	4676

Table 3 Per patient cost of prostate cancer in France, Germany, United Kingdom and Canada *(Continued)*

Study (year)	Description of cost	Cost year	Currency	Mean cost
	Early health states: hormone therapy[a]	2008	CAD	3357
	Middle health states: post-radiation therapy[a]	2008	CAD	1556
	Middle health states: post-radical prostatectomy[a]	2008	CAD	732
	Middle health states: recurrence/progression[a]	2008	CAD	1919
	Late health states: hormone therapy refractory[a]	2008	CAD	4503
	Late health states: metastatic[a]	2008	CAD	4062
	Late health states: metastatic refractory[a]	2008	CAD	6398
	Late health states: final[a]	2008	CAD	13,739
Sanyal et al. (2016) [51]	Total overall cost (overall cohort) at:			
	5 years	2014	CAD	18,503 (17,851–19,185)
	10 years	2014	CAD	28,032 (26,129–29,973)
	15 years	2014	CAD	39,143 (36,606–41,821)
Dragomir et al. (2014) [52]	Active surveillance; cost first 5 years	2012	CAD	6200 (6083 to 6317)
	Immediate treatment; cost first 5 years	2012	CAD	13,735 (13,615 to 13,855)

[a]Cost per 100 days

Quality of life in patients with prostate cancer

There are a large number of studies in the literature that either qualitatively or quantitatively assess the impact of prostate cancer on quality of life (QoL), however, the scope of the current literature review was limited to studies reporting health state utility values for men with prostate cancer. In total, nine studies were identified that examined the health status of men with prostate cancer in either France, Germany, the UK or Canada [45, 54–61]. Several different instruments were used in these studies to directly or indirectly assess QoL in men with prostate cancer including the EQ-5D, European Organization for Research and Treatment of Cancer 8-dimensional utility index (EORTC-8D), patient-oriented prostate utility scale (PORPUS-U), Health Utilities Index 2 and 3 (HUI-2; HUI-3) and the Quality of Well Being scale (QWB). Utility values were also reported for several different health states including overall men at risk for prostate cancer, overall populations of men with prostate cancer, men with localized disease and those with metastatic disease as well as pre- and post-treatment utility values. Heterogeneity in the literature in terms of the exact definitions of health states used, treatment modalities and the time period at which QoL was assessed complicates the comparison of QoL between studies. However, the literature consistently showed that QoL is reduced in men with prostate cancer relative to the general population, although the magnitude of impairment was influenced by disease stage, treatment and presence of complications in terms of urinary function, bowel function and sexual function (Table 4). In particular, men with who reported moderate or big problems with bowel function had a mean (SD) utility value (EQ-5D) of 0.653 (0.195) compared with 0.862 (0.166) for those with no problems with bowel function [56]. Other studies conducted in the general population confirm that complications of treatment, including erectile dysfunction, bowel dysfunction and urinary incontinence can have a substantial detrimental impact on QoL. For example, in one multinational study of QoL in men with erectile dysfunction, and their partners, mean utility values, elicited using standard gamble, ranged from 0.40–0.49 [62]. Similarly, QoL is also reduced relative to the general population in people with urinary incontinence [63].

One multinational study presented utility values (using the EQ-5D) for men with metastatic hormone refractory prostate cancer reported health state utility values ranging from 0.527 for men in Germany to 0.750 for men in Canada [54]. Interestingly, these values are notably lower than those reported by Krahn et al. for Canadian men with metastatic disease, who had a mean utility value (using the EQ-5D) of 0.84, which was the same as that for men with localized prostate cancer who were receiving treatment (radical prostatectomy, radiotherapy or hormonal therapy) [58]. Lloyd et al. also assessed QoL in UK-based men with metastatic castration-resistant prostate cancer using both the EQ-5D and EORTC-8D questionnaires. Using the EQ-5D Lloyd et al. report a mean (SD) utility value of 0.830 (0.126) for men who were asymptomatic or mildly symptomatic before chemotherapy, whilst for men who were symptomatic this value was substantially lower at 0.625 (0.173) [55]. However, the same study reported higher values for the same health states when utility values were elicited using the EORTC-8D questionnaire. For example, the mean (SD) utility value for men with metastatic castration resistant prostate cancer currently receiving chemotherapy was 0.692 (0.219) using the EQ-5D and 0.750 (0.117) using the EORTC-8D [55]. A Canadian study by Krahn et al. (2007) also examined QoL using several different instruments [58]. Utility values were broadly similar between the HUI-2, HUI-3 and EQ-5D, however utilities elicited using the QWB were notably lower. Krahn et al. also noted that disease-specific instruments (e.g. PORPUS), were more sensitive and had better internal responsiveness than generic QoL instruments. Lower utility scores with the QWB relative to the HUI-3 were also reported in another Canadian study by Bremner et al., who reported a mean (SD) utility for men with prostate cancer of 0.80 (0.19) using the HUI-3 but 0.65 (0.13) using the QWB [61].

Overall, literature on QoL shows that prostate cancer is associated with a decrement in QoL, but that treatment and treatment-related side effects are also associated with deficits in QoL.

Discussion

Incidence, mortality and survival

Evidence from epidemiologic studies revealed a consistent trend for a continuing increase in the incidence of prostate cancer across all four settings included in the review. The increases in incidence, particularly of low grade tumors, reported in many settings have been partly attributed to the introduction of PSA screening in the early 1990s as well as increasing life expectancy. However, the etiology of prostate cancer is unclear so other factors may be contributing to incidence trends. Age, ethnicity and family history are known to be the major risk factors for prostate cancer; the role of diet and other risk factors are thought to be only minor influencing factors in overall risk and, moreover, studies on dietary risk factors have yielded inconsistent results. Additionally, between study differences in incidence rates may also be due in part to differences in population groups in different studies and also the methods and/or quality of data collection used.

Evidence from included studies also showed that relative survival rates have improved over time, although the 5-year relative survival rate in the UK was found to be lower than in both France and Germany. Improved relative survival in the post- versus pre-PSA screening era has also been reported in other European countries,

Table 4 Quality of life in men with prostate cancer

Study (year)	Health state	Mean (SD or 95% CI) utility value					
		EQ-5D	EORTC-8D	PORPUS-U	HUI-2	HUI-3	QWB
France							
Sullivan et al. (2007) [54]	Metastatic hormone refractory prostate cancer, baseline	0.669					
Germany							
Sullivan et al. (2007) [54]	Metastatic hormone refractory prostate cancer, baseline	0.527					
UK							
Sullivan et al. (2007) [54]	Metastatic hormone refractory prostate cancer, baseline	0.715					
Hall et al. (2015) [45]	Baseline, at diagnosis	0.838					
	9 months post-diagnosis	0.868					
	15 months post-diagnosis	0.868					
Lloyd et al. (2015) [55]	MCRPC asymptomatic/mildly symptomatic before chemotherapy	0.830 (0.126)	0.856 (0.089)				
	MCRPC symptomatic before chemotherapy	0.625 (0.173)	0.697 (0.118)				
	MCRPC currently receiving chemotherapy	0.692 (0.219)	0.750 (0.117)				
	MCRPC post chemotherapy	0.700 (0.183)	0.753 (0.133)				
Watson et al. (2016) [56]	Diagnosed with prostate cancer in previous 9–24 months (overall)	0.852 (0.173)					
	No moderate/big problem with urine function	0.868 (0.160)					
	No moderate/big problem with bowel function	0.862 (0.166)					
	No moderate/big problem with sexual function	0.861 (0.176)					
	Moderate/big problem with urine function	0.773 (0.222)					
	Moderate/big problem with bowel function	0.653 (0.195)					
	Moderate/big problem with sexual function	0.838 (0.170)					
Canada							
Krahn et al. (2013) [57]	Prostate cancer survivors (overall)			0.91 (0.08)	0.85 (0.15)	0.78 (0.24)	
Krahn et al. (2007) [58]	Localized prostate cancer receiving radical prostatectomy, radiation, or hormonal therapy	0.84			0.87	0.81	0.61
	Metastatic disease	0.84			0.86	0.82	0.63
	Stable patients	0.85			0.86	0.81	0.63
Ku et al. (2009) [59]	Patients undergoing radical prostatectomy, baseline (pre-surgery)			0.94 (0.93–0.95)			
	Patients undergoing radical prostatectomy, 0–3 months post surgery			0.81 (0.79–0.82)			
	Patients undergoing radical prostatectomy, 3–9 months post surgery			0.87 (0.86–0.89)			
	Patients undergoing radical prostatectomy, 9–18 months post surgery			0.89 (0.87–0.90)			
	Patients undergoing radical prostatectomy, 18–30 months post surgery			0.90 (0.88–0.91)			

Table 4 Quality of life in men with prostate cancer *(Continued)*

Study (year)	Health state	Mean (SD or 95% CI) utility value					
		EQ-5D	EORTC-8D	PORPUS-U	HUI-2	HUI-3	QWB
Sullivan et al. (2007) [54]	Metastatic hormone refractory prostate cancer, baseline	0.750					
Gries et al. (2016) [60]	Men at risk for prostate cancer				0.83 (0.168)	0.77 (0.238)	
	Men with prostate cancer				0.83 (0–124)	0.75 (0.260)	
	General population				0.87 (0.136)	0.84 (0.178)	
Bremner et al. (2007) [61]	Men with prostate cancer (overall population)					0.80 (0.19)	0.65 (0.13)

***MCRPC* metastatic hormone resistant prostate cancer**

including one recently published study from Finland where improved 5-year relative survival was reported for both localized and metastasized prostate cancer [64, 65]. In these studies improved survival outcomes were at least partly attributed to earlier diagnosis owing to PSA screening. Although it was also noted that PSA screening can result in lead-time bias in survival estimates, where lead-time is *"the time by which PSA screening advances prostate cancer diagnosis"* [65].

Notably, in their European-wide study, Bray et al. noted a lack of correlation between incidence and mortality rates, particularly in the later years of their study, which they suggest was due to the detection and over-diagnosis of indolent tumors, which was in turn likely attributable to increasing uptake of PSA screening [23]. Similar findings have been reported in a meta-analysis of population screening studies, which showed that whilst PSA screening has led to a significant increase in prostate cancer detection as well as a significant grade shift towards lower grade tumors, it has not significantly influenced mortality rates [66].

A key limitation of this review is that although the overarching goal was to characterize the burden of prostate cancer in contemporary clinical practice a number of included articles, although published recently, did not contain recent data. The scope of the literature searches was limited to articles published after 2006. However, a substantial proportion of the articles meeting this cut-off threshold reported data from earlier, often considerably earlier, time periods. Therefore, currently available data on incidence and prostate cancer-specific mortality may not accurately reflect the current situation in contemporary clinical practice. A further limitation is that in terms of 5-year relative survival data included in the review, the most recent data are from 2010, which again may not accurately reflect the current situation in routine clinical practice. Allied to this, in the area of oncology long-term follow-up (typically 15–20 years) is required to fully investigate and elucidate the underlying mechanisms for changes in mortality rates. Only a small number of studies included in the review were conducted over time horizons of > 15 years.

Evidence from several studies showed that in the UK in particular, the incidence of prostate cancer is influenced by ethnic group and socioeconomic status. Specifically, UK-based men of African, or African-Caribbean descent have been consistently reported to have higher incidence rates whilst those of South Asian descent had consistently lower incidence rates of prostate cancer relative to those of European descent [67–69] In particular, the rate ratio for Black African and Black Caribbean men in the UK ranged from 2.4–3.1 compared with white males, whilst for South Asian males the corresponding range was 0.3–0.7 [67, 68]. However, Chingewundoh et al. reported no notable differences between ethnic groups in terms of clinical presentation of prostate cancer, with no significant differences reported in mean PSA score, stage or Gleason score at presentation [69]. Differences in incidence according to ethnic group were also reported in Canada, with Aboriginal men in Quebec having a substantially lower age-standardized incidence of prostate cancer compared with the general population (47 [38–57] per 100,000 versus 67 [67, 68] per 100,000) [36]. Additionally, evidence from a UK-based study from the West of Scotland showed that from 1998 onwards a deprivation gap appeared in the incidence of low grade, but not high grade, prostate cancer, with men in the most deprived socioeconomic group having a 37% lower incidence of low grade prostate cancer compared with men in the most affluent group [32]. However, the authors note that the reason for this deprivation gap is unclear, stating that possible explanations include a difference in causal factors and competing mortality, as incidence is strongly related to age although the difference is unlikely to have been due to PSA screening as the overall increase in incidence was not accompanied by a grade shift towards lower grade disease.

Although not included in the current review (as data were reported in graphical rather than numerical format) Collin et al. compared trends in prostate cancer mortality in the UK and the US over the period 1975–2004 [70]. In both settings, mortality rate declined from 1994 onwards, but the rate of decline in the US was four-fold greater than in the UK. This difference was attributed to a combination of several factors including much higher uptake rates of PSA screening in the US as well as a more aggressive approach towards management of early stage treatment. However, it should also be noted that there have been considerable advances in the treatment of prostate cancer since 2004 [71], which may have influenced mortality rates in both the UK and US.

Economic burden of prostate cancer

Overall, the findings from studies included in the current review suggest that the economic burden associated with the treatment and monitoring of men with prostate cancer is both substantial and increasing over time. Factors contributing to the increasing economic burden include increasing incidence, advances in treatment and advances in diagnostic and monitoring technologies such as the increased use of MRI and the introduction of genomic profiling tools. However, it should be noted that some of the cost data included in the current review may not adequately capture the direct costs, or savings, associated with the most recent advances in the treatment of prostate cancer. For example, increased use of robot-assisted radical prostatectomy is associated with increased surgical costs relative to open or laparoscopic radical prostatectomy [72]. Additionally, increasing use of advances such as prostate-specific membrane antigen based PET or CT imaging and 3 T MRI in the diagnosis of prostate cancer are also likely to have influenced the overall economic burden of disease.

One aspect of economic burden that was not well characterized in the literature was costs associated with treatment-related complications that some patients experience such as incontinence, bowel dysfunction and erectile dysfunction. However, other studies, not included in the review have examined costs in patients with these conditions. For example, one publication (excluded from the current review as is was not published in English) estimated that in Germany the direct and indirect costs associated with urinary incontinence following prostatectomy are approximately EUR 71.8 million [73]. Similarly, figures from the UK estimate that on a per patient level, the annual cost of erectile dysfunction is GBP 335 [74].

There is a general paucity of data relating to indirect costs for patients with prostate cancer, and intangible aspects such as the burden placed on informal caregivers is poorly characterized. The literature searches did not identify any studies relating to caregiver burden in the settings of interest (UK, Canada, Germany and France). However, two US-based studies have quantified caregiver burden in the partners of patients with prostate cancer. In one study Li et al. reported that in the year following diagnosis, mean partner working hours of men with localized prostate cancer (who were not receiving treatment other than hormone therapy) decreased from 14.0 to 10.9 h per week [75]. Additionally, a mean (SD) of 1.3 (3.3) hours per week was spent on providing informal care and 1.5 (3.7) hours/week were spent performing household tasks that would otherwise have been performed by the patient, leading to a total of 276 h per year of lost productivity, informal care and additional household tasks. In economic terms the authors reported that caregiving and lost productivity translated to an economic burden of USD 6063 per patient. A second US-based study estimated caregiver burden to be substantially higher in the first 2 years following diagnosis and a mean (SD) of 9.1 (8.8) hours per day was spent on providing informal care for a partner with prostate cancer. Using the human capital approach the mean (95% CI) economic value of informal care over this time period was USD 44,885 (35,389–54,381) (2006 USD) [76]. Additionally, another US-based study showed that in addition to the burden associated with informal care, the partners of men with prostate cancer had reduced QoL, with partner QoL being negatively influenced in particular by impotence, incontinence and the presence of metastatic disease [77, 78].

A key caveat of high levels of PSA screening is high levels of over-diagnosis and over-treatment. Over-treatment compounds not only the clinical burden of disease but side effects of treatment including impotence, incontinence and impaired bowel function that can compromise quality of life for both the patient and patient's partner. The economic burden of over-treatment is also considerable with the annual burden of prostate cancer in the UK, France and Germany ranging from EUR 117–385 million.

However, the burden of over treatment could be reduced by identifying and treating only those tumors that are likely to progress to clinically significant disease. Several genomic profiling tools that assess the expression of predictive and prognostic biomarkers in prostate cancer are now available. These include Decipher™, Oncotype DX®, and Prolaris®, the use of which may assist physicians with decision-making in terms of the risk/benefit profile of initiating treatment in men with low grade disease as well as potentially reducing the requirement for repeat biopsies in men with low grade disease assigned to watchful waiting or active surveillance. The use of such tools can enable a more personalized approach to treatment and the quantitative assessment of RNA levels in some genomic profiling tools also enables an assessment of the influence of epigenetics on gene expression in prostate tumors. However, there are substantial differences between the different tools in terms of the genes assayed and number of genes assays (e.g. Oncotype DX® Genomic Prostate Score™ incorporates multiple biologic pathways predictive of prostate cancer aggressiveness, whereas the 4 K score test exclusively examines plasma levels of four kallikrein proteins), the prognostic and/or predictive information provided, the quality and reproducibility of the test (e.g. Oncotype DX® is performed in central laboratory using standard operating procedures) and the weight of supporting clinical evidence available for each test. Additionally, many of these tools are relatively new and as such are not yet routinely used in routine practice, and cost may represent a barrier to uptake in some settings, but the development and increased use of such genomic profiling tools over the coming years may help to reduce rates of over-treatment.

Quality of life

The QoL studies included in the review consistently showed that QoL was reduced not only in men with prostate cancer but also in the partners of men with prostate cancer. Additionally, treatments such as radical prostatectomy, whilst curative for many patients, can lead to lifelong problems that compromise QoL including urinary incontinence and impotence. The burden on the caregivers, who are often partners, of men with prostate cancer is often overlooked in the literature, but the small amount of research on this area that does exist has shown that partners spend a considerable amount of time providing informal care as well as reducing their working hours in order to do this.

Conclusions

Prostate cancer is the most common cancer in men in Europe and North America, with incidence rates projected to continue to increase over the coming years and whilst advances in treatment have led to substantial improvements in mortality rates, the long-term burden of disease could be reduced by development and increased use of genomic profiling tools, which may help to reduce the over-treatment of indolent tumors.

Additional file

Additional file 1: Literature searches: Details of search strategies used in the literature review and number of hits returned. (DOCX 21 kb)

Acknowledgements
Not applicable.

Authors' contributions
JSP designed and performed the literature searches and prepared the first draft of the manuscript. WV and CT reviewed, provided critical input and made revisions to the first and all subsequent drafts of the manuscript. All authors have read and approved the final version of the manuscript.

Author details
[1]Ossian Health Economics and Communications GmbH, Bäumleingasse 20, 4051 Basel, Switzerland. [2]Genomic Health International, Geneva, Switzerland.

References
1. Ferlay J, Steliarova-Foucher E, Lortet-Tieulent J, Rosso S, Coebergh JW, Comber H, Forman D, Bray F. Cancer incidence and mortality patterns in Europe: estimates for 40 countries in 2012. Eur J Cancer. 2013;49(6):1374–403.
2. Cancer Research UK. Prostate cancer incidence statistics. Available at: http://www.cancerresearchuk.org/health-professional/cancer-statistics/statistics-by-cancer-type/prostate-cancer/incidence#heading-Eight. Accessed 16 June 2016.
3. Bell KJ, Del Mar C, Wright G, Dickinson J, Glasziou P. Prevalence of incidental prostate cancer: A systematic review of autopsy studies. Int J Cancer. 2015; 137(7):1749–57.
4. Lin K, Lipsitz R, Janakiraman S. Benefits and Harms of Prostate-Specific Antigen Screening for Prostate Cancer: An Evidence Update for the U.S. Preventive Services Task Force [Internet]. Rockville: Agency for Healthcare Research and Quality (US); 2008.
5. United States Preventative Services Task Force. Draft Recommendation Statement Prostate Cancer: Screening. May 8, 2017. Available at: https://www.uspreventiveservicestaskforce.org/Page/Document/RecommendationStatementFinal/prostatecancer-screening1. Accessed 13 Mar 2019.
6. Moore AL, Dimitropoulou P, Lane A, Powell PH, Greenberg DC, Brown CH, Donovan JL, Hamdy FC, Martin RM, Neal DE. Population-based prostate-specific antigen testing in the UK leads to a stage migration of prostate cancer. BJU Int. 2009;104(11):1592–8.
7. Hu JC, Gu X, Lipsitz SR, Barry MJ, D'Amico AV, Weinberg AC, Keating NL. Comparative effectiveness of minimally invasive vs open radical prostatectomy. JAMA. 2009;302(14):1557–64.
8. Hanchanale VS, McCabe JE, Javlé P. Radical prostatectomy practice in England. Urol J. 2010 Fall;7(4):243–8.
9. Kelly M, Sharp L, Dwane F, Kelleher T, Drummond FJ, Comber H. Factors predicting hospital length-of-stay after radical prostatectomy: a population-based study. BMC Health Serv Res. 2013;13:244.
10. Jeldres C, Cullen J, Hurwitz LM, Wolff EM, Levie KE, Odem-Davis K, Johnston RB, Pham KN, Rosner IL, Brand TC, L'Esperance JO, Sterbis JR, Etzioni R, Porter CR. Prospective quality-of-life outcomes for low-risk prostate cancer: Active surveillance versus radical prostatectomy. Cancer. 2015;121(14):2465–73.
11. Heidenreich A, Bastian PJ, Bellmunt J, et al. EAU guidelines on prostate cancer. part 1: screening, diagnosis, and local treatment with curative intent-update 2013. Eur Urol. 2014;65(1):124–37.
12. United Kingdom National Institute for Health and Care Excellence. NICE guidelines (CG175): Prostate cancer: diagnosis and management. Available at: https://www.nice.org.uk/guidance/cg175/chapter/1-recommendations. Accessed 7 June 2016.
13. Hamdy FC, Donovan JL, Lane JA, Mason M, Metcalfe C, Holding P, Davis M, Peters TJ, Turner EL, Martin RM, Oxley J, Robinson M, Staffurth J, Walsh E, Bollina P, Catto J, Doble A, Doherty A, Gillatt D, Kockelbergh R, Kynaston H, Paul A, Powell P, Prescott S, Rosario DJ, Rowe E, Neal DE, ProtecT Study Group. 10-Year Outcomes after Monitoring, Surgery, or Radiotherapy for Localized Prostate Cancer. N Engl J Med. 2016;375(15):1415–24.
14. Lotan TL, Carvalho FL, Peskoe SB, Hicks JL, Good J, Fedor HL, Humphreys E, Han M, Platz EA, Squire JA, De Marzo AM. Berman DM. PTEN loss is associated with upgrading of prostate cancer from biopsy to radical prostatectomy. Mod Pathol. 2015;28(1):128–37.
15. Jamal-Hanjani M, Quezada SA, Larkin J, Swanton C. Translational implications of tumor heterogeneity. Clin Cancer Res. 2015;21(6):1258–66.
16. Serefoglu EC, Altinova S, Ugras NS, Akincioglu E, Asil E, Balbay MD. How reliable is 12-core prostate biopsy procedure in the detection of prostate cancer? Can Urol Assoc J. 2013;7(5–6):E293–8.
17. Fourcade RO, Benedict A, Black LK, Stokes ME, Alcaraz A, Castro R. Treatment costs of prostate cancer in the first year after diagnosis: a short-term cost of illness study for France, Germany, Italy, Spain and the UK. BJU Int. 2010;105(1):49–56.
18. Serrao EM, Barrett T, Wadhwa K, Parashar D, Frey J, Koo BC, Warren AY, Doble A, Kastner C, Gallagher FA. Investigating the ability of multiparametric MRI to exclude significant prostate cancer prior to transperineal biopsy. Can Urol Assoc J. 2015;9(11–12):E853–8.
19. Kasivisvanathan V, Rannikko AS, Borghi M, Panebianco V, Mynderse LA, Vaarala MH, Briganti A, Budäus L, Hellawell G, Hindley RG, Roobol MJ, Eggener S, Ghei M, Villers A, Bladou F, Villeirs GM, Virdi J, Boxler S, Robert G, Singh PB, Venderink W, Hadaschik BA, Ruffion A, Hu JC, Margolis D, Crouzet S, Klotz L, Taneja SS, Pinto P, Gill I, Allen C, Giganti F, Freeman A, Morris S, Punwani S, Williams NR, Brew-Graves C, Deeks J, Takwoingi Y, Emberton M, Moore CM. PRECISION Study Group Collaborators. MRI-Targeted or Standard Biopsy for Prostate-Cancer Diagnosis. N Engl J Med. 2018;378(19):1767–77.
20. Yoo S, Kim JK, Jeong IG. Multiparametric magnetic resonance imaging for prostate cancer: A review and update for urologists. Korean J Urol 2015; 56(7):487–97.
21. Binder-Foucard F, Bossard N, Delafosse P, Belot A, Woronoff AS, Remontet L. French network of cancer registries (Francim). Cancer incidence and mortality in France over the 1980-2012 period: solid tumors. Rev Epidemiol Sante Publique. 2014;62(2):95–108.
22. Crocetti E, De Angelis R, Buzzoni C, Mariotto A, Storm H, Colonna M, Zanetti R, Serraino D, Michiara M, Cirilli C, Iannelli A, Mazzoleni G, Sechi O, Sanoja Gonzalez ME, Guzzinati S, Capocaccia R, Dal Maso L. AIRTUM Working group. Cancer prevalence in United States, Nordic Countries, Italy, Australia, and France: an analysis of geographic variability. Br J Cancer. 2013;109(1): 219–28.
23. Bray F, Lortet-Tieulent J, Ferlay J, Forman D, Auvinen A. Prostate cancer incidence and mortality trends in 37 European countries: an overview. Eur J Cancer. 2010;46(17):3040–52.
24. Belot A, Grosclaude P, Bossard N, Jougla E, Benhamou E, Delafosse P, Guizard AV, Molinié F, Danzon A, Bara S, Bouvier AM, Trétarre B, Binder-Foucard F, Colonna M, Daubisse L, Hédelin G, Launoy G, Le Stang N, Maynadié M, Monnereau A, Troussard X, Faivre J, Collignon A, Janoray I, Arveux P, Buemi A, Raverdy N, Schvartz C, Bovet M, Chérié-Challine L, Estève J, Remontet L, Velten M. Cancer incidence and mortality in France over the period 1980-2005. Rev Epidemiol Sante Publique. 2008;56(3):159–75.
25. Haberland J, Bertz J, Wolf U, Ziese T, Kurth BM. German cancer statistics 2004. BMC Cancer. 2010;22(10):52.
26. Dörr M, Hölzel D, Schubert-Fritschle G, Engel J, Schlesinger-Raab A. Changes in prognostic and therapeutic parameters in prostate cancer from an epidemiological view over 20 years. Oncol Res Treat. 2015;38(1–2):8–14.
27. Becker N, Altenburg HP, Stegmaier C, Ziegler H. Report on trends of incidence (1970-2002) of and mortality (1952-2002) from cancer in Germany. J Cancer Res Clin Oncol. 2007;133(1):23–35.
28. Rohde V, Weidner W, Katalinic A. Decrease in prostate cancer incidence and mortality in Germany - effects of opportunistic PSA screening or more? Urol Int. 2009;83(2):134–40.

29. Greenberg DC, Wright KA, Lophathanon A, Muir KR, Gnanapragasam VJ. Changing presentation of prostate cancer in a UK population--10 year trends in prostate cancer risk profiles in the East of England. Br J Cancer. 2013;109(8):2115–20.
30. Mistry M, Parkin DM, Ahmad AS, Sasieni P. Cancer incidence in the United Kingdom: projections to the year 2030. Br J Cancer. 2011;105(11):1795–803.
31. Pashayan N, Powles J, Brown C, Duffy SW. Incidence trends of prostate cancer in East Anglia, before and during the era of PSA diagnostic testing. Br J Cancer. 2006;95(3):398–400.
32. Shafique K, Oliphant R, Morrison DS. The impact of socio-economic circumstances on overall and grade-specific prostate cancer incidence: a population-based study. Br J Cancer. 2012;107(3):575–82.
33. Feletto E, Bang A, Cole-Clark D, Chalasani V, Rasiah K, Smith DP. An examination of prostate cancer trends in Australia, England, Canada and USA: Is the Australian death rate too high? World J Urol. 2015 Nov;33(11): 1677–87.
34. Westlake S. Cancer incidence and mortality in the United Kingdom and constituent countries, 2004-06. Health Stat Q. 2009 Autumn;43:56–62.
35. Kachuri L, De P, Ellison LF, Semenciw R. Advisory Committee on Canadian Cancer Statistics. Cancer incidence, mortality and survival trends in Canada, 1970-2007. Chronic Dis Inj Can. 2013;33(2):69–80.
36. Louchini R, Beaupré M. Cancer incidence and mortality among Aboriginal people living on reserves and northern villages in Quebec, 1988-2004. Int J Circumpolar Health. 2008;67(5):445–51.
37. Marshall DC, Webb TE, Hall RA, Salciccioli JD, Ali R, Maruthappu M. Trends in UK regional cancer mortality 1991-2007. Br J Cancer. 2016;114(3):340–7. https://doi.org/10.1038/bjc.2015.428.
38. Trama A, Foschi R, Larrañaga N, Sant M, Fuentes-Raspall R, Serraino D, Tavilla A, Van Eycken L, Nicolai N, EUROCARE-5 Working Group. Survival of male genital cancers (prostate, testis and penis) in Europe 1999-2007: Results from the EUROCARE-5 study. Eur J Cancer. 2015. https://doi.org/10.1016/j.ejca.2015.07.027. Epub ahead of print.
39. Jansen L, Castro FA, Gondos A, Krilaviciute A, Barnes B, Eberle A, Emrich K, Hentschel S, Holleczek B, Katalinic A, Brenner H. GEKID Cancer Survival Working Group. Recent cancer survival in Germany: an analysis of common and less common cancers. Int J Cancer. 2015;136(11):2649–58.
40. Gondos A, Arndt V, Holleczek B, Stegmaier C, Ziegler H, Brenner H. Cancer survival in Germany and the United States at the beginning of the 21st century: an up-to-date comparison by period analysis. Int J Cancer. 2007; 121(2):395–400.
41. Hiripi E, Gondos A, Emrich K, Holleczek B, Katalinic A, Luttmann S, Sirri E, Brenner H. GEKID Cancer Survival Working Group. Survival from common and rare cancers in Germany in the early 21st century. Ann Oncol. 2012; 23(2):472–9.
42. Nennecke AL, Hentschel S, Reintjes R. Cancer survival analysis in Hamburg 1995-2003: assessing the data quality within a population-based registry. Acta Oncol. 2009;48(1):34–43.
43. Cancer Research UK. Prostate cancer survival statistics. Available at: http://www.cancerresearchuk.org/health-professional/cancer-statistics/statistics-by-cancer-type/prostate-cancer/survival#heading-Three. Accessed 17 June 2016.
44. Molinier L, Castelli C, Bauvin E, Rebillard X, Soulié M, Daurès JP, Grosclaude P. Cost study of the clinical management of prostate cancer in France: results on the basis of population-based data. Eur J Health Econ. 2011;12(4): 363–71.
45. Hall PS, Hamilton P, Hulme CT, Meads DM, Jones H, Newsham A, Marti J, Smith AF, Mason H, Velikova G, Ashley L, Wright P. Costs of cancer care for use in economic evaluation: a UK analysis of patient-level routine health system data. Br J Cancer. 2015;112(5):948–56.
46. Marti J, Hall PS, Hamilton P, Hulme CT, Jones H, Velikova G, Ashley L, Wright P. The economic burden of cancer in the UK: a study of survivors treated with curative intent. Psychooncology. 2016;25(1):77–83.
47. de Oliveira C, Bremner KE, Pataky R, Gunraj N, Haq M, Chan K, Cheung WY, Hoch JS, Peacock S, Krahn MD. Trends in use and cost of initial cancer treatment in Ontario: a population-based descriptive study. CMAJ Open. 2013;1(4):E151–8.
48. Krahn MD, Zagorski B, Laporte A, Alibhai SM, Bremner KE, Tomlinson G, Warde P, Naglie G. Healthcare costs associated with prostate cancer: estimates from a population-based study. BJU Int. 2010;105(3):338–46.
49. de Oliveira C, Bremner KE, Ni A, Alibhai SM, Laporte A, Krahn MD. Patient time and out-of-pocket costs for long-term prostate cancer survivors in Ontario, Canada. J Cancer Surviv. 2014;8(1):9–20.
50. Krahn MD, Bremner KE, Zagorski B, Alibhai SM, Chen W, Tomlinson G, Mitsakakis N, Naglie G. Health care costs for state transition models in prostate cancer. Med Decis Mak. 2014;34(3):366–78.
51. Sanyal C, Aprikian AG, Cury FL, Chevalier S, Dragomir A. Management of localized and advanced prostate cancer in Canada: A lifetime cost and quality-adjusted life-year analysis. Cancer. 2016;122(7):1085–96.
52. Dragomir A, Cury FL, Aprikian AG. Active surveillance for low-risk prostate cancer compared with immediate treatment: a Canadian cost comparison. CMAJ Open. 2014;2(2):E60–8.
53. Luengo-Fernandez R, Leal J, Gray A, Sullivan R. Economic burden of cancer across the European Union: a population-based cost analysis. Lancet Oncol. 2013;14(12):1165–74.
54. Sullivan PW, Mulani PM, Fishman M, Sleep D. Quality of life findings from a multicenter, multinational, observational study of patients with metastatic hormone-refractory prostate cancer. Qual Life Res. 2007;16(4):571–5.
55. Lloyd AJ, Kerr C, Penton J, Knerer G. Health-Related Quality of Life and Health Utilities in Metastatic Castrate-Resistant Prostate Cancer: A Survey Capturing Experiences from a Diverse Sample of UK Patients. Value Health. 2015;18(8):1152–7.
56. Watson E, Shinkins B, Frith E, Neal D, Hamdy F, Walter F, Weller D, Wilkinson C, Faithfull S, Wolstenholme J, Sooriakumaran P, Kastner C, Campbell C, Neal R, Butcher H, Matthews M, Perera R, Rose P. Symptoms, unmet needs, psychological well-being and health status in survivors of prostate cancer: implications for redesigning follow-up. BJU Int. 2016;117(6B):E10–9.
57. Krahn MD, Bremner KE, Alibhai SM, Ni A, Tomlinson G, Laporte A. Naglie G. A reference set of health utilities for long-term survivors of prostate cancer: population-based data from Ontario, Canada. Qual Life Res. 2013;22(10): 2951–62.
58. Krahn M, Bremner KE, Tomlinson G, Ritvo P, Irvine J, Naglie G. Responsiveness of disease-specific and generic utility instruments in prostate cancer patients. Qual Life Res. 2007;16(3):509–22.
59. Ku J, Krahn M, Trachtenberg J, Nesbitt M, Kalnin R, Lockwood G, Alibhai SM. Changes in health utilities and health-related quality of life over 12 months following radical prostatectomy. Can Urol Assoc J. 2009;3(6):445–52.
60. Gries KS, Regier DA, Ramsey SD, Patrick DL. Preferences for Prostate Cancer Outcomes: A Comparison of the Patient Perspective, the General Population Perspective, and a Population at Risk for Prostate Cancer. Value Health. 2016;19(2):218–25.
61. Bremner KE, Tomlinson G, Krahn MD. Marker states and a health state prompt provide modest improvements in the reliability and validity of the standard gamble and rating scale in prostate cancer patients. Qual Life Res. 2007;16(10):1665–75.
62. Menegatou E, Claeys C, Wasserman D, Tomaszewski K. Assessment of Health States and Erectile Dysfunction-Associated Quality of Life Among Adult Males and Females With Male Partners in Germany, the United Kingdom and the United States. Value Health. 2014;17(7):A516.
63. Garcia-Gordillo MA, Collado-Mateo D, Olivares PR, Adsuar JC. Application of EQ-5D-5L questionnaire in patients suffering from urinary incontinence. Actas Urol Esp. 2016;40(7):457–62.
64. Marcos-Gragera R, Salmerón D, Izarzugaza I, Ardanaz E, Serdà BC, Larrañaga N, San Román E, Navarro C, Chirlaque MD. Trends in prostate cancer survival in Spain: results from population-based cancer registries. Clin Transl Oncol. 2012;14(6):458–64.
65. Seikkula HA, Kaipia AJ, Rantanen ME, Pitkäniemi JM, Malila NK, Boström PJ. Stage-specific mortality and survival trends of prostate cancer patients in Finland before and after introduction of PSA. Acta Oncol. 2017;56(7):971–7.
66. Lumen N, Fonteyne V, De Meerleert G, Ost P, Villeirs G, Mottrie A, De Visschere P, De Troyer B, Oosterlinck W. Population screening for prostate cancer: an overview of available studies and meta-analysis. Int J Urol. 2012; 19(2):100–8.
67. Maruthappu M, Barnes I, Sayeed S, Ali R. Incidence of prostate and urological cancers in England by ethnic group, 2001-2007: a descriptive study. BMC Cancer. 2015;21(15):753.
68. Bhopal RS, Bansal N, Steiner M, Brewster DH; Scottish Health and Ethnicity Linkage Study. Does the 'Scottish effect' apply to all ethnic groups? All-cancer, lung, colorectal, breast and prostate cancer in the Scottish Health and Ethnicity Linkage Cohort Study. BMJ Open 2012;2(5):e001957.
69. Chinegwundoh F, Enver M, Lee A, Nargund V, Oliver T, Ben-Shlomo Y. Risk and presenting features of prostate cancer amongst African-Caribbean, South Asian and European men in North-east London. BJU Int. 2006;98(6): 1216–20.

70. Collin SM, Martin RM, Metcalfe C, Gunnell D, Albertsen PC, Neal D, Hamdy F, Stephens P, Lane JA, Moore R, Donovan J. Prostate-cancer mortality in the USA and UK in 1975-2004: an ecological study. Lancet Oncol. 2008;9(5):445–52.
71. Attard G, Parker C, Eeles RA, Schröder F, Tomlins SA, Tannock I, Drake CG, de Bono JS. Prostate cancer. Lancet. 2016;387(10013):70–82.
72. Bolenz C, Freedland SJ, Hollenbeck BK, Lotan Y, Lowrance WT, Nelson JB, Hu JC. Costs of radical prostatectomy for prostate cancer: a systematic review. Eur Urol. 2014;65(2):316–24.
73. Lent V, Schultheis M. Economic importance of postoperative urinary incontinence. Urologe A. 2015;54(11):1564–6.
74. Goldmeier D, Malik F, Phillips R, Green J. Cost implications of sexual dysfunction: the female picture. Int J Impot Res. 2004;16(2):130–4.
75. Li C, Zeliadt SB, Hall IJ, Smith JL, Ekwueme DU, Moinpour CM, Penson DF, Thompson IM, Keane TE, Ramsey SD. Burden among partner caregivers of patients diagnosed with localized prostate cancer within 1 year after diagnosis: an economic perspective. Support Care Cancer. 2013;21(12):3461–9.
76. Yabroff KR, Kim Y. Time costs associated with informal caregiving for cancer survivors. Cancer. 2009;115(18 Suppl):4362–73.
77. Harden J, Sanda MG, Wei JT, Yarandi HN, Hembroff L, Hardy J, Northouse L. Survivorship after prostate cancer treatment: spouses' quality of life at 36 months. Oncol Nurs Forum. 2013;40(6):567–73.
78. Basu A, Dale W, Elstein A, Meltzer D. A time tradeoff method for eliciting partner's quality of life due to patient's health states in prostate cancer. Med Decis Mak. 2010;30(3):355–65.

24

Comparisons of cancer detection rate and complications between transrectal and transperineal prostate biopsy approaches

Guan-Lin Huang, Chih-Hsiung Kang, Wei-Ching Lee and Po-Hui Chiang*

Abstract

Background: Prostate biopsy remains the gold standard approach to verify prostate cancer diagnosis. Transrectal (TR) biopsy is a regular modality, while transperineal (TP) biopsy is an alternative for the patients who display persistently high levels of prostate-specific antigen (PSA) and thus have to undergo repeat biopsy. This study aimed to compare the cancer detection rates between TR and TP approaches and assess the post-bioptic complications of the two procedures. Besides, the feasibility of performing TP biopsies under local anesthesia was also evaluated.

Methods: A total of 238 outpatient visits meeting the criteria for prostate cancer biopsy were enrolled for this study. They were divided into two groups: the TP group ($n = 130$) consists of patients destined to undergo local anesthetic TP biopsy; and the TR group ($n = 108$) contained those who received TR biopsy as comparison. Age, PSA level, digital rectal exam (DRE) finding, prostate volume, and biopsy core number were used as the parameters of the multivariable analyses. The comparable items included cancer detection rate, complication rate, admission rate and visual analog scale (VAS) score.

Results: The cancer detection rates between TP and TR groups were quite comparable (45% v.s. 49%) ($p = 0.492$). However, the TP group, as compared to the TR group, had significantly lower incidence of infection-related complications (except epididymitis and prostatitis) that commonly occur after biopsies. None of the patients in the TP group were hospitalized due to the post-bioptic complications, whereas there was still a minor portion of those in the TR group (7.4%) requiring hospitalization after biopsy. Medians (25–75% quartiles) of visual analog scale (VAS) were 3 [3, 4] and 4 [3–5] respectively for the TP and TR procedures under local anesthesia, but no statistical significance existed between them ($p = 0.085$).

Conclusions: Patients receiving TP biopsy are less likely to manifest infection-related complications. Therefore, TP biopsy is a more feasible local anesthetic approach for prostate cancer detection if there are concerns for infectious complications and/or the risk of general anesthesia.

Keywords: Prostate biopsy, Transperineal (TP), Transrectal (TR), Local anesthesia

* Correspondence: tuoa480713@yahoo.com.tw
Department of Urology, Kaohsiung Chang Gung Memorial Hospital and Chang Gung University College of Medicine, No.123, Dapi Rd., Niaosong Dist., Kaohsiung, Taiwan, Republic of China

Background

The transrectal (TR) ultrasound-guided biopsy is the gold standard approach for prostate cancer diagnosis [1, 2]. Though being generally considered a relatively low-risk outpatient approach, up to 50% of the patients suffer from minor complications (e.g. hematuria, hematospermia, rectal bleeding, and acute urine retention) to severe complications (e.g. anemia and syncope) [3]. Approximately 4 to 5% of the patients who undergo this procedure require hospital admission due to infection-related complications (ranging from bacteriuria to sepsis) [4, 5]. Therefore, prostate biopsy performed through other approaches should be considered.

Transperineal (TP) biopsy is an alternative approach for patients required to undergo prostate repeat biopsy. This procedure has been shown to greatly improve the cancer detection rates in the anterior and apical areas of the prostate and also reduce the risk for infectious complications [6, 7]. Nevertheless, TP biopsy is not used as widely as TR biopsy owing to the relatively higher technical difficulty and the pain occurring without the use of anesthetics. In this study, we compared the rates of cancer detection and post-bioptic complications between the Taiwanese patients receiving transperineal (TP) and transrectal (TR) prostate biopsies, respectively. Comparisons of visual analog scale (VAS) scores between these two patient groups were done for evaluating the feasibility of TP under local anesthesia.

Methods

Patients

Three hundred and fifty-six patients were recruited to receive the prostate biopsy at our institute from May 2015 to Dec 2017. All patients enrolled in this IRB (IRB number:105-6117B)-approved study were given the informed consent. Biopsy criteria included elevated PSA level above 4.0 ng/mL, abnormal digital rectal examination findings, and clinical suspicion of prostate cancer. Exclusion criteria of the patients were listed as follows: (1) having previously undergone prostate biopsy, (2) clinically having locally advanced prostate cancer (verified by DRE) with significant bone pain or bone metastasis, (3) showing pathological evidence of metastatic prostate cancer. After excluding the non-qualifiers, 130 and 108 patients were respectively assigned to the TP and TR groups by their attending physicians (TP group: PHC; TR group: CSK & WCL). The patients were clearly and concisely informed of the benefits and the risk separately from the TP and TR bioptic procedures via an oral explanation, and the letter of their consent was acquired. Digital rectal examination, negative urinalysis, and PSA evaluation were carried out in all male patients prior to biopsy.

Biopsy protocols

For transrectal (TR) prostate biopsy: patients received the perioperative oral antibiotics (empirically using levofloxacin/ceftibuten/baktar, or others according to the culture data) for 3 days with pre-procedure 1pc Gentamicin IM injection. Biopsy gun (BARD MAXCORE/18*20; Bard, Tempe, USA) was applied through the transrectal ultrasonography (bk3000; BK Medical Aps, Copenhagen, Denmark) with full lidocaine cream lubrication.

Generally, the 10 core biopsy included 8 slices from the apex-mid plane-basal peripheral zone (PZ) containing the far lateral area as well as 2 slices from the bilateral transitional zone (TZ) via the probe guided-side hole. (Fig. 1.) The biopsy number might vary according to the prostate volume or additional suspicious transrectal ultrasound findings.

For transperineal (TP) prostate biopsy: The patient was placed in the lithotomy position with well-disinfected perineum preparation. Under the transrectal ultrasonography guidance (bk3000; BK Medical Aps, Copenhagen, Denmark), the Biplane prostate probe (Prostate Biplane E14C4t/4 M Hz; BK Medical Aps) was introduced for localization (Fig. 2). Systemic transperineal 18-gauge needle was inserted with 0–2 cores on the anterior-apical region, 2 cores on the transitional zone, and 6–8 cores on the peripheral zone (Fig. 3). Perioperative antibiotic treatment wasn't needed during the procedure.

Anesthesia procedure: Patients of the TR group were treated with a lidocaine cream lubricant through the transrectal ultrasound puncturing hole. In the TP group, the patients underwent local anesthesia or intravenous general anesthesia. Local anesthesia with a peri-prostate nerve block effect (TP: LA + PPNB) was conducted with a 21-gauge needle. 2% 10 ml lidocaine was injected into the bilateral prostate basal area where the major neurovascular bundle transverses through [8, 9] (Fig. 4). Besides, additional 10 ml lidocaine was injected around the perineum skin for local anesthesia (Fig. 5).

Data collection and analysis

All the procedures were carried out via the OPD surgery without admission by attending physicians (PHC, CSK, and WCL). Cancer detection rates and complications were independently collected and analyzed by another team member of this research (GLH).

Complication definition

Urine retention is defined as being hard to urinate with catheterization within the 7 days after biopsy. Epididymitis was diagnosed by the physical examination and testis ultrasonography. Post-procedure sepsis was defined as fever > 38.5 °C with single or multiple organ dysfunctions during hospital admission. Hematuria and perineal

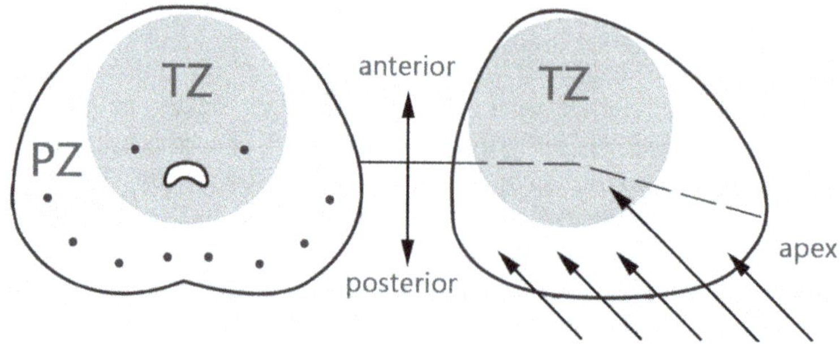

Fig. 1 Transrectal prostate biopsy mapping. A total of 10 pieces of biopsy tissue including 2 pieces focusing on transitional zone were taken. Large prostate or significant prostate lesion under transrectal ultrasound may need additional pieces by clinical judgement. TZ: transitional zone. PZ: peripheral zone

hematoma were collected by patient-reported results in 7 days after the bioptic procedure.

Pain score evaluation

An independent nurse in the operation room recorded the VAS pain scores immediately after the procedure. All patients were asked about their willingness to undergo re-biopsy if false negative findings were reported.

Statistics and analysis

IBM SPSS Statistics ver. 21.0 (SPSS Inc., Chicago, IL) was used for data analysis with Student *t*-test and Mann-Whitney U test on the basic characteristic data of the two groups. Binary outcomes of the infection-related complications were analyzed by Chi-square test. Analysis of VAS pain scores under TR and TP was performed using the Kruskal-Wallis test.

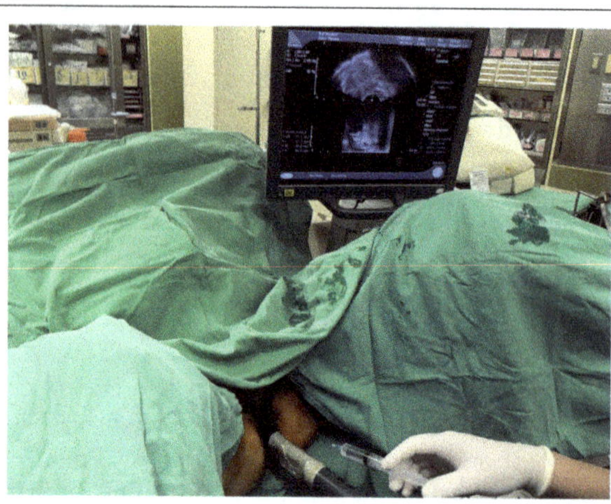

Fig. 2 Transperineal prostate biopsy. Under axial and sagittal view of ultrasonography, 2% lidocaine was infiltrated through the 21-gauge fine needle from the perineum skin to prostate capsule

Results

As shown in Table 1, the mean age of the patients in TP and TR groups was 66.6 and 67.1 years old respectively. The median PSA value for the males in TP and TR groups was 9.3 and 10.9 ng/ml, respectively. There were no statistical differences when comparing the age, PSA values, DRE positivity, and median biopsy core number of the TP group with those of the TR group (Table 1). Nevertheless, the median prostate volume of the TR patient group was significantly greater than the of the TP group (Median, 35 ml vs 32.5 ml, $p = 0.015$).

45% of the patients in the TP group ($n = 130$) and 49% of those in the TR group ($n = 108$) were separately diagnosed with prostate cancer (Table 2). The cancer detection rates, with respect to the two groups, were statistically comparable ($p = 0.492$). Regarding the post-bioptic infectious complications, 0.9, 4.6, 12, and 6.4%, 6.4% of the patients in the TR group were shown to have the following conditions: epididymitis, prostatitis, UTI, fever (> 38.5 °C), and sepsis, respectively. In the TP group, though there were 2.2 and 0.7% of patients who were further diagnosed with UTI and prostatitis, no one else was shown to get epididymitis, fever, and sepsis following the bioptic procedure. Statistically, except for prostatitis and epididymitis, all infection-related complications were lower in the TP group. (Table 2.)

As for the minor complications, gross hematuria was found in 13.8 and 5.3% of the patients in TR and TP groups ($p = 0.024$), respectively (Table 2). The portion of the patients who had urine retention after the TR procedure was mildly higher, as compared to the TP procedure (12% v.s. 3%, $p = 0.076$). Merely two of the patients in the TP group had perineal hematomas after the bioptic procedure, whereas none of the patients in the TR group had such complication ($p = 0.196$) (Table 2). Taken together, these results suggest that patients undergoing transperineal prostate biopsy are at lower risk of post-bioptic complications. Therefore, the hospitalization rate of the patients in the TP group (0%) was obviously lower than that in the TR group (7.4%) (Table 2). In addition, median

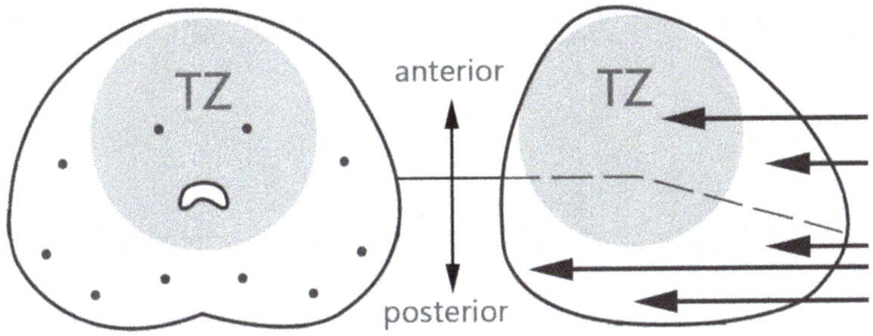

Fig. 3 Transperineal prostate biopsy mapping. Systemic biopsy includes 6 cores over the peripheral zone, 2 cores over the anterior-apical area and 2 cores over the transitional zone. Biopsy core numbers may vary according to prostate volume and additional lesions

(25–75% quartiles) of VAS scores of the patients in the TP and TR groups was 3 [3, 4] and 4 [3–5], respectively, but there was no statistically significant difference between these two groups ($p = 0.085$) (Table 3) (Fig. 6).

Discussion

Transrectal prostate biopsy has been accepted as the standard procedure for prostate cancer diagnosis and evolved into an extended prostate biopsy that includes up to ten and even twelve cores over the past decades [10]. Transperineal biopsy was initially deemed as an alternative cancer detection tool after negative TR biopsy, while the subsequent study results showed non-inferiority of TP biopsy for prostate cancer detection when either of these two approaches were solely performed [7]. For the time being, passage of the biopsy needle through the rectal wall is a mainstream procedure for prostate diagnosis in the United States, while transperineal biopsy is comparatively more accepted in Europe and Japan. A prospective study carried out by Watanabe et al. showed that the extensive 12-core approach simultaneously combining TR and TP biopsies could significantly improve the overall cancer detection rate, and was particularly effective for males with a negative DRE finding, accompanied by PSA levels of 4–10 ng/ml [11]. As an attempt for initial prostate biopsy by the transperineal approach, Kojima et al. demonstrated that extended TP biopsy up to 10–12 cores could lead to a better cancer detection rate, as compared to 6-core TP biopsy [12]. In our study, the averagely 10-core prostate biopsy was performed in the patients assigned to the TP and TR groups, respectively. The cancer detection rates, with respect to TP biopsy and TR biopsy (45 and 49%), were statistically comparable. Which suggests TP biopsy as a primary diagnostic tool not inferior to TR biopsy. Correspondingly, TP biopsy is, in general, regarded as an alternative strategy when TR biopsy fails or the quantity of obtained samples isn't sufficient [13, 14].

TR biopsy is widely used in the US, and the complications following prostate biopsy have been well documented [15]. Post-bioptic infectious complications and the ensuing mortality are nightmares to urologists serving in the areas where multi-resistant bacteria are increasing at an alarming rate [16, 17]. The incidence of infectious complications

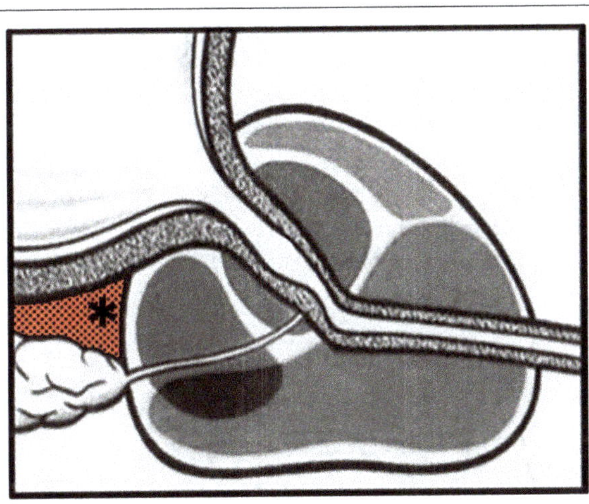

Fig. 4 Periprostatic nerve block. Under transrectal ultrasound guidance, 2% lidocaine was injected into the triangular asterisk area where prostate neurovascular bundle passes through

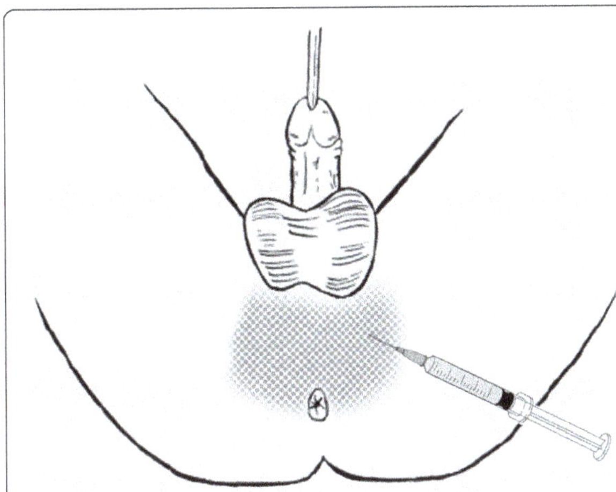

Fig. 5 Transperineal biopsy under local anesthesia. 2% lidocaine was adequately infiltrated over the perineum for multiple biopsy puncture through skin

Table 1 Characteristics in the trans-perineal (TP) and trans-rectal prostate (TR) biopsy

	TP(*n* = 130)	TR(*n* = 108)	*P* value
Age (years)	66.6 ± 8.81	67.1 ± 8.45	0.708[b]
Median PSA level (ng/ml) [25–75%]	9.3[6.3–20.3]	10.9[7.8–17]	0.099[a]
PSA < 4 ng/ml	3/130	7/108	0.11[c]
10 > PSA > 4 ng/ml	62/130	52/108	0.944[c]
PSA > 10 ng/ml	66/130	49/108	0.407[c]
DRE positive	49/130	50/108	0.18[c]
Median Biopsy core number [25–75%]	10[10–10]	10[10–10]	0.574[a]
Prostate Volume [25–75%]	32.5[27–41]	35[29–47]	0.015[a]
Prophylaxis abx use	0/130	Baktar: 28/108 Ceftibuten:25/108 Ciprofloxacin:5/108 Levofloxacin:50/108	<0.001[c]
Anesthesia procedure	IVG: 32/130 LA + PPNB: 98/130	Lidocaine Jelly lubrication	

TP trans-perineal prostate biopsy, *TR* trans-rectal prostate biopsy, *PSA* prostate specific antigen, *DRE* digital rectal examination, [a]: Mann-Whitney test. [b]: Student T test. [c]: Chi-Square test

after TR biopsy is reported to range from 0.1–7% and the rate of hospital admission due to post-bioptic infection is 0.6–4.1% [5]. *Escherichia coli* is the most common pathogen with fluoroquinolone-resistance identified in patients with post-bioptic infectious complications. Risk factors for post-bioptic infection-related complications include: (1) previous use of fluoroquinolone, (2) diabetes mellitus (3) chronic obstructive pulmonary disease, (4) hospitalization in preceding months, and (5) long-term Foley catheter in-dwelling [17, 18]. Although pre-biopsy rectal swab and use of targeted prophylaxis antibiotics are advocated for high-risk patients, the evidence for the routine implication remains inadequate [19]. Changing the prophylaxis antibiotics from fluoroquinolone to third-generation cephalosporin or in combination with gentamicin or amikacin, however, may contribute to occurrence of ESBL-producing bacteria and eventually increase bacterial resistance [5]. Post-TR-biopsy sepsis is caused by direct inoculation of bacteria from the rectal mucosa into the prostate, blood vessels and urinary tract via the biopsy needle. The alternative for preventing the post-biopsy infectious complications is to use the TP biopsy gun that punctures through the disinfected perineal skin instead of the rectal mucosa. In our study, there were only 2.2 and 0.7% of the patients in the TP group who respectively diagnosed with post-bioptic UTI and prostatitis. In the TR group, up to 12% of the patients were diagnosed with post-bioptic UTI, while 6.4% of the patients went to the emergency room (ER) due to the post-bioptic fever and sepsis. Although all the sepsis patents made an uneventful recovery after treated with IV antibiotics, the rate of post-bioptic hospitalization for infectious complications was 7.4%, which resulted in unnecessary medical costs.

Grummet et al. described that only 5 cases (0.076%) of the 6609 patients undergoing TP biopsy were admitted to hospital for post-bioptic sepsis, and no infection related

Table 2 Complications, cancer detection rate and VAS between the trans-perineal (TP) and trans-rectal prostate (TR) biopsy

	TP (*n* = 130)	TR (*n* = 108)	*P* value
Gross hematuria	7/130(5.3%)	15/108(13.8%)	0.024[#]
Urine retention	4/130(3%)	9/108(12.0%)	0.076[#]
Perineal hematoma	2/130(1.5%)	0/101	0.196[#]
Epididymitis	0/130	1/108(0.9%)	0.272[#]
Prostatitis	1/130(0.7%)	5/108(4.6%)	0.059[#]
UTI	3/130(2.2%)	13/108(12.0%)	0.003[#]
Fever > 38.5	0/130	7/108(6.4%)	0.003[#]
Sepsis	0/130	7/108(6.4%)	0.015[#]
Hospitalization for complication	0/130	8/108(7.4%)	0.008[#]
VAS [25–75%]	3[2–4]	3[3–4]	0.239[○]
Cancer detection rate	58/130(45%)	53/108(49%)	0.492[#]

UTI urinary tract infection, *VAS* Visual analog score. [#]: Chi-square test. [○]: Mann-Whitney test

Table 3 Mean VAS and error bar among the different biopsy procedures

	TR(*n* = 108)	TP:LA + PPNB(*n* = 98)
Median VAS [25–75%]	3[3–4]	4[3–5]
Independent Kruskal-Wallis test	*p* = 0.085	

TR transrectal prostate biopsy, TP: LA + PPNB: transperineal approach, local anesthesia with periprostatatic nerve block

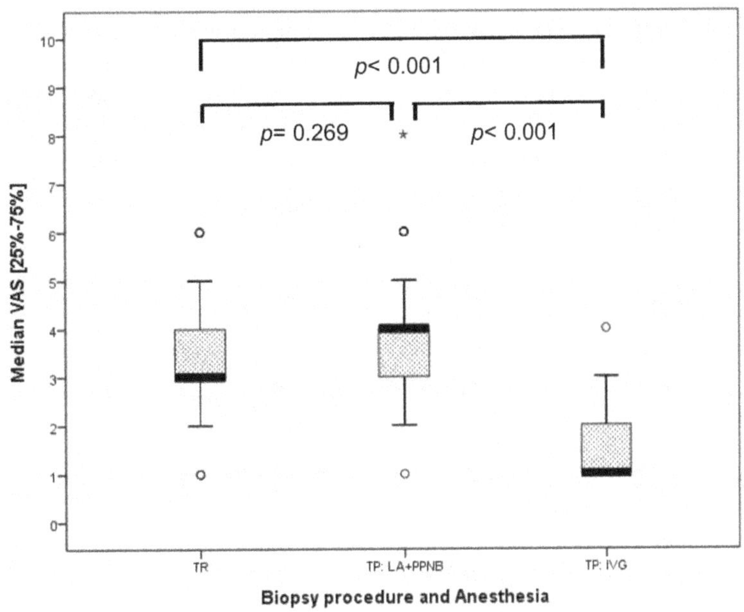

Fig. 6 Median VAS scores and error bar between transperineal and transrectal procedures. TR: transrectal prostate biopsy. TP: LA + PPNB: transperineal approach, local anesthesia & peri-prostatic nerve block; IVG: Intravenous general anesthesia. Patients assigned to the TP group were subjected to anesthesia either locally via perineal injection or generally through intravenous injection

mortality occurred as a result [16]. In terms of TR prostate biopsy, incidence of post-bioptic bacteremia is up to 3.0~6.9% and may be up to one-quarter for the patients needing ICU monitoring and treatment [17, 20–24]. In this regard, performing prostate biopsy through the TP approach should be advocated as the cancer detection rate of TP biopsy is comparable to that of TR biopsy, and, more importantly, TP biopsy demonstrates lower risk of infection-related complications [25].

One of the most common complications after prostate biopsy is hematuria, with reported incidence of 2–84% depending on the definition, follow-up duration and methods [26–29]. In our study, the incidence of hematuria was 5.3 and 13.8% respectively for patients in the TP and TR groups (7/130 vs 15/108, $p = 0.024$). This significant difference in the rate of hematuria between the TP and TR groups might be attributable to the significant difference of the prostate volume between the two groups (35.4 ml vs 40.1 ml, $p = 0.015$). In our study, there were totally 22 hematuria patients, whose symptoms were self-limited, and all of them were subjected to the conservative treatment as per previous reports [26–28].

Risk factors for post prostate biopsy urine retention have been reported, including large prostate volume, bulging prostate transitional zone and high International Prostate Symptom Score (IPSS) scores [15, 30, 31]. In our study, the rate of urine retention for the patients in the TP and TR groups was 3 and 12%, respectively ($p = 0.076$). Larger prostate volume of the patients in the TR group may be suggested as the cause of higher urine retention rate found in these patients.

Perineal hematoma was identified in two of the patients in the TP group, possibly because no perineum compression took place after the procedure. On the contrary, none of the patients in the TR group had perineal hematoma, since the compression was done after the procedure. Pepe et al. reported, according to their experience of performing more than 4000 transperineal prostate biopsies, that the incidence of perineal hematoma was around 0.3–1% [32]. In our study, most hematoma was self-limited, and no more cases were found after routine compression of the TP puncture site after the 2 episodes.

Pain is of great concern when considering different biopsy protocols. According to previous studies [33–35], TR biopsy with lidocaine cream lubrication was worldwidely conducted in many hospitals with tolerability. Other alternative anesthetic procedures, like lidocaine spray administration or replacing lidocaine cream with EMLA cream were reported for a better control of the pain during TR biopsy as well [36, 37]. In contrast, use of the TP biopsy gun to penetrate through the sensitive perineum skin and neurovascular bundles surrounding the prostate capsule is painful and intolerable. General or spinal anesthesia may be required when the procedure is carried out without adequate pain control and sedation [38–40]. However, general anesthesia is not feasible for high anesthesia-risk patients or in anesthetist resource-limited areas. Periprostatic nerve block (PPNB) has been reported as an effective method for alleviating pain and discomfort during TR biopsy and transurethral surgery [41, 42]. Local lidocaine anesthesia with sufficient perineum skin infiltration and PPNB provides an alternative for those patients. In our study, under local anesthesia, there were no significant differences in VAS scores between the patients in the TR and TP groups (TR: 3 [3, 4], TP:LA + PPNB: 3 [3–5], $p = 0.085$). Based on the experience of performing 50 TP prostate biopsies under local anesthesia, Smith et al. reported that the mean VAS scores respectively for probe insertion, LA injection, and bioptic procedure were 3.28, 3.29, and 2.88, which suggests feasibility of TP under local anesthesia [43]. Our clinical observation also demonstrated the feasibility of TP prostate biopsy under local anesthesia. In contrast, Udeh et al. reported that a much higher level of experienced pain was detected in the patients undergoing anesthetic TP biopsy, as compared those receiving TR biopsy under local anesthesia [44]. In this respect, digital-guided biopsy should be replaced with ultrasound-guided biopsy for the TP procedure, and full lidocaine cream premedication is also recommended for decreasing the discomfort during the procedure [34]. Besides, finger manipulation may exacerbate the pain when performing the biopsy. Younger patient age, which denote the higher drug metabolism and more analgesics use, may also account for the sensitiveness of the patients to pain [45]. In our study, there were 15 cases of the patients in the TP group showing the VAS score greater than 5. In our experience, adequate local anesthesia injection into the perineum skin, together with sufficient infiltration time, can alleviate pain and discomfort caused multiple punctures through the skin, and its efficiency is as important as periprostatic nerve block.

With an increase of antibiotic-resistant bacteria in developing countries, TP biopsy procedures have gained particular interest in these regions. However, most clinical studies regarding TP biopsy were carried out under general and spinal anesthesia. In this study, we utilized the LA plus PPNB approach to enhance the pain control and tolerability in TP biopsy patients. Larger sample size and randomized-design studies will be considered for validation in our future study.

Limitations of this study include lack of randomization in a relatively small study population of 238 patient cases collected in a single institute. However, double-blind designs for TP and TR procedures remain practical when performing the operation and post-operation evaluation. This prospective preliminary result provides the realistic nature for transperineal prostate biopsy implication.

Conclusions

The cancer detection rates were comparable to both transperineal (TP) and transrectal (TR) prostate bioptic approaches. However, the ratios of post-bioptic infectious complications in patients undergoing TP biopsy were much lower than those receiving conventional transrectal prostate biopsy. Besides, TP biopsy under local anesthesia is feasible for high general anesthesia-risk patients, particularly in the areas where the emergence of antibiotic-resistance is rising or the resources are limited.

Abbreviations

DRE: digital rectal exam; ESBL: extended-spectrum β-lactamase; IM: intramuscular; IPSS: International Prostate Symptom Score; LA: lidocaine anesthesia; OPD: outpatient department; PC: prostate cancer; PPNB: periprostatic nerve block; PSA: prostate-specific antigen; PZ: peripheral zone; TP: transperineal; TR: transrectal; TZ: transitional zone; UTI: urinary tract infection; VAS: visual analog scale

Acknowledgements

Not applicable

Authors' contributions

GLH was involved in literature search as well as data acquisition and analysis. PHC, CSK and WCL were the attending physicians responsible for carrying out the bioptic procedures during the OPD surgery. All authors contributed to result interpretation and manuscript drafting.

References

1. Ghafoori M, Velayati M, Aliyari Ghasabeh M, Shakiba M, Alavi M. Prostate biopsy using Transrectal ultrasonography; the optimal number of cores regarding Cancer detection rate and complications. Iran J Radiol. 2015;12(2):e13257.
2. Salomon G, Kollerman J, Thederan I, Chun FK, Budaus L, Schlomm T, Isbarn H, Heinzer H, Huland H, Graefen M. Evaluation of prostate cancer detection with ultrasound real-time elastography: a comparison with step section pathological analysis after radical prostatectomy. Eur Urol. 2008;54(6):1354–62.
3. Shahait M, Degheili J, El-Merhi F, Tamim H, Nasr R. Incidence of sepsis following transrectal ultrasound guided prostate biopsy at a tertiary-care medical center in Lebanon. Int Braz J Urol. 2016;42(1):60–8.
4. Efesoy O, Bozlu M, Çayan S, Akbay E. Complications of transrectal ultrasound-guided 12-core prostate biopsy: a single center experience with 2049 patients. Turkish journal of urology. 2013;39(1):6–11.
5. Lee S-J. Infection after transrectal ultrasound-guided prostate biopsy. Korean journal of urology. 2015;56(5):346–50.
6. Bjurlin MA, Wysock JS, Taneja SS. Optimization of prostate biopsy: review of technique and complications. The Urologic clinics of North America. 2014; 41(2):299–313.
7. Emiliozzi P, Corsetti A, Tassi B, Federico G, Martini M, Pansadoro V. Best approach for prostate cancer detection: a prospective study on transperineal versus transrectal six-core prostate biopsy. Urology. 2003;61(5):961–6.
8. Nash PA, Bruce JE, Indudhara R, Shinohara K. Transrectal ultrasound guided prostatic nerve blockade eases systematic needle biopsy of the prostate. J Urol. 1996;155(2):607–9.
9. Nazir B. Pain during transrectal ultrasound-guided prostate biopsy and the role of periprostatic nerve block: what radiologists should know. Korean J Radiol. 2014;15(5):543–53.
10. Hodge KK, McNeal JE, Terris MK, Stamey TA: Random systematic versus directed ultrasound guided transrectal core biopsies of the prostate. J Urol 1989, 142(1):71–74; discussion 74-75.
11. Watanabe M, Hayashi T, Tsushima T, Irie S, Kaneshige T, Kumon H. Extensive biopsy using a combined transperineal and transrectal approach to improve prostate cancer detection. International journal of urology : official journal of the Japanese Urological Association. 2005;12(11):959–63.
12. Kojima M, Hayakawa T, Saito T, Mitsuya H, Hayase Y. Transperineal 12-core systematic biopsy in the detection of prostate cancer. International journal of urology : official journal of the Japanese Urological Association. 2001;8(6):301–7.
13. Kawakami S, Yamamoto S, Numao N, Ishikawa Y, Kihara K, Fukui I. Direct comparison between transrectal and transperineal extended prostate biopsy for the detection of cancer. International journal of urology : official journal of the Japanese Urological Association. 2007;14(8):719–24.

14. Shen PF, Zhu YC, Wei WR, Li YZ, Yang J, Li YT, Li DM, Wang J, Zeng H. The results of transperineal versus transrectal prostate biopsy: a systematic review and meta-analysis. Asian journal of andrology. 2012;14(2):310–5.
15. Raaijmakers R, Kirkels WJ, Roobol MJ, Wildhagen MF, Schrder FH. Complication rates and risk factors of 5802 transrectal ultrasound-guided sextant biopsies of the prostate within a population-based screening program. Urology. 2002;60(5):826–30.
16. Grummet JP, Weerakoon M, Huang S, Lawrentschuk N, Frydenberg M, Moon DA, O'Reilly M, Murphy D. Sepsis and 'superbugs': should we favour the transperineal over the transrectal approach for prostate biopsy? BJU Int. 2014;114(3):384–8.
17. Williamson DA, Barrett LK, Rogers BA, Freeman JT, Hadway P, Paterson DL. Infectious complications following transrectal ultrasound-guided prostate biopsy: new challenges in the era of multidrug-resistant Escherichia coli. Clinical infectious diseases : an official publication of the Infectious Diseases Society of America. 2013;57(2):267–74.
18. Carignan A, Roussy JF, Lapointe V, Valiquette L, Sabbagh R, Pepin J. Increasing risk of infectious complications after transrectal ultrasound-guided prostate biopsies: time to reassess antimicrobial prophylaxis? Eur Urol. 2012;62(3):453–9.
19. Taylor AK, Zembower TR, Nadler RB, Scheetz MH, Cashy JP, Bowen D, Murphy AB, Dielubanza E, Schaeffer AJ. Targeted antimicrobial prophylaxis using rectal swab cultures in men undergoing transrectal ultrasound guided prostate biopsy is associated with reduced incidence of postoperative infectious complications and cost of care. J Urol. 2012;187(4):1275–9.
20. Williamson DA, Roberts SA, Paterson DL, Sidjabat H, Silvey A, Masters J, Rice M, Freeman JT. Escherichia coli bloodstream infection after transrectal ultrasound-guided prostate biopsy: implications of fluoroquinolone-resistant sequence type 131 as a major causative pathogen. Clinical infectious diseases : an official publication of the Infectious Diseases Society of America. 2012;54(10):1406–12.
21. Abughosh Z, Margolick J, Goldenberg SL, Taylor SA, Afshar K, Bell R, Lange D, Bowie WR, Roscoe D, Machan L, et al. A prospective randomized trial of povidone-iodine prophylactic cleansing of the rectum before transrectal ultrasound guided prostate biopsy. J Urol. 2013;189(4):1326–31.
22. Loeb S, Carter HB, Berndt SI, Ricker W, Schaeffer EM. Is repeat prostate biopsy associated with a greater risk of hospitalization? Data from SEER-Medicare. J Urol. 2013;189(3):867–70.
23. Loeb S, van den Heuvel S, Zhu X, Bangma CH, Schroder FH, Roobol MJ. Infectious complications and hospital admissions after prostate biopsy in a European randomized trial. Eur Urol. 2012;61(6):1110–4.
24. Unnikrishnan R, El-Shafei A, Klein EA, Jones JS, Kartha G, Goldman HB. For single dosing, levofloxacin is superior to ciprofloxacin when combined with an aminoglycoside in preventing severe infections after prostate biopsy. Urology. 2015;85(6):1241–6.
25. Loeb S, Carter HB, Berndt SI, Ricker W, Schaeffer EM. Complications after prostate biopsy: data from SEER-Medicare. J Urol. 2011;186(5):1830–4.
26. Borghesi M, Ahmed H, Nam R, Schaeffer E, Schiavina R, Taneja S, Weidner W, Loeb S. Complications after systematic, random, and image-guided prostate biopsy. Eur Urol. 2017;71(3):353–65.
27. Ehdaie B, Vertosick E, Spaliviero M, Giallo-Uvino A, Taur Y, O'Sullivan M, Livingston J, Sogani P, Eastham J, Scardino P, et al. The impact of repeat biopsies on infectious complications in men with prostate cancer on active surveillance. J Urol. 2014;191(3):660–4.
28. Ghani KR, Dundas D, Patel U. Bleeding after transrectal ultrasonography-guided prostate biopsy: a study of 7-day morbidity after a six-, eight- and 12-core biopsy protocol. BJU Int. 2004;94(7):1014–20.
29. Rosario DJ, Lane JA, Metcalfe C, Donovan JL, Doble A, Goodwin L, Davis M, Catto JW, Avery K, Neal DE, et al. Short term outcomes of prostate biopsy in men tested for cancer by prostate specific antigen: prospective evaluation within ProtecT study. BMJ (Clinical research ed). 2012;344:d7894.
30. Klein T, Palisaar RJ, Holz A, Brock M, Noldus J, Hinkel A. The impact of prostate biopsy and periprostatic nerve block on erectile and voiding function: a prospective study. J Urol. 2010;184(4):1447–52.
31. Tsivian M, Abern MR, Qi P, Polascik TJ. Short-term functional outcomes and complications associated with transperineal template prostate mapping biopsy. Urology. 2013;82(1):166–70.
32. Pepe P, Aragona F. Prostate biopsy: results and advantages of the transperineal approach--twenty-year experience of a single center. World J Urol. 2014;32(2):373 7.
33. Goluza E, Hudolin T, Kastelan Z, Peric M, Murselovic T, Sosic H. Lidocaine suppository for transrectal ultrasound-guided biopsy of the prostate: a prospective, double-blind, randomized study. Urol Int. 2011;86(3):315–9.
34. Wang J, Wang L, Du Y, He D, Chen X, Li L, Nan X, Fan J. Addition of intrarectal local analgesia to periprostatic nerve block improves pain control for transrectal ultrasonography-guided prostate biopsy: a systematic review and meta-analysis. International journal of urology : official journal of the Japanese Urological Association. 2015;22(1):62–8.
35. Borghesi M, Ahmed H, Nam R, Schaeffer E, Schiavina R, Taneja S, Weidner W, Loeb S. Complications After Systematic, Random, and Image-guided Prostate Biopsy. Eur Urol. 71(3):353–65.
36. Dell'Atti L. Lidocaine spray administration in transrectal ultrasound-guided prostate biopsy: five years of experience. *Archivio italiano di urologia, andrologia : organo ufficiale [di] Societa italiana di ecografia urologica e nefrologica*. 2014;86(4):340–3.
37. Galosi AB, Minardi D, Dell'atti L, Yehia M, Muzzonigro G. Tolerability of prostate transrectal biopsies using gel and local anesthetics: results of a randomized clinical trial. J Endourol. 2005;19(6):738–43.
38. Abdollah F, Novara G, Briganti A, Scattoni V, Raber M, Roscigno M, Suardi N, Gallina A, Artibani W, Ficarra V, et al. Trans-rectal versus trans-perineal saturation rebiopsy of the prostate: is there a difference in cancer detection rate? Urology. 2011;77(4):921–5.
39. Huang S, Reeves F, Preece J, Satasivam P, Royce P, Grummet JP. Significant impact of transperineal template biopsy of the prostate at a single tertiary institution. Urology Annals. 2015;7(4):428–32.
40. Miller J, Perumalla C, Heap G. Complications of transrectal versus transperineal prostate biopsy. ANZ J Surg. 2005;75(1–2):48–50.
41. Rabets JC, Jones JS, Patel AR, Zippe CD. Bupivacaine provides rapid, effective periprostatic anaesthesia for transrectal prostate biopsy. BJU Int. 2004;93(9):1216–7.
42. Gorur S, Inanoglu K, Akkurt BC, Candan Y, Kiper AN. Periprostatic nerve blockage reduces postoperative analgesic consumption and pain scores of patients undergoing transurethral prostate resection. Urol Int. 2007;79(4):297–301.
43. Smith JB, Popert R, Nuttall MC, Vyas L, Kinsella J, Cahill D. Transperineal sector prostate biopsies: a local anesthetic outpatient technique. Urology. 2014;83(6):1344–9.
44. Udeh EI, Amu OC, Nnabugwu II, Ozoemena O. Transperineal versus transrectal prostate biopsy: our findings in a tertiary health institution. Niger J Clin Pract. 2015;18(1):110–4.
45. Bellville JW, Forrest WH Jr, Miller E, Brown BW Jr. Influence of age on pain relief from analgesics. A study of postoperative patients. JAMA. 1971;217(13):1835–41.

Prostatic utricles without external genital anomalies in children: Our experience, literature review and pooling analysis

Bo Liu[1,2], Dawei He[1,2*], Deying Zhang[1], Xing Liu[1], Tao Lin[1,2] and Guanghui Wei[1,2]

Abstract

Background: It has been recognized that the incidence of prostatic utricle in boys is increasing and is closely associated with diseases such as hypospadias. However, the clinical features of prostatic utricle with normal external genitalia have received little attention.

Methods: Based on this, a series of 22 male children with prostatic utricles has been compiled by adding our 3 patients to 19 cases reported. All children enrolled had normal external genitalia. Clinical data of the case was reviewed.

Results: Urinary tract infection, purulent urethral discharge and pyuria were the most common presenting chief complaint (41%), irritative lower urinary tract symptoms were present in 17% of cases, obstructive lower urinary tract symptoms were noted in 14%. Urinary retention has been reported in 18% and epididymitis has been reported in 14%. Relatively rare clinical symptoms are abdominal pain, hematuria, and hematospermia. A case of calculus formation and a case of neoplasia within the prostatic utricle has been reported. A cystic mass found by digital rectal examination is the most common presenting sign. A utricular lesion posterior to the bladder was revealed by imaging examination. Unilateral renal agenesis was associated in 32% of reports. Non-surgical approach was chosen in 3 cases, transrectal ultrasonography guided aspiration has been reported in 1 case. Endoscopic techniques were used in 3 cases. Open excision was used in 11 cases. The laparoscopic excision was chosen in 3 cases and Robot-assisted laparoscopy was reported in 1 case. Symptoms and signs disappeared after treatment in all children, and no recurrence occurred during follow-up.

Conclusions: Prostate utricles without external genital anomalies are rarely reported in children, and are easily missed and misdiagnosed, often accompanied by recurrent urinary tract infections, lower urinary tract symptoms, epididymitis, dysuria and other symptoms. Imaging studies can confirm the diagnosis. Symptomatic and large utricles should be actively treated. The treatment program should be based on the age, clinical symptoms, and size and location of the utricle.

Keywords: Prostatic utricle cyst, External genital anomalies, Children

* Correspondence: 400116@hospital.cqmu.edu.cn
[1]Department of Urology, Children's Hospital of Chongqing Medical University, No. 136, Zhongshan 2 RD, Yuzhong District, Chongqing 400014, China
[2]Ministry of Education Key Laboratory of Child Development and Disorders, Chongqing Key Laboratory of Pediatrics, China International Science and Technology Cooperation base of Child Development and Critical Disorders, Chongqing Key Laboratory of Children Urogenital Development and Tissue Engineering, Chongqing 400014, China

Background

The prostatic utricle is an enlarged diverticulum in the posterior urethra, which result from incomplete degradation of the Müllerian ducts or decreased androgenic stimulation of the urogenital sinus [1]. Prostatic utricle is an uncommon congenital anomalies, with 1% incidence in autopsy findings and clinical prevalence of 5% in urologic patients [2]. Prostatic utricles are seen in young men commonly in the first and second decades and are associated with hypospadias, cryptorchidism, and pseudohermaphroditism/intersex disorders [3]. It is dived into grade 0-III according to the present feature based on voiding cystourethrogram (grade 0 - confined to the verumontanum; grade 1 - below the bladder neck; grade 2 - extend over the bladder neck; grade 3- opening distal to the external sphincter). The majority of prostatic utricles are asymptomatic. Symptomatic prostatic utricles may present with var. ious complaints including recurrent urinary tract infection, post-voiding dribbling, urethral discharge and epididymitis [4]. In particular, the presence of prostatic utricles in male patients with normal external genitalia has been reported but is exceedingly rare. Because these utricles are very rare, with few symptoms and no specific symptoms, a correct diagnosis is difficult to establish. Since no single series has been amassed for analysis, the clinical features, symptoms and signs of these patients, and how to deal with them have not been well characterized. Therefore, we combined the previously reported 19 cases with our own 3 cases for analysis to better clarify their clinical features and treatment management.

Methods

All cases of prostatic utricles published in English from PubMed were reviewed, the closing date was June 30, 2018. All patients included in our study were children (age ≤ 18 years). Four cases were excluded due to the lack of required clinical data, and the remaining 19 cases (No. 4–22) and our own 3 cases (No. 1–3) constituted the subjects of this study [1, 4–20]. Clinical data of the case was reviewed with special attention to the patient's clinical manifestations, diagnostic methods, therapeutic methods, pathological diagnosis and follow-up results.

Results

General information

The age of 22 patients with clinical symptoms ranged from 2 months to 18 years (mean age 5.8 years). Cases of the prostatic utricles have been reported in all races but are more common in white races (Table 1).

Clinical manifestation

Urinary tract infection, purulent urethral discharge and pyuria were present in 9 patients (41%). Irritative lower urinary tract symptoms (urinary frequency, urgency, dysuria and incontinence) were noted in 6 patients (17%). Obstructive lower urinary tract symptoms (Difficulty voiding, dribbling stream and poor stream of urine) were noted in 3 patients (14%). Urinary retention has been reported in 4 patients (18%) and epididymitis has been reported in 3 patients (14%). Relatively rare clinical symptoms are abdominal pain, hematuria, and hematospermia. A case of calculus formation and a case of neoplasia within the prostatic utricle has been reported. In 7 patients (32%), a digital rectal examination revealed a utricular mass above the prostate and posterior to the bladder. Less commonly reported signs include pelvic or abdominal mass and enlarged scrotal swelling.

Associated congenital anomalies

All included cases have completely normal genitalia, unilateral renal agenesis was noted in 7 patients (32%). Less frequently patients have associated with congenital obstructive posterior urethral and vesicoureteral reflux.

Diagnosis methods

Ultrasound was the most commonly used imaging method (Fig. 1), proving a correct diagnosis in 15 cases (68%). During voiding cystourethrogram (VCUG) or retrograde urethrogram (RUG) a utricular chamber filled from the posterior urethra in 13 cases (59%) (Fig. 2). Computerized tomography (CT) and magnetic resonance imaging (MRI) also made correct diagnosis in 11 cases (50%) (Figs. 3 and 4). Intravenous pyelogram (IVP) was used to auxiliary diagnosis of renal agenesis in 2 cases. Urethrocystoscopy revealed an orifice opening into a utricle in 10 cases.

Treatments and outcomes

Non-surgical approach (including antimicrobial treatment) was chosen in 3 cases, transcrectal ultrasound (TRUS) guided aspiration has been reported in 1 case. Endoscopic techniques (utricle catheterization and aspiration and endoscopic utricle orifice incision) were used in 3 cases. Open excision (suprapubic extravesical, extraperitoneal, transvesical, retrovesical, retropubic, posterior transsacral, posterior sagittal rectum retracting approach) was used in 11 cases. The laparoscopic excision was chosen in 3 cases and Robot-assisted laparoscopy was reported in 1 case. No recurrence or repeated symptoms of the prostatic utricles were reported after any treatment.

Pathology

In 15 cases of surgical excision, pathological findings were reported in 7 cases. Two of them were lined with squamous epithelium, one was lined with transitional epithelium and 1 was lined with flattened cuboidal epithelium. Two utricles were noted to have areas of squamous metaplasia. A rare clear cell adenocarcinoma was reported in a prostatic utricle.

Table 1 Characteristics of prostatic utricles with normal external genitalia

Case No.- Pt. Age	Symptoms	Physical examination	Diagnostic procedure	Associated anomalies	Treatment performed
1 - 10 m	Recurrent purulent urethral discharge, recurrent UTI	Cystic rectal mass	Ultrasound, VCUG, MRI	None	Utricle catheterization and aspiration
2 - 15y	Acute urinary retention	Cystic rectal mass	Ultrasound, VCUG, CT	None	Utricle catheterization and aspiration
3 - 8 m	Recurring epididymitis	Cystic rectal mass	Ultrasound, VCUG, CT, MRI	None	Laparoscopic excision
4–4 1/2y	Difficulty voiding, low abdominal pain	Normal	Cystogram, cystoscope,	None	Retropubic, open operation
5 - 2 m	UTI	Normal	Ultrasound, VCUG, cystoscopy	Left renal agenesis, congenital obstructive posterior urethral membrane	Antimicrobial treatment
6 - 3y	UTI	Normal	IVP, cystoscopy, RUG	Left renal agenesis	Antimicrobial treatment
7 - 4y	UTI	Low abdominal mass	Ultrasound, urethroscopy,	None	Retrovesical, open operation
8 - 9y	Frequency, dribbling stream, daytime wetting, post-void fullness	Cystic rectal mass	VCUG	Vesicoureteral reflux	Posterior transsacral, open operation
9 - 10 m	Pyuria and fever	Cystic rectal mass, pus discharge on pressure	Ultrasound, cystoscopy	None	Transvesical, open operation
10 - 7y	Recurring epididymitis	Normal	Ultrasound, IVP, VCUG, RUG, cystoscope	Right renal agenesis	Transvesical, open operation
11 - 4y	Penile pain, low grade fever, urinary frequency, recurrent UTI	Mid swelling in the right testis, reproducible tenderness in the suprapubic area	Ultrasound, VCUG	None	Transvesical, open operation
12 - 16y	Intermittent, nonpainful, gross hematuria	Cystic rectal mass	CT, urethrocystoscopy	Right renal agenesis	Open operation
13 - 10y	Acute urinary retention	Distended urinary bladder	MRI, TRUS	None	TRUS guided aspiration
14 - 3y	Fever, lower abdominal pain, dysuria, acute urinary retention	Cystic rectal mass	MRI, cystoscopy	None	Laparoscopic excision
15 - 18 m	Recurrent UTI	Normal	RUG, cystoscope	Right renal agenesis	Laparoscopic excision
16 - 6 m	Retention and poor stream of urine	Palpable bladder	Ultrasound, VCUG	None	Posterior sagittal rectum retracting approach, open operation
17 - 6 m	Persistent purulent urethral discharge, recurrent UTI	Normal	Ultrasound, RUG, urethrocystoscopy	Right renal agenesis	Endoscopic utricle orifice incision
18 - 15y	Recurrent episodes of hematospermia	Normal	TRUS, MRI with an endorectal coil	None	Non-surgical approach
19 - 16y	Recurrent UTI, scrotal pain, low-grade fever, urinary frequency	Retrovesical mass	Ultrasound, MRI	None	Suprapubic extraperitoneal, open operation
20–1 1/2y	Recurrent epididymitis	Enlarged left-sided scrotal swelling	Ultrasound, CT, barium enema, RUG	None	Suprapubic extravesical and extraperitoneal, open operation
21 - 8y	Painful micturition, fever, progressive increasing abdominal girth	Cystic pelvic mass	CT	Left renal agenesis	laparotomy
22 - 6y	Urinary incontinence	Normal	Ultrasound, VCUG, MRI	None	Robot-assisted laparoscopy

CT, computed tomography; IVP, intravenous pyelogram; MRI, magnetic resonance imaging; RUG, retrograde urethrogram; TRUS, transcrectal ultrasound; UTI, urinary tract infection; VCUG, voiding cystourethrogram

Discussion

The prostatic utricle is a rudimentary structure in the posterior urethra of males. After careful embryological investigation, the researchers believe that the cranial portion of the prostatic utricle is derived from the Müllerian ducts and the caudal segment has a mixed origin from the Müllerian ducts and Wolffian ducts and the urogenital sinus [13]. In males, the Müllerian ducts regress respond to Müllerian inhibiting factor (MIF) produced by the fetal testis, leaving them as a vestige.

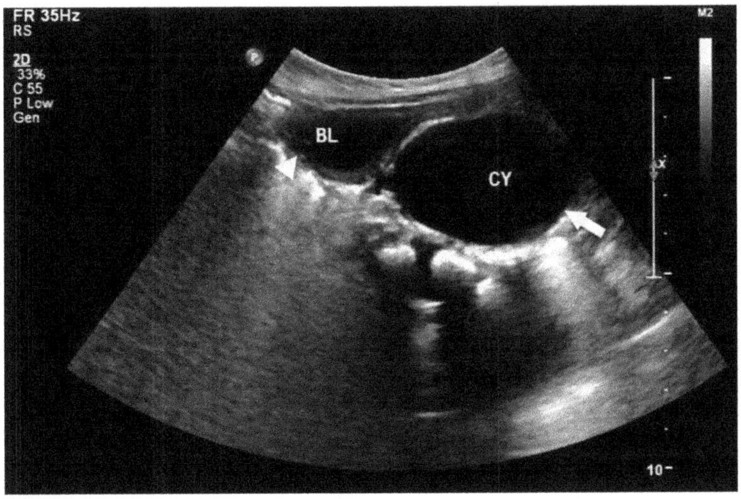

Fig. 1 Transverse ultrasound of the pelvis shows a large utricle in the midline (white arrow), posterior to the urinary bladder (white arrowhead)

The urogenital sinus, which continues to form the distal third of the vagina in female, does not respond to MIF but instead masculinizes by closing off in response to testosterone in males [21]. Therefore, it is not surprising that the utricles were lined with squamous epithelium (Müllerian ducts), cuboidal epithelium and transitional epithelium (Wolffian ducts and urogenital sinus) in our reported histological examination. We also found that 32% of the cases show an association of unilateral renal agenesis, this may be due to the metanephric bud and renal blastema are in contiguity during the stage of prostatic utricle embryogenesis (7 to 8 weeks) [7].

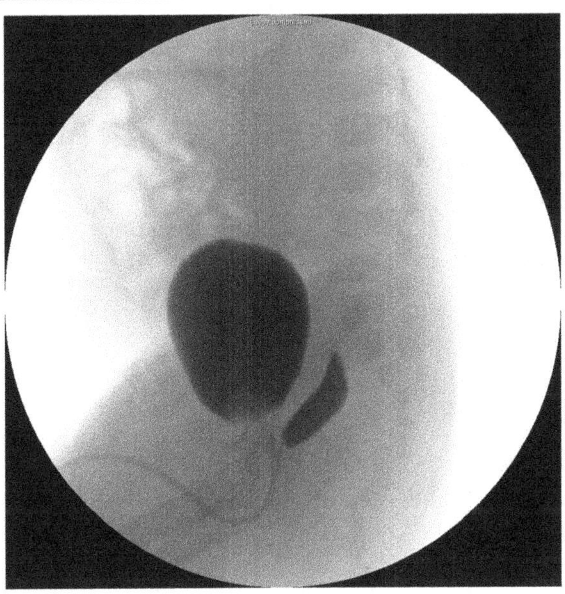

Fig. 2 VCUG image depicts a prostatic utricle manifesting as a diverticulum that arises from the posterior wall of the urethra

The differential diagnosis need to be considered include Müllerian duct cyst, bladder diverticulum, urachal cyst, or a seminal vesicle cyst [22]. Among the diseases that need to be identified, Müllerian duct cysts are the most difficult to distinguish from embryology, clinical and imaging with the prostatic utricles because both of them are median intraprostatic cysts. Some researchers believe that the Müllerian duct cyst originates from the mesoderm, while the prostatic utricles originate from the endoderm [7]. Müllerian duct cysts are generally not connected to the prostatic urethra. They are round in shape and are often found in adults (20-40y) with normal external genitalia. Prostate utricles are tubular or vesicular in shape and most commonly seen in children (<20y) with hypospadias, cryptorchidism and gender dysplasia, usually communicating with the prostatic urethra [19]. Our patient is rare and unusual because all the features are in favor of a utricle that presented in the first or second period and communicated with the urethra but at the same time our patient had normal external genitalia. Two reasons are considered for the low number of reported cases. One is that the majority of prostatic utricles are asymptomatic, especially when small, thus symptomatic prostatic utricles are easily misdiagnosed or never diagnosed. Another is that symptoms of the prostatic utricle are varied and nonspecific, and outpatients are often treated symptomatically without further examination to determine the underlying disease. When large, the clinical presentation includes recurrent urinary tract infection, urethral discharge, post void urine dribbling, urinary retention, epididymitis, calculi formation and in rare cases malignant transformation [4].

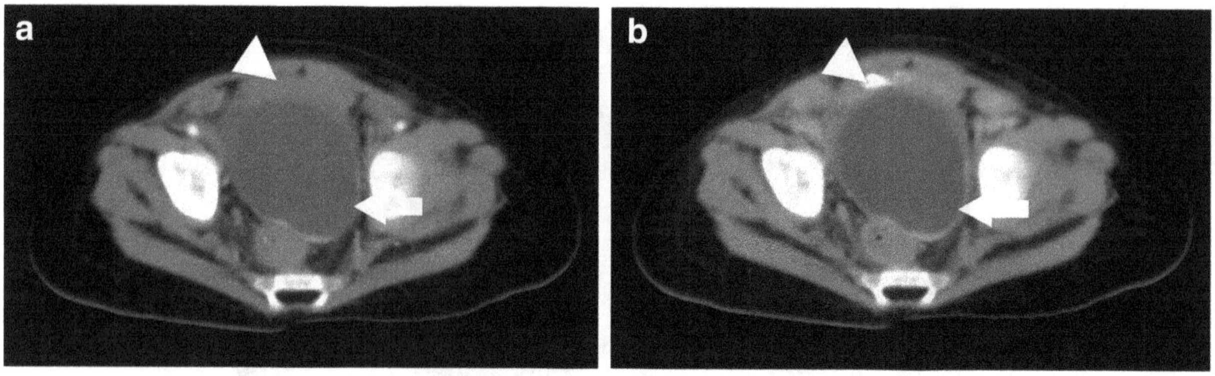

Fig. 3 Contrast-enhanced computed tomography shows a large, utricular mass (white arrow) behind the urinary bladder (white arrowhead). **a** Enhanced CT shows a utricular retrovesical mass compressing the urinary bladder. **b** Delayed enhanced CT shows the bladder filled with contrast agent, a large utricular mass located behind and in close proximity to the urinary bladder

The diagnosis is suspected when there is clinical manifestation and the mass is felt on the digital rectal examination. A pelvic ultrasound, a transrectal ultrasound or a perineal ultrasound can show cavity filled with fluid and its relationship with adjacent anatomical structures such as the prostate and urethra [23]. In VCUG or RUG, the utricles may have different sizes, showing an opacified cystic structure posterior to the prostatic urethra. However, it is worth noting that the identification of the prostate utricle by VCUG or RUG is often missed because the utricle is not fully filled, and the small prostate utricle is not easily detected by ultrasound. Fortunately, small prostate utricle (grade 0 and I) are often asymptomatic, and only need to be monitored without treatment. Enlarged prostatic utricles (grade II and III), which often requires surgical intervention, are easily detected by ultrasound, RUG and VCUG [24]. Using CT to detect these utricles is more accurate but it does not provide more help than ultrasound, RUG or VCUG. An MRI with an endorectal coil is particularly useful to delineate the utricle from the other pelvic structures due to their high resolution and multiplanar capability [25]. Certainly, the most useful investigation for a prostatic utricle is the urethrocystoscopy to identify the utricular orifice in the posterior urethra. Catheterization of the utricle with injection of contrast agent can be implemented to delineate the pouch more clearly [10]. Surgical treatment can also be performed with the aid of cystourethroscope.

Appropriate surgical procedures have been described to treat symptomatic and enlarged prostatic utricle. The first is endoscopic utricle orifice dilation, catheterization and aspiration, and resection of utricle roof. These methods have the advantage of less invasive, but also have a relatively high risk of

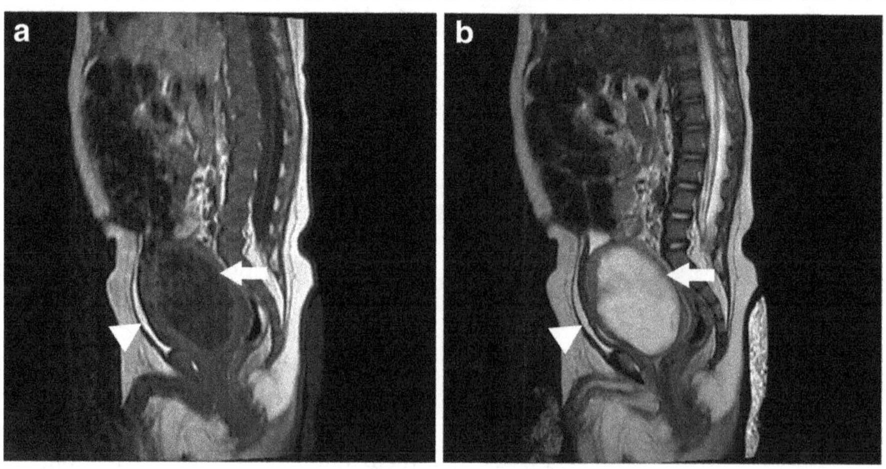

Fig. 4 Magnetic resonance image shows a large prostatic utricle (white arrow) behind the urinary bladder (white arrowhead). **a** Sagittal T1 weighted MR image showing a hypointense lesion (white arrow) with thick and irregular wall posterior to urinary bladder (white arrowhead) and anterior to the rectum. **b** Sagittal T2 weighted MR image demonstrating a thick-wall, large utricular lesion behind the urinary bladder

recurrence [26]. We treated 2 of our patient with endoscopic utricle catheterization and aspiration. The reason for choosing this option was because the symptoms of the child were first seen, and also to avoid impotency and infertility caused by surgery. There was no recurrence by the adequate drainage of the wide mouthed diverticulum into the urethra. Surgical resection is recommended for utricles with recurrent symptoms and further neoplastic changes. Many open surgical approaches have been proposed to excise prostate utricle such as posterior pararectal [15]. Traditional open surgical approaches require high operational skills and may damage adjacent tissues [26]. Laparoscopic excision of prostatic utricle is suitable for surgeons who are skilled in advanced laparoscopic techniques. This technique reduces intrusion to the retrovesical space, provides a clear vision, and reduces the time required for recovery [26]. We have successfully applied laparoscopic techniques to a child with recurrent symptoms. Recently robot-assisted laparoscopy was considered as an advantageous technique for the treatment of prostatic utricle [20].

Conclusions

The presence of a prostatic utricle in the absence of hypospadias, cryptorchidism or pseudohermaphroditism/intersex disorders is a rare finding. A combination of clinical signs and findings on physical examination guide diagnosis. Imaging test and urethrocystoscope can not only diagnose the prostatic utricle but also investigate its anatomical relationship. In general, small, asymptomatic, accidentally diagnosed prostatic utricles can be followed up without treatment. Complicated and large utricles need to be cured by surgery.

Abbreviations

CT: Computerized tomography; MRI: Magnetic resonance imaging; RUG: Retrograde urethrogram; VCUG: Voiding cystourethrogram

Acknowledgements

Not applicable.

Author contributions

BL and DWH participated in its design and coordination and helped to draft the manuscript. BL, DYZ and XL carried out the concept of the study, participated in the statistical analysis, and drafted the manuscript. DWH, TL performed relevant operations and collected patients' data. GHW participated in the statistical analysis. All authors read and approved the final manuscript.

References

1. Verma SK, Shetty BS, Kanth L. A boy with acute urinary retention: a Mullerian duct remnant (2006: 3b). Eur Radiol. 2006;16(6):1401–3.
2. Meng X, Liu J, Yu X, Wang S, Liu C, Ye Z. A giant Müllerian duct cyst in the perineum: a case report. Front Med. 2012;6(4):440 3.
3. Shebel HM, Farg HM, Kolokythas O, El-Diasty T. Cysts of the lower male genitourinary tract: embryologic and anatomic considerations and differential diagnosis. Radiographics. 2013;33(4):1125–43.
4. Ramachandra M, Bendre PS, Redkar RG, Taide DV. Isolated prostatic utricle. J Indian Assoc Pediatr Surg. 2009;14(4):228–9.
5. SPENCE HM, CHENOWETH VC. Cysts of prostatic utricle (müllerian duct cysts); report of two cases in children, each containing calculi, cured by retropubic operation. J Urol. 1958;79(2):308–14.
6. Stuppler SA, Naranjo CA, Kandzari SJ. A Müllerian duct remnant without associated stigmas of intersex: report of a case. J Urol. 1973;110(1):133–5.
7. Schuhrke TD, Kaplan GW. Prostatic utricle cysts (müllerian duct cysts). J Urol. 1978;119(6):765–7.
8. Youngson GG. Squamous metaplasia complicating a müllerian duct remnant. Br J Urol. 1990;65(2):211–2.
9. McDermott V, Orr JD, Wild SR. Duplicated müllerian duct remnants associated with unilateral renal agenesis. Abdom Imaging. 1993;18(2):193–5.
10. Meisheri IV, Motiwale SS, Sawant VV. Surgical management of enlarged prostatic utricle. Pediatr Surg Int. 2000;16(3):199–203.
11. Yeung CK, Sihoe JD, Tam YH, Lee KH. Laparoscopic excision of prostatic utricles in children. BJU Int. 2001;87(6):505–8.
12. Lopatina OA, Berry TT, Spottswood SE. Giant prostatic utricle (utriculus masculinis): diagnostic imaging and surgical implications. Pediatr Radiol. 2004;34(2):156–9.
13. Gualco G, Ortega V, Ardao G, Cravioto F. Clear cell adenocarcinoma of the prostatic utricle in an adolescent. Ann Diagn Pathol. 2005;9(3):153–6.
14. Siomou E, Papadopoulou F, Salakos C, Giapros V, Andonikou S, Siamopoulou A. Rare combination of unilateral renal agenesis, congenital obstructive posterior urethral membrane, and enlarged prostatic utricle, with absence of hydroureteronephrosis. Urology. 2007;70(5):1008.e1–3.
15. Al-Salem AH. An unusual and rare cause of recurrent epididymitis in an infant. JPSS. 2008;2(1):39–41.
16. Incedayi M, Sivrioglu AK, Sonmez G, Ozturk E. Large prostatic utricle cyst. BMJ Case Rep. 2013;2013.
17. Momin YA, Dhende NP, Ghodke BA, Ansari SA, D'Costa GF, Mahajan VR. An abnormally large prostatic utricle cyst associated with unilateral renal agenesis. Urol Ann. 2013;5(2):129–31.
18. Feutry G, De Perrot T, Wirth GJ, Montet X, Martin SP. Prostatic utricle cyst as the Most likely cause in a case of recurrent episodes of Hematospermia. Case Rep Urol. 2017;2017.
19. Lazarus J, Maison POM, Howlett J. Prostatic utricle cyst presenting with recurrent urethral discharge in the newborn: a case report. Pediatric Urology Case Reports. 2017;4(6):383–6.
20. Lima M, Maffi M, Di Salvo N, Ruggeri G, Libri M, Gargano T, Lardy H. Robotic removal of Müllerian duct remnants in pediatric patients: our experience and a review of the literature. Pediatr Med Chir. 2018;40(1).
21. Berrocal T, López-Pereira P, Arjonilla A, Gutiérrez J. Anomalies of the distal ureter, bladder, and urethra in children: embryologic, radiologic, and pathologic features. Radiographics. 2002;22(5):1139–64.
22. Johnson D, Parikh K, Schey W, Mar W. MRI in diagnosis of a giant prostatic utricle. Case Rep Radiol. 2014;2014:217563.
23. Hester AG, Kogan SJ. The prostatic utricle: an under-recognized condition resulting in significant morbidity in boys with both hypospadias and normal external genitalia. J Pediatr Urol. 2017;13(5):492.e1–5.
24. Kojima Y, Hayashi Y, Maruyama T, Sasaki S, Kohri K. Comparison between ultrasonography and retrograde urethrography for detection of prostatic utricle associated with hypospadias. Urology. 2001;57(6):1151–5.
25. Mukha R, Sriram K, Ganesh G. Prostatic utricle cyst–a case report and review of current literature. The Internet J Urol. 2009;6.
26. Luo JH, Chen W, Sun JJ, Xie D, Mo JC, Zhou L, Lu J. Laparoscopic management of Müllerian duct remnants: four case reports and review of the literature. J Androl. 2008;29(6):638–42.

26

A comparative effectiveness analysis of the PBCG vs. PCPT risks calculators in a multi-ethnic cohort

Samuel Carbunaru[1†], Oluwarotimi S. Nettey[1†], Pooja Gogana[1], Irene B. Helenowski[2], Borko Jovanovic[2], Maria Ruden[3], Courtney M. P. Hollowell[4], Roohollah Sharifi[5,6], Rick A. Kittles[7], Edward Schaeffer[1], Peter Gann[8] and Adam B. Murphy[1,4,5*]

Abstract

Background: Predictive models that take race into account like the Prostate Cancer Prevention Trial Risk Calculator 2.0 (PCPT RC) and the new Prostate Biopsy Collaborative Group (PBCG) RC have been developed to equitably mitigate the overdiagnosis of prostate specific antigen (PSA) screening. Few studies have compared the performance of both calculators across racial groups.

Methods: From 1485 prospectively recruited participants, 954 men were identified undergoing initial prostate biopsy for abnormal PSA or digital rectal examination in five Chicago hospitals between 2009 and 2014. Discrimination, calibration, and frequency of avoided biopsies were calculated to assess the performance of both risk calculators.

Results: Of 954 participants, 463 (48.5%) were Black, 355 (37.2%) were White, and 136 (14.2%) identified as Other. Biopsy results were as follows: 310 (32.5%) exhibited no cancer, 323 (33.9%) indolent prostate cancer, and 321 (33.6%) clinically significant prostate cancer (csPCa). Differences in area under the curve (AUC)s for the detection of csPCa between PCPT and PBCG were not statistically different across all racial groups. PBCG did not improve calibration plots in Blacks and Others, as it showed higher levels of overprediction at most risk thresholds. PCPT led to an increased number of avoidable biopsies in minorities compared to PBCG at the 30% threshold (68% vs. 28% of all patients) with roughly similar rates of missed csPCa (23% vs. 20%).

Conclusion: Significant improvements were noticed in PBCG's calibrations and net benefits in Whites compared to PCPT. Since PBCG's improvements in Blacks are disputable and potentially biases a greater number of low risk Black and Other men towards unnecessary biopsies, PCPT may lead to better biopsy decisions in racial minority groups. Further comparisons of commonly used risk calculators across racial groups is warranted to minimize excessive biopsies and overdiagnosis in ethnic minorities.

Keywords: Prostate biopsy collaborative group risk calculator, Prostate Cancer prevention trial risk calculator 2.0, Prostate cancer risk prediction, Risk calculator, African American validation

* Correspondence: a-murphy2@northwestern.edu
[†]Samuel Carbunaru and Oluwarotimi S. Nettey contributed equally to this work.
[1]Department of Urology, Northwestern University Feinberg School of Medicine, 303 E Chicago Avenue, Tarry 16, Chicago, IL 60611, USA
[4]Division of Urology, Cook County Health and Hospitals System, 303 E Chicago Avenue, Tarry 16, Chicago, IL 60611, USA
Full list of author information is available at the end of the article

Background

Prostate cancer (PCa) is the leading malignancy amongst men with 164,690 new diagnoses in the United States in 2018 [1]. Prostate specific antigen (PSA) screening has reduced PCa specific mortality by ~50% [2]. Approximately 1 million biopsies are performed in the US each year, however, 54% of them are negative and another 25% reveal presumably indolent PCa [3, 4]. Complications of prostate biopsy are not uncommon and should be considered. Infectious complications affect 0.1 to 7.0% of patients, followed by sepsis ranging from 0.3 to 3.1% [5]. To mitigate screening harms, several predictive risk calculators (RCs) have been developed to help men make informed decisions about biopsy and better identify men who are likely to have clinically significant PCa. However, it is unclear if commonly used RCs are appropriately calibrated to identify racial minorities who can avoid unnecessary biopsies. While racial disparities in PCa between US Blacks and Whites have diminished over the past decades, there are still considerable differences [6]. Black men present with higher PSA levels, are at higher risk of developing clinically significant PCa (csPCa), and have higher mortality rates compared to Whites [7, 8]. The commonly used Prostate Cancer Prevention Trial 2.0 (PCPT) and the new Prostate Biopsy Collaborative Group (PBCG) RCs both take race into consideration, but were developed in largely European ancestry populations [9, 10].

This study compares the PBCG and PCPT RCs across racial groups using discrimination and calibration statistics, as well as the frequency of avoided biopsies and missed csPCa in an urban, multi-racial cohort.

Methods

Study participants

Following institutional review board approval at Northwestern University, University of Chicago, University of Illinois at Chicago, Jesse Brown VA Medical Center and Cook County Health from 2009 to 2014, 954 consecutive ambulatory men from urology clinics at two privately funded and three publicly funded institutions were enrolled in a cross-sectional study evaluating the association between vitamin D status and prostate biopsy outcomes [11]. Patients were deemed eligible if they were undergoing their first prostate biopsy for an abnormal PSA level or digital rectal exam (DRE). All patients provided written informed consent.

Data collection

A self-administered questionnaire confirmed self-reported race & ethnicity, demographics, and medical history. Histologic diagnosis, DRE, and imaging reports were evaluated to determine disease stage according to American Joint Committee on Cancer TNM (tumor, node, metastasis) staging system [2]. All patients underwent a transrectal ultrasound guided biopsy with at least a 10-core biopsy with a median of 12 cores. Biopsies were read by three experienced uropathologists at Northwestern (XY) and at the University of Illinois at Chicago (ABJ and VM).

Statistical analysis

Descriptive statistics were used to characterize important covariates including age, race, PSA, PSA density, prostate volume, body mass index (BMI), alcohol and smoking use, income, family history of PCa, marital status, abnormal DRE, college completion, 5 alpha-reductase inhibitor (5-ARI) use, and the clinical diagnosis of benign prostatic hyperplasia (BPH). To compare groups, Student's t-tests or nonparametric Wilcoxon-Mann tests were performed for continuous variables, and Pearson-χ^2 tests were used for categorical variables.

The PCPT RC 2.0 [10] and PBCG [9] were applied, as provided in R package, to estimate the risk of overall PCa and csPCa (defined as Gleason ≥3 + 4) for each participant using PSA, DRE, first-degree family history of PCa (father, brother or son ever diagnosed with PCa) and history of a prior negative prostate biopsy. All patients had no prior prostate biopsy as they were recruited at time of initial biopsy. Categories for self-reported race included Black/African American, White/Caucasian, Hispanic and Other. Because published logistic regression coefficients in the PCPT RC [10] computed probabilities by race similarly for 'Hispanic' and 'Other', we categorized all participants who were non-Black and non-White as 'Other' in our analysis. For participants with unknown family history or DRE status, "Do not know" and "Not performed or not sure", respectively, were used following the recommendation by the online RCs. Percent free PSA, PCA3, and TMPRSS ERG were not included in the risk calculations since the test was not routinely ordered for all participants. The primary endpoints were the presence of any prostate adenocarcinoma and the presence of Gleason ≥3 + 4 PCa on prostate biopsy. Of the Gleason 6 tumors, 77% were very low to low risk according to NCCN guidelines [12].

Discrimination was calculated by quantifying the non-parametric area under the receiver operating characteristics curve (AUC). AUC was calculated for PBCG and PCPT by race (Black, White, Other). We were powered to detect a 7% AUC difference between PCPT and PBCG in Blacks and Whites at alpha = 5% with greater than 99% power. For Other men we achieved a 76% power. We assumed a PCPT AUC of 0.60 with a one-sided alpha of 0.05, and a 0.95 correlation between PCPT and PBCG for both positive and negative results.

Calibration curves were generated by plotting the predictions generated by the PBCG and PCPT RC on the x-axis in deciles and the observed outcomes for men in that decile on the y-axis. In the calibration plot, the 45-degree line represents perfectly calibrated predictions. A Hosmer-Lemeshow test for goodness-of-fit was performed to assess the quality of the calibration of each risk calculator.

Decision curve analysis (DCA) is a graphical statistical method that plots a population's net benefit from a RC on the y-axis over a variety of probabilities for the calculator detecting true disease on the x-axis [13]. Patients and providers usually have individual *probability thresholds* of disease detection above which they would undergo or recommend the biopsy that range between 5 and 40% [14–17]. The probability threshold can be used to estimate how a decision maker might weigh the relative benefit of appropriate treatment compared to the potential harms of undergoing unnecessary biopsy. The net benefit of PBCG and PCPT has not been compared across race previously.

The net benefits were compared using the following biopsy strategies: Biopsy All men, Biopsy based on PBCG Thresholds, and Biopsy based on PCPT Thresholds. For the Biopsy All men curve, an exchange rate of 1/9 was used (as in Vickers et al.'s analysis of PCa biomarkers [18]), meaning we are willing to perform nine unnecessary biopsies to detect one case of csPCa.

Statistical analyses were performed using Excel, SPSS 24 (IBM Corporation 2016, United States), R 3.3.3., SAS v9.4 (SAS Institute, Cary, NC, USA), and Stata 12.1 (StataCorp, 2011, College Station, TX).

Results

Demographics

In total, 954 men with elevated PSA levels or abnormal DRE results underwent an initial transrectal ultrasound guided prostate biopsy during 2009–2014 (see Table 1). The sample included men who self-reported as Black (463, 48.5%), White (355, 37.2%), and Other races (136, 14.2%). The Other racial group included Hispanic (n = 103, 75.7%), Asian (n = 28) and Middle Eastern men

Table 1 Patient sociodemographic characteristics and clinical risk factors by race

Continuous Variables	Black (n = 463) Median [IQR]	White (n = 355) Median [IQR]	Other (n = 136) Median [IQR]	p Value [1]
Age, years	61.0 [57.0, 67.0]	62.0 [58.0, 67.0]	62.0 [57.0, 67.0]	0.47
BMI, kg/m ^{2}	27.8 [24.5, 31.8]	27.5 [25.0, 30.6]	27.4 [24.2, 30.3]	0.56
PSA, ng/ml	7.8 [5.3, 15.5]	4.8 [3.6, 7.3]	7.2 [5.1, 12.4]	**< 0.001**
Prostate Volume, cm ^{3}	39.5 [28.8, 55.4]	39.5 [29.7, 51.0]	48.7 [30.0, 69.4]	**< 0.001**
PSA density, ng/cm^3	0.23 [0.12,0.43]	0.13 [0.09, 0.20]	0.18 [0.11, 0.32]	**< 0.001**
PCPT csPCa Risk, %	25.0 [17.0, 40.0]	7.0 [5.0, 12.0]	11.5 [7.0, 18.0]	**< 0.001**
PBCG csPCa Risk, %	45.0 [31.0, 65.0]	26.0 [18.0, 41.0]	37.5 [22.0, 54.2]	**< 0.001**
Categorical Variables	**Black n (%)**	**White n (%)**	**Other n (%)**	***p* Value[2]**
Clinical Risk Factors				
Family History of PCa	93 (20.1)	88 (24.8)	21 (15.4)	0.055
Abnormal DRE	140 (30.3)	112 (31.5)	43 (31.3)	0.92
BPH/LUTS	151 (32.6)	135 (38.0)	66 (48.5)	**0.003**
5-ARI Use (current)	43 (9.3)	19 (5.4)	26 (19.1)	**< 0.001**
Substance Use History				
Heavy Smoking (>1ppd)	29 (6.4)	19 (5.4)	1 (0.7)	**0.034**
Heavy Alcohol Use (> 10 drinks/week)	30 (6.6)	46 (13.0)	5 (3.7)	**< 0.001**
Demographic Factors				
Married	192 (42.1)	269 (76.2)	105 (77.2)	**< 0.001**
College Completion	165 (36.2)	248 (70.3)	46 (33.8)	**< 0.001**
Income < $30,000	161 (43.9)	39 (12.0)	42 (55.2)	**< 0.001**
Biopsy Outcomes				**< 0.001[3]**
Indolent Cancer	167 (36.1)	118 (33.2)	38 (27.9)	0.20
Clinically Significant Cancer	175 (37.8)	120 (33.8)	26 (19.1)	**< 0.001**
No Cancer	121 (26.1)	117 (33.0)	72 (52.9)	**< 0.001**

[1]Using Kruskal-Wallis tests; [2]Using Pearson-χ^2 tests; [3]χ^2 trend test. Bold type indicates p values < 0.05. Abbreviations: *BMI* body mass Index, *PSA* prostate specific antigen, *BPH/LUTS* clinical diagnosis of Benign Prostatic Hyperplasia/Lower Urinary Tract Symptoms, *DRE* digital rectal examination, *csPCa* clinically significant prostate cancer, *PBCG* Prostate Biopsy Collaborative Group, *PCPT* Prostate Cancer Prevention Trial, *ppd* pack per day

($n = 5$). All groups had a comparable age ($p = 0.47$) and BMI ($p = 0.56$). Black men had higher pre-biopsy PSA values and density (both $p < 0.001$).

Of the 954 biopsies, 310 (32.5%) were negative for PCa, 323 (33.9%) were positive for indolent PCa, and 321 (33.6%) demonstrated csPCa. Black men were more often diagnosed with overall PCa (73.9%) and csPCa (37.8%) on biopsy than White or Other men (both $p < 0.001$). A comparison of median risk scores shows that Blacks had higher risk scores for csPCa compared to White and Other men in both PCPT and PBCG ($p < 0.001$).

Discrimination/calibration

Statistically, there was no difference in the AUCs between PBCG and PCPT for overall PCa when all men are included. The AUC for csPCa was 0.64 (95% CI: 0.61–0.68) for PCPT and 0.65 (95% CI: 0.62–0.68) for PBCG ($p = 0.27$). The AUCs slightly improved with PBCG in Whites (0.64 vs. 0.66; $p = 0.07$) and Blacks (0.67 vs. 0.68; $p = 0.25$), but not in Others (0.64 vs. 0.64; $p = 0.81$); yet, none of these differences were statistically significant.

Figure 1 depicts the calibration and distribution plots for csPCa by racial group. The PBCG calculator results in a broader distribution of men in all racial groups, as opposed to the PCPT RC where most men are clustered in the lower risk deciles (< 30%). The PBCG calibration in all men outperforms PCPT at the < 30% range, while the PCPT is better calibrated at ≥30% risk deciles. It is unclear if the improved calibration at probabilities ≥30% is clinically significant since most men will opt for biopsy at > 30% risk [16]. For Blacks and Others PCPT seems to be better calibrated, as PBCG over-predicts csPCa across most risk thresholds. In Whites, however, the opposite is seen with PBCG being better calibrated, since PCPT underestimates the risk of csPCa in the 10–60% range. After performing a Hosmer-Lemeshow test for goodness-of-fit, no statistically significant changes were detected in calibration plots between PCPT and PBCG in any racial group: Blacks ($p = 0.15$), Whites ($p = 0.08$), and Others ($p = 0.07$).

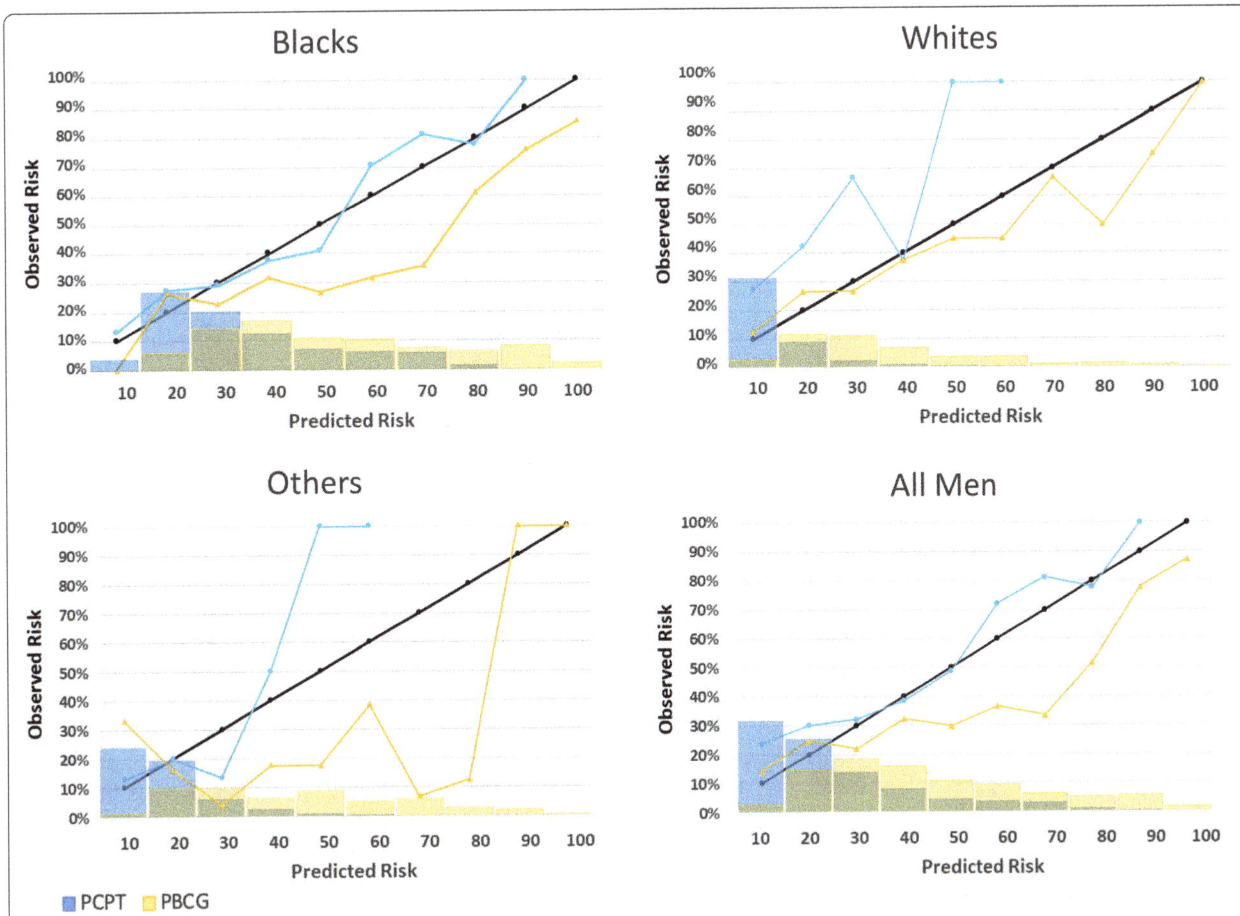

Fig. 1 Race-stratified calibration curves and the risk probability distribution histograms for clinically significant prostate cancer for PBCG and PCPT risk calculators. PCPT = Prostate Cancer Prevention Trial risk calculator; PBCG = Prostate Biopsy Collaborative Group risk calculator; Blue lines and histograms = PCPT; Yellow lines and histograms = PBCG; Black lines = 45-degree line representing perfect calibration

Number of avoided biopsies and missed clinically significant prostate cancer

Figure 2 presents the theoretical number of biopsies avoided and missed csPCa at the ≥10% and ≥ 30% risk thresholds.

At the ≥10% threshold, assuming no biopsies are performed below this threshold, the number of biopsies avoided with the PCPT RC for All men is 336/954 (35%) compared to 28/954 (3%) with PBCG. The PCPT RC, however, missed 80 (24%) csPCas compared to 4 (14%) csPCas when using PBCG. Few Black men fall below the 10% risk threshold, so the number of avoided biopsies is small with both calculators. The difference is particularly prominent in Whites where the percentage of biopsies avoided is ten-fold higher with PCPT relative to PBCG (71% vs 7%).

At the ≥30% threshold in All men, 748 (78%) biopsies are avoided using PCPT compared to 376 (39%) with PBCG, and the number of missed csPCa is 207 (28%) and 85 (23%), respectively. Black and Other men demonstrate a similar trend, where more than twice as many biopsies are avoided using PCPT with similar rates of missed csPCa (27% vs. 24% in Blacks; and 16% vs. 11% in Others).

Unnecessary biopsies in low risk men

The proportion of low risk men (i.e. men with PSA < 10 ng/mL and either Gleason 6 tumors or no cancer) who underwent unnecessary biopsies was assessed by racial group. At a threshold of ≥10%, assuming that men with higher scores are biopsied, 250/487 (51%) low risk men would have undergone a biopsy with PCPT and 466 (96%) with PBCG. Almost all low risk Black men are biopsied with both PCPT (92%) and PBCG (99.5%). For Whites and Others, the proportion of low risk men biopsied with PCPT is much lower relative to PBCG (see Additional file 1).

At the ≥30% threshold, PCPT would spare most low risk men a biopsy and only subject 5% to a prostate biopsy, while 42% are still biopsied with PBCG. In Blacks, the number of low risk men biopsied substantially decreases to 25 (12%) with PCPT, but continues to remain high with PBCG at 121 (59%). There were no White and Other men biopsied with PCPT, while 27 and 38% were biopsied using PBCG, respectively. The increase in risk scores seen in PBCG does not spare low risk men, resulting in many unnecessary biopsies performed in men with indolent or no PCa.

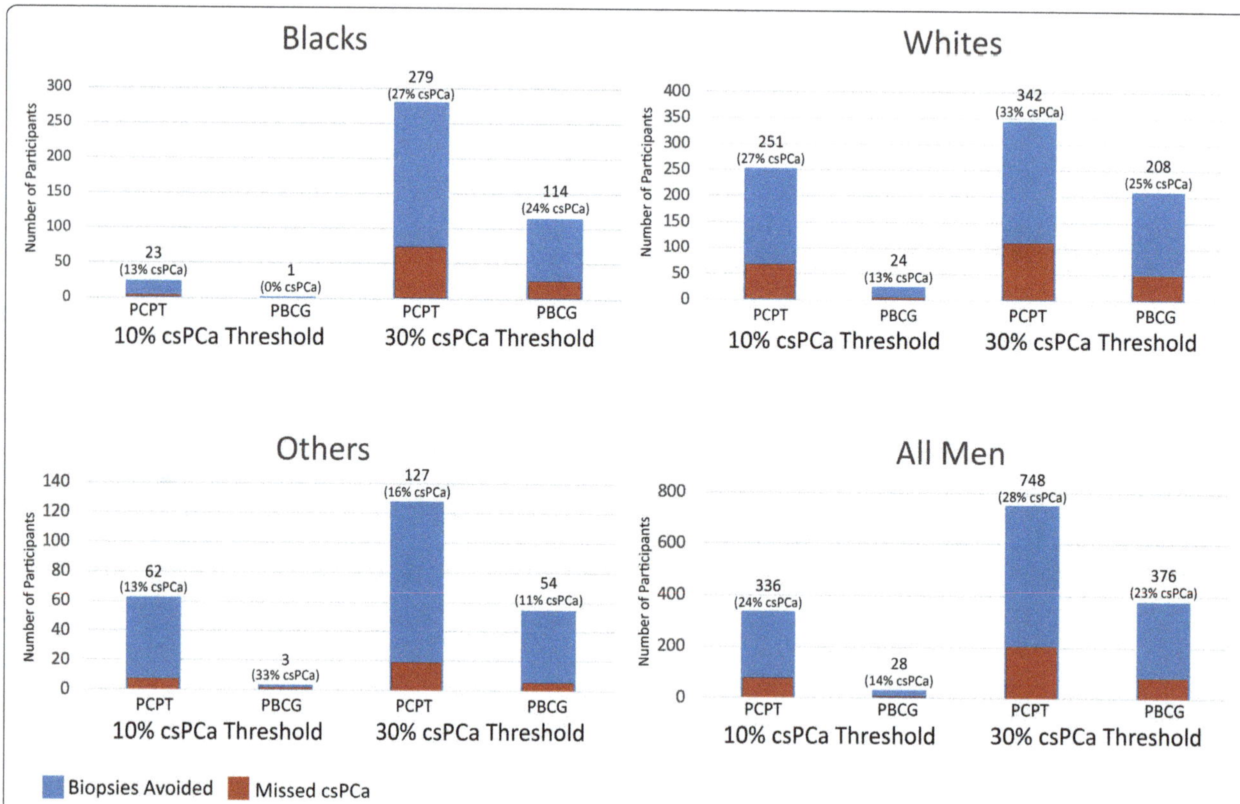

Fig. 2 Theoretical number of avoided biopsies and missed clinically significant cancers at the 10 and 30% predictive thresholds by race. PCPT = Prostate Cancer Prevention Trial risk calculator; PBCG = Prostate Biopsy Collaborative Group risk calculator; csPCa = clinically significant prostate cancer. Blue bar: Total number of biopsies avoided; Red bar: Missed clinically significant prostate cancer

Decision curve analysis: net benefit

The net benefit of each risk model is displayed graphically in Fig. 3. When calculating the net benefit analysis for All men, we note that the net benefit for PBCG is higher than PCPT at low threshold probabilities; however, neither RC shows higher net benefit than the Biopsy All men strategy at thresholds below 25%. At the higher risk thresholds (> 30%), PCPT surpasses the net benefit of PBCG.

These results differ vastly by race. Black men show similar trends as the ones described above with PBCG having higher net benefits than PCPT at lower thresholds, but not at thresholds above 30%. White men show a more pronounced improvement with PBCG across all thresholds. In Other men, the opposite is seen with PCPT showing higher net benefit than PBCG throughout all thresholds. Overall, PBCG demonstrates improved net benefits below the 30% threshold in Whites and, to lesser extent, in Blacks, but not in Others.

Discussion

Discrimination between PBCG and PCPT was not statistically different for overall or csPCa ($p = 0.27$). Although Ankerst et al. did show a statistically significant 3% improvement in PBCG over PCPT on both the internal and external validation [9], our study was not powered to detect this difference. The PCPT RC has been mostly validated in populations of European descent, which might not be representative of the demographics in the United States. The PCPT 2.0 risk calculator development cohort included 219 (3.3%) Blacks, but did not report the AUCs for csPCa by race. This study includes a multi-racial cohort of men recruited from five institutions in a large metropolitan city. Few studies have evaluated the performance of the PCPT RC in diverse populations. The Durham VA (North Carolina) cohort enrolled high numbers of Black men (45%) and demonstrated an AUC of 0.74 [19]. The Cleveland Clinic cohort was composed of 13% Black men and had an AUC of 0.64 [19]. Lastly, the SABOR Cohort from San Antonio, Texas compared PCPT across racial groups and showed that PCPT performs best in Black men compared to other races (AUC 0.80 vs. 0.66, $p = 0.02$) [20]. The AUC for Blacks in our study (0.67) was notably lower than SABOR's and Durham's, and similar to the Cleveland Clinic's cohort.

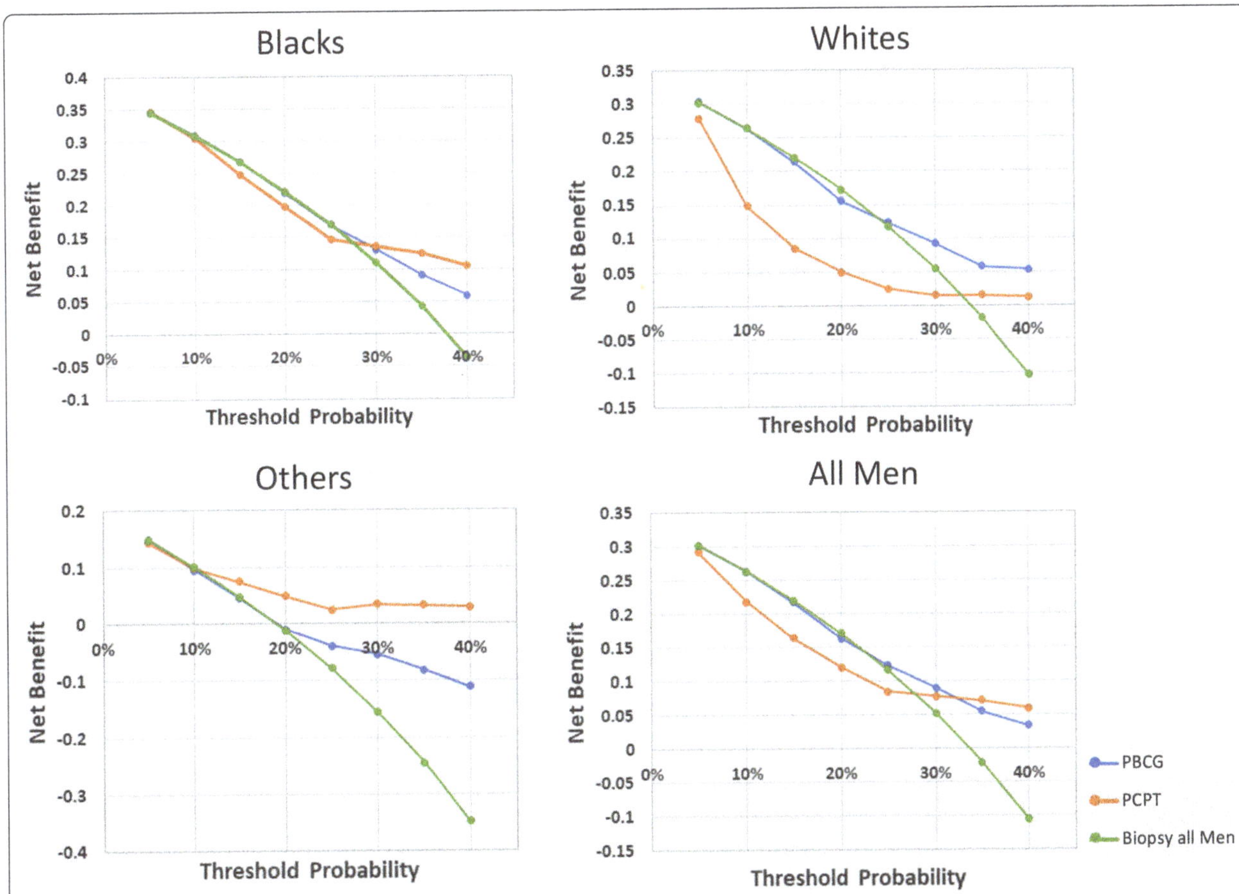

Fig. 3 Net Benefit curves for clinically significant prostate cancer prediction comparing PBCG to PCPT and the Biopsy all Men strategy by race. PCPT = Prostate Cancer Prevention Trial risk calculator; PBCG = Prostate Biopsy Collaborative Group risk calculator. Green line = Biopsy All men (assuming an exchange rate = 1/9); Orange line = Biopsy based on the probability risk thresholds of the PCPT risk calculator; Blue line = Biopsy based on the probability risk thresholds of the PBCG risk calculator

Like SABOR's, the AUC for Blacks in our cohort was slightly higher than Whites' (0.64), although this was not statistically significant.

In terms of the calibration curves, PBCG's calibrations in White men appear to be superior to PCPT. Blacks and Others show a different trend, where PCPT appears better calibrated since PBCG overestimates the rates of csPCa. Ankerst et al.'s validations also show a widened distribution for PBCG across all thresholds [9]. Their results are similar to the calibration plots we obtained for csPCa in our White population, but not in our minority groups. Since their internal and external validations had a non-Black population of 87% and 99.7%, their results come from a more racially homogeneous sample [9], which might explain these discrepancies. To our knowledge, no other studies have validated PBCG in a racially diverse cohort.

The cutoff most urologists use to decide if a patient should undergo a biopsy lies somewhere between the 5–30% threshold [18]. Therefore, this range is where nomograms serve the greatest clinical utility. At the 30% threshold, PCPT results in more than twice the amount of avoided biopsies with similar rates of missed csPCa in Blacks and Others (see Fig. 2). In addition, despite similar frequencies of indolent PCa and negative biopsy in Blacks and Whites (62.2% vs. 66.2%, $p = 0.24$), PBCG disproportionally biases more low risk Black men towards unnecessary biopsies (59% low risk men missed) relative to White men (27% missed).

The net benefits and clinical utility of different strategies vary widely by race, as seen in Fig. 3. In our data, White men and Black men seem to have higher net benefit with PBCG at relevant thresholds between 0 and 25%. For Others, PCPT has higher net benefit across all thresholds, which might be due their lower prevalence of csPCa compared to Blacks and Whites. Below the 30% threshold, the PBCG RC shows no greater benefit than the "Biopsy All strategy" in Black and White men, indicating that the conservative cutoff of 10% might not have any clinical benefit to avoid unnecessary biopsies.

Our comparison of PBCG vs. PCPT concurs with the study published by Ankerst et al. in that PBCG has higher discrimination [9], though not statistically significant in our smaller sample. However, we find that the performance of both calculators varies widely by race. Unfortunately, Ankerst et al. did not include an analysis on how the calibration or net benefit plots differ by racial groups. Although the PBCG RC was developed in a cohort with 13% Blacks, the validation study only included 33 (0.3%) Blacks in the cohort. Our results coincide with Ankerst et al. in that PBCG results in significant improvements compared to PCPT in Whites; yet, we find that the PBCG RC results in overprediction of PCa and a significant increase in the number of unnecessary biopsies in racial minorities. Given that PCPT was of higher accuracy in Blacks in prior validations, it may be prudent to continue to use it in biopsy decision making for Blacks. This should be compared in future studies using other diverse cohorts.

With the increasing popularity of multiparametric magnetic resonance imaging (mpMRI) as a PCa detection method, many are doubting the current need for risk calculators or are incorporating mpMRI PIRADS scores into them [21]. There is substantial evidence supporting the advantage of mpMRI, as it has been shown to avoid biopsies in around 28% of men and subsequently decrease the overdiagnoses of indolent PCa [15]. However, the adoption of mpMRI would add approximately $3 billion annually, meaning that this diagnostic test would account for 15% of all PCa related cost [22]. The use of mpMRI has become common practice in large academic institutions; however, 70% of community hospitals have not adopted such practice and 75% of hospitals perform few mpMRI (< 20 mpMRI/month) [22]. Currently, a patient's geographic location (non-urban settings) and insurance type (health maintenance organizations) greatly reduce their chances of having access to a mpMRI [22, 23]. The accuracy of mpMRI in community settings is also risky with only 55% concordance between community and expert academic radiologists [24]. While mpMRIs show promising results, the need for predictive nomograms is still warranted in areas of the country that face barriers in the implementation of mpMRIs.

This study has several limitations that should be noted. The recruitment was done in tertiary and publicly funded medical centers in a large metropolitan city. Our population was recruited from the outpatient Urology clinics between 2009 and 2014 and Gleason grading has shifted several Gleason 6's to Gleason 7 tumors limiting generalizability to our contemporary patients [25]. Our Gleason 6 tumors were consistent with NCCN very low or low risk group in 77% of cases. There were low numbers of non-Black minorities enrolled, which limits power and prevents subgroup analyses of Hispanics, Asians and other ethnic groups. The PCPT RC can accommodate biomarkers that we did not account for like PCA3, free PSA, and TMPRSS2–ERG [26].

Conclusions

Since PBCG's improvements in Blacks are disputable and potentially biases a greater number of low risk Black and Other men towards unnecessary biopsies, PCPT may lead to better biopsy decisions in racial minority groups. Further validation studies in racially diverse cohorts are warranted to mitigate the harms of PSA screening in ethnic minorities.

Supplementary information

Additional file 1. Percentage of low risk men who underwent an unnecessary prostate biopsy at the 10 and 30% risk thresholds stratified by race. Low risk Men includes men with PSA < 10 ng/mL and either a negative biopsy ($n = 238$) or Gleason 3 + 3 prostate cancer and less than clinical T3a ($n = 249$); PCPT = Prostate Cancer Prevention Trial Risk Calculator; PBCG = Prostate Biopsy Collaborative Group Risk Calculator.

Abbreviations

5-ARI: 5 alpha-reductase inhibitor; AUC: Area Under the Receiver Operating Characteristics Curve; BMI: Body Mass Index; BPH: Benign Prostatic Hyperplasia; csPCa: Clinically Significant Prostate Cancer; DCA: Decision Curve Analysis; DRE: Digital Rectal Exam; PBCG: Prostate Biopsy Collaborative Group; PCa: Prostate Cancer; PCPT: Prostate Cancer Prevention Trial 2.0; PSA: Prostate Specific Antigen; RC: Risk Calculators

Acknowledgements

We would like to thank the participating urologists, study participants, and the staff at each clinic for contributing to the research.

Authors' contributions

SC, OSN, ABM were major contributors in writing the manuscript. SC, OSN, IBH, BJ analyzed and interpreted the data. PG1 aided in the acquisition of data and data analysis plan. MR aided in data acquisition and data quality control. CMPH, RAK aided in editing the manuscript and data acquisition. RS aided in data acquisition and patient recruitment. ES made contributions in the design of the study, acquiring study funding, and drafting the data analysis plan. PG2 substantially developed the data analysis plan and revised the manuscript. All authors read and approved the final version of the submitted manuscript.

Author details

[1]Department of Urology, Northwestern University Feinberg School of Medicine, 303 E Chicago Avenue, Tarry 16, Chicago, IL 60611, USA. [2]Department of Preventive Medicine, Northwestern University Feinberg School of Medicine, Chicago, IL, USA. [3]Department of Medicine, University of Illinois at Chicago, Chicago, IL, USA. [4]Division of Urology, Cook County Health and Hospitals System, 303 E Chicago Avenue, Tarry 16, Chicago, IL 60611, USA. [5]Section of Urology, Jesse Brown VA Medical Center, 303 E Chicago Avenue, Tarry 16, Chicago, IL 60611, USA. [6]Department of Urology, University of Illinois at Chicago School of Medicine, Chicago, IL, USA. [7]Division of Health Equities, Department of Population Sciences, City of Hope Cancer Center, Duarte, CA, USA. [8]Department of Pathology, University of Illinois at Chicago School of Medicine, Chicago, IL, USA.

References

1. Key Statistics for Prostate Cancer Date. Available from: https://www.cancer.org/cancer/prostate-cancer/about/key-statistics.html2019. Accessed 3 Jan 2019.
2. Bokhorst LP, Bangma CH, van Leenders GJ, Lous JJ, Moss SM, Schröder FH, et al. Prostate-specific antigen–based prostate Cancer screening: reduction of prostate cancer mortality after correction for nonattendance and contamination in the Rotterdam section of the European randomized study of screening for prostate Cancer. Eur Urol. 2014;65(2):329–36.
3. Loeb S, Carter HB, Berndt SI, Ricker W, Schaeffer EM. Complications after prostate biopsy: data from SEER-Medicare. J Urol. 2011;186(5):1830–4.
4. Siddiqui MM, Rais-Bahrami S, Turkbey B, George AK, Rothwax J, Shakir N, et al. Comparison of MR/ultrasound fusion–guided biopsy with ultrasound-guided biopsy for the diagnosis of prostate cancer. JAMA. 2015;313(4):390 7.
5. Liss MA, Ehdaie B, Loeb S, Meng MV, Raman JD, Spears V, et al. An update of the American urological association white paper on the prevention and treatment of the more common complications related to prostate biopsy. J Urol. 2017;198(2):329 34.
6. Zeng C, Wen W, Morgans AK, Pao W, Shu X-O, Zheng W. Disparities by race, age, and sex in the improvement of survival for major cancers: results from the National Cancer Institute surveillance, epidemiology, and end results (SEER) program in the United States, 1990 to 2010. JAMA Oncol. 2015;1(1):88–96.
7. Moyer VA. Screening for prostate cancer: US preventive services task force recommendation statement. Ann Intern Med. 2012;157(2):120–34.
8. Shao Y-H, Demissie K, Shih W, Mehta AR, Stein MN, Roberts CB, et al. Contemporary risk profile of prostate cancer in the United States. J Natl Cancer Inst. 2009;101(18):1280–3.
9. Ankerst DP, Straubinger J, Selig K, Guerrios L, De Hoedt A, Hernandez J, et al. A contemporary prostate biopsy risk calculator based on multiple heterogeneous cohorts. Eur Urol. 2018;74(2):197–203.
10. Ankerst DP, Hoefler J, Bock S, Goodman PJ, Vickers A, Hernandez J, et al. Prostate Cancer prevention trial risk calculator 2.0 for the prediction of low- vs high-grade prostate cancer. Urology. 2014;83(6):1362–8.
11. Murphy AB, Kelley B, Nyame YA, Martin IK, Smith DJ, Castaneda L, et al. Predictors of serum vitamin D levels in African American and European American men in Chicago. Am J Mens Health. 2012;6(5):420–6.
12. Mohler JL, Antonarakis ES, Armstrong AJ, D'Amico AV, Davis BJ, Dorff T, et al. Prostate Cancer, version 2.2019, NCCN clinical practice guidelines in oncology. J Natl Compr Cancer Netw. 2019;17(5):479–505.
13. Vickers AJ, Elkin EB. Decision curve analysis: a novel method for evaluating prediction models. J Med Decis Making. 2006;26(6):565–74.
14. Chiu PK, Alberts AR, Venderbos LD, Bangma CH, Roobol MJ. Additional benefit of using a risk-based selection for prostate biopsy: an analysis of biopsy complications in the Rotterdam section of the European randomized study of screening for prostate Cancer. BJU Int. 2017;120(3):394–400.
15. Mehralivand S, Shih JH, Rais-Bahrami S, Oto A, Bednarova S, Nix JW, et al. A magnetic resonance imaging–based prediction model for prostate biopsy risk stratification. JAMA Oncol. 2018;4(5):678–85.
16. Vickers AJ, Van Calster B, Steyerberg EW. Net benefit approaches to the evaluation of prediction models, molecular markers, and diagnostic tests. BMJ. 2016;352:i6.
17. Roobol MJ, Verbeek JF, van der Kwast T, Kümmerlin IP, Kweldam CF, van Leenders GJ. Improving the Rotterdam European randomized study of screening for prostate Cancer risk calculator for initial prostate biopsy by incorporating the 2014 International Society of Urological Pathology Gleason Grading and Cribriform growth. J Eur Oncol. 2017;72(1):45–51.
18. Vickers AJ. Decision analysis for the evaluation of diagnostic tests, prediction models and molecular markers. Am Stat. 2008;62(4):314–20.
19. Ankerst DP, Boeck A, Freedland SJ, Thompson IM, Cronin AM, Roobol MJ, et al. Evaluating the PCPT risk calculator in ten international biopsy cohorts: results from the prostate biopsy collaborative group. World J Urol. 2012; 30(2):181–7.
20. Parekh DJ, Ankerst DP, Higgins BA, Hernandez J, Canby-Hagino E, Brand T, et al. External validation of the prostate Cancer prevention trial risk calculator in a screened population. Urology. 2006;68(6):1152–5.
21. Alberts AR, Roobol MJ, Verbeek JF, Schoots IG, Chiu PK, Osses DF, et al. Prediction of high-grade prostate cancer following multiparametric magnetic resonance imaging: improving the Rotterdam european randomized study of screening for prostate cancer risk calculators. Eur Urol. 2019;75(2):310–8.
22. Kim SJ, Vickers AJ, Hu JC. Challenges in adopting level 1 evidence for multiparametric magnetic resonance imaging as a biomarker for prostate cancer screening. JAMA Oncol. 2018;4(12):1663–4.
23. Liu W, Patil D, Howard DH, Moore RH, Wang H, Sanda MG, et al. Adoption of prebiopsy magnetic resonance imaging for men undergoing prostate biopsy in the United States. Urology. 2018;117:57–63.
24. Hansen NL, Koo BC, Gallagher FA, Warren AY, Doble A, Gnanapragasam V, et al. Comparison of initial and tertiary Centre second opinion reads of multiparametric magnetic resonance imaging of the prostate prior to repeat biopsy. Eur Radiol. 2017;27(6):2259–66.
25. Epstein JI, Egevad L, Amin MB, Delahunt B, Srigley JR, Humphrey PA. The 2014 International Society of Urological Pathology (ISUP) consensus conference on Gleason grading of prostatic carcinoma. Am J Surg Pathol. 2016;40(2):244–52.
26. Prostate Cancer Prevention Trial Risk Calculator Version 2.0. Available from: http://riskcalc.org/PCPTRC/.

Impact of bilateral biopsy-detected prostate cancer on an active surveillance population

Jonathan H. Wang[1†], Pablo Sierra[1,2†], Kyle A. Richards[1,3], E. Jason Abel[1,3], Glen O. Allen[1], Tracy M. Downs[1,3] and David F. Jarrard[1,3,4*]

Abstract

Background: To assess factors that can predict active surveillance (AS) failure on serial transrectal ultrasound guided biopsies in patients with low-risk prostate cancer.

Methods: We evaluated the records of 144 consecutive patients enrolled in AS between 2007 and 2014 at a single academic institution. Low risk inclusion criteria included PSA < 10 ng/ml, cT1c or cT2a, Grade Group (GG) 1, < 3 positive cores, and < 50% tumor in a single core with the majority having a PSA density of < 0.15. AS reclassification was defined as progression to GG ≥2, 3 or more cores, or core tumor volume ≥ 50%. Univariate and multivariate Cox proportional hazards regression analysis was used to determine predictors of reclassification and a match-pair analysis performed on a control group of patients choosing surgery.

Results: Inclusion criteria were met by 130 men with a median follow-up of 52 months. The reclassification or AS failure rate was 38.5%, with the majority 41/50 (82%) finding GG ≥ 2 cancer. Most patients had unilateral disease on diagnostic biopsy (94.6%), but 40.7% had bilateral cancer detected during follow-up. Men with bilateral detected tumor were more likely to ultimately fail AS than patients with unilateral tumors (HR 4.089; $P < 0.0001$) and failed earlier with a reclassification-free survival of 32 vs 119 months respectively. In a matched-pair analysis using a population of 211 concurrent patients that chose radical prostatectomy rather than AS, 76% of patients with unilateral cancer on biopsy had bilateral cancer on final pathology.

Conclusions: The finding of bilateral prostate cancer on biopsy is associated with earlier AS reclassification. Finding bilateral disease may not represent disease progression, but rather enhanced detection of more extensive disease highlighting the importance of confirmatory biopsy.

Keywords: Active surveillance, Prostate biopsy, Bilateral disease, Grade group

Background

Currently 15% men are diagnosed with prostate cancer (PC) during their lifetime but the risk of death due to the disease is only 3% [1]. The average expected years of life lost due to PC is 1.8 years, compared to other common malignancies such as breast cancer, at 16.7 years [2]. To further emphasize this long natural history, up to 45% of patients are diagnosed with low risk PC [3].

The rationale for active surveillance (AS) is that many patients have indolent tumors and would not benefit from immediate definitive treatment. However, there is always concern from both the patient and urologist that undiagnosed, aggressive disease exists. Indeed 30–50% of patients that meet AS criteria with Gleason Score 6 cancers are upgraded at radical prostatectomy with Gleason Score pattern 4 or higher being found [4–8]. Subsequently, larger cohorts have shown that 10–38% of patients are reclassified on follow-up during AS due to Gleason Score upgrading or increased tumor volume (no. cores, maximal core involvement (MCI)) [9–14]. It is imperative to improve the ability to identify those patients at higher risk for failing AS, either due to disease progression or reclassification, in order to provide better counseling regarding treatment options and to adjust surveillance schedules. In addition, it is not clear

* Correspondence: jarrard@urology.wisc.edu
†Jonathan H. Wang and Pablo Sierra contributed equally to this work.
[1]Department of Urology, University of Wisconsin School of Medicine and Public Health, Madison, WI, USA
[3]University of Wisconsin Carbone Cancer Center, Madison, WI, USA
Full list of author information is available at the end of the article

whether or not patients that fail AS do so as a result of finding previously undetected disease or disease progression.

The objective of the study was to analyze clinical and pathologic variables available at diagnosis to determine factors that could predict reclassification and AS failure. Our hypothesis is that having a biopsy showing bilateral tumor would indicate multifocal PC, which may be associated with higher volume and higher stage disease compared to those with unilateral tumors on initial biopsy.

Methods

Cohort definition

A retrospective review of a previously described protocol driven cohort [15] of patients in the AS program at our institution was performed from 2007 to 2014. This was prior to the wider use of MRI for additional evaluation. Criteria utilized for AS were based on the National Comprehensive Cancer Network definition for very low risk disease including PSA < 10 ng/ml, Grade Group 1 (Gleason grade 6), ≤2 biopsy cores with cancer, and maximal core involvement (MCI) with cancer < 50%. PSA density was < 0.15 in 86% of patients, but density was not part of our exclusion criteria. Patients were followed with serial biopsies annually and delayed intervention using pre-identified clinical and pathologic cut-offs as trigger points to indicate disease progression. This study was approved by our Institutional Review Board.

Of 144 low risk patients in the AS program, 14 patients were excluded from analysis: 9 without a confirmatory biopsy, and 5 patients were T1a or T1b diagnosed after a transurethral resection of the prostate. In all patients a confirmatory biopsy was performed within 3–12 months after initial transrectal ultrasound guided (TRUS) biopsy was performed. Twelve to 16 core biopsies were obtained at each procedure. PSA was tested every 3–6 months per protocol and a follow-up biopsy was done within 1 year of diagnosis and then every 1–2 years. Patients who did not fail AS due to biopsy criteria, continued until they were reassigned to a watchful waiting (WW) non-intervention protocol due to advanced age or other significant comorbidities.

Patients were reclassified (e.g. failed AS criteria) and offered definitive therapy (radical prostatectomy or radiotherapy) if they met the following criteria on repeat biopsy: Grade Group upgrade, ≥3 cores positive for cancer, > 50% cancer core involvement or clinical progression defined as a palpable nodule greater than previously found or a change in the TNM classification.

We then performed a separate secondary analysis of 211 patients that met the same AS criteria over a similar time period (2007–2014) who declined AS and elected upfront radical prostatectomy. All pathology was read by a fellowship-trained urologic pathologist.

Statistical methods

Kaplan-Meier method was used to estimate time to reclassification (AS failure). Univariate and multivariate Cox proportional hazards regression analysis was performed to evaluate predictors of reclassification and AS failure. All analyses were performed using software SAS 9.4 (SAS institute Inc., Cary, NC, US). Matched pair analysis was performed for the radical prostatectomy and AS populations controlling for age, PSA < BMI, Prostate Volume, and PSA Density. Statisical support was provided by Dr. Glen Leverson, PhD.

Results

Characteristics of patient population

The clinical features of the 130 sequential patients with low risk PC on AS after exclusions are presented in Table 1. Characteristics include a mean age at diagnosis of 61 y (range 40–75) and a follow-up from initial cancer diagnosis of 52.4 m (range 3–196) with 66% observed for more than 3 years. Among the cohort, two patients died from unrelated causes and no patients developed metastatic disease.

Table 1 Clinicopathologic features of patients on active surveillance at diagnosis

Variables	n (%)	Median (IQR)
Follow-up (m)	130	42.5 (24–74)
Age (years)	130	61 (57–66)
< 50 y	5 (4)	48
50–60 y	56 (43)	57
> 60 y	69 (53)	66
PSA (ng/ml)	130	5.08 (4.2–7)
< 4 ng/ml	26 (20)	3.21
≥ 4 ng/ml	104 (80)	5.9
PSA density	130	0.13 (0.09–0.16)
≤ 0.15	112 (86)	0.12
BMI (kg/m^2)	130	27.5 (25.6–31.7)
≤ 30	89 (68.5)	26.2
> 30	41 (31.5)	32.8
Prostate Volume (cc)	130	42 (32–57)
< 30	23 (17.7)	24
30–60	82 (63.1)	42
> 60	25 (19.2)	73
Follow-up biopsies	130	2.5 (2–4)
2	65 (50)	2
3	29 (22.3)	3
> 4	36 (27.7)	4.5
Max Core Involvement %[a]	130	5 (3–10)

[a]Maximal Percentage of the most involved core
Prostate Specific Antigen (PSA), Body Max Index (BMI)

The majority of the cohort is staged as cT1c (126 pts., 97%), with 4 (3%) diagnosed due to an abnormal DRE (cT2a). Baseline PSA was < 4 ng/ml in 20% and median PSA was 5.08 ng/ml (0.52–9.8). Fifty-percent of the patients had 2 follow-up biopsies, 22% had 3, and 36 patients (28%) had 4 or more biopsies. At the time of analysis, 77/130 patients (59%) remained on AS with 53 patients (41%) undergoing treatment. Of this group, 16 patients chose to electively stop AS and pursue definitive treatment, rather than having treatment due to reclassification on surveillance biopsies.

Reclassification/AS failure

Reclassification on follow-up biopsies occurred in 50/130 patients (38.5%) the majority consisting of grade progression (82%). Failure occurred solely due to the identification of cancer in > 2 cores in 9 patients, GG ≥ 2 in 12 patients and in 29 due to both. No patients were reclassified based solely on the finding of > 50% core involvement. Of our 50 AS failures, 74% (37) proceeded to treatment, and the remaining 26% [13] of reclassified patients did not receive treatment and remained on AS because of personal preference (8 patients) or switched to WW do to new comorbidities or advancing age (5 patients). Of the reclassified patients, 40% (20/50) occurred in the first 12 months, 22% during the second year and 10, 8, and 6% during years 3, 4, 5 respectively. Of note, 12% (7 pts) failed surveillance beyond 5 years.

Reclassification according to lateralization at biopsy

At initial biopsy, 123 patients (94.6%) had unilateral tumor burden; the distribution for left versus right-sided disease was similar (59 and 64, respectively) and seven patients had bilateral tumor on initial biopsy (5.4%). On subsequent biopsies, 46 of the patients initially diagnosed with unilateral disease were found to have bilateral cancer. In total during AS follow-up, 77/130 patients (59.2%) continued to have tumor solely in the same lobe of the prostate on follow-up biopsies (unilateral tumor), but 53/130 (40.7%) had bilateral tumor discovered. Of these, 53 patients that initially had or developed bilateral disease, 35(66%) experienced reclassification during subsequent biopsies compared to 19.4% (15/77) those with only unilateral disease (Fig. 1). Of note, the 7 patients who initially presented with bilateral disease, 5 were reclassified during the course of our study (71%). In comparison, 29 of 46 men (63%) who initially had unilateral disease but then developed bilateral disease, while still meeting active surveillance criteria, eventually failed active surveillance.

On Cox proportional hazards regression analysis, patients with bilateral disease were more likely to reclassify and fail AS than patients with unilateral disease (HR 4.09; 95% CI (2.22–7.53); $P < 0.0001$) (Table 2). Patients with the finding of bilateral disease when subsequently followed over time (Kaplan Meier analysis, Fig. 2) were reclassified earlier than those with unilateral disease (32 months compared to 119 months respectively). The reclassification-free survival probability at 1 year, 2 years and 5 years was 0.71, 0.55 and 0.34 for patients with bilateral disease compared to 0.93, 0.88 and 0.78 for patients with unilateral tumor. The presence of bilateral cancer was the strongest predictor of reclassification leading to AS failure compared to all other clinicopathologic features examined.

Very low-risk patients choosing radical prostatectomy with an initial unilateral positive biopsy commonly have bilateral tumor on final specimen

We then performed an additional analysis on a separate cohort of 211 patients that met low risk, AS criteria over a similar time (2007–2014), but elected radical prostatectomy as primary treatment (Table 3). At time of diagnostic biopsy, 186 of these patients had a unilateral tumor while 25 had a bilateral tumor (88.2 and 11.8% respectively). Of the patients who had unilateral disease on diagnostic biopsy, 73.1% (136/186), were found to have pT2c (bilateral disease on final pathology) while 24.7% of the patients were found to have true unilateral disease, pT2a/b. The majority of patients who had bilateral disease on biopsy, were also found to have bilateral tumor on final pathology (88%). After surgery, 90 patients (42.6%) were upgraded on the final pathologic specimen, most being upgraded to 3 + 4 (80/90). Patients that had a bilateral tumor on biopsy did not have higher rates of positive margins at radical prostatectomy compared to patients with unilateral tumor ($p = 0.37$).

To control for an age bias, a matched-pair analysis was performed between low risk patients who underwent surgery and the AS cohort based on age, PSA, BMI, PSA density, and prostate volume (Table 4). Comparing the 111 matched pairs, the majority of patients (75.8%) with unilateral disease at biopsy, would have had at diagnosis pT2c disease on final pathology (Tables 5 and 6).

Discussion

The selection of patients for AS according to current recommendations is guided by clinical and pathologic features that indicate the patient has a small, organ confined, well-differentiated tumor [9–14]. Patients are labeled as having failed AS if they are found to have a pathological indication to suggest that the tumor is progressing (reclassification), including increasing tumor volume (increasing number of cores with cancer or increasing volume of cancer within a biopsy core) or Gleason score upgrading [9–11, 13, 16]. Regular repeated biopsies play a pivotal role in redefining risk and

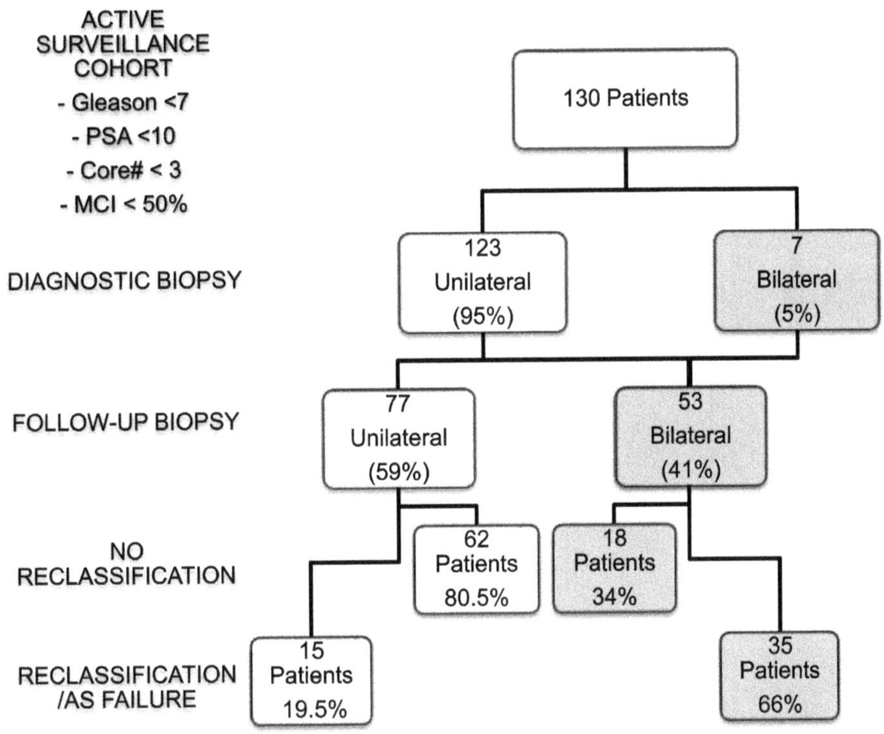

Fig. 1 Reclassification to bilateral-biopsy detected cancer on patient follow-up. The flow chart demonstrates 41% of patients had bilateral cancer on repeated biopsies of which 66% had reclassification of their disease versus 19.5% of patients with unilateral cancer

reclassifying patients. Negative biopsies during surveillance follow-up occurs in 21–52% of patients and previous studies have shown these patients with no cancer on follow-up biopsies have a 53% reduction in risk of disease progression [17, 18]. There are ongoing efforts to both improve the diagnostic yield of prostate biopsies and identify factors that may predict patients who are at higher risk for failing AS in order to provide better counseling regarding treatment options and avoid unnecessary interventions.

In our AS cohort, we found that patients with bilateral tumor on initial or surveillance biopsies were reclassified during AS follow-up over time earlier and more frequently compared to those with unilateral disease (66% vs 19.5% respectively). This risk increases over time (Fig. 2). The finding of bilateral disease has a higher rate of active surveillance failure than other clinical features including PSA density. PSA density was low (< 0.15) for the majority of the population making it a less powerful indicator of failure in this population. This finding is supported by a study in which the presence of bilateral prostate cancer on biopsy was exchanged with > 50% MCI as a reason for excluding AS excusion criteria, demonstrating good performace in predicting clinically significant prostate cancer [19]. These findings suggest that the presence of bilateral disease is a clinically significant and inexpensive way to risk stratify patients enrolled in AS

Table 2 Regression analysis of clinical and pathologic features predicting active surveillance failure

Variables	Univariable COX regression			Multivariable COX regression		
	HR	95% CI	*p*-Value	HR	95% CI	*p*-Value
Bilateral tumor on Bx	4.09	2.22–7.53	< 0.0001*	3.8	2.05–7.06	< 0.0001*
MCI	1.01	0.98–1.05	0.418			
PSA	1.02	0.90–1.16	0.747			
PSA density	1.32	0.88–1.98	0.186	1.34	0.85–2.11	0.21
BMI	1	0.94–1.07	0.995			
Prostate Volume	0.99	0.97–1.00	0.131			
Previous (–) Biopsy	0.91	0.48–1.75	0.78			

Prostate Specific Antigen (PSA), Body Max Index (BMI), Maximal Percentage of the most involved core (MCI), Prostate Biopsy (Bx)

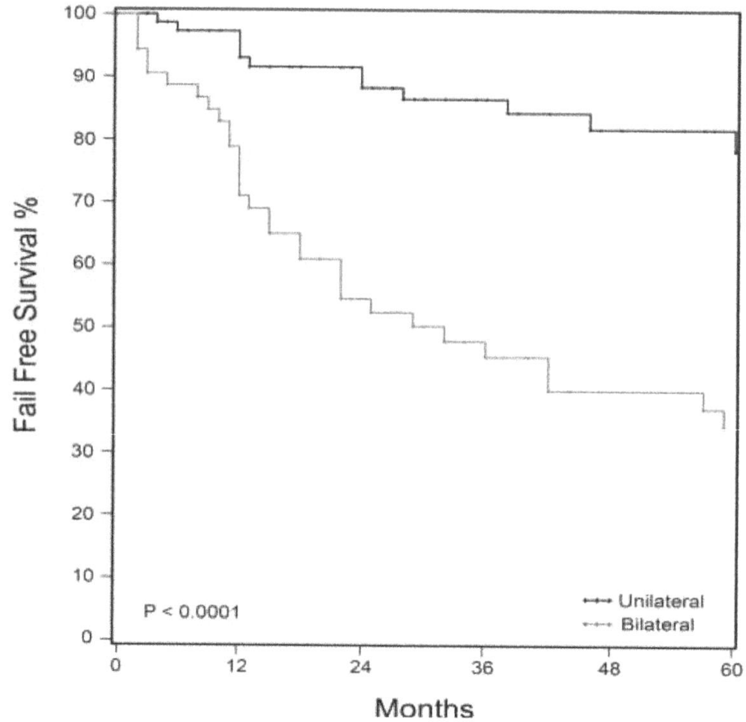

Time(mos.)		12	24	36	48	60
# unilateral		4	3	2	2	1
# bilateral		11	9	3	2	2

Time(mos.)		12	24	36	48	60
# At Risk Unilateral		72	69	68	66	63
# At Risk Bilateral		38	30	25	22	20

Fig. 2 Active surveillance reclassification-free survival analysis using Kaplan Meier analysis: comparison between patients with unilateral versus bilateral cancer on prostate biopsy. Number of patients at risk shown. Patients with bilateral disease were reclassified on subsequent biopsy earlier than those with unilateral disease

(Fig. 2). The presence of bilateral tumor can be used in counseling patients and as a trigger for further evaluation due to high failure rate in this group of patients.

In our analysis, bilateral disease on biopsy was the strongest parameter in predicting AS failure, outperforming other factors including the number of cores with cancer, MCI and PSA density. Other studies have assessed PSA kinetics to determine if this parameter can be used as a trigger for intervention. For example, in the PRIAS [9] study, the largest ongoing prospective study, PSA doubling time < 3y was a trigger for intervention. However, Klotz et al. [11] discontinued its use in 2009 and is not being used in other larger cohorts such as the John Hopkins AS group [11] or UCSF. There is also suggestive data that PSA density can be a strong predictor for reclassification over longer term time periods, however more studies are needed to confirm these findings [9, 20, 21]. In our data PSA density did not perform as well as the detection of bilateral cancer likely due to the fact that the majority (86%) of patients had a PSA density of < 0.15 and thus only a limited range was evaluated.

An important question is whether patients fail AS due to disease progression or due to detection at subsequent biopsy. Conceptually TRUS biopsy, although templated, is a procedure with a relatively low negative predictive value. In our separate analysis of a concurrent cohort of 211 patients eligible for AS but elected for upfront radical prostatectomy, 73% of these patients had bilateral, pT2c disease on final pathology. This was confirmed with our matched pair analysis. Studies have demonstrated that 71–80% of low risk patients have bilateral

Table 3 Clinical and pathologic features in patients with low risk prostate cancer, eligible for active surveillance, who elected treatment with radical prostatectomy (2007–2014)

Variable	Unilateral at biopsy (*n* = 186)	Bilateral at biopsy (*n* = 25)	*p* value
Clinical Presentation	median (IQR)	median (IQR)	–
Age (years)	58 (54–64)	58 (55–61)	0.78
PSA (ng/ml)	5 (4–6.6)	4.6 (4.2–5.9)	0.51
PSAD	0.12 (0.088–0.17)	0.14 (0.1–0.18)	0.48
BMI (kg/m^2)	29 (25.8–31.8)	28.3 (25–33)	0.86
US Vol (mL)	41.7 (32.6–53.2)	35 (25–42)	**0.03**
Max core inv.%	8 (5–20)	8 (5–10)	0.95
Grade Group	1	1	–
Stage			1
T1c	172 (92.5%)	24 (96%)	
T2a	14 (7.5%)	1 (4%)	
RP Pathology			–
Prostate weight (g)	45.4 (26–56.3)	42.5 (34.1–52.9)	0.28
Grade Group (Gleason)			0.37
GG1 (3 + 3)	106 (57%)	15 (60%)	
GG2 (3 + 4)	72 (39%)	8 (32%)	
GG3 (4 + 3)	6 (3%)	1 (4%)	
GG4 (4 + 4)	1 (0.5%)	1 (4%)	
GG5 (4 + 5)	1 (0.5%)	0	
Upgrading	80 (43%)	10 (40%)	–
% of tumor	4%	5%	0.11
Pathologic Stage			0.49
pT2a	44 (23.7%)	3 (12%)	
pT2b	2 (1.1%)	0	
pT2c	136 (73.1%)	22 (88%)	
pT3a	4 (2.1%)	0	
pT3b	0	0	

Prostate Specific Antigen (PSA), Prostate Specific Antigen Density (PSAD) Body Max Index (BMI), Radical Prostatectomy (RP)

Table 4 Comparison of baseline demographics at time of diagnosis between patients on active surveillance (AS) and patients who met active surveillance criteria but chose upfront radical prostatectomy (RP)

Variable	Active Surveillance	Radical Prostatectomy	
	Median (IQR)	Median (IQR)	*p*-value
Age (years)	61 (57–66)	58 (54–62)	< 0.01*
PSA (ng/ml)	5.08 (4.2–7)	5 (4–6.6)	0.39
BMI (kg/m^2)	27.52 (25.63–31.74)	28.98 (25.78–32)	0.27
Prostate vol (mL)	42 (32–57)	40 (31–53)	0.39
PSA density	0.13 (0.09–0.16)	0.12 (0.09–0.18)	0.58

*All patients Gleason 6 at diagnosis
Prostate Specific Antigen (PSA), Body Max Index (BMI)

Table 5 Matched pair analysis between patients with low risk prostate cancer undergoing active surveillance or prostatectomy, controlling for age, PSA < BMI, Prostate Volume, and PSA Density. *N* = 222, (111 pairs)

Variable	Active Surveillance	Radical Prostatectomy	
	Median (IQR)	Median (IQR)	*p*-value
Age (Years)	60 (57–65)	60 (57–64)	0.9
PSA (ng/L)	5 (4.1–7)	5.3 (4.3–6.7)	0.54
BMI (kg/m^2)	27.7 (25.7–32)	29 (26–31.2)	0.82
Prostate Volume (mL)	42 (32–57)	42 (34–56)	0.74
PSA density	0.12 (0.09–0.15)	0.12 (0.09–0.18)	0.26

tumor on final specimen when taken for upfront radical prostatectomy [22–24]. This suggests that the majority of the patients with PC have multifocal, bilateral tumors that are missed during TRUS biopsy even in a selected low risk population.

While it is important to fine tune the ability of urologists to use standard TRUS biopsy information to guide treatment counseling, MRI increasingly is being employed. In our active surveillance cohort, 42/130 (32%) patients had a prostate MRI either prior to diagnosis of prostate cancer, or as part of their follow-up. Recent improvements in MRI technology increase the yield of prostate biopsy, but not all practitioners worldwide have access to high quality imaging. To illustrate the limits of access to this technology, Japan has the most MRI units per million population (47) with the US second (38 upm). This is compared to countries like Germany (12 upm), France (11 upm), Canada (9 upm), UK (6 upm), and Mexico (2 upm) [25]. MRI has a lower sensitivity of 63% in detecting lower volume (< 0.5 ml) and intermediate grade (Gleason 7) PC, but does have up to 80% detection rate for higher grade Gleason > 8 PC [26]. There has been an increased use of MRI during AS to help determine eligibility and disease progression [27]. These technologies are not yet widely adopted due to cost and access especially in underserved populations. MRI guided, targeted prostate biopsies may improve our management of AS patients and could be important in driving changes in biopsy schedules or AS criteria with additional data. With limited MRI access, these data demonstrating greater risk with bilateral positive

Table 6 Biopsy results of matched pair cohort correlated with pathologic stage

Biopsy Laterality	Pathological Stage		
	pT2a	pT2c	pT3a
Bilateral n(%)	1 (6.7)	14 (93.3)	0
Unilateral n(%)	20 (21.1)	72 (75.8)	3 (3.2)

biopsies may help direct those patients who need further radiologic evaluation.

Our AS failure rate is 38.5% is slightly higher compared to other cohorts as reported by Klotz et al. [11], PRIAS [9], Tosoian et al. [10], Preston et al. [12], Dall'Era et al. [13], (22.6, 28, 30.6, 34.7, 38%). These variations in failure rates may result from different criteria or the population utilized for the study. Our study is limited in its retrospective nature and single institution, but it is strengthened by our assessment of a concurrent group of patients who met AS criteria and elected definitive treatment. A matched-pair analysis was performed in an effort to limit treatment bias in this population.

Conclusions

Finding bilateral PC on TRUS biopsy is an important predictor of reclassification or AS failure. Our data supports the use of identification of bilateral disease on prostate biopsy to guide patient counseling on AS, as these patients are more likely to require reevaluation with MRI or repeat biopsy at an earlier time. Given the high rate of bilateral PC seen in a concurrent low risk AS-eligible population with unilaterally positive biopsies, the development of bilateral disease represents improved detection rather than progression for many of these patients.

Abbreviations

AS: Active Surveillance; GG: Grade Group; MCI: Maximal core involvement; PC: Prostate Cancer; PSA: Prostate Specific Antigen

Acknowledgements

Thanks to Glen Leverson for statistical support.

Author details

[1]Department of Urology, University of Wisconsin School of Medicine and Public Health, Madison, WI, USA. [2]Universidad CES, Medellin, Colombia. [3]University of Wisconsin Carbone Cancer Center, Madison, WI, USA. [4]Wisconsin Institute for Medical Research, 1111 Highland Avenue, Madison, WI 53705-2281, USA.

References

1. Siegel RL, Miller KD, Jemal A. Cancer statistics, 2015. CA Cancer J Clin. 2015; 65(1):5–29.
2. Liu P-H, Wang J-D, Keating NL. Expected years of life lost for six potentially preventable cancers in the United States. Prev Med. 2013;56(5):309–13.
3. Bangma CH, Bul M, van del Kwast TH, et al. AS for low-risk prostate cancer. Crit Rev Oncol Hematol. 2013;85(3):295–302.
4. Chun FK, Steuber T, Erbersdobler A, et al. Development and internal validation of a nomogram predicting the probability of prostate cancer Gleason sum upgrading between biopsy and radical prostatectomy pathology. Eur Urol. 2006;49:820–6.
5. Pinthus JH, Witkos M, Fleshner NE, et al. Prostate cancers scored as Gleason 6 on prostate biopsy are frequently Gleason 7 tumors at radical prostatectomy: implication on outcome. J Urol. 2006;176:979–84.
6. Epstein JI, Feng Z, Trock BJ, Pierorazio PM. Upgrading and down- grading of prostate cancer from biopsy to radical prostatectomy: incidence and predictive factors using the modified Gleason grading system and factoring in tertiary grades. Eur Urol. 2012;61:1019–24.
7. Schiffmann J, Wenzel P, Salomon G, et al. Heterogeneity in D'Amico classification-based low-risk prostate cancer: differences in upgrading and upstaging according to AS eligibility. Urol Oncol. 2015;33:329.e13–9.
8. Dinh KT, Mahal BA, Zier DR, et al. Incidence and predictors of upgrading and up staging among 10,000 contemporary patients with low risk prostate cancer. J Urol. 2015;194:343–9.
9. Bul M, Zhu X, Valdagni R, et al. AS for low-risk prostate Cancer worldwide: the PRIAS study. Eur Urol. 2013;63:597–603.
10. Tosoian JJ, Trock BJ, Landis P, et al. AS program for prostate cancer: an update of the Johns Hopkins experience. J Clin Oncol. 2011;29:2185–90.
11. Klotz L, Vesprini D, Sethukavalan P, Jethava V, Zhang L, Jain S, et al. Long-term follow-up of a large AS cohort of patients with prostate Cancer. J Clin Oncol. 2015;33(3):272–7.
12. Preston MA, Feldman AS, Coen JJ, McDougal WS, Smith MR, Paly JJ, et al. AS for low-risk prostate cancer: need for intervention and survival at 10 years. Urol Oncol. 2015;33(9):383.e9–383.e16.
13. Dall'Era MA, Konety BR, Cowan JE, Shinohara K, Stauf F, Cooperberg MR, et al. AS for the management of prostate cancer in a contemporary cohort. Cancer. 2008;112(12):2664–70.
14. NCCN Clinical Practice guidelines in oncology. Prostate Cancer (Version 4. 2018). https://www.nccn.org/professionals/physician_gls/pdf/prostate.pdf. Accessed 7 Oct 2018.
15. King AC, Livermore A, Laurila TAJ, Huang W, Jarrard DF. Impact of immediate TRUS rebiopsy in a patient cohort considering AS for favorable risk prostate cancer. Urol Oncol. 2013;31(6):739–43.
16. Selvadurai ED, Singhera M, Thomas K, et al. Medium-term outcomes of AS for localised prostate cancer. Eur Urol. 2013;64:981–7.
17. Dall'Era MA, Albertsen PC, Bangma C, et al. AS for prostate cancer: a systematic review of the literature. Eur Urol. 2012;62:976–83.
18. Wong L-M, Alibhai SMH, Trottier G, Timilshina N, Van der Kwast T, Zlotta A, et al. A negative confirmatory biopsy among men on AS for prostate Cancer does not protect them from histologic grade progression. Eur Urol. 2014;66(3):406–13.
19. Kryvenko ON, Carter HB, Trock BJ, Epstein JI. Biopsy criteria for determining appropriateness for active surveillance in the modern era. Urology. 2014;83: 869–74.
20. San Francisco IF, Werner L, Regan MM, et al. Risk stratification and validation of prostate specific antigen density as independent predictor of progression in men with low risk prostate cancer during AS. J Urol. 2011;185:471.
21. Cary KC, Cowan JE, Sanford M, Shinohara K, Perez N, Chan JM, et al. Predictors of pathologic progression on biopsy among men on AS for localized prostate Cancer: the value of the pattern of surveillance biopsies. Eur Urol. 2014;66(2):337–42.
22. Gallina A, Maccagnano C, Suardi N, Capitanio U, Abdollah F, Raber M, et al. Unilateral positive biopsies in low risk prostate cancer patients diagnosed with extended transrectal ultrasound-guided biopsy schemes do not predict unilateral prostate cancer at radical prostatectomy. BJU Int. 2012; 110(2b):E64–8.
23. Briganti A, Tutolo M, Suardi N, Gallina A, Abdollah F, Capitanio U, et al. There is no way to identify patients who will harbor small volume, unilateral prostate cancer at final pathology. Implications for focal therapies. Prostate. 2012;72(8):925–30.
24. Mouraviev V, Mayes JM, Sun L, Madden JF, Moul JW, Polascik TJ. Prostate cancer laterality as a rationale of focal ablative therapy for the treatment of clinically localized prostate cancer. Cancer. 2007;110(4):906–10.
25. OECD. Health at a Glance 2015: OECD Indicators. Paris: OECD publishing; 2015. https://doi.org/10.1787/health_glance-2015-en.
26. Turkbey B, et al. Multiparametric 3T prostate magnetic resonance imaging to detect cancer: histopathological correlation using prostatectomy specimens processed in customized magnetic resonance imaging based molds. J Urol. 2011;186:1818.
27. Diaz AW, Shakir NA, George AK, et al. Use of serial multiparametric magnetic resonance imaging in the management of patients with prostate cancer on AS. Urol Onc Sem. 2015;33:202.e1–7.

Improving ultrasound-based prostate volume estimation

Saro Aprikian[1], Murilo Luz[1,2], Fadi Brimo[1,3], Eleonora Scarlata[1], Lucie Hamel[1], Fabio L. Cury[1,4], Simon Tanguay[1,2,5], Armen G. Aprikian[1,2,5], Wassim Kassouf[1,2,5] and Simone Chevalier[1,2,5,6*]

Abstract

Background: To define a new coefficient to be used in the formula (Volume = L x H x W x Coefficient) that better estimates prostate volume using dimensions of fresh prostates from patients who had transrectal ultrasound (TRUS) imaging prior to prostatectomy.

Methods: The prostate was obtained from 153 patients, weighed and measured to obtain length (L), height (H), and width (W). The density was determined by water displacement to calculate volume. TRUS data were retrieved from patient charts. Linear regression analyses were performed to compare various prostate volume formulas, including the commonly used ellipsoid formula and newly introduced bullet-shaped formula.

Results: By relating measured prostate volumes from fresh prostates to TRUS-estimated prostate volumes, 0.66 was the best fitting coefficient in the (L x H x W x Coefficient) equation. This newfound coefficient combined with outlier removal yielded a linear equation with an R^2 of 0.64, compared to 0.55 and 0.60, for the ellipsoid and bullet, respectively. By comparing each of the measured vs. estimated dimensions, we observed that the mean prostate height and length were overestimated by 11.1 and 10.8% using ultrasound ($p < 0.05$), respectively, while the mean width was similar ($p > 0.05$). Overall, the ellipsoid formula underestimates prostate volumes by 18%, compared to an overestimation of 4.6 and 5.7% for the bullet formula and the formula using our coefficient, respectively.

Conclusions: This study defines, for the first time, a coefficient based on freshly resected prostates as a reference to estimate volumes by imaging. Our findings support a bullet rather than an ellipsoid prostate shape. Moreover, substituting the coefficient commonly used in the ellipsoid formula by our calculated coefficient in the equation estimating prostate volume by TRUS, provides a more accurate value of the true prostate volume.

Keywords: Prostate volume, Trans-rectal ultrasound, Ellipsoid, Bullet, Formula, Coefficient

Background

Prostate volume is an important parameter used by clinicians to better manage patients with lower urinary tract symptoms (LUTS) or cancer. The increase in prostate volume with age is correlated with the development of benign prostatic hyperplasia (BPH), which can potentially obstruct the bladder outlet, and necessitate interventions [1]. Knowing the volume of the prostate can help surgeons decide on pharmacological treatments or possibly optimal surgical modalities to resect sufficient prostatic tissue to relieve or improve LUTS. Moreover, the prostate volume is of utility in prostate cancer detection and management as it can be used in conjunction with serum prostatic specific antigen (PSA) to define the PSA density, a clinically relevant parameter for decision-making [2]. In addition, the measurement of prostatic volume is also required in other fields such as radiation oncology, as patients might not be deemed candidates for brachytherapy or stereotactic body radiotherapy (SBRT) if prostate volumes are > 60 cc and > 80 cc, respectively. Hence, estimating the actual prostate volume with accuracy is required for proper medical and surgical management of prostatic diseases as well as for ablative procedures.

* Correspondence: simone.chevalier@mcgill.ca
[1]Urologic Oncology Research Group, Cancer Research Program, Research Institute (RI) of McGill University Health Center (MUHC), Glen Campus, E M2.2210, 1001 Blvd Décarie, Montréal, Qc H4A 3J1, Canada
[2]Department of Surgery (Urology Division), MUHC and McGill University, Montreal, Canada
Full list of author information is available at the end of the article

Ultrasonography, and more specifically transrectal ultrasonography (TRUS), is the most commonly used tool to estimate prostate volume [3]. The ultrasonograph computes the total volume by measuring the length (L), height (H) and width (W) of the gland and multiplying the product by a coefficient of $\pi/6$ (0.52), also known as the prolate ellipsoid formula [4]. The same formula can also be used in Magnetic Resonance Imaging (MRI) modalities for the estimation of prostate volume [4]. Another geometrical model known as the bullet formula (L x H x W × 5π/24) or (L x H x W × 0.65) was proposed in 2009 as a potentially superior formula in estimating prostatic volume [5]. Interestingly, existing studies examining the accuracy of these methods in measuring true prostate volume have reported conflicting evidence as to which formula is more accurate. For instance, Lee et al. had concluded that the ellipsoid formula is adequate and accurate enough in estimating prostatic volume using either TRUS or MRI [4]. However, Rodriguez et al. rather concluded that the ellipsoid formula consistently underestimates prostate size by more than 10% at least 80% of the time [6]. Furthermore, and in support of the latter findings, MacMahon et al. have demonstrated that the ellipsoid formula, on average, underestimated prostate volume by 17% [5].

These conflicting studies, along with the lack of comparison to true prostate volumes measured from fresh prostate-based studies, prompted the present investigation aiming to determine the best possible coefficient to be used in imaging-based volume estimation obtained from the dimensions of fresh prostates.

Methods

Patient cohort

Radical prostatectomy was performed at the McGill University Health Center on 153 patients with localized prostate cancer between the ages of 44 to 76. All had undergone standardized TRUS examination of the prostate by experienced ultrasonographers prior to surgery. Patients had signed consent forms approved by the McGill Ethics Committee for the use of their data for research.

Prostate measurements

Within 10 min of surgical removal, each prostate was trimmed to remove seminal vesicles and surrounding fat tissues, weighed, and measured by two examiners with a 15 cm ruler using standard operating procedures in Pathology to obtain the prostate dimensions, L (apex to base), H (anterior to posterior) and W (lateral to lateral). The prostate was subsequently inked and further processed fresh for banking and formaldehyde-fixed for pathological examination. All parameters were measured prospectively by the same two individuals over time.

A series of 8 fresh prostates were used in water displacement experiments, according to Archimedes' Principle, to determine the mean density. With this newfound density, prostate weights were directly converted to volumes and considered as *measured* volumes.

TRUS measurement data were retrieved from patient medical files. They comprised the individual L, H, and W dimensions as well as the *estimated* volume determined using the standard prolate ellipsoid formula. The true prostate dimensions were used in relation with the true measured volumes post-surgery in order to determine a new coefficient that best relates the two volumes. The measured dimensions by TRUS were then incorporated in all three different formulas (ellipsoid, bullet and our newfound formula) to compare volumes.

Statistical analyses

Multiple linear regression analyses, Bland-Altman and box plots as well as Student t-tests were performed to compare prostate measured volumes with estimated volumes in addition to comparing the individual dimensional measurements from TRUS with the ones measured after surgical resection of the prostate. Differences were considered significant at $p \leq 0.05$.

Results

Basic characteristics of freshly resected prostates

The mean prostate weight was 47.1 g, ranging from 22.2 g to 115.9 g for the 153-patient cohort. The weight range of the series of 8 prostates used in the water displacement experiments, that are representative of radical prostatectomy cohorts, was from 21.0 g to 82.2 g, with a mean weight of 50.2 g and diverging from the overall cohort by 6.6%. Based on the new ISUP Grade Grouping (GG) [7] the 8 prostates were classified as: 2 GG 1; 5 GG 2; and 1 GG 3; pT2c to pT3b; 5 to 10% tumor volume. Using Archimedes' Principle, we determined the density of the average prostate to be 1.02 ± 0.01 g/cc.

Relationship between measured and estimated prostate volumes

The estimated volume from TRUS imaging assumes an ellipsoid geometrical shape of the prostate using the formula (V = L x H x W x Coefficient). In order to identify the best coefficient for this series of 153 fresh prostate specimens, we used the measured prostate weight converted to measured prostate volume by using 1.02 g/cc as the density, as defined above. Thus, the mean measured volume of our cohort was 48.1 cc (range 22.6-118.3 cc).

Measured prostate volumes along with TRUS-obtained prostate dimensions were then used to calculate a new coefficient from the rearranged algebraic formula: Coefficient = V/L x H x W, where L, H and W were all obtained by TRUS, and V is the measured prostatic volume of fresh prostates, obtained just after surgery, as mentioned above. This calculation was performed for each of the 153 prostates, which led to a calculated mean coefficient of 0.66.

Linear regression plots were created in order to compare the newfound coefficient of 0.66 with the ellipsoid coefficient of 0.52. Figure 1a (solid line) shows that plotting estimated prostate volumes against measured prostate volumes using 0.66 as a coefficient yielded an equation of y = 0.892x + 8.8829 with an R^2 value of 0.42 (p-value = 0.043; lower 95% confidence interval/CI = 0.27 and upper 95% CI = 17.49). By performing the same analysis using 0.52 as the coefficient, the equation generated was y = 0.5652x + 13.028 with R^2 = 0.32 (Fig. 1b).

While values were relatively well fitting in the regression, outliers were observed. Bland-Altman analyses (Fig. 2a and b) were used to keep values within 1.5 standard deviations. This type of analysis has as purpose to assess the agreement between two quantitative methods of measurement [8]. This resulted in 18 out of 153 (11.7%) outliers, which were consequently removed. The new mean measured prostate volume of the updated cohort of 135 cases was 46.2 cc (range 22.6–118.0 cc).

New regression analyses were performed with the reduced cohort, using 0.66 and 0.52 as coefficients. Figure 2c shows that the updated equation with 0.66 as the coefficient was improved to y = 0.9309x + 5.6897 with an R^2 of 0.64, compared to the analysis using the ellipsoid coefficient, which yielded an equation of 0.7278x + 5.1463 and an R^2 of 0.55 (Fig. 2d), thereby demonstrating the superiority of 0.66 as the coefficient to better estimate prostate volumes using TRUS dimensions.

The second step was to assess the accuracy of our coefficient compared to the bullet formula, L x H x W × 5π/24, as proposed by MacMahon et al. [5]. In Fig. 3a, we repeated the same type of regression analyses using the bullet

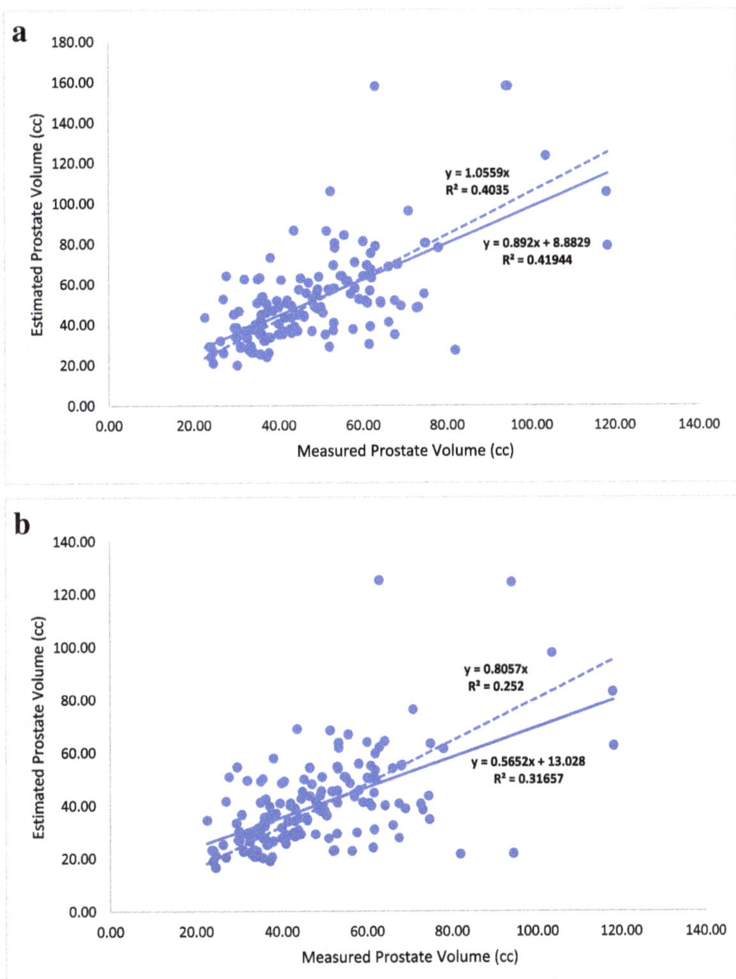

Fig. 1 Linear regression analyses of estimated vs. measured prostate volumes using (**a**) the new formula with 0.66 as a coefficient and (**b**) the ellipsoid formula. Solid line represents the linear regression with a constant term. Dashed line represents the linear regression passing through the intercept

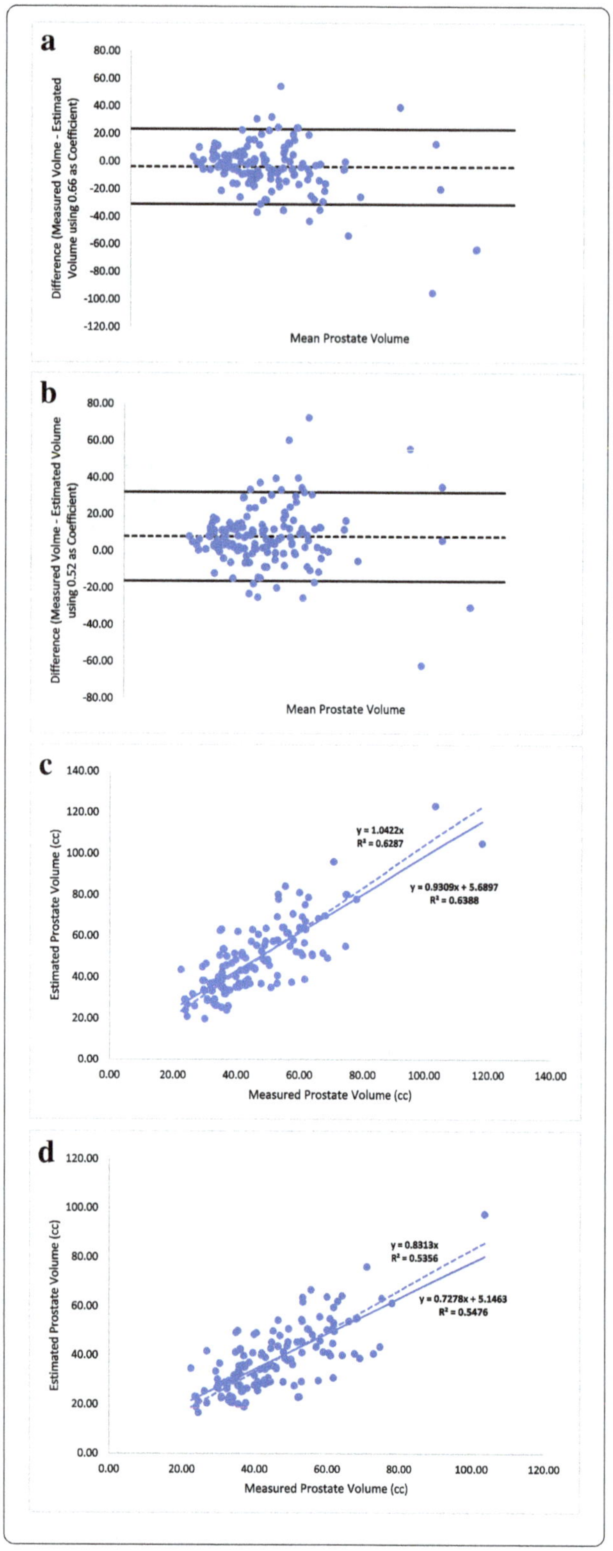

Fig. 2 Bland-Altman plots for outlier removal when using (**a**) the new formula with 0.66 as a coefficient and (**b**) the ellipsoid formula. Linear regression analyses of estimated vs. measured prostate volumes using (**c**) the new formula with 0.66 as a coefficient, after outlier removal and (**d**) the ellipsoid formula, after outlier removal. In (**c**) and (**d**), solid line represents the linear regression with a constant term. Dashed line represents the linear regression passing through the intercept

formula for the entire cohort ($n = 153$; as in Fig. 1a). The equation generated was $y = 0.8784x + 8.7483$ with an R^2 value of 0.42. The Bland-Altman analysis was also performed (Fig. 3b) as above, allowing removal of outliers, reducing the cohort to 138 prostates. The new regression analysis yielded an equation of $y = 0.8867x + 7.1574$ with an R^2 value of 0.60 (Fig. 3c), a value closer to the one obtained in Fig. 2c using 0.66 as a coefficient, but with a lower slope value 0.8784 for the bullet coefficient 0.65 vs. 0.9309 for the new coefficient 0.66.

Altogether these findings suggest that our prostate-derived coefficient of 0.66 is more accurate than that of the ellipsoid formula (0.52) and slightly better than the coefficient of the bullet formula (0.65) in estimating true prostate volume.

Comparison of measured and TRUS-estimated prostate dimensions

The next step was to examine differences in individual prostate dimensions according to the method used to obtain them. We compared each dimension (L, H, W) estimated by ultrasound prior to surgery vs. the same respective prostate dimensions measured post-surgery from our initial cohort of 153 patients. This comparison is shown in Fig. 4. We observed that the mean length of the prostate was overestimated by 10.8% using ultrasound (4.1 cm vs. 3.7 cm) ($p < 0.05$). The mean height was overestimated using TRUS by 11.1% (4.0 cm vs. 3.6 cm) ($p < 0.05$). Finally, the width of the gland estimated by TRUS was fairly similar to the measured value (4.7 cm vs. 4.8 cm) ($p > 0.05$).

Comparison of measured prostate volume and TRUS – estimated prostate volume

We further examined the percent-difference in volumes between measured and estimated volumes using the three formulas for our primary cohort ($n = 153$). In comparison to the measured volume, the ellipsoid formula revealed an underestimation of the volume by a mean of 8.80 cc (18%), whereas the bullet formula overestimated prostate volumes by 1.97 cc (4.6%). Finally, when comparing measured prostate volumes to TRUS-estimated volumes using our new formula with 0.66 as the coefficient, there was an overestimation by a mean of 2.76 cc (5.7%).

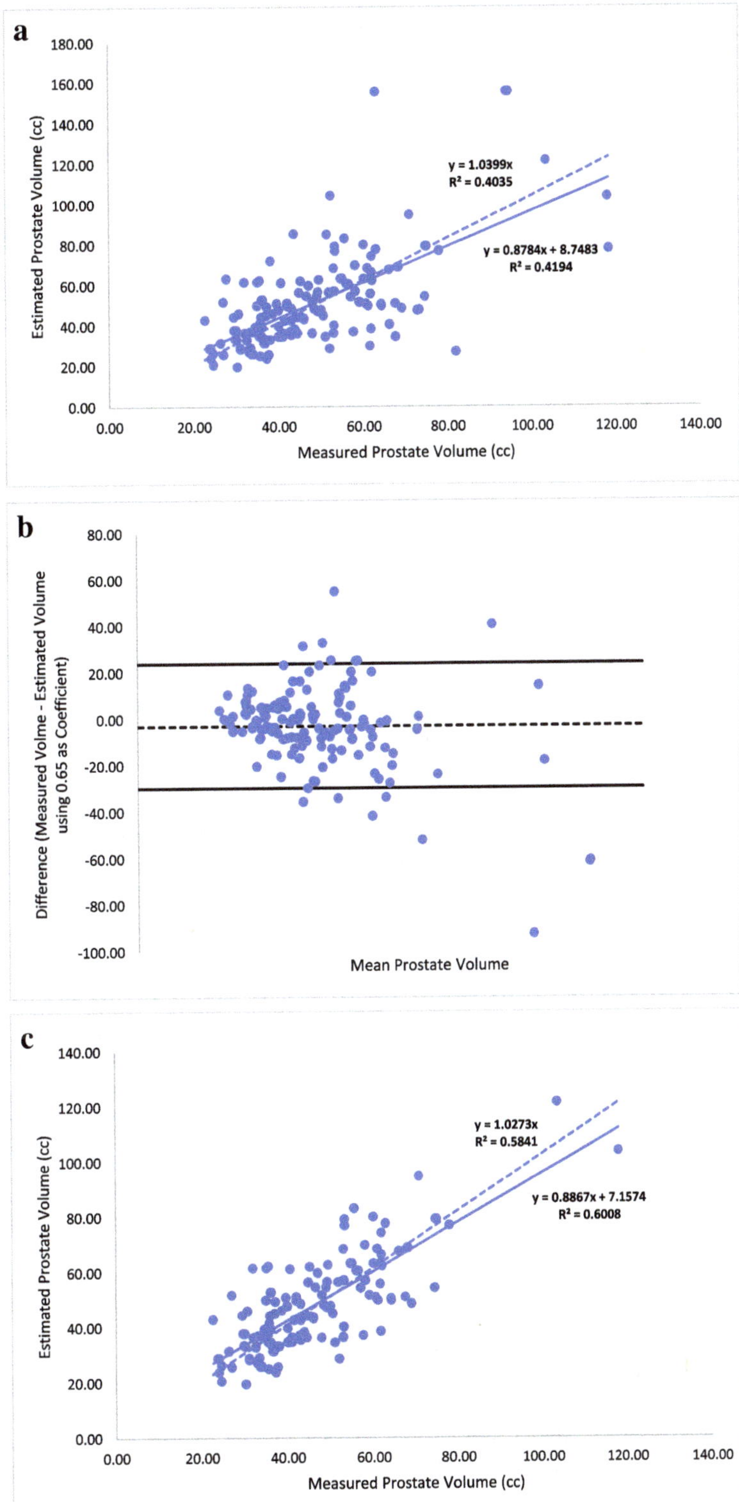

Fig. 3 Linear regression analysis of estimated vs. measured prostate volumes using the bullet formula (**a**) with the full cohort. **b** Bland-Altman plot for outlier removal when using the bullet formula. **c** Linear regression analysis of estimated vs. measured prostate volumes using the bullet formula with the updated cohort, after outlier removal. In (**a**) and (**c**), solid line represents the linear regression with a constant term. Dashed line represents the linear regression passing through the intercept

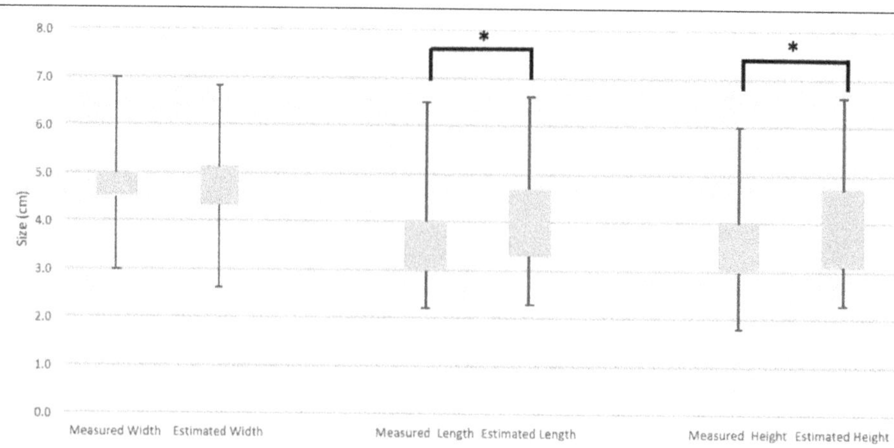

Fig. 4 Box plot of individual prostate dimensions, estimated vs. measured. * $p \leq 0.05$

Prostates were next grouped by size to compare the performance of the three coefficients in estimating prostate volumes. For the 37 larger prostates with measured volumes greater than 60 cc (mean = 76.0 cc), the volume differences between measured vs. TRUS-calculated by ellipsoid, bullet, or with 0.66 as the coefficient were − 22.74 cc (− 30%), − 6.07 cc (− 8%), and − 5.00 cc (− 6.6%), respectively. Performing the same analysis for the 13 smaller prostates (< 30 cc) (mean = 26.7 cc), differences were 3.36 cc (12.6%) for the ellipsoid, 8.6 cc (32.2%) for the bullet, and 9.14 cc (34.2%) using 0.66 as the coefficient. For the medium sized prostates (between 30 and 60 cc) (mean = 42.7 cc), differences for ellipsoid, bullet, and with 0.66 as the coefficient were 5.78 cc (14%), − 3.57 cc (− 8.3%) and − 4.31 cc (− 10%), respectively. These results suggest that the ellipsoid formula is more conformant to smaller prostates below 30 cc, while the bullet and our new formula with 0.66 as the coefficient conform better to medium- to larger-sized prostates of over 30 cc and as observed in most patients consulting for BPH and prostate cancer.

Discussion

The estimation of prostate volume is valuable for clinicians seeing patients with potential prostatic diseases, helping them in both diagnosis and treatment. As such, TRUS remains the main method applied routinely in the clinic to assess prostate volumes. Thus far, geometrical models were used to describe prostate shape, assuming the gland to be a prolate ellipsoid and more recently, a bullet. The present study is the first to prospectively use fresh prostate specimens as a reference to define a new coefficient of 0.66, which performed better than the universally adopted coefficient of 0.52 from the ellipsoid formula to estimate prostate volumes. Moreover, the new coefficient predicts a model closer to a bullet-shaped prostate based on 0.65 as its coefficient. Therefore, we suggest using 0.66 as the coefficient in the eq. (V = L x H x W x Coefficient) for image-based prostate volume estimation.

Among reasons in support of this proposition is that the coefficient derived from freshly obtained and trimmed prostates in our study is quite representative of patients consulting clinicians in general. For instance, this cohort was part of a larger cohort of 604 consecutive patients with a similar age distribution (mean = 61.3 years old, range = 44–76 years old) undergoing radical prostatectomy for localized prostate cancer at our centre. Unfortunately, TRUS measurement data were not available for most patients who were often referred for surgery from other centres. Nevertheless, all prostates were similarly processed, and their mean weight was similar: 45.1 g (range = 17.1 g–165.6 g). Among additional factors supporting the adoption of the prostate-derived 0.66 coefficient is the fresh status of specimens, rapidly processed and measured prospectively after excision, which is close to the in vivo situation. Often times in other studies, measurements are done after formaldehyde fixation, a process known to affect the prostate weight and volume [9].

The comparison of the 0.66 coefficient with the ellipsoid and bullet coefficients showed superiority of the prostate-derived coefficient, performing better than the universally-adopted 0.52 value and being closer to the bullet formula using 0.65 as the coefficient. Indeed, the equation obtained between measured and estimated prostate volumes always yielded a higher slope and a better correlation with the 0.66 coefficient over the two others, before and after the removal of outliers. Our results are somewhat similar to a study performed on 73 prostate samples using the ellipsoid formula, showing an almost identical slope value, 0.933 vs. 0.931 in the present study, but differing by the previously reported higher R^2 value of 0.847 [4]. This discrepancy may be related to cohort size which was significantly larger in our study ($n = 153$ vs. 73), and was composed of a greater number of prostates with larger volumes, 48.1 cc in our study vs. 39.2 cc in the study done by Lee et al. As mentioned above, the average volume of the prostate in patients undergoing radical prostatectomy for localized prostate cancer at our center is approximately 50.0 cc.

Our study showed that measurements done by experienced ultrasonographers using TRUS as compared to our pathologists' measurements by ruler on the same prostate in the fresh setting, underestimated height (4.0 cm vs. 3.6 cm) as well as length (4.1 cm vs. 3.7 cm), while the width was similar in both cases (4.7 cm vs. 4.8 cm). These findings are slightly different than that of an earlier report carried out on 87 prostates, which indicated an underestimation of height using TRUS vs. pathological dimensions (3.2 cm vs. 3.7 cm), and width (4.8 cm vs. 5.2 cm) but no difference in length [6].

Our study also demonstrated that the ellipsoid formula underestimates prostate volume by a mean of 18% when using TRUS imaging. The extent of underestimation of TRUS-measured prostate volume using the ellipsoid formula has been reported in a prior study to be greater than 10% and shown to underestimate true prostate volumes 80% of the time [6]. In comparison, analyses with our coefficient in the formula ($V = H \times L \times W \times 0.66$) provides a more accurate estimate of prostate volumes with an overestimation of 5.7%. In addition, a larger study comparing TRUS estimation of prostate volumes using the ellipsoid formula with 318 prostatectomy specimens showed a 9.1% underestimation for prostates with a mean volume of 37.3 cc [10]. Once more, the prostates in the latter study were smaller than in our series, 11 cc less than the average 48.1 cc prostates we studied. Also, it is important to emphasize that in that study the measurements of the prostatectomy specimens were retrieved retrospectively from pathology reports as opposed to the prospective nature in our study focused on true prostate volume determination. Furthermore, it is unclear whether seminal vesicles were removed, measurements were done on fresh vs. fixed specimens, or if there were one or several health care professionals measuring prostate dimensions and recording data. A main limitation in all studies, including our own, is that TRUS data for prostate dimensions and volumes were retrieved from patient medical charts since it was part of routine tests done in the clinic and not part of a prospective research project. Finally, Scott et al. evaluated the reliability of total prostate and transition zone volume measurements by TRUS among three examiners with various levels of experience and, as expected, found that more experienced examiners had better reproducibility [11].

Our new coefficient estimates a model closer to a bullet-shaped prostate, with its formula developed via ultrasound planimetry creating 3D images for brachytherapy [5]. The comparison of prostate volumes using the $5\pi/24$ coefficient (0.65) of the bullet formula with our coefficient of 0.66 supports a slightly higher accuracy with our prostate-derived 0.66 coefficient, with a better slope value (0.931 vs. bullet slope of 0.887) and correlation coefficient ($R^2 = 0.64$ vs. 0.60 for the bullet). The bullet formula was reported to yield a R^2 of 0.935 when comparing planimetry-based volumes but for smaller prostates (mean of 29.4 cc) in a smaller sample set (60 cases) [5]. More importantly, our study is the first to validate the bullet formula with prospectively measured fresh prostate specimens.

By comparing all formulas in three different prostate volume subgroups: small (< 30 cc), medium (> 30 cc < 60 cc) and large (> 60 cc), we observed that the ellipsoid formula estimates measured volume better when studying smaller prostates, while the bullet formula and our prostate-derived formula using 0.66 as the coefficient better estimates true volume in the case of medium to large prostates, as observed in the majority of men consulting for BPH or prostate cancer. Nevertheless, an external validation study should be conducted in order to confirm our findings before it can be used clinically.

Although we believe that our new coefficient is better suited for clinical use in men consulting for BPH and prostate cancer, we appreciate and understand the challenges in changing the standard practice of the universally accepted, geometrically defined ellipsoid formula and its coefficient of 0.52. This is highlighted by the fact that the bullet formula and its superior coefficient of 0.65, as established in 2009, and which has been shown to be superior to the ellipsoid formula has not been adopted in clinical practice. The adoption of our coefficient, the first to be prostate-derived, will depend on the diffusion of the present findings in the medical community and its testing and applicability by specialists advocating for the integration of our coefficient in medical devices or equipments designed for prostate volume estimation.

Conclusions

Our prospective study on freshly obtained prostates as the reference defines a coefficient of 0.66 to be superior in estimating prostate volume in the eq. $V = L \times H \times W \times$ Coefficient when using TRUS. This new coefficient not only provides a more accurate estimation of true prostate volumes than the universally established ellipsoid coefficient, but also supports the suggestion that the prostate shape is closer to that of a bullet.

Abbreviations

BPH: Benign prostatic hyperplasia; CI: Confidence interval; GG: ISUP Grade Grouping; H: Height; L: Length; LUTS: Lower urinary tract symptoms; MRI: Magnetic Resonance Imaging; PSA: Prostatic specific antigen; SBRT: Stereotactic body radiotherapy; TRUS: Transrectal Ultrasound; W: Width

Acknowledgements
The authors acknowledge the technical help of Ms. JS Chen in the processing and measurements of prostates, Mr. G Kalloghlian for his contribution in statistical analyses and Drs R Kool and M. Anidjar in the retrieving of pathological data.

Authors' contributions
SA: Research trainee who contributed significantly towards the project (retrieval, verification, and organization of all datasets). He generated equations and derived the coefficient, performed statistical analyses, created the Figures, reviewed the literature, wrote and revised the manuscript. ML: Fellow initially involved and who performed experiments to determine the prostate density. He contributed to the retrieval of ultrasound data from patient files and performed preliminary analyses of data. FB: Genito-urinary pathologist responsible of prostate processing and overlooking procedures related to the prostate from the operation room to the pathology laboratory. ES: Obtained and processed the fresh prostate specimens, took prostate dimensions or parameters, involved in writing the Methods section on prostate samples. LH: Built the dataset referring to patient pathological measurements and ultrasound measurements from clinical files. FLC: Clinician involved when the project was proposed. Co-supervision of research fellow helping in the retrieval of data and doing preliminary analyses. ST: Urologist who recruited and consented patients, performed the radical prostatectomies, collected the clinical and pathologic data from his individual patients, critically revised the manuscript and provided final approval. AGA: Urologist part of the study design, who recruited and consented patients, performed the radical prostatectomies, collected the clinical and pathologic data from his individual patients, drafted and critically revised the manuscript and provided final approval. WK: Urologist who recruited and consented patients, performed the radical prostatectomies, collected the clinical and pathologic data from his individual patients, critically revised the manuscript and provided final approval. WK is also the Editorial Board Member of BMC Urology. SC: Generated the idea and planned the project, overlooked the work done by team members, meeting them and discussing progress. Covered part of expenses and involved in the drafting, writing and revision of the manuscript. All authors have read and approved the manuscript.

Author details
[1]Urologic Oncology Research Group, Cancer Research Program, Research Institute (RI) of McGill University Health Center (MUHC), Glen Campus, E M2.2210, 1001 Blvd Décarie, Montréal, Qc H4A 3J1, Canada. [2]Department of Surgery (Urology Division), MUHC and McGill University, Montreal, Canada. [3]Department of Pathology, MUHC and McGill University, Montreal, Canada. [4]Department of Radiation Oncology, MUHC and McGill University, Montreal, Canada. [5]Department of Oncology, MUHC and McGill University, Montreal, Canada. [6]Department of Medicine, MUHC and McGill University, Montreal, Canada.

References
1. Nickel JC. Benign prostatic hyperplasia: does prostate size matter? Rev Urol. 2003;5(Suppl 4):S12–7.
2. Jue JS, Barboza MP, Prakash NS, Venkatramani V, Sinha VR, Pavan N, Nahar B, Kanabur P, Ahdoot M, Dong Y, et al. Re-examining prostate-specific antigen (PSA) density: defining the optimal PSA range and patients for using PSA density to predict prostate Cancer using extended template biopsy. Urology. 2017;105:123–8.
3. Harvey CJ, Pilcher J, Richenberg J, Patel U, Frauscher F. Applications of transrectal ultrasound in prostate cancer. Br J Radiol. 2012;85 Spec No(1):S3–17.
4. Lee JS, Chung BH. Transrectal ultrasound versus magnetic resonance imaging in the estimation of prostate volume as compared with radical prostatectomy specimens. Urol Int. 2007;78(4):323–7.
5. MacMahon PJ, Kennedy AM, Murphy DT, Maher M, McNicholas MM. Modified prostate volume algorithm improves transrectal US volume estimation in men presenting for prostate brachytherapy. Radiology. 2009;250(1):273–80.
6. Rodriguez E Jr, Skarecky D, Narula N, Ahlering TE. Prostate volume estimation using the ellipsoid formula consistently underestimates actual gland size. J Urol. 2008;179(2):501 3.
7. Epstein JI, Egevad L, Amin MB, Delahunt B, Srigley JR, Humphrey PA. The 2014 International Society of Urological Pathology (ISUP) consensus conference on Gleason grading of prostatic carcinoma: definition of grading patterns and proposal for a new grading system. Am J Surg Pathol 2016;40:244–52.
8. Giavarina D. Understanding bland Altman analysis. Biochem Med (Zagreb). 2015;25(2):141–51.
9. Schned AR, Wheeler KJ, Hodorowski CA, Heaney JA, Ernstoff MS, Amdur RJ, Harris RD. Tissue-shrinkage correction factor in the calculation of prostate cancer volume. Am J Surg Pathol. 1996;20(12):1501–6.
10. Paterson NR, Lavallee LT, Nguyen LN, Witiuk K, Ross J, Mallick R, Shabana W, MacDonald B, Scheida N, Fergusson D, et al. Prostate volume estimations using magnetic resonance imaging and transrectal ultrasound compared to radical prostatectomy specimens. Can Urol Assoc J. 2016;10(7–8):264–8.
11. Sech S, Montoya J, Girman CJ, Rhodes T, Roehrborn CG. Interexaminer reliability of transrectal ultrasound for estimating prostate volume. J Urol. 2001;166(1):125–9.

29

Pelvic plexus block to provide better anesthesia in transperineal template-guided prostate biopsy

Xue-fei Ding[1], Tian-bao Huang[1], Sheng-ming Lu[1], Hua-zhi Tao[1], Xiao-fang Ye[1], Fei Wang[1], Yao-zong Xu[1], Jia-nan Xu[1], Yu-quan Zhou[1] and Yang Luan[1,2*]

Abstract

Background: To evaluate the efficacy of pelvic plexus block (PPB) in relief pain during transperineal template-guided prostate biopsy (TTPB), compared with conventional periprostatic nerve block (PNB).

Methods: From July 2016 to August 2017, 245 patients who were performed TTPB in Clinical Medical College of Yangzhou University were recruited. The patients were randomized into three groups using a random number table. Group-1 received prostate capsule local anesthesia with 22 ml of 1% lidocaine. Group-2 additionally received PNB on the basis of Group-1. To perform PNB, 5 ml 1% lidocaine was injected into the region of prostatic neurovascular bundle situated in the angle of prostate-bladder-seminal vesicle. Group-3 received prostate capsule local anesthesia plus PPB (5 ml of 1% lidocaine injection into the pelvic plexus which located on lateral to the bilateral seminal vesicle apex). The patients' pain and satisfaction were evaluated by visual analogue scale and visual numerical scale, respectively.

Results: The age, total prostate volume, PSA and the number of cores were comparable among the three groups. The visual analog scale scores of group-3 were significantly lower than group-2 during biopsy ($P = 0.003$). Conversely, the visual numeric scale scores were higher in group-3 ($P = 0.039$). Both the group-2 and group-3 outperformed the group-1 in alleviating pain and had a higher quantification of satisfaction. There were no significant differences in the pain scores or the satisfaction scores at 30 min after the procedure among the three groups.

Conclusions: The analgesic efficacy of PPB guided by Doppler ultrasound in TTPB was better than that of PNB and both were superior to no nerve block.

Keywords: Prostate, Biopsy, Nerve block, Pain

* Correspondence: Luan_Y@163.com
[1]Department of Urology, Clinical Medical College, Yangzhou University, No. 98 West Nantong Road, Yangzhou, Jiangsu Province 225001, China
[2]Department of Urology, Taihe County People's Hospital, Fuyang 226600, Anhui Province, China

Background

Early screening for prostate cancer (PCa) can significantly lower disease-related morbidity and even prolong life expectancy [1]. Transperineal template-guided prostate biopsy (TTPB) is one of most effective procedures for detection of prostate cancer [2, 3]. However, compared with the transrectal biopsy, transperineal route may cause more pain [4]. In the absence of anesthesia, about 20% of patients refused to undergo prostate biopsy [5]. Therefore, effective anesthesia is a important precondition for successful prostate biopsy [6]. Periprostatic nerve block (PNB) has attracted more and more attention due to its excellent analgesic effect and high safety. At present, PNB is regarded as the "golden standard" of analgesia during prostate biopsy [7–10]. In 1996, Nash et al. [11] were the first to introduce PNB, and found that it can relieve the pain during transrectal ultrasound (TRUS) -guided prostate biopsy. Conde et al. [12] found that the anesthesia effect of PNB was superior to oral morphine. Hergan et al. [13] conducted a meta analysis of fourteen trials and found that PNB had better anesthesia effect than that of local anesthesia or placebo. However, some patients have poor response to PNB in clinical practice. Apart from sensitivity to pain, most of these patients were with larger prostate volume [14]. It may be that, due to the increase in prostate volume may lead to a decrease in prostate cancer detection rate [15]. Hence, in order to improve the positive rate, it is necessary to increase the number of needles, which aggravates the pain of patients. Kevar et al. [16] called the condition as "cumulative pain". Besides, the irregular growth of prostate cancer [17] increases the difficulty of locating the angle prostate-bladder-seminal vesicle. In addition, Nguyen et al. [18] found that apical biopsies were more painful than were biopsies from other areas of the prostate under PNB.

Hence, PNB cannot completely eliminate discomfort. A small number of nerve fibers are located on the anterior and superolateral parts of the prostate, and PNB does not block these nerve fibers, which is the limitation of PNB. Recently, some studies have shown that direct blocking of the origin of the prostatic nerves, the pelvic plexus, may obtained better analgesia [19–22].

In this study, we compared pelvic plexus block (PPB) with conventional PNB to evaluate whether PPB has better anesthetic efficacy in the process of TTPB.

Methods

Clinical data

The prospective, randomized controlled study was done in our hospital from July 2016 to August 2017. Ethics clearance was obtained from the Clinical Medical College of the Yangzhou University.

Study inclusion criteria included: digital rectal examination findings nodules; and/or ultrasound or magnetic resonance imaging revealings suspicious of prostate cancer; and/or PSA4 ~ 10 ng/ml with an abnormal free/total PSA or PSA density; and/or PSA > 10 ng/ml. Exclusion criteria were chronic pelvic pain syndrome, chronic prostatitis, previous prostate biopsies, allergy to local anesthetic, bleeding disorder, pathological rectum, active urinary tract infection and taking analgesic medications. All patients signed a written informed consent before prostate biopsy. Assisted by a computer program, an independent researchers used a random number table to randomly divide the patients into three groups. The patients of group-1 received prostate capsule local anesthesia (PLA), group-2 received PNB in addition to PLA, and group-3 received PLA along with a PPB. Regarding the grouping assignment, the patients were unaware the details.

Biopsy procedure

The biopsy device included: A biplanar TRUS probe (Flex focus 1202; BK, Naerum, Denmark), brachytherapy stepping unit (Fixer, template, stepper) (Mick Radio-Nuclear Instruments, Mount Vernon, NY, USA), Bard biopsy gun (Bard MCl 820) and an 18-gauge biopsy needle.

Before prostate biopsy, complete blood cell count with differentiation, coagulation test and comprehensive metabolic panel were routinely performed. The patients were given oral intestinal clearance drugs one day before operation and emptied their stools on the morning of operation.

The patients were placed in a lithotomy position and underwent a conventional digital rectal examination. The TRUS probe was fixed on the brachytherapy stepping unit and was placed into the rectum. Then, the patients received the following anesthesia:

Group-1 (PLA): under the guidance of TRUS, the projection range of prostate in perineal skin was observed. In an area larger 0.5 cm than this range, infiltration anesthesia of perineal skin used 10 ml of 1% lidocaine. Then infiltration anesthesia was performed on the apex of the prostate. At the 1, 3, 5, 7, 9 and 11 o'clock of the area which prostate apex projected in the perineal skin, the syringe enters from these points and injected 12 ml of 1% lidocaine near the apex of the prostate.

Group-2 (PLA + PNB): for PNB, by rotating the TRUS probe, the vessels in the prostatic neurovascular bundle (NVB) can be observed at the prostate-bladder-seminal vesicle angle. Therefore, the NVB can be located by blood vessels. In the region of NVB, ANSll 0.5 mm * 112 mm spinal needle was used to inject 5 ml of 1% lidocaine to perform PNB. The same was done for the other side (Fig. 1).

Group-3 (PLA + PPB): for PPB, under color Doppler ultrasound guidance, pelvic plexus was positioned which situated in the lateral to the apex of bilateral seminal vesicles. Then, in the area of the pelvic plexus, 5 ml 1% lidocaine was injected (Fig. 2).

To avoid injecting local anesthetic into the vessels, the syringe was aspirated before injecting local anesthetic in the three groups. After 5 min, prostate biopsies were performed.

Pain and complication assessment

Pain was evaluated by the visual analog scale (VAS; 0, none; 10, intolerable pain), and satisfaction was quantified using a visual numeric scale (VNS; 0, terrible; 4, perfect); only integers were allowed [23, 24]. Another independent resident and the patients were 'blinded' to the type of anesthesia given. The resident explained the VAS and VNS to the patients and requested them to rate their level of pain or satisfaction. VAS scores and VNS scores had two time points: VAS-1 and VNS-1 during the biopsy procedure, and VAS-2 and VNS-2 at 30 min after the procedure. The patients recorded the VAS and VNS scores without any other assistance.

Patients were given a nonvalidated self-administered questionnaire about complications such as hematuria, hemospermia, urinary retention and infection.

Statistical analysis

Epi Info™ 7 (WHO, Geneva, Switzerland) was used for sample size calculation. 95% CI, 5% α error, 80% power and 90% population proportion were set. It was estimated that at least 42 men would be needed for each of the three groups. And according to the 20% predicted clinical missed follow-up rate, at least 51 patients in each group were required.

Data analysis was performed using SPSS (version 19.0; IBM Corp, Armonk, NY) statistical software. The VAS scores and VNS scores were shown as mean ± SD and were compared using the one-way ANOVA test. And the rates of complications were compared using χ^2 test. $P < 0.05$ was considered statistically significant.

Results

From July 2016 to August 2017, 271 patients were performed TTPB in Clinical Medical College of Yangzhou University. Of these, 21 patients did not fulfil inclusion criteria and 5 did not provide consent. Ultimately, 245 patients were randomized into three groups. Groups-1, 2 and 3 included 81, 83 and 81 patients, respectively (Fig. 3). The age, prostate volume, serum PSA level and the number of cores showed no significant differences among these three groups, as presented in Table 1.

In groups-1, 2 and 3, VAS-1 was 3.3 ± 1.6, 2.7 ± 1.3 and 2.1 ± 1.1, and VNS-1 was 2.8 ± 0.9, 3.1 ± 0.8 and 3.3 ± 0.2, respectively. The pain scores in group-3 were significantly lower than in group-2 ($P = 0.003$). Both the group-2 and group-3 outperformed the group-1 in alleviating pain. Satisfaction scores in group-3 were significantly higher than in group-2 ($P = 0.039$). Group-2 and group-3 were higher than group-1 in terms of satisfaction. In groups-1, 2 and 3, VAS-2 was 0.7 ± 0.4, 0.6 ± 0.5 and 0.5 ± 0.3, and VNS-2 was 3.5 ± 0.6, 3.5 ± 0.6 and 3.7 ± 0.8, respectively. At 30 min after the procedure,

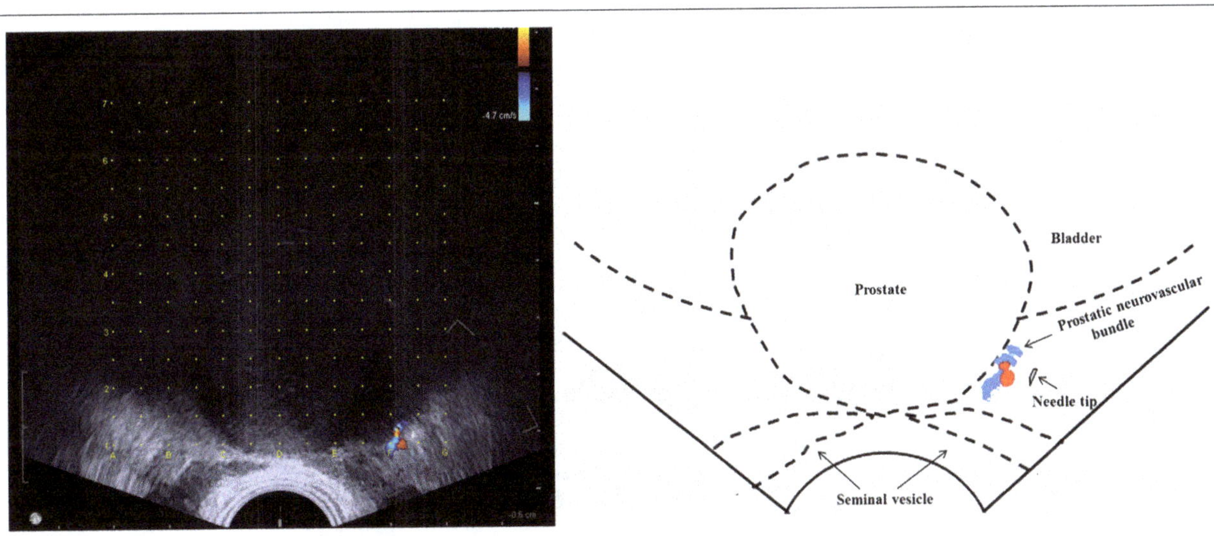

Fig. 1 PNB: 5 ml of 1% lidocaine was injected into the position adjacent to the prostatic neurovascular bundle, location at the prostate-bladder-seminal vesicle angle

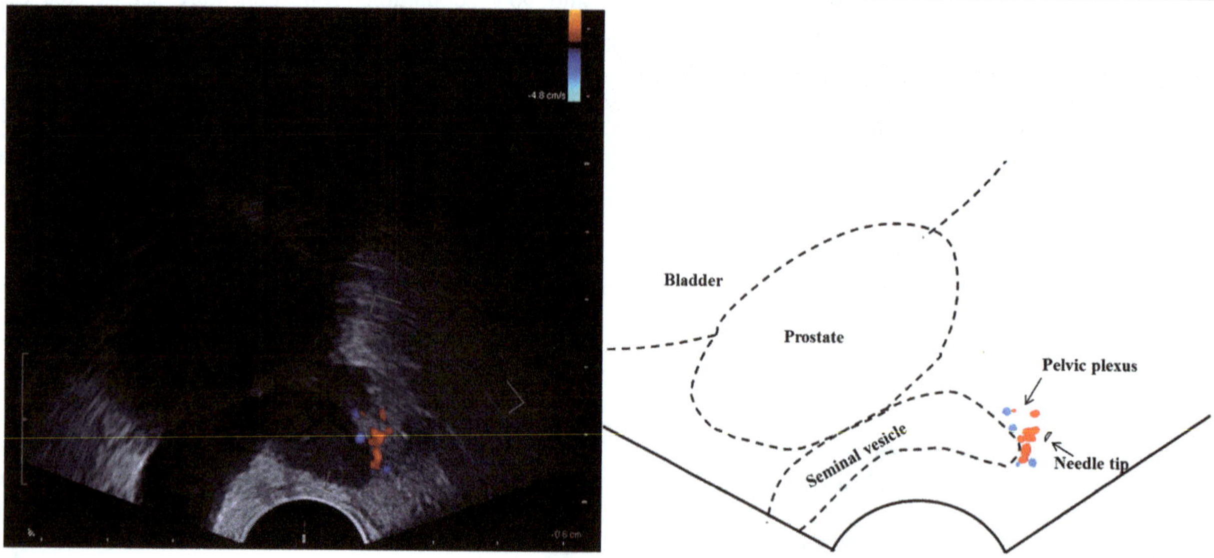

Fig. 2 PPB: 5 ml of 1% lidocaine was injected into the region of the pelvic plexus, situated lateral to the apex of the seminal vesicles

there were no statistically significant differences in VAS scores or VNS scores among the three groups (Table 2).

There was no significant difference in complications including hematospermia, hematuria, infection and urinary retention among the three groups (Table 3).

Discussion

TTPB has become one of the most commonly methods for the diagnosis of Pca. As an invasive operation, TTPB is related to obvious discomfort and pain.

Currently, PNB is safe, easily performed and high-efficiency, and it is generally regarded as the preferred method for analgesia during biopsy needles inserting into the prostatic tissue [7–10]. Recently, PPB was reported to have a definitive theoretical advantage for decreasing pain, challenging conventional PNB [19–22].

The nerves of the prostate come from the pelvic plexus, including the sympathetic and parasympathetic nerves. The sympathetic nerve fibers are mainly transmitted to the pelvic plexus through the superior hypogastric plexus.

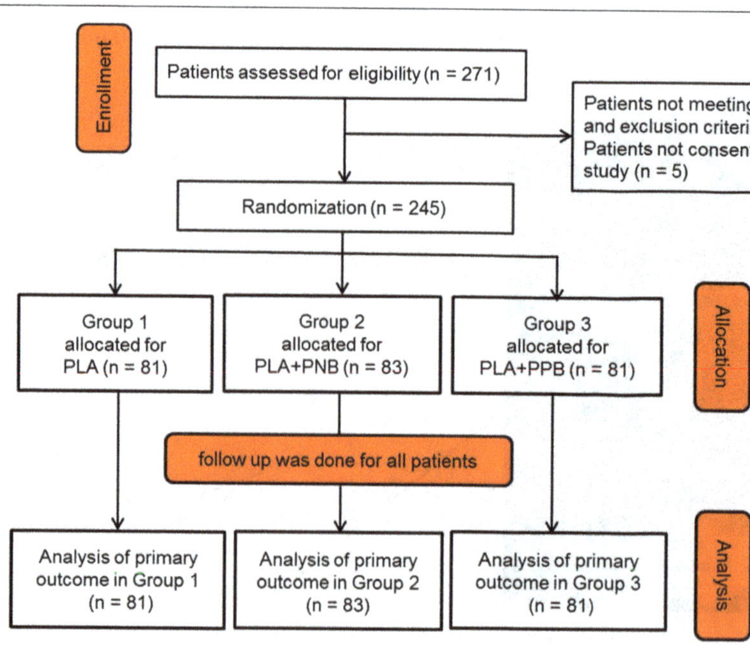

Fig. 3 The flow diagram of the study as per the Consolidated Standard of Reporting Trials guidelines

Table 1 The patients' characteristics in the three groups

Groups	*N*	Age(years)	Prostate volume (ml)	PSA level (ng/ml)	Number of cores
Group-1	81	67.2 ± 9.5	47.7 ± 19.3	33.1 ± 23.1	23.3 ± 8.5
Group-2	83	68.2 ± 8.6	46.7 ± 20.4	30.9 ± 21.7	22.9 ± 8.2
Group-3	81	67.9 ± 9.1	48.2 ± 19.2	35.3 ± 22.6	23.1 ± 8.2
P value		0.790	0.885	0.475	0.945

Parasympathetic fibers originate from the 2–4 sacral spinal nerves and are transmitted through them. These nerves unite to form the pelvic plexus [21, 25]. And which is rectangular and 4 to 5 cm in length. The midpoint of pelvic plexus is located on the lateral to the apex of bilateral seminal vesicles. The pelvic plexus is penetrated by many vessels that supply the the prostate, seminal vesicles, bladder and rectum. At the most caudal portion of the pelvic plexus, the nerve innervating the prostate and the cavernosal nerves, the prostatic plexus, is generated [26, 27]. Subsequently, the prostatic plexus and the vessels of the prostate form the NVB, which is distributed along the posterolateral margin of the prostate and is considered to be the primary nerves innervating the prostate. However, there are a few other nerve fibers also running on the anterior and superolateral surfaces of the prostate [11, 19, 27, 28].

PNB mainly blocks the prostatic plexus located on the posterolateral side of the prostate, which is the primary nerve that supplies the prostate [19–22]. However, a small number of nerve fibers located on the anterior and superolateral parts of the prostate were omitted and thus not blocked. This may be the reason why a research has found that biopsies at the apex of the prostate were more painful than those at other sites [18]. PPB directly injects lidocaine into the pelvic plexus, and all nerve fibers supplying to the prostate are blocked. Hence, compared with PNB, PPB have theoretical advantages.

Wu et al. [22] first reported PPB. Under grayscale ultrasound guidance, they injected 5 ml of 1% lidocaine into lateral to the seminal vesicles apex. However, they didn't find any reduce the pain associated with biopsy. Conversely, Akpinar et al. [21] found that compared with PNB, the analgesic efficacy of PPB (2 ml 2% lidocaine for each pelvic plexus) was better. Cantiello et al. [19] mixed 1% lidocaine with 0.75% Naropin and injected 2.5 ml mixture into each pelvic plexus lateral to the apex of the seminal vesicles under the guidance of color Doppler ultrasound. Jindal et al. [20] injected 2.5 ml 2% lidocaine into the bilateral pelvic plexus. In studies of Cantiello et al. and Jindal et al., they reported PPB had a better anesthetic effect than did PNB. The results of the last three researches are different from those of Wu et al., and the reason may be related to the use of color Doppler ultrasound, which can provide more accurate positioning of pelvic plexus.

All of the above studies were meant to explore the anesthetic efficacy of PPB in the transrectal prostate biopsy. Owing to the high positive rate and few complications, The value of TTPB in the diagnosis of Pca is becoming more and more important [2, 3]. Hence, we evaluated the anesthetic efficacy of PPB in TTPB in this study. Our present outcomes showed that the PPB group had higher satisfaction and lower pain scores than did the PNB group. Both these groups had higher levels of satisfaction, and pain control was better than that in the group without any nerve block. After 30 min of the biopsy, most patients returned to normal without pain. There were no differences in pain scores or satisfaction scores at 30 min after the procedure among the three groups.

Doppler ultrasound can avoid damage to the vessels and accurately inject the local anesthetics into the region of the pelvic plexus, thus reducing the incidence of complications related to the nerve block anesthesia technique, especially vascular complications. In our study, there was no significant difference in complications including hematospermia, hematuria, infection and urinary retention among the three groups .

Our study has several limitations. We assessed pain scores and satisfaction scores after biopsy. This might lead to 'recall bias'. Nevertheless, we chose this method for avoiding any possible factors for disturbing biopsy

Table 2 The VAS scores and VNS scores in the three groups

Groups	Group-1 $n = 81$	Group-2 $n = 83$	Group-3 $n = 81$	*P* value		
				Group-1 vs 2	Group-1 vs 3	Group-2 vs 3
VAS-1	3.3 ± 1.6	2.7 ± 1.3	2.1 ± 1.1	0.007	0.000	0.003
VAS-2	0.7 ± 0.4	0.6 ± 0.5	0.5 ± 0.3	0.169	0.071	0.572
VNS-1	2.8 ± 0.9	3.1 ± 0.8	3.3 ± 0.2	0.027	0.000	0.039
VNS-2	3.5 ± 0.6	3.6 ± 0.3	3.7 ± 0.8	0.511	0.071	0.323

Table 3 The complications of prostate biopsy [% (cases)]

Groups	*N*	hematuria	urinary retention	infection	hemospermia
Group-1	81	32.1 (26)	3.7 (3)	2.5 (2)	3.7 (3)
Group-2	83	33.7 (28)	2.4 (2)	2.4 (2)	3.6 (3)
Group-3	81	30.9 (25)	2.5 (2)	1.2 (1)	4.9 (4)
P value		0.925	0.860	0.579	0.895

performed by the resident, which may affect the scores. Although VAS and VNS are relatively objective indicators of pain detection, the evaluation of pain is still dominated by the subjective feelings of patients, and there is a lack of objective quantitative indicators, which needs further study. And in the future, we would study whether PPB results in more adhesions, making the surgical steps more difficult. We also need to explore whether it affects erectile function and urinary continence.

Conclusions

Under the guidance of color Doppler ultrasound, PPB has better analgesic efficacy than did PNB in TTPB process and both were superior to no nerve block.

Abbreviations

Pca: Prostate cancer; PLA: Prostate-coated local anesthesia; PPB: Pelvic plexus block; PSA: Prostate specific antigen; PSAD: Prostate specific antigen density; TRUS: Transrectal ultrasound; TTPB: Transperineal template-guided prostate biopsy; VAS: Visual analogue scale; VNS: Visual numeric scale

Acknowledgments

None.

Authors' contribution

XFD: Project development, Data Collection, Study design, Manuscript editing; YL: Manuscript writing, Study design, Data Collection, Statistical analysis; TBH: Manuscript editing, Data Collection; SML, FW, and JNX: Data Collection, Statistical analysis; HZT, XFY, YZX and YQZ: Data Collection, Data interpretation. All authors read and approved the final manuscript.

References

1. Heijnsdijk EA, Wever EM, Auvinen A, Hugosson J, Ciatto S, Nelen V, Kwiatkowski M, Villers A, Paez A, Moss SM, et al. Quality-of-life effects of prostate-specific antigen screening. N Engl J Med. 2012;367(7):595–605.
2. Muthuveloe D, Telford R, Viney R, Patel P. The detection and upgrade rates of prostate adenocarcinoma following transperineal template-guided prostate biopsy - a tertiary referral Centre experience. Central European journal of urology. 2016;69(1):42–7.
3. Mai Z, Xiao Y, Yan W, Zhou Y, Zhou Z, Liang Z, Ji Z, Li H. Comparison of lesions detected and undetected by template-guided transperineal saturation prostate biopsy. BJU Int. 2017.
4. Udeh EI, Amu OC, Nnabugwu II, Ozoemena O. Transperineal versus transrectal prostate biopsy: our findings in a tertiary health institution. Niger J Clin Pract. 2015;18(1):110–4.
5. Bingqian L, Peihuan L, Yudong W, Jinxing W, Zhiyong W. Intraprostatic local anesthesia with periprostatic nerve block for transrectal ultrasound guided prostate biopsy. J Urol. 2009;182(2):479–83 discussion 483-474.
6. Ukimura O, Coleman JA, de la Taille A, Emberton M, Epstein JI, Freedland SJ, Giannarini G, Kibel AS, Montironi R, Ploussard G, et al. Contemporary role of systematic prostate biopsies: indications, techniques, and implications for patient care. Eur Urol. 2013;63(2):214 30.
7. Anup K, Pawan V, Niraj K, Biswajit N, Nayan MK. A prospective randomized trial comparing three different analgesic techniques for pain control during transrectal ultrasound guided prostate biopsy: a single center experience. Minerva urologica e nefrologica = The Italian journal of urology and nephrology. 2013;65(1):77–82.
8. Otunctemur A, Dursun M, Besiroglu H, Can Polat E, Cakir SS, Ozbek E, Karadeniz T. The effectivity of periprostatic nerve blockade for the pain control during transrectal ultrasound guided prostate biopsy. Archivio italiano di urologia, andrologia : organo ufficiale [di] Societa italiana di ecografia urologica e nefrologica / Associazione ricerche in urologia. 2013; 85(2):69–72.
9. Wang J, Wang L, Du Y, He D, Chen X, Li L, Nan X, Fan J. Addition of intrarectal local analgesia to periprostatic nerve block improves pain control for transrectal ultrasonography-guided prostate biopsy: a systematic review and meta-analysis. Int J Urol. 2015;22(1):62–8.
10. Wang N, Fu Y, Ma H, Wang J, Gao Y. Advantages of caudal block over intrarectal local anesthesia plus periprostatic nerve block for transrectal ultrasound guided prostate biopsy. Pakistan journal of medical sciences. 2016;32(4):978–82.
11. Nash PA, Bruce JE, Indudhara R, Shinohara K. Transrectal ultrasound guided prostatic nerve blockade eases systematic needle biopsy of the prostate. J Urol. 1996;155(2):607–9.
12. Conde Redondo C, Alonso Fernandez D, Robles Samaniego A, Del Valle Gonzalez N, Castroviejo Royo F, Delgado Marcos C, Rodriguez Toves A, Martinez-Sagarra Oceja JM. TRUS-guided biopsy: comparison of two anesthetic methods. Actas Urol Esp. 2006;30(2):134–8.
13. Hergan L, Kashefi C, Parsons JK. Local anesthetic reduces pain associated with transrectal ultrasound-guided prostate biopsy: a meta-analysis. Urology. 2007;69(3):520–5.
14. Luan Y, Huang TB, Gu X, Zhou GC, Lu SM, Tao HZ, Liu BD, Ding XF. Effect of prostate volume on the peripheral nerve block anesthesia in the prostate biopsy: a strobe-compliant study. Medicine. 2016;95(28):e4184.
15. Leibovici D, Shilo Y, Raz O, Stav K, Sandbank J, Segal M, Zisman A. Is the diagnostic yield of prostate needle biopsies affected by prostate volume? Urol Oncol. 2013;31(7):1003–5.
16. Kaver I, Mabjeesh NJ, Matzkin H. Randomized prospective study of periprostatic local anesthesia during transrectal ultrasound-guided prostate biopsy. Urology. 2002;59(3):405–8.
17. Konyalioglu E, Tarhan H, Cakmak O, Pala EE, Zorlu F. Prostate cancer volume estimations based on transrectal ultrasonography-guided biopsy in order to predict clinically significant prostate cancer. Int Braz J Urol. 2015;41(3):442–8.
18. Nguyen CT, Jones JS. Comparison of traditional basal and apical periprostatic block: impact on injection pain and biopsy pain. BJU Int. 2007; 99(3):575–8.
19. Cantiello F, Cicione A, Autorino R, Cosentino C, Amato F, Damiano R. Pelvic plexus block is more effective than periprostatic nerve block for pain control during office transrectal ultrasound guided prostate biopsy: a single center, prospective, randomized, double arm study. J Urol. 2012;188(2):417–21.
20. Jindal T, Mukherjee S, Sinha RK, Kamal MR, Ghosh N, Saha B, Mitra N, Sharma PK, Mandal SN, Karmakar D. Transrectal ultrasonography (TRUS)-guided pelvic plexus block to reduce pain during prostate biopsy: a randomised controlled trial. BJU Int. 2015;115(6):892–6.
21. Akpinar H, Tufek I, Atug F, Esen EH, Kural AR. Doppler ultrasonography-guided pelvic plexus block before systematic needle biopsy of the prostate: a prospective randomized study. Urology. 2009;74(2):267–271 e261.
22. Wu CL, Carter HB, Naqibuddin M, Fleisher LA. Effect of local anesthetics on patient recovery after transrectal biopsy. Urology. 2001;57(5):925–9.
23. Robins D, Lipsky M, RoyChoudry A, Wenske S. Assessment of discomfort and pain in patients undergoing fusion magnetic resonance imaging-guided vs TRUS-guided prostate biopsy. Urology. 2018;116:30–4.
24. Doganca T, Savsin A, Erdogan S, Altindas F, Ozdemir F, Ekici B, Obek C. Procedural sedation and analgesia as an adjunct to periprostatic nerve block for prostate biopsy: a prospective randomized trial. J Clin Ultrasound. 2015;43(5):288–94.
25. Choi JW, Kim WH, Lee CJ, Sim WS, Park S, Chae HB. The optimal approach for a superior hypogastric plexus block. Pain practice : the official journal of World Institute of Pain. 2017.
26. Schlegel PN, Walsh PC. Neuroanatomical approach to radical cystoprostatectomy with preservation of sexual function. J Urol. 1987;138(6): 1402–6.

30

Meta-analysis of the efficacy and safety of combination of tamsulosin plus dutasteride compared with tamsulosin monotherapy in treating benign prostatic hyperplasia

Zhongbao Zhou[1,2†], Yuanshan Cui[2†], Jitao Wu[2], Rui Ding[2], Tong Cai[1] and Zhenli Gao[2*]

Abstract

Background: We performed a meta-analysis to confirm the efficacy and safety of the combination of tamsulosin plus dutasteride compared with tamsulosin monotherapy in treating benign prostatic hyperplasia (BPH) during a treatment cycle of at least 1 year.

Methods: Randomized controlled trials were searched by using MEDLINE, EMBASE, and the Cochrane Controlled Trials Register. Systematic review was carried out using the Preferred Reporting Items for Systematic Reviews and Meta-analyses. The data was evaluated and statistically analyzed by using RevMan version 5.3.0.

Results: Five studies including 4348 patients were studied. The analysis found that the combination group was significantly greater effect in international prostate symptom score (mean difference [MD], − 1.43; 95% confidence interval [CI], − 2.20 to − 0.66; $P = 0.0003$), prostate volume (MD, − 10.13; 95% CI, − 12.38 to − 7.88; $P < 0.00001$), transitional zone volume (MD, − 3.18; 95% CI, − 3.57 to − 2.79; $P<0.0001$), maximum urine flow rate (MD, 1.05; 95% CI, 0.82 to 1.29; $P < 0.00001$), prostate specific antigen (MD, − 0.54; 95% CI, − 0.80 to − 0.29; $P < 0.0001$) and post-void residual volume (MD, − 3.85; 95% CI, − 4.95 to − 2.76; $P < 0.00001$) compared with the tamsulosin group. In terms of safety, including adverse events (odds ratio [OR], 2.06; 95% CI, 1.34 to 3.17; $P = 0.001$), erectile dysfunction (OR, 2.24; 95% CI, 1.73 to 2.92; $P < 0.00001$), ejaculation disorder (OR, 3.37; 95% CI, 1.97 to 5.79; $P < 0.0001$), retrograde ejaculation (OR, 2.30; 95% CI, 1.08 to 4.93; $P = 0.03$), decreased libido (OR, 2.25; 95% CI, 1.53 to 3.31; $P < 0.0001$) and loss of libido (OR, 3.38; 95% CI, 1.94 to 5.88; $P<0.0001$), the combination group showed poor tolerance than the tamsulosin group with the exception of dizziness (OR, 1.16; 95% CI, 0.75 to 1.80; $P = 0.50$). The combination group significantly reduced the risk of clinical progression than the tamsulosin group especially in incidence of BPH-related symptom progression (OR, 0.56; 95% CI, 0.46 to 0.67; $P < 0.00001$) and acute urinary retention (OR, 0.61; 95% CI, 0.38 to 0.98; $P = 0.04$).

Conclusion: The combination of tamsulosin plus dutasteride provides a preferable therapeutic effect for BPH with a higher incidence of sexual side effects, but combination-therapy can markedly reduce risk of BPH-related symptom progression and acute urinary retention relative to tamsulosin monotherapy.

Keywords: Benign prostatic hyperplasia, Meta-analysis, Randomized controlled trials, Tamsulosin, Dutasteride

* Correspondence: 3446395106@qq.com
†Zhongbao Zhou and Yuanshan Cui are contributed equally to this work as co-first authors.
[2]Department of Urology, The Affiliated Yantai Yuhuangding Hospital of Qingdao University, Yantai, NO. 20 East Yuhuangding Road, Yantai 264000, Shandong, China
Full list of author information is available at the end of the article

Background

Benign Prostatic Hyperplasia (BPH) is a progressive disease that causes lower urinary tract symptoms (LUTS) which substantially affect quality of life for many patients [1, 2]. Men with BPH can result in more severe LUTS, as well as other symptoms and episodes such as reduction of urinary flow rate, increased incidence of urinary infection, acute urinary retention and increased incidence of surgery for BPH, which have a greater unpleasant impact on the patient's quality of life [3, 4].

Dihydrotestosterone (DHT) is the primary androgen responsible for the excessive growth of the prostate that is characteristic of BPH, which is converted from testosterone by the catalysis of 5α-reductase (5AR) in the prostate gland [5, 6]. Besides, 5AR can take part in steroid metabolism and have a tight interaction with the androgen receptor than testosterone [7]. The excessive expression of DHT would trigger the proliferation of prostate epithelial and mesenchymal cells and lead to the development of BPH [8].

5AR inhibitors (5ARI) can lower the serum concentration of DHT and control the development of prostate and the progression of BPH by inhibiting this enzyme [9]. Dutasteride, a selective inhibitor of the type 1 and type 2 5ARI, is the most frequently prescribed 5ARI [10]. However, the latest clinical trials have found that the effectiveness of dutasteride was limited by its side effects, mainly involving erectile dysfunction, ejaculation disorder and decreased libido [11]. Tamsulosin, as an efficient α1-blockers, improves dysuria and other BPH symptoms by selectively blocking α_1A-adrenergic receptor in the prostate to relax the smooth muscles of the prostate [12]. In view of the unique mechanism of tamsulosin and dutasteride, the combination of these two drugs was feasible and have already been examined in some clinical studies [13, 14]. At present, there is no evidence of evidence-based medicine to explain the advantages and disadvantages of the combination of tamsulosin plus dutasteride compared with tamsulosin monotherapy.

We performed a meta-analysis to confirm the efficacy and safety of the combination of tamsulosin plus dutasteride compared with tamsulosin monotherapy in treating BPH during a treatment cycle of at least 1 year.

Methods

Study design

Systematic review of randomized controlled trials (RCTs) was carried out using the preferred reporting items for systematic reviews and meta-analyses (PRISMA) checklist [15].

Search strategy

WE searched MEDLINE (1992 to Jul 2018), EMBASE (1995 to Jul 2018) and the Cochrane Controlled Trials Register to collect studies investigating the combination of tamsulosin plus dutasteride versus tamsulosin alone in treating BPH. The search formula was as follows: "tamsulosin, dutasteride, BPH and RCT". All articles were browsed and read independently by two authors, and if there was any objections, it was referred to the third person for examination. The study was limited to published research with no restrictions on language. If the study was a review or summary presented at the meeting, it would be excluded. Authors were contacted to offer further information from their research if necessary. Furthermore, the search was also performed to investigate relevant references from the retrieved studies.

Inclusion criteria and trial selection

RCTs that met the following criteria were included: (1) The combination of tamsulosin plus dutasteride versus tamsulosin alone in treating BPH were evaluated; (2) Full-text content and related data can be obtained; (3) The study provided accurate data that could be analyzed, mainly including the total number of subjects and the valuable results of each indicator; (4) The article was a randomized controlled study; (5) Treatment duration is greater than or equal to 1 year. If the identical experiment was published in different journals or at different time, the latest study was included in the meta-analysis. If the same group of researchers studied a group of subjects with multiple experiments, then each study was included. The PRISMA flow diagram of study selection and elimination is shown in Fig. 1.

Quality assessment

The Jadad Scale was used to assess the quality of each RCT [16]. Additionally, the methods of quality assessment, including method of patient allocation, concealment of allocation, blinding method and number of lost to follow-up, were used to analyze the quality of individual study. Individual studies were assessed on the basis of guidelines published in the *Cochrane Handbook for Systematic Reviews of Interventions v5.10* [17]. Every article was evaluated and classified based on quality assessment criteria: (A) Satisfying almost all of the quality criteria, it would be considered to have a low probability of bias; (B) Ambiguous about one or more quality criteria, the study was considered to have a secondary probability of bias; or (C) Barely met the quality criteria, the study was considered to have a high probability of bias. All authors participated in the quality assessment of RCTs retrieved, eventually everyone agree with the results of the assessment. All authors participated in the quality assessment of RCTs retrieved. Differences regarding the quality assessment were resolved by discussion among the researchers.

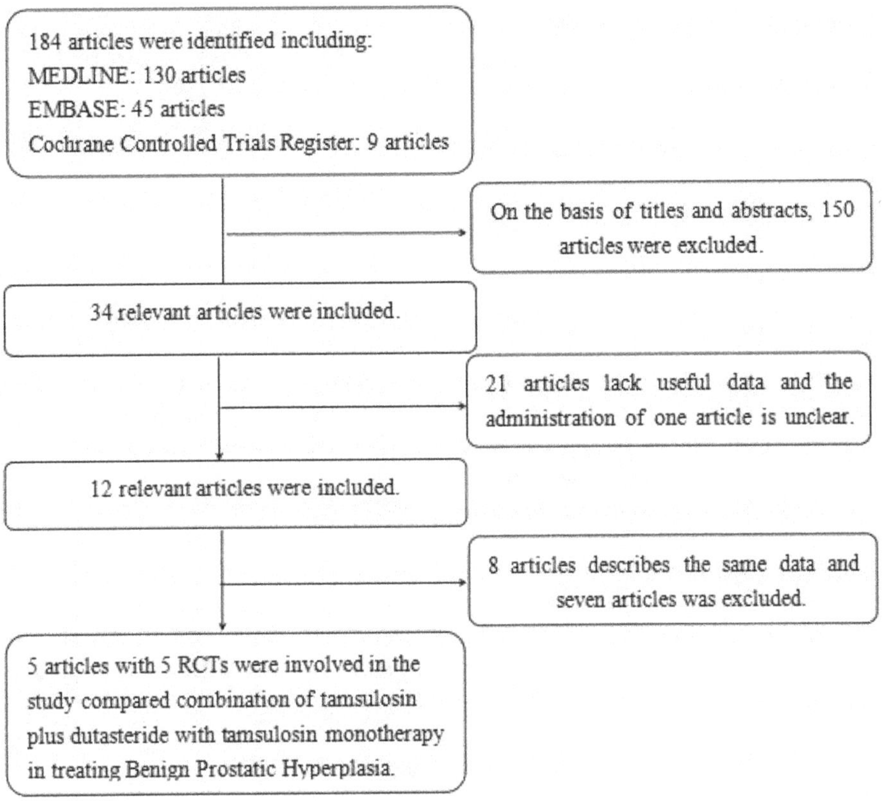

Fig. 1 Flowchart of the study selection process. RCT, randomizeda controlled trials

Data extraction

Two authors independently collected data from the articles based on predetermined criteria. The following information was collected for each study: (A) Publication time; (B) Name of first author; (C) Patient's received therapy; (D) Capacity of sample; (E) Data on international prostate symptom score (IPSS), prostate volume (PV), transitional zone volume (TZV), maximum urine flow rate (Qmax), prostate specific antigen (PSA), post-void residual volume (PVRV), adverse events (AEs), erectile dysfunction, ejaculation disorder, retrograde ejaculation, decreased libido, loss of libido, dizziness, BPH-related symptom progression, BPH-related acute urinary retention, BPH-related urinary incontinence, BPH-related urinary tract infection and BPH-related renal insufficiency. These results had clinical significance because they made a measurable impact at patients. No ethical approval was required for our study.

Statistical analyses and meta-analysis

The data was calculated by using RevMan version 5.3.0 (Cochrane Collaboration, Oxford, UK) [18]. We analyzed the data of the change of IPSS, PV, TZV, Qmax, PVRV and PSA between the combination of tamsulosin plus dutasteride and tamsulosin monotherapy in treating BPH. In addition, we also analyzed the number of AEs, erectile dysfunction, ejaculation disorder, retrograde ejaculation, decreased libido, loss of libido, dizziness, BPH-related symptom progression, BPH-related acute urinary retention, BPH-related urinary incontinence, BPH-related urinary tract infection and BPH-related renal insufficiency. Fixed and random effects models were used to evaluate the study. Mean difference (MD) was used to access continuous data and the odds ratio (OR) for dichotomous results with the corresponding 95% confidence interval [CI] [18]. The result of analysis showed p-value>0.05, we considered the study to be homogeneous and fixed-effect model was used to the analysis. We analyzed inconsistency using the I^2 statistic which reflected the proportion of heterogeneity across trails. A random effect model is used for results where the I^2 value is greater than 50%. If p-value was less than 0.05, we thought it's statistically significant.

Results

Characteristics of individual studies

Our search strategy found 184 articles. Reviewing abstracts and titles, we excluded 150 articles. With the remaining 34 articles, 21 articles were excluded due to lack of effective data and one article [19] on drug management is not clear. 8 articles described the same data and 7 articles was excluded. Finally, 5 articles containing

5 RCTs [20–24] were included in our study to analyze the combination of tamsulosin plus dutasteride versus tamsulosin alone in treating BPH during a treatment cycle of at least 1 year. The details of individual study were counted in Table 1. Patients with symptomatic BPH included in each study showed similar evaluation indicators. The baseline characteristics of the population included were showed in Table 2.

Quality of the individual studies

All studies included in the analysis were the random control study, and two studies [21, 24] specified a random protocol. Four studies [20–23] had a appropriate calculation of sample size and one study [24] did not calculate the sample size. Two studies [22, 23] showed an intention-to-treat analysis. However, in all studies, the specific methods of blind did not explicitly explaining with their Jadad scores rating B. All studies were included in the analysis regardless of the grade of quality (Table 3). The plot was highly symmetrical and five squares were contained in the large triangle, and no evidence of bias was found (Fig. 2).

Efficacy

IPSS

Four RCTs enrolling 4274 participants were used to analyze the change of IPSS. The higher heterogeneity was found among studies ($P = 0.0003$, I2 = 77%). The forest plots indicated a greater decrease for IPSS in the combination group compared with the tamsulosin group (MD -1.43, 95% CI -2.20 to – 0.66, $P = 0.0003$) (Fig. 3a).

PV

Three RCTs enrolling 3532 participants were used to analyze the change of PV. The higher heterogeneity was found among studies ($P<0.00001$, $I^2 = 94\%$). The combination group was significantly superior to the tamsulosin group in reducing PV (MD -10.13, 95% CI -12.38 to – 7.88, $P<0.00001$) (Fig. 3b).

TZV

Two RCTs enrolling 311 participants were chosen in the analysis of the change of TZV. The combination group was significantly superior to the tamsulosin group in reducing TZV (MD -3.18, 95% CI -3.57 to – 2.79, $P<0.00001$) (Fig. 3c).

Qmax

Three RCTs enrolling 3532 participants contained data on the Qmax. A fixed-effects model showed a marked differences between the combination group and the tamsulosin group in improving Qmax (MD 1.05, 95% CI 0.82 to 1.29, $P<0.00001$) with the lower risk of heterogeneity ($P = 0.63$, $I^2 = 0\%$) (Fig. 4a).

PSA and PVRV

Two RCTs enrolling 311 participants was extracted on data related to PSA and PVRV. The combination group was obviously superior to the tamsulosin group in lowering PSA (MD -0.54, 95%CI -0.80 to – 0.29, $P<0.0001$) (Fig. 4b) and PVRV (MD -3.85, 95%CI -4.95 to – 2.76, $P<0.00001$) (Fig. 4c).

Safety

AEs

Four RCTs containing a sample size of 4230 participants evaluated the incidence of AEs. The meta-analysis showed a significant distinction between the combination group and tamsulosin group in the rate of AEs across four studies (OR 2.06, 95% CI 1.34 to 3.17, $P = 0.001$) (Fig. 5a).

Erectile dysfunction

Four RCTs including 4230 participants accessed the severity of erectile dysfunction. A fixed-effects model showed a obvious significance between the combination group and tamsulosin group in the rate of erectile dysfunction (OR 2.24, 95% CI 1.73 to 2.92, $P<0.00001$) (Fig. 5b).

Ejaculation disorder

Three RCTs including 4037 participants analyzed the severity of ejaculation disorder. A fixed-effects model showed a statistical significance between the combination group and tamsulosin group in the occurrence rate of ejaculation disorder (OR 3.37, 95% CI 1.97 to 5.79, $P<0.0001$) (Fig. 6a).

Retrograde ejaculation

Three RCTs including 4156 participants contained data on retrograde ejaculation. A random-effects model showed a larger number in the combination group compared with tamsulosin group in the occurrence of retrograde ejaculation (OR 3.37, 95% CI 1.97 to 5.79, $P<0.0001$) (Fig. 6b).

Decreased libido

Four RCTs including 4230 participants contained data on decreased libido. The combination group had a larger number in the decreased libido (OR 2.25, 95% CI 1.53 to 3.31, $P<0.0001$) (Fig. 7a) compared with tamsulosin group.

Loss of libido

Two RCTs containing a sample size of 3963 participants accessed the severity of loss of libido. A fixed-effects model showed a significantly higher incidence in the combination group compared with tamsulosin group in the occurrence of loss of libido (OR 3.38, 95% CI 1.94 to 5.88, $P<0.0001$) (Fig. 7b).

Table 1 The details of individual study

Study	Therapy in experimental group	Therapy in control group	Sample size		method	Follow-up time (month)	Dosage (mg/mg)	Main inclusion criteria	Main exclusion criteria
			experimental	control					
Hong et al. (2010) [20]	tamsulosin plus dutasteride	tamsulosin	37	37	Oral	12	0.2mg + 0.5mg/ 0.2mg	Men aged 45–75 years with moderate to severe symptomatic BPH, IPSS > 7, Qmax < 15 mL/s, PV ≥30 mL on TRUS, PSA < 10 ng/mL.	Previous treatment with a 5ARI or other hormonal drugs, endocrine disorder including diabetes mellitus, previous prostatic surgery within the past year.
Joo et al. (2012) [21]	tamsulosin plus dutasteride	tamsulosin	98	95	Oral	12	0.2mg + 0.5mg/ 0.2mg	Age ≥ 40 years with diagnosis of BPH, IPSS ≥13, Qmax of 4–15 ml/s in a total voided volume ≥ 150 ml.	Patients had been treated previously for BPH, diagnosed with prostate cancer, bladder cancer or other progressive diseases that could cause LUTS; PVR > 200 ml.
Roehrborn et al. (2014) [22]	tamsulosin plus dutasteride	tamsulosin	1610	1611	Oral	48	0.4mg + 0.5mg/ 0.4mg	Patients ≥50 years of age with diagnosis of BPH, IPSS ≥12, PV ≥30 mL, serum PSA ≥1.5 ng/mL, and Qmax > 5 mL/s and ≤ 15 mL/s with a minimum voided volume ≥ 125 mL.	Serum PSA > 10 ng/mL, history of prostate cancer and previous prostatic surgery, history of AUR within 3 months before entry, 5ARI use within 6 months before entry, or use of α-blocker within 2 weeks before entry.
Roehrborn et al. (2015) [23]	tamsulosin plus dutasteride	tamsulosin	369	373	Oral	24	0.4mg + 0.5mg/ 0.4mg	Men aged ≥50 years with diagnosis of BPH and moderate LUTS, IPSS of 8–19, PV ≥30 cc by TRUS and serum PSA ≥1.5 ng/ml.	Serum PSA > 10.0 ng/ml, history or evidence of prostate cancer and any current or prior treatment related to BPH.
Choi et al. (2016) [24]	tamsulosin plus dutasteride	tamsulosin	59	59	Oral	12	0.2mg + 0.5mg/ 0.2mg	Age ≥ 40, PV > 30 ml, IPSS ≥13, Qmax of 4–15 ml/s for a total voided volume of ≥150 ml, and no medical history relating to BPH during the previous 12 months.	Patients had allergies to α-blocker, conditions other than BPH that could induce LUTS, progressive diseases, or severe hepatic or renal dysfunction, PVR > 200 ml or serum PSA > 4 ng/ml.

BPH Benign Prostatic Hyperplasia, *IPSS* International Prostate Symptom Score, *5ARI* 5-Alpha Reductase Inhibitor, *Qmax* maximum urine flow rate, *PSA* Prostate Specific Antigen, *PV* Prostate Volume, *PVR* Post-Void Residual, *TRUS* Transrectal ultrasonography, *LUTS* Lower Urinary Tract Symptoms, *AUR* Acute Urinary Retention

Table 2 The baseline characteristics of individual study

Study	Group	Age (years)	BMI (kg/m^2)	PV (ml)	PSA (ng/ml)	IPSS	Qmax (ml/s)	PVR (ml)
Hong et al. (2010) [20]	Combination	66.60 ± 7.10	24.90 ± 3.00	≥ 30	3.0 ± 3.90	> 7	< 15	unmentioned
	Tamsulosin	65.70 ± 8.50	24.60 ± 2.30		2.6 ± 2.30			
Joo et al. (2012) [21]	Combination	65.85 ± 7.77	unmentioned	37.26 ± 13.22	1.77 ± 1.40	19.94 ± 6.14	11.13 ± 5.08	49.16 ± 23.52
	Tamsulosin	65.79 ± 8.87		36.63 ± 13.16	1.70 ± 1.23	19.95 ± 5.54	11.32 ± 5.77	49.19 ± 22.04
Roehrborn et al. (2014) [22]	Combination	66.00 ± 7.05	unmentioned	54.7 ± 23.51	4.00 ± 2.05	16.60 ± 6.35	10.90 ± 3.61	68.20 ± 66.12
	Tamsulosin	66.20 ± 7.00		55.8 ± 24.18	4.00 ± 2.08	16.40 ± 6.10	10.70 ± 3.66	67.70 ± 65.14
Roehrborn et al. (2015) [23]	Combination	66.30 ± 7.78	27.28 ± 3.53	51.0 ± 18.17	3.90 ± 2.00	13.20 ± 4.06	unmentioned	unmentioned
	Tamsulosin	66.20 ± 7.34	27.94 ± 3.77	52.6 ± 19.57	3.70 ± 1.91	12.90 ± 3.95		
Choi et al. (2016) [24]	Combination	61.86 ± 1.26	unmentioned	41.05 ± 2.67	1.31 ± 0.15	20.04 ± 0.62	11.81 ± 0.29	31.08 ± 2.76
	Tamsulosin	61.94 ± 1.23		40.34 ± 1.43	1.35 ± 0.12	19.09 ± 0.60	11.40 ± 0.38	31.00 ± 3.44

Data presented as mean ± SD
IPSS International Prostate Symptom Score, *Qmax* maximum urine flow rate, *PSA* Prostate Specific Antigen, *PV* Prostate Volume, *PVR* Post-Void Residual, *BMI* Body Mass Index

Dizziness

Three RCTs with a sample of 4156 participants accessed the incidence of dizziness. The combination group had a similar number on the dizziness (OR 1.16, 95% CI 0.75 to 1.80, $P = 0.50$) (Fig. 7c) compared with tamsulosin group.

BPH clinical progression after drug administration

Two RCTs with a enough sample size of 3963 participants accessed the extent of BPH clinical progression after drug administration. In view of BPH-related symptom progression, which was the most common progression event in each group, the study found the tamsulosin group had a larger number (OR 0.56, 95%CI 0.46 to 0.67, $P<0.00001$) (Fig. 8a) compared with the combination group.

In terms of BPH-related acute urinary retention, the tamsulosin group had a higher incidence than the combination group (OR 0.61, 95% CI 0.38 to 0.98, $P = 0.04$) (Fig. 8b). In other aspects of BPH-related clinical progression, mainly containing urinary incontinence, urinary tract infection and renal insufficiency, no significant differences were found between the two treatment groups (Fig. 8c, d, e).

Discussion

BPH is a progressive condition characterized by prostate growth accompanying LUTS and sexual dysfunction [25, 26]. Clinical treatment of BPH with 5ARIs and/or α1-blockers has been front-line treatment, and the two drugs showed different mechanisms of action to influence the progression of prostate [27]. Currently, European Association of Urology (EAU) guidelines recommend to offer combination treatment with an α1-blocker and a 5ARI to men with moderate-to-severe LUTS and an increased risk of disease progression (e.g. prostate volume > 40 mL) [28]. The latest prospective study found that the combination of tamsulosin plus dutasteride was more efficient than placebo in treating LUTS and may contribute to ejaculation disorders especially in sexually active men with BPH [14].

We performed this meta-analysis for five studies including 4348 participants to compare the efficacy and safety of the combination of tamsulosin plus dutasteride compared with tamsulosin monotherapy in treating BPH

Table 3 Quality assessment of individual study

Study	Allocation sequence generation	Allocation concealment	Blinding	Loss to follow-up	Calculation of sample size	Statistical analysis	Level of quality	ITT analysis
Hong et al. (2010) [20]	A	A	B	3	Yes	Mann-Whitney U-test; Chi-square test	A	No
Joo et al. (2012) [21]	A	A	B	unmentioned	Yes	Student's t-test; Pearson's x^2-test	A	No
Roehrborn et al. (2014) [22]	A	A	B	unmentioned	Yes	Mann-Whitney U-test; Chi-square test; T-tests	A	Yes
Roehrborn et al. (2015) [23]	A	A	B	16	Yes	T-tests	A	Yes
Choi et al. (2016) [24]	A	A	B	17	No	Mann-Whitney U-test	A	No

A, almost all quality criteria met: low risk of bias, B, one or more quality criteria met:moderate risk of bias; C, one or more criteria not met: high risk of bias; ITT, intention-to-treat

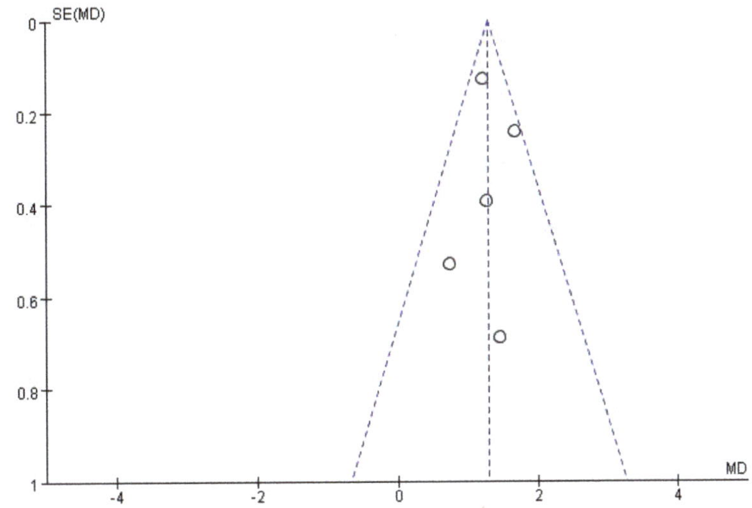

Fig. 2 Funnel plot of the studies included in our meta-analysis. MD, mean difference; SE, standard error

during a treatment cycle of at least 1 year. The analysis demonstrated that the combination-therapy had greater decrease than the monotherapy in aspects of IPSS, PV, TZV and PVRV. Three RCTs containing data on Qmax showed a marked improvement in the combination therapy relative to the tamsulosin group. Overall, the results suggested that combination therapy of tamsulosin plus dutasteride was more effective than tamsulosin monotherapy in patients seeking improvement in symptoms.

Deslypere et al. [29] found that the progress of BPH were inseparable from the vary of DHT which has a high affinity for androgen receptor and an inhibitory effect on testosterone. Previous studies have suggested that the most popular combination therapy which was found to

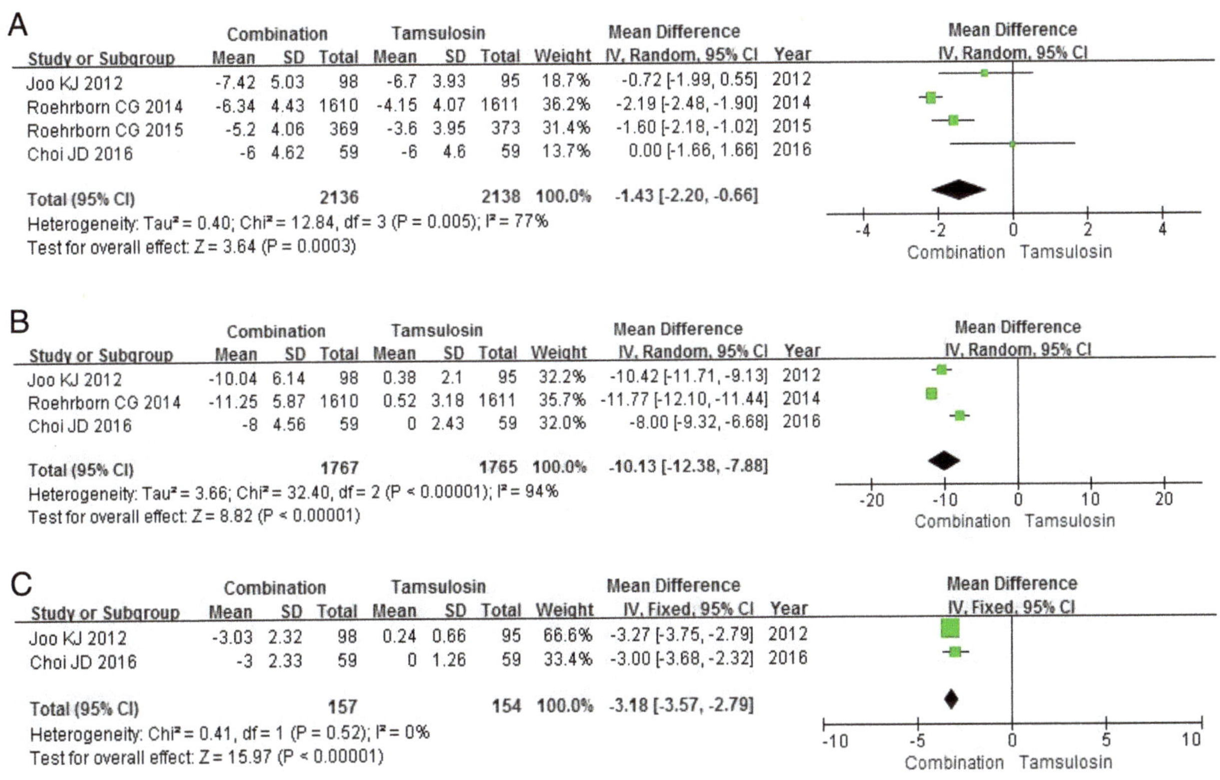

Fig. 3 Forest plots showing changes in (**a**) international prostate symptom score; (**b**) prostate volume; (**c**) transitional zone volume; SD, standard deviation; IV, inverse variance; CI, confidence interval; df, degrees of freedom

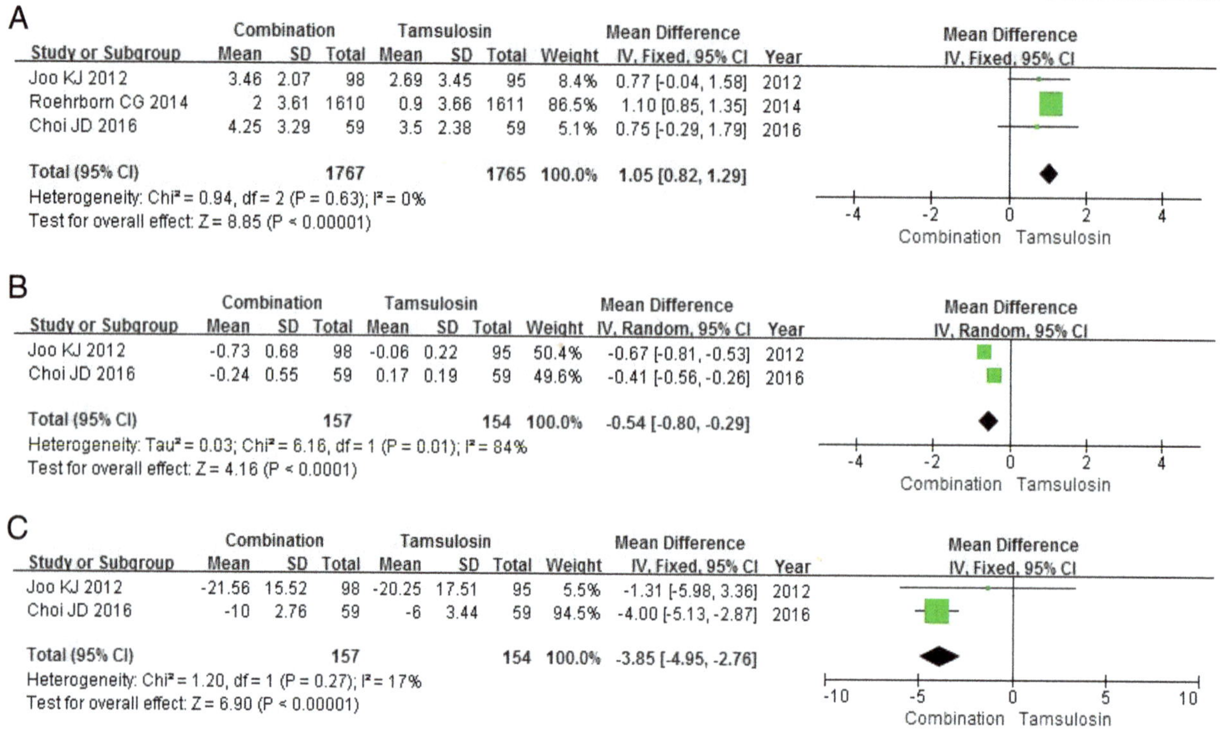

Fig. 4 Forest plots showing changes in (**a**) maximum urine flow rate; (**b**) prostate specific antigen; (**c**) post-void residual volume; SD, standard deviation; IV, inverse variance; CI, confidence interval; df, degrees of freedom

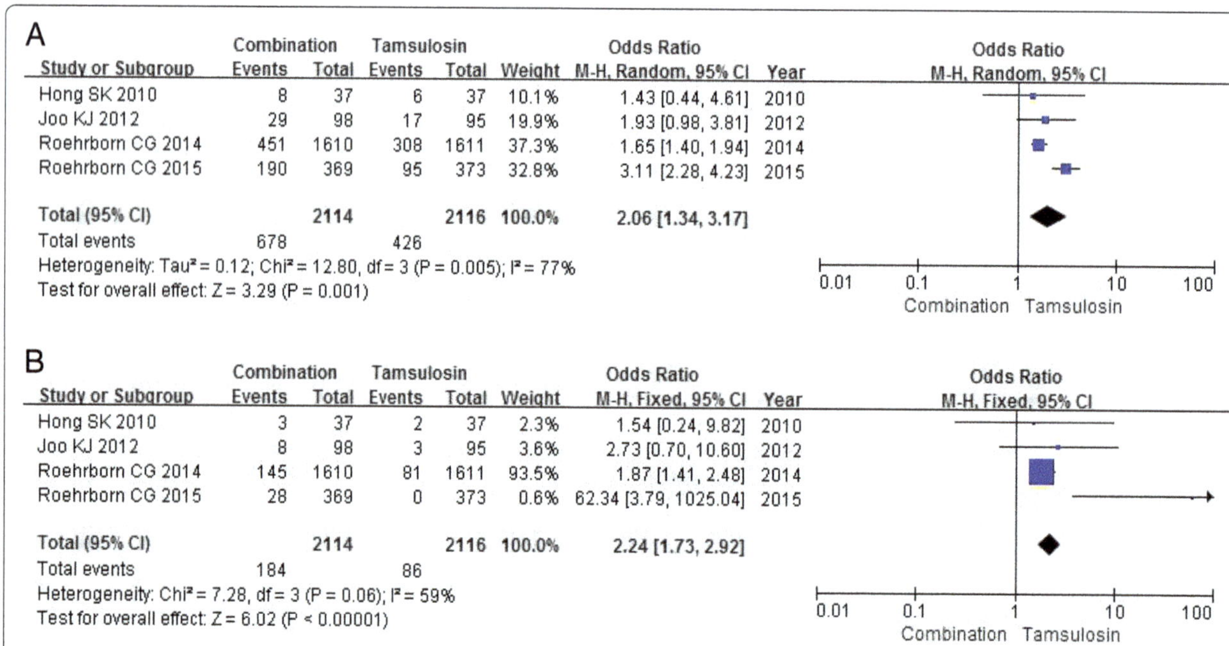

Fig. 5 Forest plots showing numbers in (**a**) adverse Events; (**b**) erectile dysfunction; M-H, Mantel-Haenszel; CI, confidence interval; df, degrees of freedom

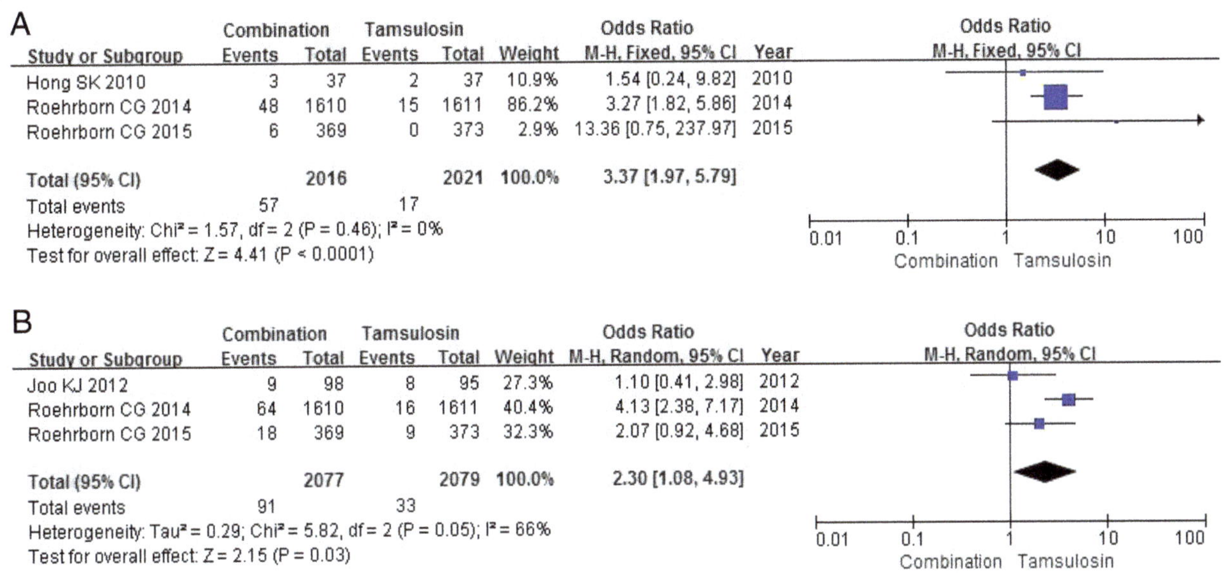

Fig. 6 Forest plots showing numbers in (**a**) ejaculation disorder; (**b**) retrograde ejaculation; M-H, Mantel-Haenszel; CI, confidence interval; df, degrees of freedom

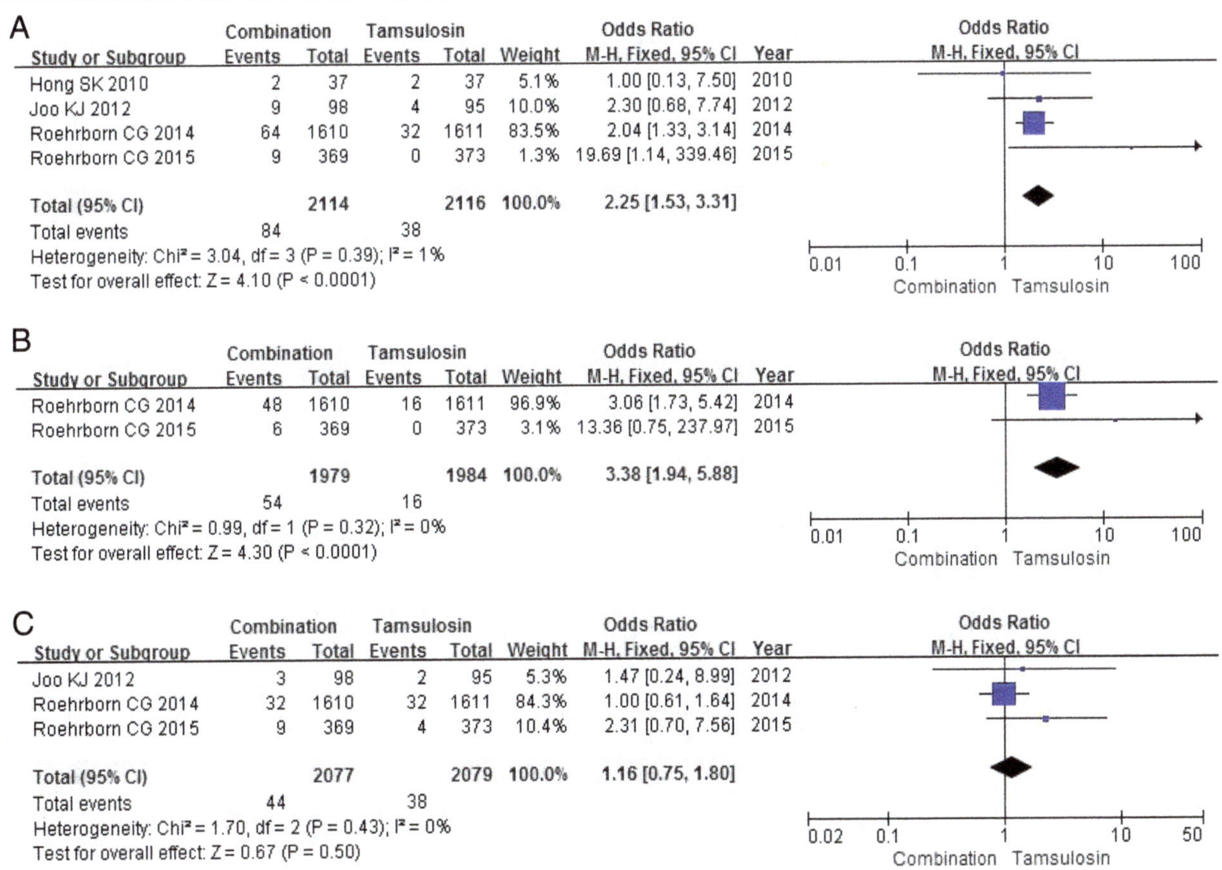

Fig. 7 Forest plots showing numbers in (**a**) decreased libido; (**b**) loss of libido; (C) dizziness; M-H, Mantel-Haenszel; CI, confidence interval; df, degrees of freedom

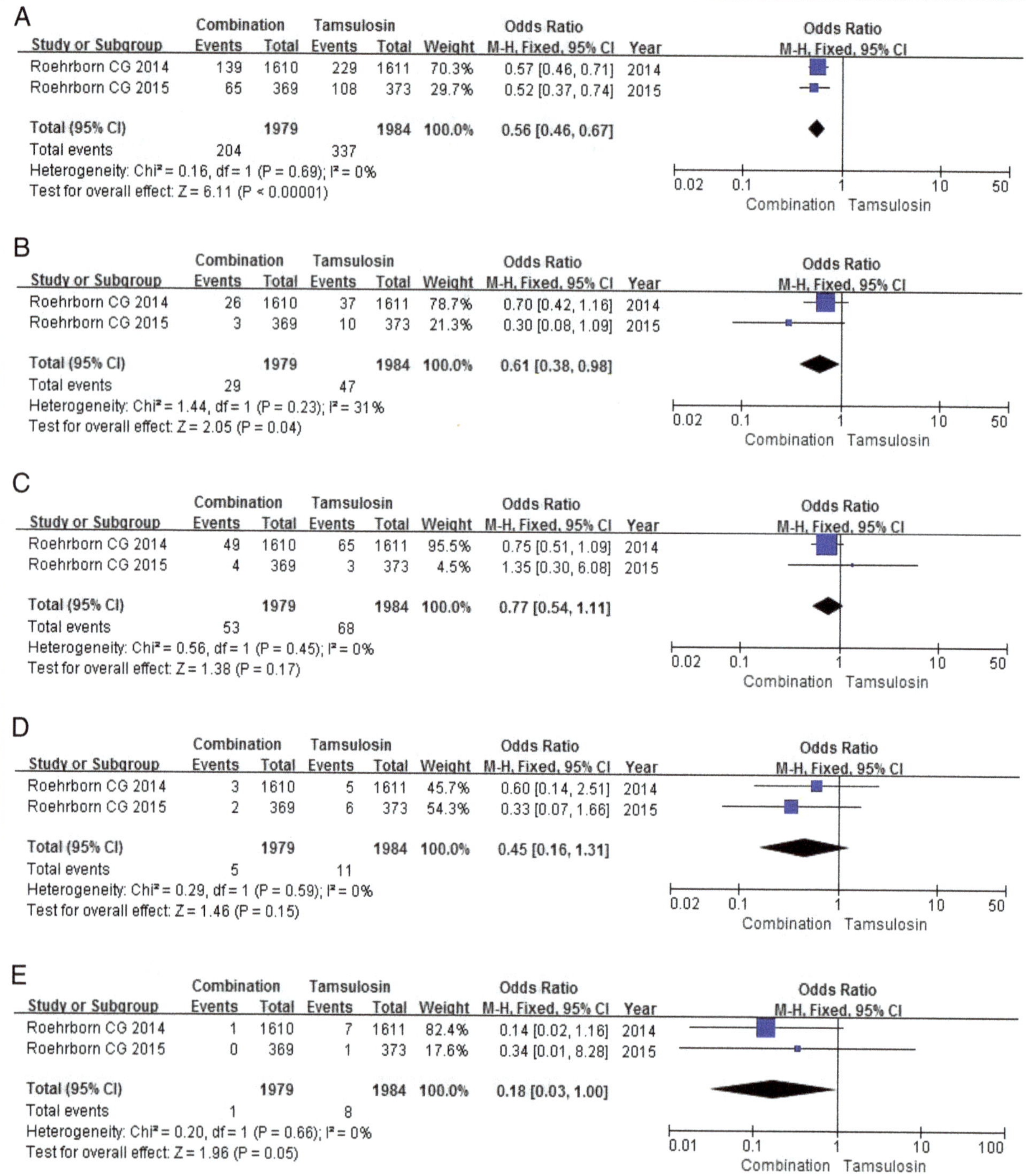

Fig. 8 Forest plots showing numbers in (**a**) BPH-related symptom progression; (**b**) BPH-related acute urinary retention; (**c**) BPH-related urinary incontinence; (**d**) BPH-related urinary tract infection; (**e**) BPH-related renal insufficiency; M-H, Mantel-Haenszel; CI, confidence interval; df, degrees of freedom

offer a statistically significant improvement than monotherapy was finasteride plus tamsulosin [30]. Currently, dutasteride inhibits two subtypes of 5AR, and has a 45 times greater affinity for type I and a 2.5 times greater affinity for type II than finasteride. As a result of this higher affinity, dutasteride effectively inhibits DHT much more rapidly than finasteride [31, 32]. Our study found that dutasteride can also be used as an effective ingredient in combination medication, which may be even superior to past management. Further clinical studies are needed to explain the effect of different combination of drug on treating BPH.

For safety, including AEs, erectile dysfunction, ejaculation disorder, retrograde ejaculation, decreased libido, loss of libido, the combination group had a higher incidence than the tamsulosin group with the exception of dizziness. These results stated that the physician should explain to patients potential side effects of long-term combination of tamsulosin plus dutasteride treatment before adopting this treatment. One study showed that long-term dutasteride therapy produced worsening of erectile dysfunction, reduced testosterone levels, increased glucose and altered lipid profiles, suggesting induced imbalance of metabolic function and deterioration of gonadal function [33]. Manohar et al. demonstrated that tamsulosin had a better effective in alleviating BPH symptoms and frequently produced a variety of adverse reactions, such as dizziness, decreased blood pressure, increased heart rate, occasional abdominal pain, nausea and allergic reactions [34].

Two RCTs containing data on PSA demonstrated the combination group was obviously superior to the tamsulosin group in reducing serum PSA level. Reviewing pharmacological effect, 5ARI may cause the degradation of prostate tissue which is the major source of serum PSA, and inhibition of DHT by 5ARI indirectly lowered serum PSA levels [35]. Usually, PSA is a commonly used screening indicator for the diagnosis of prostate cancer. Schröder et al. have shown that long-term use of 5ARI can result in low PSA levels, which can lead to a significant reduction in the relevance ratio of prostate cancer and increase the rate of misdiagnosis [36]. Our analysis found that the combination group may be noteworthy in reducing diagnostic ratio of prostate cancer. If PSA has a significant change during the treatment of combination for patients suffering from BPH, we need to think about more possibilities.

About clinical progression after drug administration, the combination therapy can markedly lower risk of BPH-related symptom progression and acute urinary retention than tamsulosin monotherapy. In other BPH-related clinical progression, involving urinary incontinence, urinary tract infection and renal insufficiency, no significant differences were found among two treatment groups. Tamsulosin can selectively block α1-adrenergic receptor in the prostate to relax the smooth muscles of the prostate, expanding the prostatic part of the urethra, changing the symptoms of urinary and reducing the possibility of acute urinary retention [12]. Correspondingly, 5ARI inhibits the growth of PV by suppressing the generation of DHT and relieves pressure on the urethra from the large prostate gland [31]. Eventually, The corporate action of the two drugs results in a reduced risk of clinical progression.

Besides, the CombAT study [22] showed that the combination of tamsulosin plus dutasteride is more effective to monotherapy in improving clinical symptoms (IPSS difference 0.4) and urine flow rate starting from the treatment of nine months, and superior to tamsulosin in reducing the incidence of urinary retention (68%) and surgery (71%) starting from the treatment of eight months. Above all, the combination of tamsulosin plus dutasteride provides a preferable therapeutic effect for BPH with a higher incidence of sexual side effects, but the combination therapy can markedly reduce risk of BPH-related symptom progression and acute urinary retention relative to tamsulosin monotherapy.

Our meta-analysis involved five RCTs and the quality of each RCT was high. We could not acquire the long-term efficacy and tolerance of combination therapy, and selection bias, subjective factors and publication bias may also affect the final results of our study. So it still needs a lot of RCTs including sufficient sample size and statistics to confirm our findings. More high-quality RCTs with suitable study cohorts are needed to ascertain the efficacy and tolerance of combination of tamsulosin plus dutasteride and tamsulosin monotherapy in treating BPH.

Conclusions

This meta-analysis suggests that the combination of tamsulosin plus dutasteride provides a preferable therapeutic effect for BPH with a higher incidence of sexual side effects, but the combination therapy can markedly reduce risk of BPH-related symptom progression and acute urinary retention relative to tamsulosin monotherapy.

Abbreviations

5AR: 5α-reductase; 5ARI: 5α-reductase inhibitors; AEs: Adverse events; BPH: benign prostatic hyperplasia; CI: Confidence interval; DHT: Dihydrotestosterone; EAU: European Association of Urology; IPSS: International prostate symptom score; LUTS: Lower urinary tract symptoms; MD: Mean difference; OR: Odds ratio; PRISMA: Preferred reporting items for systematic reviews and meta-analyses; PSA: Prostate specific antigen; PV: Prostate volume; PVRV: Post-void residual volume; Qmax: Maximum urine flow rate; RCTs: Randomized controlled trials; TZV: Transitional zone volume

Acknowledgements

Not applicable.

Authors' contributions

GZL designed the research, interpreted the data and revised the paper. ZZB, CYS, WJT, DR and CT performed the data extraction, carried out the meta-analysis and drafted the paper. All authors contributed substantial intellectual contributions and approved the final version of the manuscript.

Author details

[1]Binzhou Medical University, Yantai, Shandong, China. [2]Department of Urology, The Affiliated Yantai Yuhuangding Hospital of Qingdao University, Yantai, NO. 20 East Yuhuangding Road, Yantai 264000, Shandong, China.

References

1. Bushman W. Etiology, epidemiology, and natural history of benign prostatic hyperplasia. Urol Clin North Am. 2009;36(4):403–15.
2. Woodard TJ, Manigault KR, McBurrows NN, et al. Management of Benign Prostatic Hyperplasia in older adults. Consult Pharm. 2016;31(8):412–24.
3. Anderson JB, Roehrborn CG, Schalken JA, et al. The progression of benign prostatic hyperplasia: examining the evidence and determining the risk. Eur Urol. 2001;39:390–9.
4. AUA Practice Guidelines Committee. AUA guideline on management of benign prostatic hyperplasia. J Urol. 2003;170:530–47.
5. Banerjee PP, Banerjee S, Brown TR, et al. Androgen action in prostate function and disease. Am J Clin Exp Urol. 2018;6(2):62–77.
6. Finn DA, Beadles-Bohling AS, Beckley EH, et al. A new look at the 5alpha-reductase inhibitor finasteride. CNS Drug Rev. 2006;12:53–76.
7. Welen K, Damber JE. Prostate diseases--role of sex steroids and their inhibitors. Best Pract Res Clin Endocrinol Metab. 2011;25(2):355–67.
8. Griffiths K, Eaton CL, Harper ME, et al. Steroid hormones and the pathogenesis of benign prostatic hyperplasia. Eur Urol. 1991;20(Suppl 1):68–77.
9. Naslund M, Regan TS, Ong C, et al. 5-alpha reductase inhibitors in men with an enlarged prostate: an evaluation of outcomes and therapeutic alternatives. Am J Manag Care. 2008;14(5 Suppl 2):S148–53.
10. Roehrborn CG, Boyle P, Nickel JC, et al. Efficacy and safety of a dual inhibitor of 5-alpha-reductase types 1 and 2 (dutasteride) in men with benign prostatic hyperplasia. Urology. 2002;60:434–41.
11. Kiguradze T, Temps WH, Yarnold PR, et al. Persistent erectile dysfunction in men exposed to the 5α-reductase inhibitors, finasteride, or dutasteride. Peer J. 2017;5:e3020.
12. Yanase H, Wang X, Momota Y, et al. The involvement of urothelial alpha1A adrenergic receptor in controlling the micturition reflex. Biomed Res. 2008;29(5):239–44.
13. Fossler MJ, Collins DA, Thompson MM, et al. Pharmacokinetic bioequivalence studies of a fixed-dose combination of tamsulosin and dutasteride in healthy volunteers. Clin Drug Investig. 2014;34(5):335–49.
14. Roehrborn CG, Manyak MJ, Palacios-Moreno JM, et al. A prospective randomised placebo-controlled study of the impact of dutasteride/tamsulosin combination therapy on sexual function domains in sexually active men with lower urinary tract symptoms (LUTS) secondary to benign prostatic hyperplasia (BPH). BJU Int. 2018;121(4):647–58.
15. Moher D, Liberati A, Tetzlaff J, et al. Preferred reporting items for systematic reviews and meta-analyses: the PRISMA statement. Ann Intern Med. 2009;151:264–9.
16. Jadad AR. Randomised controlled trials. London: BMJ Publishing Group; 1998.
17. Higgins JP, Green S, editors. Cochrane handbook for systematic reviews of interventions. version 5.1.0 [Internet]. The Cochrane Collaboration, 2011 [uptated 2011 Mar; cited 2017 May 10]. Available from: https://onlinelibrary.wiley.com/doi/book/10.1002/9780470712184.
18. DerSimonian R, Laird N. Meta-analysis in clinical trials. Control Clin Trials. 1986;7(3):177–88.
19. Alcaraz A, Carballido-Rodríguez J, Unda-Urzaiz M, et al. Quality of life in patients with lower urinary tract symptoms associated with BPH: change over time in real-life practice according to treatment-the QUALIPROST study. Int Urol Nephrol. 2016;48(5):645–56.
20. Hong SK, Min GE, Ha SB, et al. Effect of the dual 5alpha-reductase inhibitor, dutasteride, on serum testosterone and body mass index in men with benign prostatic hyperplasia. BJU Int. 2010;105(7):970–4.
21. Joo KJ, Sung WS, Park SH, et al. Comparison of α-blocker monotherapy and α-blocker plus 5α-reductase inhibitor combination-therapy based on prostate volume for treatment of benign prostatic hyperplasia. J Int Med Res. 2012;40(3):899–908.
22. Roehrborn CG, Barkin J, Tubaro A, et al. Influence of baseline variables on changes in international prostate symptom score after combined therapy with dutasteride plus tamsulosin or either monotherapy in patients with benign prostatic hyperplasia and lower urinary tract symptoms: 4-year results of the CombAT study. BJU Int. 2014;113(4):623–35.
23. Roehrborn CG, Oyarzabal Perez I, Roos EP, et al. Efficacy and safety of a fixed dose combination of dutasteride and tamsulosin treatment (Duodart(®)) compared with watchful waiting with initiation of tamsulosin therapy if symptoms do not improve, both provided with lifestyle advice, in the management of treatment-naïve men with moderately symptomatic benign prostatic hyperplasia: 2-year CONDUCT study results. BJU Int. 2015;116(3):450–9.
24. Choi JD, Kim JH, Ahn SH. Transitional zone index as a predictor of the efficacy of α-blocker and 5α-reductase inhibitor combination therapy in Korean patients with benign prostatic hyperplasia. Urol Int. 2016;96(4):406–12.
25. Girman CJ. Population-based studies of the epidemiology of benign prostatic hyperplasia. Br J Urol. 1998;82(Suppl 1):34–43.
26. EmbertonM AGL, de la Rosette J, et al. Benign prostatic hyperplasia: a progressive disease of aging men. Urology. 2003;61:267–73.
27. Madersbacher S, Marszalek M, Lackner J, et al. The long-term outcome of medical therapy for BPH. Eur Urol. 2007;51:1522–33.
28. Oelke M, Bachmann A, Descazeaud A, et al. EAU guidelines on the treatment and follow-up of non-neurogenic male lower urinary tract symptoms including benign prostatic obstruction. Eur Urol. 2013;64(1):118–40.
29. Deslypere JP, Young M, Wilson JD, et al. Testosterone and 5alpha-dihydrotestosterone interact differently with the androgen receptor to enhance transcription of the MMTV-CAT reporter gene. Mol Cell Endocrinol. 1992;88:15–22.
30. Hutchison A, Farmer R, Verhamme K, et al. The efficacy of drugs for the treatment of LUTS/BPH, a study in 6 European countries. Eur Urol. 2007;51(1):207–15.
31. Shibata Y, Arai S, Miyazawa Y, et al. Effects of steroidal antiandrogen or 5-alpha-reductase inhibitor on prostate tissue hormone content. Prostate. 2017;77(6):672–80.
32. Evans HC, Goa KL. Dutasteride. Drugs Aging. 2003;20:905–18.
33. Traish A, Haider KS, Doros G, et al. Long-term dutasteride therapy in men with benign prostatic hyperplasia alters glucose and lipid profiles and increases severity of erectile dysfunction. Horm Mol Biol Clin Investig. 2017;30(3).
34. Manohar CMS, Nagabhushana M, Karthikeyan VS, et al. Safety and efficacy of tamsulosin, alfuzosin or silodosin as monotherapy for LUTS in BPH- a double-blind randomized trial. Cent European J Urol. 2017;70(2):148–53.
35. Guess HA, Gromley GJ, Stoner E, et al. The effect of finasteride on prostate specific antigen: review of available data. J Urol. 1996;155:3–9.
36. Schröder FH. Review of diagnostic markers for prostate cancer. Recent Results Cancer Res. 2009;181:173–82.

31

Where is the limit of prostate cancer biomarker research? Systematic investigation of potential prognostic and diagnostic biomarkers

Anika Kremer[1], Tobias Kremer[2], Glen Kristiansen[1†] and Yuri Tolkach[1*†]

Abstract

Background: The identification of appropriate biomarkers is essential to support important clinical decisions in patients with prostate cancer. The aim of our study was a systematic bioinformatical analysis of the mRNA expression of all genes available for the prostate adenocarcinoma cohort of The Cancer Genome Atlas (TCGA), regarding their potential prognostic and diagnostic role.

Methods: The study cohort comprises 499 patients (TCGA prostate cancer cohort). mRNA expression data were available for approx. 20,000 genes. The bioinformatical statistical pipeline addressed gene expression differences in tumor vs. benign prostate tissue (including gene set enrichment analysis, GSEA) in samples from tumors with different aggressivenesses (Gleason score), as well as prognostic values in multistep survival analyses.

Results: Among all genes analyzed, 1754 were significantly downregulated and 1553 genes were significantly upregulated in tumor tissue. In GSEA, 16 of 30 top enriched biological processes were alterations of epigenetic regulation at different levels. Significant correlation with Gleason Score was evident for 8724 genes (range of Pearson r-values 0.09–0.43; all $p < 0.05$). In univariate Cox regression analyses, mRNA expression of 3571 genes showed statistically significant association with biochemical recurrence-free survival with a range of hazard ratios 0.3–3.8 (p-value 7.4e− 07 to 0.05). Among these, 571 genes were independently associated with biochemical recurrence in multivariate analysis. Access to the full database including results is provided as supplement.

Conclusions: In our systematic analysis we found a big number of genes of potential diagnostic and prognostic value, many of which have not been studied in prostate cancer to date. Due to the comprehensive nature of this analysis and free access to the results, this study represents a reference database for prostate cancer researchers which can be used as a powerful tool for validation purposes and planning of new studies.

Keywords: Prostate cancer, Biomarkers, Bioinformatics, mRNA expression, Prognostic, Diagnostic

Background

Prostate cancer (PCa) is one of the most common cancers in men worldwide [1]. Once the prostate carcinoma is diagnosed, it is considered well treatable if recognized at an early stage. Though, over the past years, PCa therapy came into the focus of criticism due to its potential for overtreatment by e.g. radical prostatectomy [2, 3]. However, rendering reliable diagnoses and prognoses of the progression of the disease based on tumor grading and modern classifications is impeded by its high degree of morphological and molecular genetic heterogeneity [4, 5]. Therefore, its high rate of occurrence and frequent heterogeneity make PCa not only a crucial but also a complex and challenging research target in clinical and research settings.

The identification of appropriate biomarkers is therefore essential to drive important clinical decisions in patients with prostate cancer [6]. Hundreds

* Correspondence: yuri.tolkach@ukbonn.de
†Glen Kristiansen and Yuri Tolkach shared senior authors.
[1]Institute of Pathology, University Hospital of Bonn, Bonn, Germany
Full list of author information is available at the end of the article

of studies focusing on new biomarkers are being published every year for more than 40 years now [7]. Three main biomarker branches have been established: diagnostic markers, that identify patients at risk of prostate cancer using serum/ urine as substrate, or diagnostic immunohistochemistry during biopsy evaluation, prognostic markers, which give an idea of a certain clinical outcome, e.g. biochemical recurrence after radical treatment and predictive markers, predicting a response to specific, usually medicament-based therapy.

Prognostic biomarkers, even after their almost 40-year-long research way, are still not recommended for utilization in clinical routine although several of them (in form of commercial gene expression signatures) are considered as potential candidates. However, with no data currently available about their clinical relevance at long term, also prospective validation is lacking [8].

Given that after 40 years of research multiple studies appear constantly in the literature addressing single genes or their combinations in the prognostic setting, the aim of our study was to define the limits of biomarker research in patients with prostate cancer, primarily through the identification of potential targets not yet investigated. This comprehensive, holistic approach cannot only serve as an outline of the immense possibilities that are still left for prognostic and diagnostic biomarker research but could also be used as a starting point for important discussions such as the prioritization of research targets and changes in research methodology for future prostate cancer research.

Methods

Patient cohort

This study comprised a total of 499 patients from the prostate adenocarcinoma cohort of The Cancer Genome Atlas (TCGA). Mean age of the patients was 61.0 years (range 41–78 years). Clinicopathological information was available for all patients (Fig. 1). Follow-up information with biochemical recurrence as an endpoint was available for 452 patients, 83 of which have developed a biochemical recurrence. Median follow-up time was 16.9 months (range 1–153 months).

Quality control of clinical data

The raw clinical data (version 28.01.2016) was preprocessed and organized in a database as follows: 1) selection of relevant clinicopathological parameters (age, serum PSA level, pathological staging and grading, follow-up information); 2) All parameters were controlled for consistency, duplicates were removed.

mRNA expression data

mRNA expression data were generated using the Illumina HiSeq 2000 RNA Sequencing platform (Version 2; data version 28.01.2016). RNA expression was available for tumor samples of all patients and for additional 53 samples with normal tissue normalize according to TCGA protocol. Using barcode as an identifier, tumor and normal tissue samples were extracted separately with further merging of RNA expression data for tumor samples to clinical data. After excluding the genes with duplicate names and missing expression, mRNA expression of 20,500 genes was available for analysis. From this list, further 2819 genes were excluded due to absent or very low mRNA expression values (median = 0 reads), leaving 17,681 genes in the final analysis.

Bioinformatical approach / statistics

All statistical analyses were performed using R (R Foundation for Statistical Computing; version 3.5.0). The packages used were pastecs, TCGAbiolinks, limma, edgeR, KMsurv, survMisc, rms, stringi, Hmisc, tidyverse and doParallel.

The fully automatized bioinformatical pipeline is outlined in Fig. 2. In brief, for survival analyses, dichotomization of mRNA expression was carried out using 1) median level of mRNA expression and 2) cut-off optimization (best cut-off). The best cut-off was selected using the survMisc package (automatized systematic univariate Cox regression-based analysis of all available cut-offs for mRNA expression of single genes). Survival analyses were conducted using univariate and multivariate Cox proportional hazards regression. Kaplan-Meier estimates were calculated using both the best cut-off and median for each gene with accompanying log-rank test and automatic generation of Kaplan-Meier curves for all genes. The inclusion criterion for multivariate analysis was a p-value < 0.05 in univariate analysis.

Correlation analyses were performed to identify the associations of clinical variables (Gleason Score) with the mRNA expression of single genes (Pearson correlation coefficient (r) and p-level). Pairwise comparison of the gene expression of normal and tumor tissue was carried out using a negative binomial generalized log-linear model and correction for false discovery rate (FDR).

Gene set enrichment analysis (GSEA)

GSEA for tumor versus normal tissue was performed using the GSEAPreranked tool in javaGSEA Application (The Broad Institute, Inc., Massachusetts Institute of Technology and Regents of the University of California). Single genes were ranked based on the logFC parameter stemming from differential gene expression analysis. Gene sets from the Hallmark collection (well-defined biological states or processes, $n = 50$) and the Gene

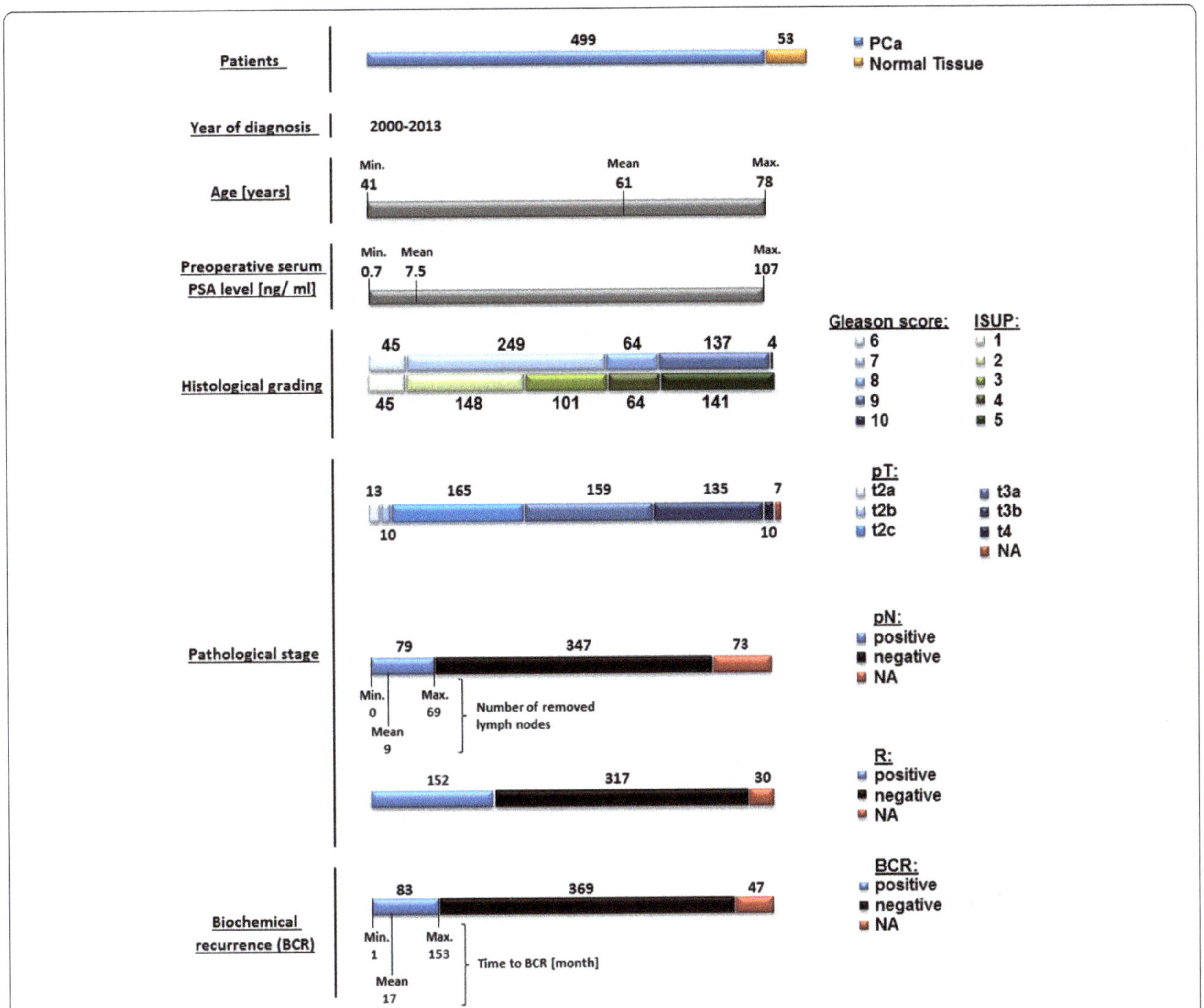

Fig. 1 Clinicopathological characteristics of patients

Ontology database (GO biological processes, $n = 4436$) were used for GSEA as provided by Molecular Signatures Database (MSigDB) v6.2 (The Broad Institute, Inc., Massachusetts Institute of Technology and Regents of the University of California). GSEA was performed using the following setup: number of permutations – 1000, enrichment statistic – weighted, gene set size restriction – 15-500 genes, FDR cut-off – 0.25.

Results

Tumor vs normal tissue

Among all genes analyzed, 1754 were significantly downregulated in tumor tissue (fold change (FC) > 2, logFC < − 1.0; FDR range from 0.05 to 3.3e-275). 133 of these genes showed profound downregulation with logFC < − 3.0 (maximal logFC -9.7; FDR 1.4e- 09 – 3.3e-275).

Another 1553 genes were significantly upregulated in tumor tissue (FC > 2, logFC > 1; FDR range from 0.047 to 1.6e-51) with very high levels of upregulation (logFC > 3; maximal logFC 9.9) in 123 genes (FDR 0.02–4.1e-36). For full information see Additional file 2: Table S1.

In GSEA analysis, 10 Hallmark gene sets and 809 gene sets from the GO Biological Processes collection were enriched in tumor tissue with FDR < 0.25 (Fig. 3, Additional file 3: Table S2). Multiple Biological Processes enriched in tumor tissue were related to altered epigenetic regulation (chromatin organization, gene silencing).

Correlation with Gleason score (tumor aggressiveness)

Of 17,681 genes, 8724 genes showed significant correlation levels to the International Society of Urological Pathology (ISUP) histological grading group of the tumor (based on the Gleason Score) with p-values

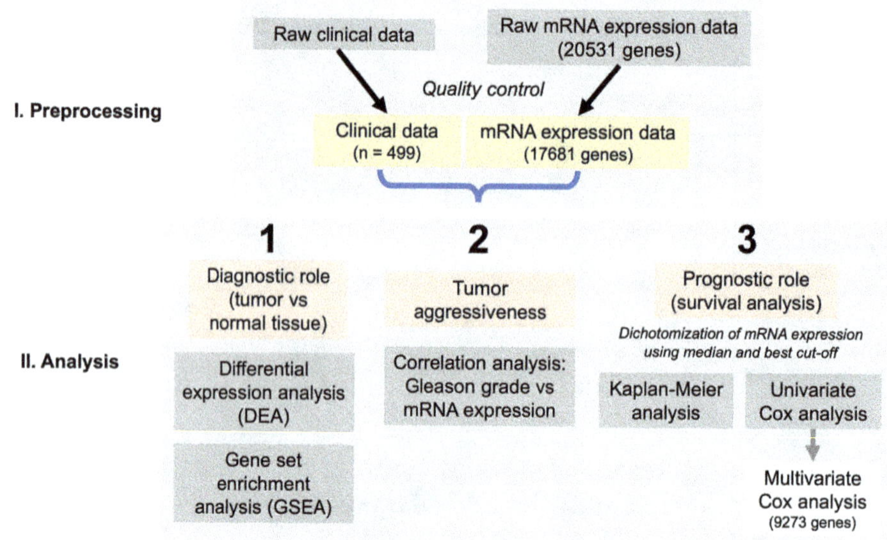

Fig. 2 Bioinformatical pipeline for the analysis of the prognostic role of gene expression

ranging from 10e-24 up to 0.05 and range of Pearson r-values of 0.09–0.43. From this list, 5557 genes were positively correlated to ISUP grouping, while 3167 genes were negatively correlated. Top 20 genes with the highest levels of positive and negative correlation are presented in Table 1 (for full analysis see Additional file 4: Table S3; for correlation analysis high grade (≥4 + 4) vs low grade tumors see Additional file 5: Table S4).

Prognostic role of mRNA expression (survival analyses)

Univariate cox regression

In univariate Cox regression analyses (Fig. 4), 3571 of 17, 681 genes showed a statistically significant association with biochemical recurrence (BCR)-free survival of patients with a range of hazard ratios (HR) 0.3–3.8 (p-values 7.4e- 07 to 0.05), when dichotomized using median of expression (additional 5719 genes demonstrated statistical significance with $p < 0.05$ using best cut-off for dichotomization). Of 3571

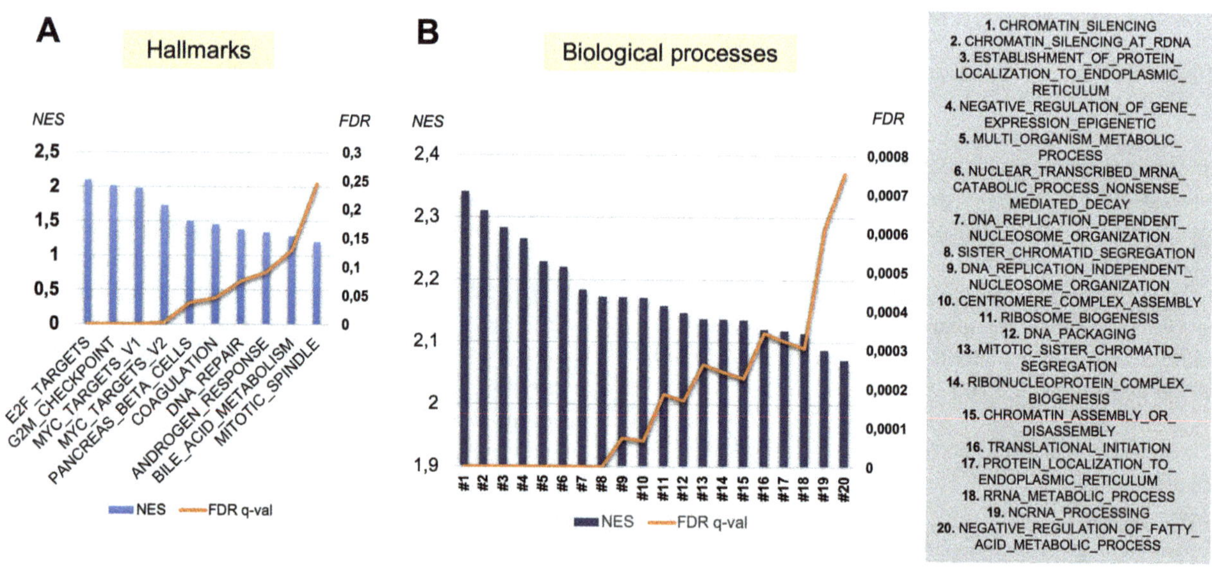

Fig. 3 The results of Gene Set Enrichment Analysis (GSEA) in tumor tissue compared to normal tissue. Two collections of gene sets from Molecular Signatures Database (MSigDB) were analyzed: **a**) Hallmarks of well-defined biological states of processes (10/10 enriched signatures for tumor tissue are shown). **b** Gene Ontology database: biological processes (top 20/809 enriched signatures are shown). False discovery rate was set at a cut-off of 0.25; 1000 permutations were made for every analysis. Abbreviations: NES – normalized enrichment score (main metrics of GSEA); FDR – false discovery rate

Table 1 Top 20 genes with the highest levels of mRNA expression correlation to ISUP grading group of the tumor

Positive correlation			Negative correlation		
Gene	ISUP / Pearson r	ISUP / p-value	Gene	ISUP / Pearson r	ISUP / *p*-value
TROAP	0,408	2,21e-21	SH3RF2	−0,429	9,99e-2
CBX1	0,408	2,55e-21	RNF185	−0,405	4,85e-21
ABCC5	0,404	6,19e-21	VPS36	−0,400	1,74e-20
DONSON	0,403	8,80e-21	ACP2	−0,397	3,60e-20
SMC4	0,400	1,55e-20	GEMIN4	−0,388	2,70e-19
KIF20A	0,400	1,65e-20	KIAA0319L	−0,387	3,03e-19
SPAG5	0,399	2,29e-20	KCNK6	-0,384	6,28e-19
NCAPG2	0,396	4,57e-20	DPP4	-0,383	7,49e-19
KIF23	0,395	5,42e-20	CCDC149	-0,381	1,33e-18
FAM72D	0,394	6,57e-20	EPHX2	-0,380	1,65e-18

genes significantly associated with BCR (dichotomization using median), 827 were not significantly correlated with the ISUP grading group of the tumor. Higher mRNA expression was prognostically unfavorable for 2390 genes and favorable for 1181 genes (top 20 genes outlined in Fig. 4). Full information about the prognostic significance of mRNA expression of single genes in univariate analysis using median and best cut-off for dichotomization is available as Additional file 4: Table S3.

Multivariate cox regression

Pathological staging of the tumor (pT: pooled pT3/4 vs pT2), ISUP histological grade group of the tumor, presence of lymph nodes metastases (pN1 vs pN0) and status of the resection margins (R1 vs R0) were included into multivariate Cox regression models, together with the expression of single genes which showed statistically significant association with BCR-free survival in univariate Cox regression analysis (3571 genes with dichotomization using median of expression and 9273 genes with dichotomization using the optimized cut-off).

Among 3571 (median as cut-off) / 9273 (best cut-off) included genes, 571 / 2435 genes, respectively, showed statistically significant association with biochemical recurrence (Fig. 5). With median as cut-off, multivariate Cox regression *p*-values for single genes ranged from

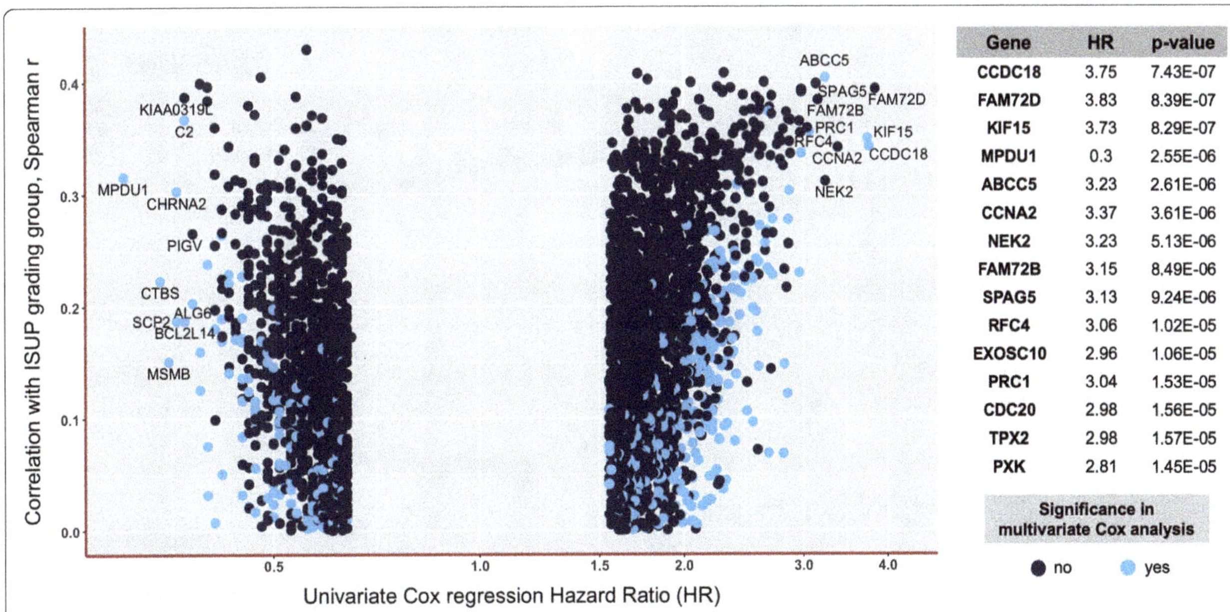

Fig. 4 All genes with statistically significant association of mRNA expression with biochemical recurrence in univariate Cox regression analysis (all $p < 0.05$, median of expression as dichotomization cut-off) stratified according to univariate Hazard Ratio (HR) and correlation level between ISUP grad group of the tumor and mRNA-expression of the gene. Blue spots represent the genes which are independently associated with biochemical recurrence-free survival in multivariate Cox regression analysis. Top 15 genes with highest levels of statistical significance in univariate Cox analysis are highlighted with detailed outputs from univariate Cox regression analysis

0.0005 to 0.05 and hazard ratios from 0.40 to 2.47 (best cut-off p-value range 2.1e- 05 – 0.05, HR range 0.10–12.31). Kaplan-Meier curves for genes most significantly and independently associated with BCR-free survival in multivariate analysis are presented in Fig. 6. Full information about the prognostic significance of mRNA expression of all single genes in the multivariate analysis with dichotomization using median and best cut-off is available as additional file 6: Table S5.

Of 571 genes independently associated with BCR-free survival (median as cut-off), mRNA expression of 276 genes was significantly correlated with the ISUP grade group of the tumor (Pearson r > 0.10, $p < 0.05$).

Characterization of the top 50 genes independently associated with BCR-free survival with analysis of their potential for further investigations in patients with prostate cancer is presented in Additional file 7: Table S6.

Discussion

The identification of appropriate biomarkers is essential to drive important clinical decisions in patients with prostate cancer [7]. Hundreds of studies focusing on new biomarkers are being published every year since the 1980th, addressing three main biomarker branches (diagnostic, prognostic, and predictive). Even though diagnostic markers have found their niche in the clinical practice (selection of patients at risk of prostate cancer for biopsy based on serum (e.g. prostate-specific antigen, four kallikrein score) or urine analysis (RNA expression of PCA3 [9], or of gene pair HOXC6 / DLX1 [10]) [8], immunohistochemistry during primary diagnosis or metastatic disease [11], theranostic targets for imaging, such as prostate-specific antigen [12]), prognostic biomarkers are still not recommended by professional guidelines, despite 40 years of intensive research in patients with prostate cancer.

The aim of our study was to delineate the limits of prostate cancer prognostic and diagnostic biomarker research and to show the extent of perspective targets have not been studied in prostate cancer yet. For this purpose, we used a well-characterized primary hormone-naïve prostate cancer cohort from TCGA with 499 patients, representing 499 tumor and 53 normal tissue samples. The limits of diagnostic and prognostic biomarker research could be investigated with the use of this cohort as it includes data regarding the status of almost all genes. We have selected RNA expression data of all genes called using RNAseq approach as a surrogate for their functional relevance, and systematically approached the questions of the diagnostic and prognostic role of single genes using our automatized bioinformatical pipeline (Fig. 2).

As for the prognostic role of these genes during the statistical stages of Kaplan-Meier, univariate and multivariate Cox-regression analysis, we have cleared out 571 genes with independent prognostic significance for biochemical recurrence after radical prostatectomy using strict rules prescribed by REMARK criteria [13] (especially, using the median of expression as cut-off for dichotomization). Even more genes (overall 2435 genes) carried independent prognostic value under relaxed

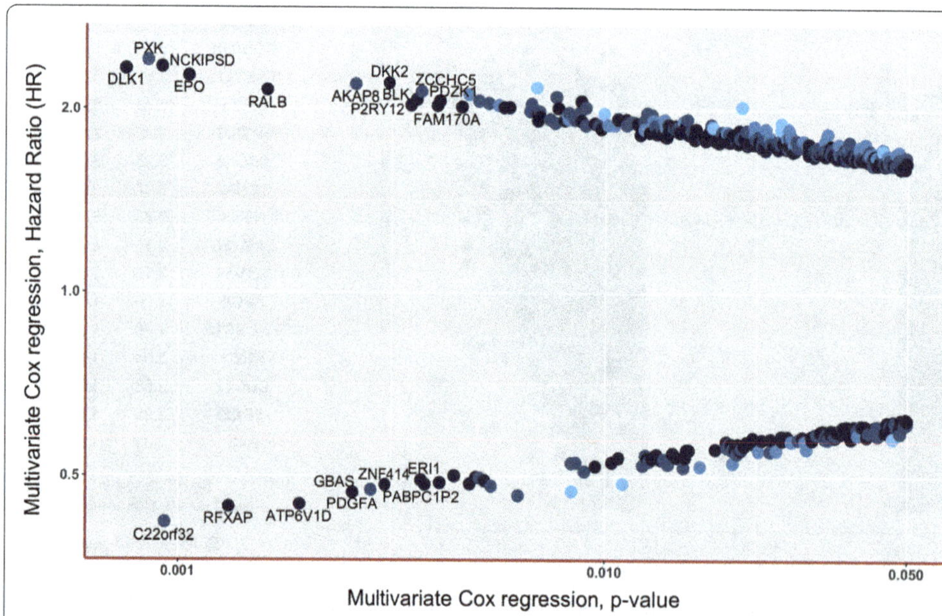

Gene	HR	p-value
DLK1	2.33	0.0008
PXK	2.41	0.0008
NCKIPSD	2.35	0.0009
C22orf32	0.42	0.0009
EPO	2.27	0.001
RFXAP	0.45	0.001
RALB	2.15	0.002
ATP6V1D	0.45	0.002
PDGFA	0.47	0.003
AKAP8	2.20	0.003
GBAS	0.48	0.003
ZNF414	0.48	0.003
DKK2	2.21	0.003
P2RY12	2.03	0.004
BLK	2.08	0.004

Fig. 5 All genes with statistically significant association of mRNA expression with biochemical recurrence in multivariate Cox regression analysis (all p < 0.05, median of expression as dichotomization cut-off) stratified according to multivariate Hazard Ratio (HR) and multivariate analysis p-level. Colors represent correlation levels to the ISUP grade group of the tumor (from dark blue = Spearman r < 0.1 and no significant correlation up to light blue = Spearman r > 0.3, $p > 0.05$). Detailed outputs for top 15 genes from multivariate Cox regression analysis are provided on the right side

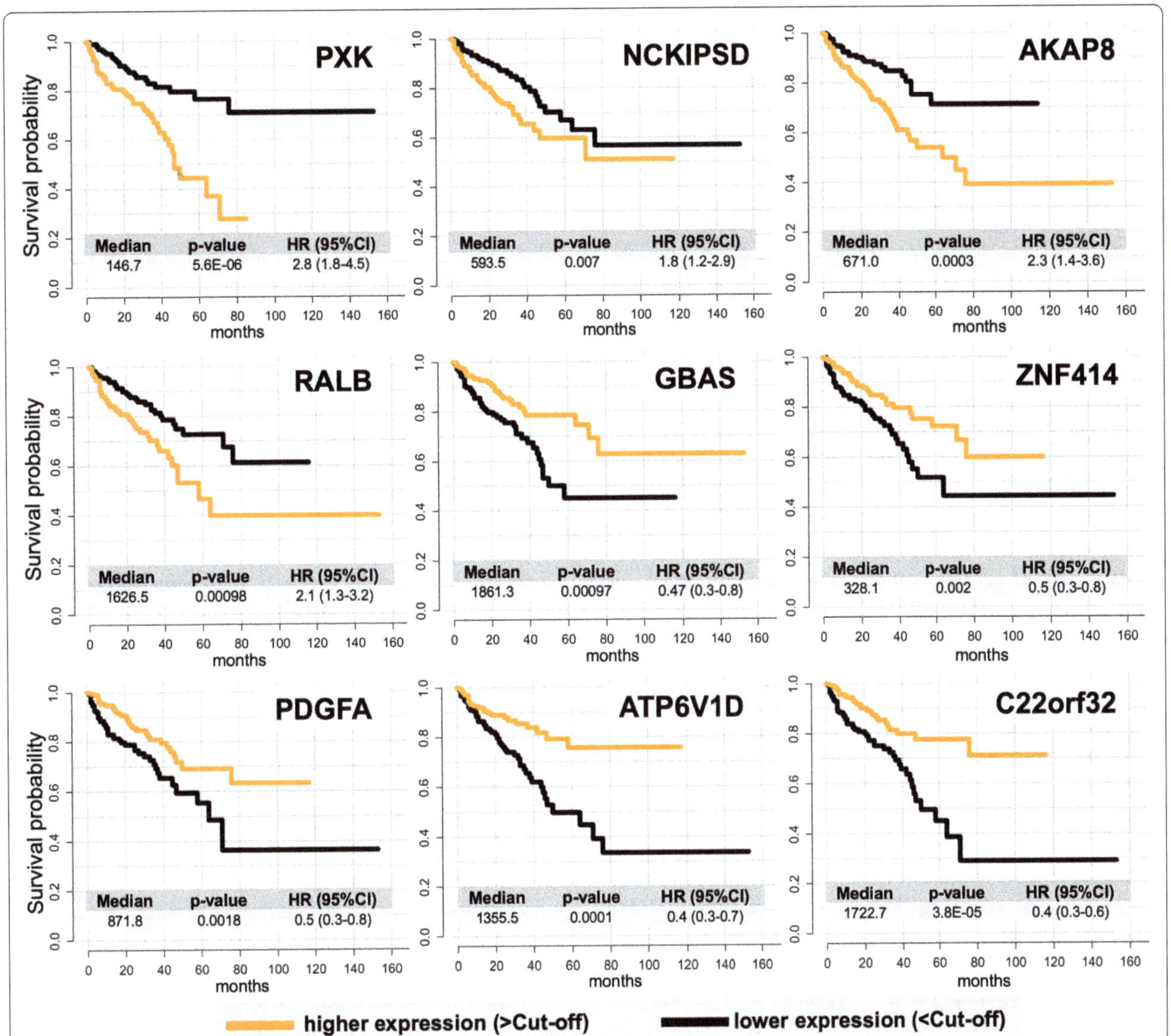

Fig. 6 Kaplan-Meier curves for nine top-ranked genes with substantial expression in prostate cancer, statistically significant and independently associated with biochemical recurrence-free survival of the patients with prostate cancer in multivariate Cox regression analysis (median of expression as dichotomization cut-off). Abbreviations: Median – median of mRNA expression, HR – hazard ratio, l95% CI and u95% CI – lower and upper 95% percentile of the confidence interval (CI), low expression – expression levels below cut-off, high expression – expression levels above cut-off

criteria (optimized cut-off for dichotomization). Although prone to statistical bias, using the best cut-off for dichotomization is logical from a biological point of view (e.g., only a small part (not the half) of carcinomas could have special aggressiveness features delineated by gene expression). Therefore, these genes also could and should be considered as potential candidates for further characterization.

Interestingly, when performing a detailed analysis of the top 50 genes showing independent prognostic value (Additional file 7: Table S6), 40 of them (80%), as for the actual state of published research, have not been studied in prostate cancer, yet. 31 of these genes were shown to be of some significance for other cancer types. This gives us a broad perspective of how much research effort and time we should invest to cover all potentially relevant targets which have not been in the scope of prostate cancer researchers yet.

As for the diagnostic role of these genes, we hereby provide a comprehensive analysis based on two approaches: 1) differential expression in tumor vs. normal tissue, and 2) correlation of mRNA expression with Gleason-Score / ISUP-grade group of the tumor. The first part of this analysis provides a big number of potential targets which are highly upregulated ($n = 123$) or downregulated ($n = 133$) in tumor tissue with fold change (FC) more than 8 (logFC > 3) with multiple genes showing less pronounced, however, still significant up- and downregulation.

Some of these genes were already extensively studied in prostate cancer, mostly those upregulated in tumor tissue: SPINK1 [14] (Top17, logFC 4.8), ETV4 [15] (Top63, logFC 3.6), PCA3 [9] (Top79, logFC 3.5), TDRD1 [16, 17] (Top86, logFC 3.4), AMACR [18] (Top105, logFC 3.2), DLX1 [10] (Top110, logFC 3.1), HOXC6 [10] (Top268, logFC 2.3). However, others are still representing potential diagnostic targets at different stages of clinical decision making (before diagnosis, after first negative biopsy, control of recurrence, immunohistochemical diagnosis of prostate cancer on biopsy, theranostic targets). Between the above mentioned highly upregulated genes and several genes used as targets in clinical practice such as FOLH1 coding PSMA (logFC 1.7, Top622 among all upregulated genes), there is a gap of approx. 500 genes which could represent potential diagnostic targets.

Interestingly, several well-known genes, despite being recommended for their utility in the identification of patients at risk of prostate cancer at RNA expression level, are by far not in the top of this list (e.g. in urine; PCA3, HOXC6, DLX1 [9, 10]). Hence, these results once again outline the need for further research on diagnostic biomarkers.

Gene set enrichment analysis (GSEA) for differentially expressed genes allowed us to detect many biological processes/pathways altered in tumor tissue. Interestingly, among the top 30 biological processes altered in prostate cancer, 16 (53.3%) were related to epigenetic mechanisms, such as chromatin functioning/ organization, and epigenetic gene silencing (Fig. 3, Additional file 3: Table S2). The epigenetics of prostate cancer are well studied at the level of DNA methylation [19], however, more studies investigating broader epigenetic mechanisms related to chromatin organization and functioning are warranted for a further comprehension of the prostate cancer biology.

In general, our study and associated supplementary materials including full results of the performed analyses represent are a very useful reference database for those researchers willing to validate the results of their studies involving different levels of gene expression (mRNA, methylation analysis, protein expression) in patients with prostate cancer.

The limitations of our study are mainly associated with the inherent limitations of the TCGA cohort and should be considered using this material as a reference point. Due to the relatively short follow-up period (median 17 months, range 1–153 months), the findings of our analyses are more useful for patients with higher Gleason scores, as they develop BCR earlier. Among 45 patients with Gleason Score 3 + 3 = 6, only 3 patients have developed BCR to the end of follow-up compared to 80 patients with BCR among patients with other Gleason scores. To address this point, we have carried out a multivariate Cox regression analysis separately for patients of all ISUP grade groups and for patients of ISUP grade groups ≥2 (Additional file 8: Table S7). In conclusion, the results showed minimal discrepancies in the resulting set of independent prognostic biomarkers and therefore, the robustness of our initial findings.

Furthermore, despite the high quality of the TCGA cohort, a validation cohort would be needed to verify the results, as it was shown earlier that a significant number of genes (mainly from small studies) do not pass the validation landmark [20]. Also, it is important to mention, that the patient cohort that was used in this study is a post-prostatectomy cohort of patients with primary hormone-naïve prostate cancer and the results, therefore, could be only in the restrictive manner extended to the patients with metastatic and castration-resistant prostate cancer.

Moreover, the analyses carried out involved only RNA expression levels of the genes. In the modern era of multi-omics and presence of multiple aspects of alternative regulation of gene function from transcription to protein function, this should be respectively interpreted. Only one tumor sample per patient was analyzed by TCGA which can introduce a bias related to undersampling of the tumor, given high levels of prostate cancer morphological and molecular genetic heterogeneity [5]. Accordingly, validation studies should address this important aspect of prostate cancer biology.

We believe that our study should also be a starting point for an important discussion. Although the particular advantage of our study is a comprehensive outline of the immense possibilities that are still left for prognostic and diagnostic biomarker research, it poses one important question (taking in account the almost 40-year-long portfolio of translational biomarker research which still didn't find its way into clinical practice): what should be the priority of the future prostate cancer research and how do we need to change our research methodology to overcome the above mentioned issues of failing clinical relevance of biomarkers (especially prognostic) studied before? There is still no definitive answer to this question. However, it is more or less clear that single targets will probably only make sense in a diagnostic, but not in a prognostic setting. The optimal methodological approach for the development of prognostic biomarkers remains to be established and probably will account for pathway-oriented genetic and epigenetic changes at different levels (mutations, copy-number rearrangements, DNA methylation, chromatin remodeling, mRNA and ncRNA expression, posttranslational modifications, protein expression) and at different time points to account for tumor evolution and tumor heterogeneity [4, 21–23].

Conclusions

Our study provides a comprehensive overview of the prognostic and diagnostic mRNA biomarkers in patients with primary prostate cancer, both already studied and, more importantly, not yet addressed in prostate cancer. Interestingly, several of them show a great potential for further research. These findings could be used as a reference point for further biomarker research and validation data for ongoing projects by most prostate cancer researchers. A full database including the results is provided as Supplement to be used as an everyday tool.

Additional files

Additional file 1: Supplementary Data. List of abbreviations. (PDF 29 kb)

Additional file 2: Table S1 Pairwise comparison of the gene expression of normal and tumor tissue using negative binomial generalized log-linear model and correction for false discovery rate (FDR). (TXT 2100 kb)

Additional file 3: Table S2 Full results of Gene Set Enrichment Analysis (GSEA) for tumor vs normal tissue using Gene Ontology Biological Processes database. (TXT 131 kb)

Additional file 4: Table S3 Correlation between ISUP histological grade group of the tumor (Grade groups 1–5) and mRNA expression of single genes, univariate Cox-regression analysis with biochemical recurrence as an endpoint. Full list of genes ($n = 17{,}681$). (TXT 3078 kb)

Additional file 5: Table S4 Correlation between ISUP histological grade group of the tumor (dichotomized as high-grade, ≥4 + 4, vs low-grade tumors) and mRNA expression of single genes. Correlation analysis for ISUP grade groups (Groups 1–5) is provided in parallel for comparison. Delta of Pearson *r* correlation levels is calculated for these 2 different settings. (TXT 2104 kb)

Additional file 6: Table S5 Full results of the multivariate Cox regression analysis for single genes. (TXT 1949 kb)

Additional file 7: Table S6 Top 50 genes with statistically significant and independent association with biochemical recurrence-free survival in multivariate Cox regression analysis (dichotomization using median) in patients with prostate cancer. Estimates of their perspectivity for further research are provided. (PDF 65 kb)

Additional file 8: Table S7 Results of the multivariate Cox regression analysis for single genes separately for patients of ISUP grade groups 2–5. (TXT 1940 kb)

Abbreviations

BCR: Biochemical recurrence; FC: Fold change; FDR: False discovery rate; ISUP: International Society of Urological Pathology; PCa: Prostate cancer; TCGA: The Cancer Genome Atlas

Acknowledgements

None.

Authors' contributions

Data curation / Bioinformatics: YT, AK, TK. Data analysis: AK, TK, YT. Visualization: AK, YT. Writing - original draft: AK, YT. Writing - review & editing: GK. Supervision: YT, GK. Critical revision for important intellectual content: all authors. The authors have read and approved this information. All authors read and approved the final manuscript.

Author details

[1]Institute of Pathology, University Hospital of Bonn, Bonn, Germany. [2]Institute of Computer Science, Johannes Gutenberg-University Mainz, Mainz, Germany.

References

1. Ferlay J, Soerjomataram I, Dikshit R, et al. Cancer incidence and mortality worldwide: sources, methods and major patterns in GLOBOCAN 2012. Int J Cancer. 2015;136:E359–86.
2. Esserman LJ, Thompson IM, Reid B, et al. Addressing overdiagnosis and overtreatment in cancer: a prescription for change. Lancet Oncol. 2014;15:e234–42.
3. Wilt TJ, Jones KM, Barry MJ, et al. Follow-up of prostatectomy versus observation for early prostate Cancer. N Engl J Med. 2017;377:132–42.
4. Boutros PC, Fraser M, Harding NJ, et al. Spatial genomic heterogeneity within localized, multifocal prostate cancer. Nat Genet. 2015;47:736–45.
5. Tolkach Y, Kristiansen G. The heterogeneity of prostate Cancer: a practical approach. Pathobiology. 2018;85:108–16.
6. Kretschmer A, Tolkach Y, Ellinger J, Kristiansen G. Molecular biomarkers and prognostic factors for prostate cancer. Urologe. 2017;56:933–44.
7. Kristiansen G. Markers of clinical utility in the differential diagnosis and prognosis of prostate cancer. Mod Pathol. 2018;31:S143–55.
8. EAU - ESTRO - ESUR - SIOG Guidelines on Prostate Cancer. Update March 2018. Accessed at uroweb.org. Accessed 25 Jan 2019.
9. Nicholson A, Mahon J, Boland A, et al. The clinical effectiveness and cost-effectiveness of the PROGENSA® prostate cancer antigen 3 assay and the prostate health index in the diagnosis of prostate cancer: a systematic review and economic evaluation. Health Technol Assess (Rockv). 2015;19:1–192.
10. Van Neste L, Hendriks RJ, Dijkstra S, et al. Detection of high-grade prostate Cancer using a urinary molecular biomarker–based risk score. Eur Urol. 2016;70:740–8.
11. Kristiansen I, Stephan C, Jung K, et al. Sensitivity of HoXB13 as a diagnostic immunohistochemical marker of prostatic origin in prostate cancer metastases: comparison to PSA, protein, androgen receptor, ERG, NKX3.1, PSAP, and PSMA. Int J Mol Sci. 2017;18. https://doi.org/10.3390/ijms18061151.
12. Berger I, Annabattula C, Lewis J, et al. 68Ga-PSMA PET/CT vs. mpMRI for locoregional prostate cancer staging: correlation with final histopathology. Prostate Cancer Prostatic Dis. 2018;21:204–11.
13. McShane LM, Altman DG, Sauerbrei W, et al. REporting recommendations for tumour MARKer prognostic studies (REMARK). Br J Cancer. 2005;93:387–91.
14. Brooks JD, Wei W, Hawley S, et al. Evaluation of ERG and SPINK1 by Immunohistochemical staining and Clinicopathological outcomes in a multi-institutional radical prostatectomy cohort of 1067 patients. PLoS One. 2015;10:e0132343.
15. TCGA. The molecular taxonomy of primary prostate Cancer. Cell. 2015;163:1011–25.
16. Leyten GHJM, Hessels D, Smit FP, et al. Identification of a candidate gene panel for the early diagnosis of prostate Cancer. Clin Cancer Res. 2015;21:3061–70.
17. Litovkin K, Joniau S, Lerut E, et al. Methylation of PITX2, HOXD3, RASSF1 and TDRD1 predicts biochemical recurrence in high-risk prostate cancer. J Cancer Res Clin Oncol. 2014;140:1849–61.
18. Tischler V, Fritzsche FR, Gerhardt J, et al. Comparison of the diagnostic value of fatty acid synthase (FASN) with alpha-methylacyl-CoA racemase (AMACR) as prostatic cancer tissue marker. Histopathology. 2010;56:811–5.
19. Chao C, Chi M, Preciado M, Black MH. Methylation markers for prostate cancer prognosis: a systematic review. Cancer Causes Control. 2013;24:1615–41.
20. Huber F, Montani M, Sulser T, et al. Comprehensive validation of published immunohistochemical prognostic biomarkers of prostate cancer—what has gone wrong? A blueprint for the way forward in biomarker studies. Br J Cancer. 2015;112:140–8.
21. Armenia J, Wankowicz SAM, Liu D, et al. The long tail of oncogenic drivers in prostate cancer. Nat Genet. 2018;50:645–51.
22. Linch M, Goh G, Hiley C, et al. Intratumoural evolutionary landscape of high-risk prostate cancer: the PROGENY study of genomic and immune parameters. Ann Oncol. 2017;28:2472–80.
23. Li S, Garrett-Bakelman FE, Chung SS, et al. Distinct evolution and dynamics of epigenetic and genetic heterogeneity in acute myeloid leukemia. Nat Med. 2016;22:792–9.

Permissions

All chapters in this book were first published by BioMed Central; hereby published with permission under the Creative Commons Attribution License or equivalent. Every chapter published in this book has been scrutinized by our experts. Their significance has been extensively debated. The topics covered herein carry significant findings which will fuel the growth of the discipline. They may even be implemented as practical applications or may be referred to as a beginning point for another development.

The contributors of this book come from diverse backgrounds, making this book a truly international effort. This book will bring forth new frontiers with its revolutionizing research information and detailed analysis of the nascent developments around the world.

We would like to thank all the contributing authors for lending their expertise to make the book truly unique. They have played a crucial role in the development of this book. Without their invaluable contributions this book wouldn't have been possible. They have made vital efforts to compile up to date information on the varied aspects of this subject to make this book a valuable addition to the collection of many professionals and students.

This book was conceptualized with the vision of imparting up-to-date information and advanced data in this field. To ensure the same, a matchless editorial board was set up. Every individual on the board went through rigorous rounds of assessment to prove their worth. After which they invested a large part of their time researching and compiling the most relevant data for our readers.

The editorial board has been involved in producing this book since its inception. They have spent rigorous hours researching and exploring the diverse topics which have resulted in the successful publishing of this book. They have passed on their knowledge of decades through this book. To expedite this challenging task, the publisher supported the team at every step. A small team of assistant editors was also appointed to further simplify the editing procedure and attain best results for the readers.

Apart from the editorial board, the designing team has also invested a significant amount of their time in understanding the subject and creating the most relevant covers. They scrutinized every image to scout for the most suitable representation of the subject and create an appropriate cover for the book.

The publishing team has been an ardent support to the editorial, designing and production team. Their endless efforts to recruit the best for this project, has resulted in the accomplishment of this book. They are a veteran in the field of academics and their pool of knowledge is as vast as their experience in printing. Their expertise and guidance has proved useful at every step. Their uncompromising quality standards have made this book an exceptional effort. Their encouragement from time to time has been an inspiration for everyone.

The publisher and the editorial board hope that this book will prove to be a valuable piece of knowledge for researchers, students, practitioners and scholars across the globe.

List of Contributors

Wendy L. Johnston
Radiation Medicine Program, Princess Margaret Cancer Centre, University Health Network, Toronto, ON, Canada

Charles N. Catton
Radiation Medicine Program, Princess Margaret Cancer Centre, University Health Network, Toronto, ON, Canada
Department of Radiation Oncology, University of Toronto, Toronto, ON, Canada

Carol J. Swallow
Lunenfeld-Tanenbaum Research Institute, Mount Sinai Hospital, Toronto, ON, Canada
Department of Surgery, University of Toronto, Toronto, ON, Canada
Institute of Medical Science, University of Toronto, Toronto, ON, Canada
Laboratory Medicine and Pathobiology, University of Toronto, Toronto, ON, Canada

Ching-Hsin Chang
Taipei Medical University Hospital, Taipei, Taiwan
Institute of Microbiology and Immunology, National Yang-Ming University, Taipei, Taiwan

Tzu-Ping Lin
Taipei Veterans General Hospital, Taipei, Taiwan

Jung-Yao Huang
Shutien Uro Clinic, Taipei, Taiwan

Caren Hilger and Friederike Kendel
Institute of Medical Psychology, Charité Universitätsmedizin Berlin, D-10117 Berlin, Germany

Martin Schostak
Department of Urology and Pediatric Urology, Otto von Guericke University Magdeburg, Magdeburg, Germany

Stephan Neubauer
Department of Urology, Klinik am Ring Cologne, Cologne, Germany

Ahmed Magheli
Department of Urology, Vivantes Klinikum am Urban Berlin, Berlin, Germany

Thomas Fydrich
Institute of Psychology, Humboldt-Universität zu Berlin, Berlin, Germany

Silke Burkert
Institute of Medical Psychology, Charité Universitätsmedizin Berlin, D-10117 Berlin, Germany
Department of Psychology, University of Applied Sciences Europe, Berlin, Germany

Yu-Li Jiang and Lu-Jie Qian
Department of Urology, The Affiliated Hospital of Hang Zhou Normal University, Hangzhou 310015, China
School of Medicine, Hang Zhou Normal University, Hangzhou 310016, China

Ulrika Rönningås
Division of Insurance Medicine, Department of Clinical Neuroscience, Karolinska Institutet, 171 77 Stockholm, Sweden
Department of Oncology, Sundsvall County Hospital, 851 86 Sundsvall, Sweden
Department of Nursing Science, Sophiahemmet University, 114 86 Stockholm, Sweden

Maja Holm
Department of Nursing Science, Sophiahemmet University, 114 86 Stockholm, Sweden

Agneta Wennman-Larsen
Division of Insurance Medicine, Department of Clinical Neuroscience, Karolinska Institutet, 171 77 Stockholm, Sweden
Department of Nursing Science, Sophiahemmet University, 114 86 Stockholm, Sweden

Per Fransson
Department of Nursing, Umeå University, 901 87 Umeå, Sweden
Cancercentrum, Norrlands University Hospital, 901 85 Umeå, Sweden

Yuki Kyoda, Koji Ichihara, Kohei Hashimoto, Ko Kobayashi, Fumimasa Fukuta and Naoya Masumori
Department of Urology, Sapporo Medical University School of Medicine, S. 1, W. 16, Chuo-ku, Sapporo 060-8543, Japan

Qing-Tong Yi, Min Gong, Chu-Hong Chen, Wei Hu and Ru-Jian Zhu
Department of Urology, Shanghai Pudong Hospital, Fudan University Pudong Medical Center, Shanghai, China

Bo-Wen Xia, Si-Cong Zhao, Zong-Ping Chen, Chao Chen, Tian-Shu Liu, Fan Yang and Yong Yan
Department of Urology, Beijing Shijitan Hospital, Capital Medical University, 10th Tieyi Road, Haidian District, Beijing 100038, China

Rafael Castilho Borges, Marcos Tobias-Machado, Estefânia Nicoleti Gabriotti, Carlos Alberto Bezerra and Sidney Glina
Department of Urology, Faculdade de Medicina do ABC, No.2000, Avenue Lauro Gomes, Santo André 09051-040, Brazil

Francisco Winter dos Santos Figueiredo
Department of Epidemiology and Data Analysis, Faculdade de Medicina do ABC, No.2000, Avenue Lauro Gomes, Santo André 09051-040, Brazil

Kerri Beckmann
Translational Oncology & Urology Research, Comprehensive Cancer Centre, King's College London, 3rd Floor, Bermondsey Wing, Guy's Hospital, London SE1 9RT, UK
University of South Australia, Centre for population Health Research Adelaide Australia, Adelaide, Australia

Netty Kinsella
Translational Oncology & Urology Research, Comprehensive Cancer Centre, King's College London, 3rd Floor, Bermondsey Wing, Guy's Hospital, London SE1 9RT, UK
Department of Urology, The Royal Marsden Hospital, London, UK

Henrik Olsson, Anna Wallerstedt Lantz, Martin Eklund and Tobias Nordstrom
Department of Medical Epidemiology and Biostatistics, Karolinska Institutet, Stockholm, Sweden

Markus Aly
Department of Medical Epidemiology and Biostatistics, Karolinska Institutet, Stockholm, Sweden
Department of Molecular Medicine and Surgery, Karolinska Institutet, Stockholm, Sweden

Jan Adolfsson
Department of Medical Epidemiology and Biostatistics, Karolinska Institutet, Stockholm, Sweden
CLINTEC-Department, Karolinska Institutet, Stockholm, Sweden

Mieke Van Hemelrijck
Translational Oncology & Urology Research, Comprehensive Cancer Centre, King's College London, 3rd Floor, Bermondsey Wing, Guy's Hospital, London SE1 9RT, UK
Unit of Epidemiology, Institute of Environmental Medicine, Karolinska Institutet, Stockholm, Sweden

Yong Soo Cho, Hyun Ju Seon and Jin Woong Kim
Department of Radiology, Chosun University Hospital and Chosun University College of Medicine, 365 Pilmun-daero, Dong-gu, Gwangju 61453, South Korea

Young Hoe Hur
Department of Hepato-Biliary-Pancreas Surgery, Chonnam National University Hwasun Hospital and Chonnam National University Medical School, Gwangju 61469, South Korea

Hyung Joong Kim
Department of Biomedical Engineering, Kyung Hee University, 23 Kyungheedaero, Dongdaemungu, Seoul 02447, South Korea

L. Käsmann and D. Rades
Department of Radiation Oncology, University of Luebeck, Luebeck, Germany

F. B. Fahlbusch
Department of Pediatrics and Adolescent Medicine, Friedrich-Alexander-University Erlangen-Nuernberg, Erlangen, Germany

D. Vordermark
Department of Radiation Oncology, University Hospital Halle (Saale), Halle, Germany

S. Janssen
Department of Radiation Oncology, University of Luebeck, Luebeck, Germany
Medical Practice for Radiotherapy and Radiation Oncology, Hannover, Germany

Sacha L. Moore
Department of Urology, Wrexham Maelor Hospital, Wrexham, Wales, UK

Chris Bell, Amarit Gill and Iqbal S. Shergill
Department of Urology, Wrexham Maelor Hospital, Wrexham, Wales, UK
North Wales Clinical Research Centre, Gwenfro, Wrexham Technology Park, Wrexham LL13 7YP, UK

Obinna Obi-Njoku and Stephen F. Hughes
North Wales Clinical Research Centre, Gwenfro, Wrexham Technology Park, Wrexham LL13 7YP, UK

Asad Saleemi, Gidon Ellis and Farooq Khan
Department of Urology, Luton and Dunstable University Hospital, Lewsey Road, Luton LU4 0DZ, UK

Lei Wang, Xiaofei Wang, Wenfeng Zhao, Zichen Zhao, Zhihu Li, He Zhu, Xiang Ji, Bing Yang, Ningchen Li and Yanqun Na
Department of urology, Peking University Shougang Hospital, Peking University Health Science Center, Beijing 100144, China
Peking University Wu Jieping Urology Center, Peking University Shougang Hospital, Peking University Health Science Center, 9# Jinyuanzhuang Road, Shijingshan district, Beijing 100144, China

Shengmin Fei
Department of medical imaging, Peking University Shougang Hospital, Peking University Health Science Center, Beijing 100144, China

Yu Hu and Qiong Wu
Department of Pathology, China-Japan Union Hospital, Jilin University, Changchun, Jilin, China

Jialin Gao, Yongrui Zhang and Yuantao Wang
Department of Urology, The First Hospital of Jilin University, No. 71 Xinmin Street, Changchun 130021, Jilin, China

Pieter Minnee
Department of Urology, LangeLand Ziekenhuis, Zoetermeer, The Netherlands

Daphne Hessels
MDxHealth BV, Nijmegen, The Netherlands

Jack A. Schalken
Department of Urology, Radboud University Nijmegen Medical Centre, Nijmegen, The Netherlands

Wim Van Criekinge
Department of Mathematical Modelling, Statistics and Bioinformatics, Ghent University, Ghent, Belgium

Barthold Philip Schrier
Department of Urology, Jeroen Bosch Hospital, 's-Hertogenbosch 5200 ME, The Netherlands

Johannes Cornelis van der Linden
Department of Pathology, Jeroen Bosch Hospital, 's-Hertogenbosch, The Netherlands

J. P. Michiel Sedelaar
Department of Urology, Radboud University Medical Centre, Nijmegen, The Netherlands

Massimo Mischi
Electrical Engineering, Eindhoven University of Technology, Eindhoven, The Netherlands

Anouk Anna Maria Arnoldus van der Aa and Maudy C. W. Gayet
Department of Urology, Jeroen Bosch Hospital, 's-Hertogenbosch 5200 ME, The Netherlands
Electrical Engineering, Eindhoven University of Technology, Eindhoven, The Netherlands

Christophe Koenraad Mannaerts
Department of Urology, AMC University Hospital, Amsterdam, The Netherlands

Harrie P. Beerlage and Hessel Wijkstra
Electrical Engineering, Eindhoven University of Technology, Eindhoven, The Netherlands
Department of Urology, AMC University Hospital, Amsterdam, The Netherlands

Mikio Sugimoto, Xia Zhang, Nobufumi Ueda, Hiroyuki Tsunemori, Rikiya Taoka, Yusi Hayashida, Hiromi Hirama, Yasuyuki Miyauchi, Yuki Matsuoka, Hirohito Naito, Yu Osaki and Yosiyuki Kekehi
Department of Urology, Kagawa University Faculty of Medicine, 1750-1 Ikenobe, Miki-cho, Kita-gun, Kagawa 761-0793, Japan

Zhao Wang
Department of Urology, Xiangya Hospital, Central South University, Changsha, Hunan, China

Zhangcheng Liao
Department of Urology, Xiangya Hospital, Central South University, Changsha, Hunan, China
Provincial Laboratory for Diagnosis and Treatment of Genitourinary System Disease, Changsha, China

Zhongyuan Jin
Department of Pathology, Xiangya Hospital, Central South University, Changsha, Hunan, China

Zhengyan Tang
Department of Urology, Xiangya Hospital, Central South University, Changsha, Hunan, China
Provincial Laboratory for Diagnosis and Treatment of Genitourinary System Disease, Changsha, China
National Clinical Research Center for Geriatric Disorders, Changsha, Hunan, China

Isaac E. Kim Jr
The Warren Alpert Medical School of Brown University, Providence, RI, USA

Sinae Kim
Department of Biostatistics, Rutgers School of Public Health, The State University of New Jersey, New Brunswick, NJ, USA

Arnav Srivastava and Isaac Yi Kim
Section of Urologic Oncology, Division of Urology, Rutgers Cancer Institute of New Jersey and Rutgers Robert Wood Johnson Medical School, Rutgers, The State University of New Jersey, 195 Little Albany Street, #4565, New Brunswick, NJ 08903, USA

Biren Saraiya and Tina Mayer
Department of Internal Medicine, Rutgers Robert Wood Johnson Medical School, Rutgers, The State University of New Jersey, New Brunswick, NJ, USA

Wun-Jae Kim
Department of Urology, Chungbuk National University College of Medicine, Cheongju, South Korea

Christina Sze
Urologic Surgery, Duke University Medical Center and the Duke Cancer Institute, Durham, NC, USA
Division of Urology, Department of Surgery, Duke University Medical Center, Yellow Zone, Durham, NC 27710, USA

Efrat Tsivian, Ariel A. Schulman, Leah G. Davis and Thomas J. Polascik
Urologic Surgery, Duke University Medical Center and the Duke Cancer Institute, Durham, NC, USA

Kae Jack Tay
Urologic Surgery, Duke University Medical Center and the Duke Cancer Institute, Durham, NC, USA
Singapore General Hospital, Singapore

Rajan T. Gupta
Urologic Surgery, Duke University Medical Center and the Duke Cancer Institute, Durham, NC, USA
Department of Radiology, Duke University Medical Center, Durham, NC, USA

Sang Eun Yoon, Youjin Kim, Jangho Cho, Su Jin Lee and Se Hoon Park
Division of Hematology-Oncology, Department of Medicine, Samsung Medical Center, Sungkyunkwan University School of Medicine, 81 Irwon-ro, Gangnam-gu, Seoul 06351, South Korea

Minyong Kang, Hyun Hwan Sung, Hwang Gyun Jeon, Byoung Chang Jeong, Seong Il Seo, Seong Soo Jeon and Hyun Moo Lee
Department of Urology, Samsung Medical Center, Sungkyunkwan University School of Medicine, Seoul, South Korea

Han Yong Choi
Department of Urology, Samsung Medical Center, Sungkyunkwan University School of Medicine, Seoul, South Korea
Department of Urology, Kangbuk Samsung Hospital, Sungkyunkwan University School of Medicine, Seoul, South Korea

J. Smith-Palmer and W. Valentine
Ossian Health Economics and Communications GmbH, Bäumleingasse 20, 4051 Basel, Switzerland

C. Takizawa
Genomic Health International, Geneva, Switzerland

Guan-Lin Huang, Chih-Hsiung Kang, Wei-Ching Lee and Po-Hui Chiang
Department of Urology, Kaohsiung Chang Gung Memorial Hospital and Chang Gung University College of Medicine, No.123, Dapi Rd., Niaosong Dist., Kaohsiung, Taiwan, Republic of China

Deying Zhang and Xing Liu
Department of Urology, Children's Hospital of Chongqing Medical University, No. 136, Zhongshan 2 RD, Yuzhong District, Chongqing 400014, China

Bo Liu, Dawei He, Tao Lin and Guanghui Wei
Department of Urology, Children's Hospital of Chongqing Medical University, No. 136, Zhongshan 2 RD, Yuzhong District, Chongqing 400014, China
Ministry of Education Key Laboratory of Child Development and Disorders, Chongqing Key Laboratory of Pediatrics, China International Science and Technology Cooperation base of Child Development and Critical Disorders, Chongqing Key Laboratory of Children Urogenital Development and Tissue Engineering, Chongqing 400014, China

Samuel Carbunaru, Oluwarotimi S. Nettey, Edward Schaeffer and Pooja Gogana
Department of Urology, Northwestern University Feinberg School of Medicine, 303 E Chicago Avenue, Tarry 16, Chicago, IL 60611, USA

Irene B. Helenowski and Borko Jovanovic
Department of Preventive Medicine, Northwestern University Feinberg School of Medicine, Chicago, IL, USA

Maria Ruden
Department of Medicine, University of Illinois at Chicago, Chicago, IL, USA

Courtney M. P. Hollowell
Division of Urology, Cook County Health and Hospitals System, 303 E Chicago Avenue, Tarry 16, Chicago, IL 60611, USA

Adam B. Murphy
Department of Urology, Northwestern University Feinberg School of Medicine, 303 E Chicago Avenue, Tarry 16, Chicago, IL 60611, USA
Division of Urology, Cook County Health and Hospitals System, 303 E Chicago Avenue, Tarry 16, Chicago, IL 60611, USA
Section of Urology, Jesse Brown VA Medical Center, 303 E Chicago Avenue, Tarry 16, Chicago, IL 60611, USA

Roohollah Sharifi
Section of Urology, Jesse Brown VA Medical Center, 303 E Chicago Avenue, Tarry 16, Chicago, IL 60611, USA
Department of Urology, University of Illinois at Chicago School of Medicine, Chicago, IL, USA

Rick A. Kittles
Division of Health Equities, Department of Population Sciences, City of Hope Cancer Center, Duarte, CA, USA

Peter Gann
Department of Pathology, University of Illinois at Chicago School of Medicine, Chicago, IL, USA

Jonathan H. Wang and Glen O. Allen
Department of Urology, University of Wisconsin School of Medicine and Public Health, Madison, WI, USA

Pablo Sierra
Department of Urology, University of Wisconsin School of Medicine and Public Health, Madison, WI, USA
Universidad CES, Medellin, Colombia

Kyle A. Richards, Tracy M. Downs and E. Jason Abel
Department of Urology, University of Wisconsin School of Medicine and Public Health, Madison, WI, USA
University of Wisconsin Carbone Cancer Center, Madison, WI, USA

David F. Jarrard
Department of Urology, University of Wisconsin School of Medicine and Public Health, Madison, WI, USA
University of Wisconsin Carbone Cancer Center, Madison, WI, USA
Wisconsin Institute for Medical Research, 1111 Highland Avenue, Madison, WI 53705-2281, USA

Saro Aprikian, Eleonora Scarlata and Lucie Hamel
Urologic Oncology Research Group, Cancer Research Program, Research Institute (RI) of McGill University Health Center (MUHC), Glen Campus, E M2.2210, 1001 Blvd Décarie, Montréal, Qc H4A 3J1, Canada

Murilo Luz
Urologic Oncology Research Group, Cancer Research Program, Research Institute (RI) of McGill University Health Center (MUHC), Glen Campus, E M2.2210, 1001 Blvd Décarie, Montréal, Qc H4A 3J1, Canada
Department of Surgery (Urology Division), MUHC and McGill University, Montreal, Canada

Fadi Brimo
Urologic Oncology Research Group, Cancer Research Program, Research Institute (RI) of McGill University Health Center (MUHC), Glen Campus, E M2.2210, 1001 Blvd Décarie, Montréal, Qc H4A 3J1, Canada
Department of Pathology, MUHC and McGill University, Montreal, Canada

Fabio L. Cury
Urologic Oncology Research Group, Cancer Research Program, Research Institute (RI) of McGill University Health Center (MUHC), Glen Campus, E M2.2210, 1001 Blvd Décarie, Montréal, Qc H4A 3J1, Canada
Department of Radiation Oncology, MUHC and McGill University, Montreal, Canada

Simon Tanguay, Armen G. Aprikian and Wassim Kassouf
Urologic Oncology Research Group, Cancer Research Program, Research Institute (RI) of McGill University Health Center (MUHC), Glen Campus, E M2.2210, 1001 Blvd Décarie, Montréal, Qc H4A 3J1, Canada
Department of Surgery (Urology Division), MUHC and McGill University, Montreal, Canada
Department of Oncology, MUHC and McGill University, Montreal, Canada

Simone Chevalier
Urologic Oncology Research Group, Cancer Research Program, Research Institute (RI) of McGill University Health Center (MUHC), Glen Campus, E M2.2210, 1001 Blvd Décarie, Montréal, Qc H4A 3J1, Canada
Department of Surgery (Urology Division), MUHC and McGill University, Montreal, Canada
Department of Oncology, MUHC and McGill University, Montreal, Canada
Department of Medicine, MUHC and McGill University, Montreal, Canada

Xue-fei Ding, Tian-bao Huang, Sheng-ming Lu, Hua-zhi Tao, Xiao-fang Ye, Fei Wang, Yao-zong Xu, Jia-nan Xu and Yu-quan Zhou
Department of Urology, Clinical Medical College, Yangzhou University, No. 98 West Nantong Road, Yangzhou, Jiangsu Province 225001, China

Yang Luan
Department of Urology, Clinical Medical College, Yangzhou University, No. 98 West Nantong Road, Yangzhou, Jiangsu Province 225001, China
Department of Urology, Taihe County People's Hospital, Fuyang 226600, Anhui Province, China

Tong Cai
Binzhou Medical University, Yantai, Shandong, China

Yuanshan Cui, Jitao Wu, Rui Ding and Zhenli Gao
Department of Urology, The Affiliated Yantai Yuhuangding Hospital of Qingdao University, Yantai, NO. 20 East Yuhuangding Road, Yantai 264000, Shandong, China

Zhongbao Zhou
Binzhou Medical University, Yantai, Shandong, China
Department of Urology, The Affiliated Yantai Yuhuangding Hospital of Qingdao University, Yantai, NO. 20 East Yuhuangding Road, Yantai 264000, Shandong, China

Anika Kremer, Glen Kristiansen and Yuri Tolkach
Institute of Pathology, University Hospital of Bonn, Bonn, Germany

Tobias Kremer
Institute of Computer Science, Johannes Gutenberg-University Mainz, Mainz, Germany

Index

Printed in the USA
CPSIA information can be obtained
at www.ICGtesting.com
LVHW080036211023
761596LV00010BA/1789

9 781646 466337